HEALTH BEHAVIOR AND HEALTH EDUCATION

Theory, Research, and Practice

THIRD EDITION

Karen Glanz
Barbara K. Rimer
Frances Marcus Lewis
Editors

Foreword by Noreen M. Clark

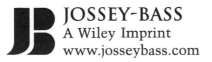

JOSSEY-BASS
A Wiley Imprint
www.josseybass.com

Published by Jossey-Bass
A Wiley Imprint
989 Market Street, San Francisco, CA 94103-1741   www.josseybass.com

Limit of Liability/Disclaimer of Warranty: While the publisher and author have used their best efforts in preparing this book, they make no representations or warranties with respect to the accuracy or completeness of the contents of this book and specifically disclaim any implied warranties of merchantability or fitness for a particular purpose. No warranty may be created or extended by sales representatives or written sales materials. The advice and strategies contained herein may not be suitable for your situation. You should consult with a professional where appropriate. Neither the publisher nor author shall be liable for any loss of profit or any other commercial damages, including but not limited to special, incidental, consequential, or other damages.

Readers should be aware that Internet Web sites offered as citations and/or sources for further information may have changed or disappeared between the time this was written and when it is read.

Jossey-Bass books and products are available through most bookstores. To contact Jossey-Bass directly call our Customer Care Department within the U.S. at 800-956-7739, outside the U.S. at 317-572-3986, or fax 317-572-4002.

Jossey-Bass also publishes its books in a variety of electronic formats. Some content that appears in print may not be available in electronic books.

Library of Congress Cataloging-in-Publication Data

Health behavior and health education: theory, research, and practice /
  Karen Glanz, Barbara K. Rimer, Frances Marcus Lewis, editors; foreword
  by Noreen M. Clark.—3rd ed.
      p.   cm.
  Includes bibliographical references and indexes.
  ISBN 0–7879–5715–1 (alk. paper)
  1. Health behavior. 2. Health education. 3. Health promotion.
  [DNLM: 1. Health Behavior. 2. Health Education. W 85 H43415 2002]
  I. Glanz, Karen. II. Rimer, Barbara K. III. Lewis, Frances Marcus.
  RA776.9 .H434 2002
  613—dc21
2002010028

Printed in the United States of America
THIRD EDITION
HB Printing   10 9 8 7 6

CONTENTS

PART FIVE: USING THEORY IN RESEARCH AND PRACTICE 405

TABLES AND FIGURES

Tables

Figures

FOREWORD

Noreen M. Clark

Why do people behave as they do? How does what they do affect their health? What causes them to change their health-related behavior? These are intriguing questions for just about everyone but most especially for public health professionals.

Research findings provide undeniable evidence of the central role of behavior in the world's major health problems. The same research has frequently elucidated the difficulty associated with understanding and changing behavior, and the complex array of factors that combine to produce behavior is fascinating to consider. Think for a moment about the multiple influences that cause one to become a smoker, or to eat in ways deleterious to health, or to engage in unprotected sex. Think, too, of the range of factors that enable people to continue such behaviors or deter them from giving them up. Having information about potential ill effects is usually insufficient in itself to trigger change. Tobacco use and overeating both provide examples of cases in which most people who smoke or are overweight know their behavior isn't good for them. Achieving behavior change is one of the knottiest and most interesting processes associated with being fully healthy.

With the recent surge in DNA-related research, many people have come to believe that genomic science will uncover the gene responsible for each extant health condition and obviate the need to tackle behavior. Scientists working in gene-based research, however, are the first to say this is wishful thinking. Certainly, most diseases will be associated with several genes and, in the opinion of genetic experts as well as behavioral scientists, behavior will continue to account for the greatest variance in disease onset and progression.

When discussing improvements in health status, the reciprocal influence of individual and collective behavior can't be overstated. More and more evidence points to how collective health behavior shapes the individual and individual behavior influences dimensions of collective health. Promoting well being, therefore, requires as much focus on communities as on individuals and, as important, on the complex interaction between the two. The dramatic decrease in smoking in the last quarter of a century is often attributed to combined efforts to assist individuals to quit and to help create new communitywide behavioral norms and expectations. The dramatic rise in smoking in cohorts of the population (for example, young women) is often attributed to the failure both to reach particular subgroups of individuals and to influence their reference communities. Behavior evident communitywide is greatly influenced by the resources and social capital available within the community and how these can be accessed by residents. No one could fail to notice, for example, the blending of community and individual actions that enabled New Yorkers to weather the 2001 terrorist attacks. Community infrastructure and material resources coupled with motivation, skills, and social connectivity of individuals led to rapid action under the most dire circumstances.

As research and practice related to behavior and behavior change grow in sophistication, work has been increasingly marked by efforts to make sense of a variety of associated causal factors. Models have evolved that attempt to account for the range of psychological, social, structural, and other salient elements that predict behavior. More advanced analytical techniques are enabling assessment of intricate and complicated relationships. The need for evermore robust methods has greatly increased with recent advances in both genomic and behavioral science. Consider that with the mapping of the human genome, twenty thousand data points at least will describe the DNA of a single individual. How will we combine these data with behavioral data, with demographic information, and with community descriptors to anticipate behavior or health status? What happens when we wish to look at a whole community of people using such complex data sets? In the coming decades, the growing capacity for data analysis will enable behavioral researchers to move health education theory, research, and practice light years forward in their contribution to improving health.

The characteristic that has always separated the successful health education researcher and practitioner from those less effective is the use of theory; that is, the capacity to translate it into interventions. This ability is gaining even more currency as more theoretical models are available and receive more testing. The third edition of *Health Behavior and Health Education: Theory, Research, and Practice* has been compiled precisely to help the health education community understand how theory informs both research and practice and how these in turn inform theory. The text has been updated to reflect the most recent work. The authors have extensive research and practice experience and use it to assess applications and to speculate on future directions for health education. The revised text is timely and welcome particularly as it arrives at a period of rapid maturation of the field. Health education has a great deal to offer worldwide health improvement, and this volume has much to offer health education.

Ann Arbor, Michigan
June 2002

PREFACE

Programs to influence health behavior, including health promotion and education programs and interventions, are most likely to benefit participants and communities when the program or intervention is guided by a theory of health behavior. Theories of health behavior identify the targets for change and the methods for accomplishing changes. Theories also inform the evaluation of change efforts by helping to identify the outcomes to be measured, as well as the timing and methods of study to be used. Such theory-driven health promotion and education efforts stand in contrast to programs based primarily on precedent, tradition, intuition, or general principles.

Theory-driven health behavior change interventions and programs require an understanding of the components of health behavior theory, as well as the operational or practical forms of the theory. The first edition of *Health Behavior and Health Education: Theory, Research, and Practice*, published in 1990, was the first text to provide in a single volume an in-depth analysis of a variety of theories of health behavior relevant to health education. It brought together dominant health behavior theories, research based on those theories, and examples of health education practice derived from theory that had been tested through evaluation and research processes. The second edition of *Health Behavior and Health Education*, published in 1996, updated and improved upon the earlier volume.

It has been over five years since the release of the second edition of this book, and the third edition of *Health Behavior and Health Education* once again updates and improves on the preceding edition. Its main purpose is the same: to advance the science and practice of health behavior and health education through the informed application of theories of health behavior. Likewise, this book serves in three ways as the definitive text for students, practitioners, and scientists in these areas and in education: by analyzing the key components of theories of health behavior relevant to health education, by evaluating current applications of these theories in selected health promotion programs and interventions, and by identifying important future directions for research and practice in health promotion and health education.

The third edition responds to new developments in health behavior theory and the application of theory in new settings, to new populations, and in new ways. This edition includes an enhanced focus on the application of theories in diverse settings; an expanded section on using theory, including its translation for program planning; and chapters on additional theories of health behavior. One new chapter addresses the challenges and opportunities afforded by the rapid growth in new communication technologies. Another presents the RE-AIM Model, an evaluation model that is compatible with increasing the yield of research on theory-driven interventions.

Audience

Health Behavior and Health Education speaks to graduate students, practitioners, and scientists who spend part or all of their time in the broad arenas of health behavior change, health promotion, and health education; the text will help them both to understand the theories and to apply them in practical settings. Practitioners as well as students will find this text a major reference for the development and evaluation of theory-driven health promotion and education programs and interventions. Researchers should emerge with a recognition of areas in which empirical support is deficient and theory-testing is required, helping to set the research agenda for health behavior and health education.

This book is intended to assist all professionals who value the need to influence health behavior positively. Their fields include health promotion and education, medicine, nursing, health psychology, behavioral medicine, health communications, nutrition and dietetics, dentistry, pharmacy, social work, exercise science, clinical psychology, and occupational and physical therapy.

Overview of the Book

The authors of this text bring to their chapters an understanding of both theory and its application in a variety of settings that characterize the diverse practice of public health education, for example, worksites, hospitals, ambulatory care settings, schools, and communities. The chapters, written or updated expressly for the third edition of this book, address theories and models of health behavior at the level of the individual, dyad, group, organization, and community.

The book is organized into five parts. Part One defines key terms and concepts. The next three parts reflect important units of health behavior and education practice: the individual, the interpersonal or group level, and the community or aggregate level. Each of these parts has several chapters, and ends with a perspectives chapter that synthesizes the preceding chapters. Part Two focuses on theories of individual health behavior, and its chapters focus on variables *within individuals* that influence their health behavior and response to health promotion and education interventions. Four bodies of theory are reviewed in separate chapters: the Health Belief Model, the Theory of Reasoned Action and the Theory of Planned Behavior, The Transtheoretical Model, and the Precaution Adoption Process Model. Part Three examines interpersonal theories, which emphasize elements in the *interpersonal* environment that affect individuals' health behavior. Chapters focus on Social Cognitive Theory, social networks and social support, stress and coping, and social influence and interpersonal communication. Part Four covers models for the community or aggregate level of change and includes chapters on community organization, adoption and diffusion of innovations, organizational change, and media communications. Part Five explores "using theory," which presents the key components and applications of overarching planning and process models and a discussion of the application of theory in culturally unique and other unique populations. It includes chapters on the PRECEDE-PROCEED model of health promotion planning; social marketing; ecological models; cultural, ethnic, and socioeconomic factors; theoretical bases for communication technology; and the RE-AIM evaluation model.

The major emphasis of *Health Behavior and Health Education* is on the analysis and application of health behavior theories to health promotion and education practice. Each core chapter in Parts Two, Three, and Four begins with a discussion of the background of the theory or model and a presentation of the theory, reviews empirical support for it, and concludes with one or two applications. Synthesis chapters review related theories and summarize their potential application to the development of health education interventions. Strengths, weaknesses, areas for future development and research, and promising strategies are highlighted.

Chapter authors are established researchers and practitioners who draw on their experience in state-of-the-art research to critically analyze the theories and apply them to health education. This text makes otherwise lofty theories accessible and practical and advances health education in the process.

No single book can be truly comprehensive and still be concise and readable. Decisions about which theories to include were made with both an appreciation of the evolution of the study of health behavior and a vision of its future (see Chapter Two). We purposely chose to emphasize theories and conceptual frameworks that encompass a range from the individual to the societal level. We acknowledge that there is substantial variability in the extent to which various theories and models have been codified, tested, and supported by empirical evidence. Of necessity, some promising evolving theories were not included.

The first two editions of *Health Behavior and Health Education* grew out of the editors' own experiences, frustrations, and needs, as well as their desire to synthesize the diverse literatures and to draw clearly the linkages between theory, research, and practice in health behavior and education. We have sought to show how theory, research, and practice interrelate and to make each accessible and practical. In this edition we have attempted to respond to changes in the science and practice of health promotion and to update the coverage of these areas in a rapidly evolving field. Substantial efforts have been taken to present findings from health behavior change interventions based on the theories that are described and to illustrate the adaptations needed to successfully reach diverse and unique populations. *Health Behavior and Health Education* has now been established as a widely used text and reference book. We hope the third edition will continue to be relevant and useful and to stimulate readers' interest in theory-based health behavior and health education. We aspire to provide readers with the information and skills to ask critical questions, think conceptually, and stretch their thinking beyond using formulaic strategies to improve health.

Acknowledgments

We owe deep gratitude to all the authors whose work is represented in this book. They worked diligently with us to produce an integrated volume, and we greatly appreciate their willingness to tailor their contributions to realize the vision of the book. Their collective depth of knowledge and experience across the broad range of theories and topics far exceeds the expertise that the editors can claim. We also wish to acknowledge authors who contributed to the first and second editions of this text; although some of them did not write chapters for this edition, their intellectual contributions form an important foundation for the present volume.

Lori Crane and Linda Baumann provided timely and insightful reviews of the chapters at a crucial stage in the book's development. The staff at Jossey-Bass provided valuable support to us for development, production, and marketing from the time that the first edition was released through completion of this edition. Our editor at Jossey-Bass, Andy Pasternack, provided encouragement, assistance, and exceptional guidance throughout.

The editors are indebted to their colleagues and students who, over the years, have taught them the importance of both health behavior theories and their cogent and precise representation. They have challenged us to stretch, adapt, and continue to learn through our years of work at Stanford University, the University of Michigan, The Johns Hopkins University, Temple University, the University of Washington, Fox Chase Cancer Center, Duke University, the University of Hawai'i, and the National Cancer Institute (NCI).

We particularly want to acknowledge Bill Rakowski for his insightful comments and reflections on theory. We appreciate the staff and colleagues at NCI whose dedication to their jobs made it possible for Barbara Rimer to remain a part of the editorial team: Arline Sanchez, Tina Felix, Stacy Vandor, Bob Croyle, and Bob Hiatt.

Completion of this manuscript would not have been possible without the continuous and dedicated assistance of Gwen Ramelb, Rochelle Fujisawa, Kathy Doering, Jared Kuroiwa, Elly Mar Aganon, Linda Nguyen, and Nanette Camacho.

We also wish to express our thanks to our colleagues, friends, staffs, and families, whose patience, good humor, and encouragement sustained us through our work on this book.

June 2002

Karen Glanz
Honolulu, Hawai'i

Barbara K. Rimer
Bethesda, Maryland

Frances Marcus Lewis
Seattle, Washington

THE EDITORS

Karen Glanz is professor and director of the Social and Behavioral Sciences Program at the Cancer Research Center of Hawai'i at the University of Hawai'i in Honolulu. From 1979 to 1993, she was professor in the Department of Health Education at Temple University in Philadelphia. She received her B.A. degree (1974) in Spanish and her M.P.H. (1977) and Ph.D. (1979) degrees in health behavior and health education, all from the University of Michigan.

Glanz's research and academic interests have been in the area of health behavior change program development and evaluation, cancer prevention and control, ethnic differences in health behavior, and risk communication. She is currently principal investigator on four federally funded research grants that test health behavior change interventions for skin cancer prevention, colorectal cancer risk counseling, and youth tobacco prevention. Glanz's scholarly contributions consist of more than two hundred journal articles and book chapters.

In 1984 Dr. Glanz received the Early Career Award of the Public Health Education Section of the American Public Health Association (APHA), and in 1992 she was a co-recipient (with Frances Lewis and Barbara Rimer) of the Mayhew Derryberry Award for outstanding contributions to theory and research in health education, also from the Public Health Education and Health Promotion Section of APHA. She received the Mohan Singh Award for contributions to humor in health education in 1996, and her recent community health education programs have received several national awards for innovative programs and program excellence.

Glanz was a member of the Behavioral Medicine Study Section of the National Institutes of Health from 1995 to 2000, and serves on numerous advisory boards and committees for scientific and health organizations in the United States and abroad. Dr. Glanz currently or recently has served on the editorial boards of several journals including the *American Journal of Health Promotion; Health Education Research; Patient Education and Counseling; Cancer Epidemiology, Biomarkers, and Prevention;* and *Health Psychology.*

Glanz was visiting professor at Teachers College, Columbia University, in 1982 and spent 1987 to 1988 as a visiting scholar in the division of epidemiology at the University of Minnesota School of Public Health. She was visiting professor at the School of Public Health at Queensland University of Technology in Brisbane, Australia, in 1994 and 1995.

Barbara K. Rimer is professor of Health Behavior and Health Education at the University of North Carolina School of Public Health, Chapel Hill. From 1997 to 2002, she was director of Cancer Control and Population Sciences at the National Cancer Institute, and from 1991 to 1997, she was director of Cancer Prevention, Detection and Control Research and professor of community and family medicine at Duke University Medical Center.

Dr. Rimer received her B.A. degree (1970) and her M.P.H. degree (1973) from the University of Michigan, and her Dr.P.H. degree in Health Education (1981) from the Johns Hopkins School of Hygiene and Public Health. Dr. Rimer's research has focused on several broad areas of cancer control. These include developing and testing targeted and tailored strategies for behavior change and informed decision making. Most recently, these strategies have included "expert-system-like interventions" created especially for the recipients. Dr. Rimer's research has included the following topic areas, among others: smoking cessation, mammography decision making and screening for women of different ages, and informed decision making about genetic testing for cancer susceptibility. She was a continuously funded NIH grantee from 1982 to 1997 and is the author of more than two hundred scientific articles.

From 1994 to 1997, Dr. Rimer was the presidentially appointed chair of the National Cancer Advisory Board. In 1997 she was given the Distinguished Achievement Award from the American Society for Preventive Oncology, and the Herbert J. Block Leadership Award from Ohio State University; she received the John P. McGovern Award in Health Promotion from the University of Texas School of Public Health in 1998 and the American Cancer Society Distinguished Service Award in 2000. Dr. Rimer is a member of several editorial boards, including those of *Effective Clinical Practice; Breast Diseases; Cancer Causes and Control; Cancer Epidemiology, Biomarkers, and Prevention; Patient Education and Counseling; Preventive Medicine;* and the *American Journal of Health Promotion.*

Frances Marcus Lewis is the Elizabeth Sterling Soule Distinguished Professor of Health Promotion and Nursing at the University of Washington. She received her B.S.N. degree and graduated summa cum laude (1967) from Loretto Heights College in Denver and received her M.N. degree (1968) from the University of Washington. She received her Ph.D. degree (1977) in sociology of education from Stanford University and completed her postdoctoral training (1978) in health education at the Johns Hopkins University School of Hygiene and Public Health.

Since 1983 she has devoted much of her research career to the development and testing of theoretical predictive models of health behavior and health outcomes in persons and family members affected by cancer and other life-threatening, chronic illnesses. Currently, Dr. Lewis is principal investigator of a National Cancer Institute-funded multistate clinical trial to enhance the functioning of family members, including children, affected by cancer in the mother.

Dr. Lewis is a member of the Public Health Sciences Division of the Fred Hutchinson Cancer Research Center, where she is a Full Affiliate Fellow appointment. She has recently delivered several distinguished lectureships, including the Bice Memorial Lectureship, University of Virginia; the Potter Memorial Lectureship, Emory University; and the Marion Woodruff Memorial Lectureship, University of British Columbia. Dr. Lewis has received a number of national awards, including the Distinguished Researcher Award of the Oncology Nursing Society, and was named a Fellow of the Japanese Society for the Promotion of Science. Most recently, she served for four years as one of the four technical lead consultants for a U.S. A.I.D. grant, during which the team developed regional breast cancer screening programs and behavioral-theory-based training for multiple medical workers, including physicians and psychologists. Currently, Dr. Lewis sits as a member and recent cochair for the California Breast Cancer Research Program, University of California, as well as a grant reviewer for the National Institutes of Health. She is a review board, reviewer, or editorial board member for *Journal of Marriage and the Family, Journal of Psychosocial Oncology, Health Education Research, Health Psychology, American Journal of Health Behavior, Social Science and Medicine,* and *Nursing Research,* among others.

THE CONTRIBUTORS

Tom Baranowski is professor at the Children's Nutrition Research Center in the Department of Pediatrics at Baylor College of Medicine.

Ronald L. Braithwaite is professor in the Department of Behavioral Sciences and Health Education at Rollins School of Public Health at Emory University in Atlanta.

Victoria L. Champion is Distinguished Professor and associate dean for research at the Indiana University School of Nursing.

Brenda M. DeVellis is professor in the Department of Health Behavior and Health Education at the School of Public Health, University of North Carolina at Chapel Hill.

Colleen DiIorio is professor in the Department of Behavioral Sciences and Health Education at Rollins School of Public Health at Emory University in Atlanta.

Kerry E. Evers is director of Health Behavior Change Projects at Pro-Change Behavior Systems in Rhode Island.

John R. Finnegan Jr. is professor in the Division of Epidemiology and associate dean for academic affairs at the University of Minnesota School of Public Health.

Michael J. Fotheringham is a NHMRC Public Health Research Fellow at Deakin University and the VicHealth Centre for Tobacco Control at the Anti-Cancer Council of Victoria in Melbourne, Australia.

Andrea Carlson Gielen is professor of Social and Behavioral Sciences in the Department of Health Policy and Management at the Bloomberg School of Public Health at Johns Hopkins University in Baltimore.

Russell E. Glasgow is senior scientist in Behavioral and Community Studies at the AMC Cancer Research Center in Denver.

Robert M. Goodman is the Usdin Family Professor in Community Health Sciences at the Tulane University School of Public Health and Tropical Medicine.

Catherine A. Heaney is associate professor in the Division of Health Behavior and Health Promotion at the School of Public Health at Ohio State University.

Barbara A. Israel is professor in the Department of Health Behavior and Health Education in the School of Public Health, University of Michigan.

Nancy K. Janz is associate professor in the Department of Health Behavior and Health Education at the University of Michigan School of Public Health.

Danuta Kasprzyk is senior research scientist at the Centers for Public Health Research and Evaluation, Battelle Memorial Institute, in Seattle.

Michelle Crozier Kegler is assistant professor in the Department of Behavioral Sciences and Health Education at Rollins School of Public Health at Emory University in Atlanta.

Caryn Lerman is professor of psychiatry and associate director for population sciences at the Comprehensive Cancer Center at the University of Pennsylvania in Philadelphia.

Megan A. Lewis is assistant professor in the Department of Health Behavior and Health Education at the School of Public Health, University of North Carolina at Chapel Hill.

Edward W. Maibach is worldwide director of social marketing for Porter Novelli.

Bess H. Marcus is professor of psychiatry and human behavior at Brown Medical School and director of physical activity research at the Centers for Behavioral and Preventive Medicine at The Miriam Hospital in Providence, Rhode Island.

Eileen M. McDonald is assistant scientist in the Department of Health Policy and Management at the Bloomsberg School of Public Health, Johns Hopkins University in Baltimore.

Meredith Minkler is professor of Community Health Education and Health and Social Behavior in the School of Public Health at the University of California, Berkeley.

Daniel E. Montaño is senior research scientist at the Centers for Public Health Research and Evaluation, Battelle Memorial Institute in Seattle.

William D. Novelli is the executive director of AARP.

Brian Oldenburg is professor and head of the School of Public Health at the Queensland University of Technology in Brisbane, Australia.

Neville Owen is professor in the School of Population Health and director of the Health Promotion and Cancer Prevention Research Centre at the University of Queensland in Brisbane, Australia.

Guy S. Parcel is acting dean and John P. McGovern Professor in Health Promotion at the University of Texas School of Public Health, where he is also director of the Center for Health Promotion Research and Development.

Cheryl L. Perry is professor in the Division of Epidemiology, School of Public Health, at the University of Minnesota.

James O. Prochaska is professor of Clinical and Health Psychology and director of the Cancer Prevention Research Center at the University of Rhode Island.

Colleen A. Redding is associate research professor at the Cancer Prevention Research Center and adjunct professor of psychology at the University of Rhode Island.

Ken Resnicow is professor in the Department of Behavioral Sciences and Health Education at Rollins School of Public Health at Emory University in Atlanta.

Michael L. Rothschild is emeritus professor in the School of Business at the University of Wisconsin-Madison.

James F. Sallis is professor in the Department of Psychology at San Diego State University.

Peter M. Sandman is a consultant in risk communication, professor of human ecology at Rutgers University, and professor of environmental and community medicine at the Robert Wood Johnson Medical School in New Jersey.

Betsy Sleath is associate professor in the School of Pharmacy, University of North Carolina at Chapel Hill.

Allan Steckler is professor of health behavior and health education at the School of Public Health, University of North Carolina at Chapel Hill.

Victor J. Strecher is director of Cancer Prevention and Control at the University of Michigan Comprehensive Cancer Center and professor in the Department of Health Behavior and Health Education at the University of Michigan School of Public Health.

K. Viswanath is a senior health communication scientist with the Health Communication and Informatics Research Branch in the Division of Cancer Control and Population Sciences at the National Cancer Institute.

Nina B. Wallerstein is associate professor and director of the Master's in Public Health Program in the Department of Family and Community Medicine at the School of Medicine, University of New Mexico in Albuquerque.

Neil D. Weinstein is professor in the Department of Human Ecology at Rutgers, The State University of New Jersey.

Lari Wenzel is adjunct associate professor in the Division of Epidemiology at the University of California at Irvine.

In memory of Godfrey Hochbaum and Rusty Rosenstock—pioneers in the field—whose guidance, inspiration, and humor taught us much about health behavior and about life

For my grandfather, Sam Glanz, who showed me NYC
and the world in more innocent times

K. G.

To my husband, Bernard Glassman, for his support, wit, and wisdom

B.K.R.

To my beloved family: Steven, David, John, Samuel,
Deloris, Alex, Laurel, and Julia Catherine

F.M.L.

PART ONE

HEALTH EDUCATION AND HEALTH BEHAVIOR

THE FOUNDATIONS

CHAPTER ONE

THE SCOPE OF HEALTH BEHAVIOR AND HEALTH EDUCATION

The Editors

The range of health education and health behavior change strategies today is nearly limitless. Health professionals and health education specialists may counsel people at risk for AIDS about safe sex; help children avoid tobacco, alcohol, and drugs; help adults to stop smoking; help patients to manage and cope with their illnesses; and organize communities or advocate policy changes aimed at fostering health improvement. Health education professionals work all over the world in a variety of settings including schools, worksites, voluntary health organizations, medical settings, and communities. They are challenged to disseminate the best of what is known in new situations. They may also forge and test fundamental theories that drive research and practice in public health, health education, and health care. A premise of *Health Behavior and Health Education* is that a dynamic exchange between theory, research, and practice is most likely to produce effective health education.

Perhaps never before have those concerned with health behavior and health education been faced with more challenges and opportunities than they are today. Kanfer and Schefft (1988) observed that "as science and technology advance, the greatest mystery of the universe and the least conquered force of nature remains the human being and his actions and human experiences." The body of research in health behavior and health education has grown rapidly over the past two decades, and health education is recognized increasingly as a way to meet public health objectives and improve the success of public health and medical interventions.

Although this increasing literature improves the science base of health behavior and health education, it also challenges those in the field to master and be facile with an almost overwhelming body of knowledge.

The science and art of health behavior and health education are eclectic, rapidly evolving, and reflective of an amalgamation of approaches, methods, and strategies from social and health sciences. They draw on the theoretical perspectives, research, and practice tools of such diverse disciplines as psychology, sociology, anthropology, communications, nursing, and marketing. Health education is also dependent on epidemiology, statistics, and medicine. There is increasing emphasis on identifying evidence-based interventions and disseminating them widely (Rimer, Glanz, and Rasband, 2001). This often requires individual health education and health behavior professionals to synthesize large and diverse literatures.

Many types of professionals contribute to and conduct health education and health behavior (HEHB) programs and research. Health education practice is strengthened by the close collaboration among professionals of different disciplines, each concerned with the behavioral and social intervention process, and each contributing a unique perspective. Psychology brings to health education a rich legacy of over a hundred years of research and practice on individual differences, motivation, learning, persuasion, and attitude and behavior change (Matarazzo, Weiss, Herd, Miller, and Weiss, 1984). Physicians are important collaborators and are in key positions to effect change in health behavior. Likewise, nurses and social workers bring to health education their particular expertise in working with individual patients and patients' families to facilitate learning, adjustment, and behavior change, and to improve quality of life. Other health, education, and human service professionals contribute their special expertise as well. Increasingly, there will be partnerships with genetic counselors and other specialists in this rapidly developing field.

Health, Disease, and Health Behavior: The Changing Context

The major causes of death in the United States and other developed countries are now chronic diseases, such as heart disease, cancer, and stroke (National Center for Health Statistics, 2000). Behavioral factors, particularly tobacco use, diet and activity patterns, alcohol consumption, sexual behavior, and avoidable injuries are among the most prominent contributors to mortality (McGinnis and Foege, 1993). The resurgence of infectious diseases, including foodborne illness and tuberculosis, and the emergence of new infectious diseases such as antibiotic-resistant infections, HIV/AIDS, Hepatitis C, and human papillomavirus (HPV) are also largely affected by human behaviors (Lederberg, Shope, and Oakes, 1992; Glanz and Yang, 1996). Substantial suffering, premature mortality, and medical costs can be avoided by positive changes in behavior. Most recently, there has been a renewed focus on public health as a result of anthrax exposure due to terrorism.

During the past twenty years, there has been a dramatic increase in public, private, and professional interest in preventing disability and death through changes in lifestyle and participation in screening programs. Much of this interest in disease prevention and early detection has been stimulated by the epidemiologic transition from infectious to chronic diseases as leading causes of death, the aging of the population, rapidly escalating health care costs, and data linking individual behaviors to increased risk of morbidity and mortality. More recent developments, such as the AIDS epidemic, have also contributed. Even as epidemiologists' efforts to better specify the links between diet, lifestyle, genetic predisposition, and environmental factors and disease approach the limits of science, they continue to generate headlines (Taubes, 1995) and influence public policy (Marshall, 1995).

Landmark reports in Canada and the United States during the 1970s and 1980s heralded the commitment of governments to health education and promotion (Lalonde, 1974; U.S. Department of Health, Education, and Welfare, 1979; Epp, 1986). In the United States, federal initiatives for public health education and monitoring populationwide behavior patterns were spurred by the development of the health objectives published in *Promoting Health and Preventing Disease: Health Objectives for the Nation* (U.S. Department of Health and Human Services, 1980) and their successors, outlined in *Healthy People 2000: National Health Promotion and Disease Prevention Objectives* and *Healthy People 2010* (U.S. Department of Health and Human Services, 1991 and 2000). Increased interest in behavioral and social determinants of health behavior change spawned numerous training programs and public and commercial service programs.

Data systems now make it possible to track trends in risk factors, health behaviors, and healthy environments and policies in the United States and, in some cases, to tie these changes to disease incidence and mortality. Indeed, there have been positive changes in several areas. A major accomplishment has been surpassing the targets for reducing deaths from coronary heart disease and cancer (National Center for Health Statistics, 2001). Blood pressure control has improved and mean population blood cholesterol levels have declined. Alcohol-related motor vehicle deaths and deaths due to automobile crashes and drowning have continued to decrease. Fewer adults are using tobacco products, and more are engaging in moderate physical activity. More adults are meeting dietary guidelines for consumption of fruits, vegetables, and grain products and for dietary fat as a percentage of calories (National Center for Health Statistics, 2001). Rates of HIV/AIDS have leveled off and transfusion-related HIV infections have decreased markedly. The proportion of women age fifty and older who have had breast examinations and mammograms has exceeded the goal of 60 percent in forty-seven states. The United States has made progress toward the goal of reducing health disparities for more than half the objectives identified in *Healthy People 2000* (National Center for Health Statistics, 2001). Major litigation against the tobacco industry and a multi-state settlement have resulted in increased restrictions on tobacco advertising and enforcement of laws against selling tobacco to minors. The collective efforts of those in health education and public health have indeed made a difference. While this progress is encouraging, much work remains to be done in these areas.

Not all the news is favorable, though. More adults and children are overweight. Diabetes is increasing in near-epidemic proportions. More adolescents are sexually active. After major increases in seatbelt use in the early 1990s, rates have declined slightly and remain at 67 percent, well below the target rate of 85 percent (National Center for Health Statistics, 2001). One-fifth of children under three years old have not received a basic series of vaccinations for polio, measles, diphtheria, and other diseases. Sixteen percent of adults under sixty-five years of age have no health insurance coverage. More than 70 percent of adults over age fifty have not been screened for colorectal cancer (National Center for Health Statistics, 2001). Ethnic minorities and those in poverty still experience a disproportionate burden of preventable disease and disability, and for many conditions the gap between disadvantaged and affluent groups is widening (House and Williams, 2000).

Changes in the health care system provide new supports and opportunities for health education. Respect for patients' rights is now recognized as fundamental to the practice of medicine (Levinsky, 1996). Moreover, there is increased attention to issues of shared decision making (Edwards and Elwyn, 1999). At the same time, patients' access to information about their health care institutions and providers remains limited. Insurance carriers and managed care systems can impose barriers that impede patients' exercise of their rights to make treatment decisions (Weston and Lauria, 1996; Levinsky, 1996). The advent of managed health care and health care financing reform pose new challenges as the drive for cost containment affects the entire health care system. While increased accountability often results in cost savings and fewer unnecessary services, little is known about its effects on the health of patients and the overall quality of care (Iglehart, 1996). Clinical prevention and behavioral interventions may grow in importance under managed care when their cost-effectiveness is demonstrated and recognized (Center for the Advancement of Health, 2000; Rimer, Glanz, and Rasband, 2001), but the climate of fiscal constraint will probably slow adoption of efficacious behavioral strategies in the short run.

The rapid emergence of new communication technologies and new uses of older technologies, such as the telephone, also provide new opportunities and dilemmas. A new chapter has been added to *Health Behavior and Health Education* to reflect the importance of new communication technologies (see Chapter Twenty-Two). A variety of electronic media for interactive health communication (for example, the internet, CD-ROMs, personal digital assistants) can serve as sources of both general and individualized health information, reminders, and social support for health behavior change.

Since the last edition of this book, use of the Internet has grown dramatically. E-health strategies are becoming an important part of the armamentarium of strategies for those in health education and health behavior. Internet and computer-based applications can support many of the strategies that evolve naturally from the theories presented in this book. It is important that use of the new technologies be based and evaluated on theories of health behavior. Otherwise, we risk being technology driven instead of outcomes driven.

New technologies have the potential to cause harm through misleading or deceptive information, promotion of inappropriate self-care, and interference in the patient-provider relationship (Science Panel on Interactive Communication and Health, 1999). Interactive health communications provide new options for behavioral medicine and preventive medicine (Noell and Glasgow, 1999; Fotheringham, Owies, Leslie, and Owen, 2000) and are altering the context of health behavior and health education as they unfold and as their effects are studied.

Health Education and Health Behavior

The Scope and Evolution of Health Education

In the fields of health education and health behavior, the emphasis during the 1970s and 1980s on individuals' behaviors as determinants of health status eclipsed attention to the broader social determinants of health. Advocates of system-level changes to improve health called for renewal of a broad vision of health education and promotion (Minkler, 1989; see Chapter Twenty). These calls for moving health education toward social action heralded a renewed enthusiasm for holistic approaches rather than an entirely new worldview. They are well within the tradition of health education and are consistent with its long-standing concern with the impact of social, economic, and political forces on health.

Over the past fifty years, outstanding leaders in health education repeatedly stressed the importance of political, economic, and social factors as determinants of health. Mayhew Derryberry (1960) noted that "health education . . . requires careful and thorough consideration of the present knowledge, attitudes, goals, perceptions, social status, power structure, cultural traditions, and other aspects of whatever public is to be addressed." In 1966, Dorothy Nyswander spoke of the importance of attending to social justice and individuals' sense of control and self-determination (Nyswander, 1966). These ideas were reiterated later when William Griffiths (1972) stressed that "health education is concerned not only with individuals and their families, but *also with the institutions and social conditions* that impede or facilitate individuals toward achieving optimum health" (emphasis added).

The view of health education as an instrument of social change has been renewed and invigorated during the past decade. Policy, advocacy, and organizational change have been adopted as central activities of public health and health education. Most recently, experts have explicitly recommended that interventions on social and behavioral factors related to health should link multiple levels of influence, including the individual, interpersonal, institutional, community, and policy levels (Smedley and Syme, 2000). This volume purposefully includes chapters on community and societal influences on health behavior and strategies to effect community and social policy changes. In this context, definitions of health education and health promotion can be recognized and discussed as overlapping and intertwined.

Definitions of Health Education

According to Griffiths (1972), "health education attempts to close the gap between what is known about optimum health practice and that which is actually practiced." Simonds (1976) defined health education as aimed at "bringing about behavioral changes in individuals, groups, and larger populations from behaviors that are presumed to be detrimental to health, to behaviors that are conducive to present and future health."

Subsequent definitions of health education emphasized voluntary, informed behavior changes. In 1980, Green defined health education as "any combination of learning experiences designed to facilitate voluntary adaptations of behavior conducive to health (Green, Kreuter, Partridge, and Deeds, 1980). The Role Delineation Project defined health education as "the process of assisting individuals, acting separately or collectively, to make informed decisions about matters affecting their personal health and that of others" (National Task Force on the Preparation and Practice of Health Educators, 1985).

Health education evolved from three settings: communities, schools, and patient care sites. Kurt Lewin's pioneering work in group process and his developmental field theory during the 1930s and 1940s form the intellectual roots of much of today's health education practice. One of the earliest models developed to explain health behavior, the Health Belief Model, was developed during the 1950s to explain behavior related to tuberculosis screening (Hochbaum, 1958).

Health education includes not only instructional activities and other strategies to change individual health behavior but also organizational efforts, policy directives, economic supports, environmental activities, mass media, and community-level programs. Two key ideas from an ecologic perspective help direct the identification of personal and environmental leverage points for health promotion and education interventions (Glanz and Rimer, 1995). First, behavior is viewed as being affected by, and affecting, *multiple levels of influence.* Five levels of influence for health-related behaviors and conditions have been identified. They are (1) intrapersonal, or individual factors; (2) interpersonal factors; (3) institutional, or organizational factors; (4) community factors; and (5) public policy factors (McLeroy, Bibeau, Steckler, and Glanz, 1988). The second key idea relates to the possibility of *reciprocal causation* between individuals and their environments; that is, behavior both influences *and* is influenced by the social environment (Stokols, 1992).

Health education covers the continuum from disease prevention and promotion of optimal health to the detection of illness to treatment, rehabilitation, and long-term care. Health education is delivered in almost every conceivable setting— universities, schools, hospitals, pharmacies, grocery stores and shopping centers, recreation settings, community organizations, voluntary health agencies, worksites, churches, prisons, health maintenance organizations, migrant labor camps, advertising agencies, the Internet, people's homes, and health departments at all levels of government. These diverse settings are discussed later in this chapter.

Health promotion is a term of more recent origin than *health education.* As defined by Green, it is "any combination of health education and related organizational, economic, and environmental supports for behavior of individuals, groups, or communities conducive to health" (Green and Kreuter, 1991). Another, slightly different definition is suggested by O'Donnell (1989): "Health promotion is the science and art of helping people change their lifestyle toward a state of optimum health . . . Lifestyle change can be facilitated by a combination of efforts to enhance awareness, change behavior, and create environments that support good health practices." Definitions arising in Europe and Canada have another emphasis again (Kolbe, 1988; Hawe, Degeling, and Hall, 1990). For example, the *Ottawa Charter for Health Promotion* defines health promotion as "the process of enabling people to increase control over, and to improve, their health . . . a commitment to dealing with the challenges of reducing inequities, extending the scope of prevention, and helping people to cope with their circumstances . . . creating environments conducive to health, in which people are better able to take care of themselves" (Epp, 1986).

While some may argue that greater precision of terminology can be achieved by drawing a clear distinction between health education and health promotion, to do so is to ignore long-standing tenets of health education and its broad social mission. Clearly, health educators have long used more than "educational" strategies. In fact, the terms *health promotion* and *health education* are often used interchangeably in the United States (Breckon, Harvey, and Lancaster, 1994). In some countries, such as Australia, health education is considered a much narrower endeavor than health promotion. Nevertheless, although the term *health promotion* emphasizes efforts to influence the broader social context of health behavior, the two terms remain closely linked and overlapping, share a common historical and philosophical foundation, and are often used in combination. In most cases, we consider the two terms too closely related to distinguish between them. In this book, the term *health education* is used most often. It is to be understood in the historical sense, as a broad and varied set of strategies to influence both individuals and their social environments, to improve health behavior, and to enhance health and quality of life.

Health Behavior

The central concern of health education is *health behavior*. It is included or suggested in every definition of health education and is the crucial dependent variable in most research on the impact of health education intervention strategies. Positive informed changes in health behavior are typically the ultimate aims of health education programs; if behaviors change but health is not subsequently improved, the result is a paradox that must be resolved by examining other issues, such as the link between behavior and health status or the ways in which behavior and health are measured. Informed decision making is a desirable endpoint for problems involving medical uncertainty, and studies suggest that shared decision making may lead to improved patient satisfaction and health outcomes (Frosch and Kaplan, 1999). Likewise, environmental or structural interventions to change presumed social environmental determinants of health behavior are intended to improve health by changing behavior. Thus, efforts to improve environments, policies, and so on should ultimately be evaluated for their effects on health behavior; if policy changes but it does not lead to measurable changes in behavior, it may be either too weak, too short-lived, or only a limited determinant of behavior.

In the broadest sense, *health behavior* refers to the actions of individuals, groups, and organizations as well as their determinants, correlates, and consequences, including social change, policy development and implementation, improved coping skills, and enhanced quality of life (Parkerson and others, 1993). This is similar to the working definition of health behavior that Gochman proposed (though his definition emphasized individuals): it includes not only observable, overt actions but also the mental events and feeling states that can be reported and measured. He defined health behavior as: "those personal attributes such as beliefs, expectations, motives, values, perceptions, and other cognitive elements; personality characteristics, including affective and emotional states and traits; and overt behavior patterns, actions, and habits that relate to health maintenance, to health restoration, and to health improvement" (Gochman, 1982; Gochman, 1997).

Gochman's definition is consistent with and embraces the definitions of specific categories of overt health behavior proposed by Kasl and Cobb in their seminal articles (1966a, 1966b). Kasl and Cobb define three categories of health behavior as follows:

> *Preventive health behavior.* Any activity undertaken by an individual who believes himself to be healthy, for the purpose of preventing or detecting illness in an asymptomatic state.
>
> *Illness behavior.* Any activity undertaken by an individual who perceives himself to be ill, to define the state of health, and to discover a suitable remedy [Kasl and Cobb, 1966a].
>
> *Sick-role behavior.* Any activity undertaken by an individual who considers himself to be ill, for the purpose of getting well. It includes receiving treatment from medical providers, generally involves a whole range of dependent behaviors, and leads to some degree of exemption from one's usual responsibilities [Kasl and Cobb, 1966b].

Settings and Audiences for Health Education

During the past century and more specifically during the past few decades, the scope and methods of health education have broadened and diversified dramatically. This section briefly reviews the range of settings and audiences of health education today.

Settings: Where Is Health Education Provided?

Today, health education can be found nearly everywhere. The settings for health education are important because they provide channels for delivering programs, provide access to specific populations and gatekeepers, usually have existing communication systems for diffusion of programs, and facilitate development of policies and organizational change to support positive health practices (Mullen and others, 1995). Six major settings are particularly relevant to contemporary health education: schools, communities, worksites, health care settings, homes, and the consumer marketplace.

Schools. Health education in the schools includes classroom teaching, teacher training, and changes in the school environment that support healthy behaviors (Luepker and others, 1996). To support long-term health enhancement initiatives, theories of organizational change are used to encourage adoption of comprehensive smoking control programs in schools (see Chapter Fifteen). Diffusion Theory and the Theory of Reasoned Action have been used to analyze factors associated with adoption of AIDS prevention curricula in Dutch schools (Paulussen, Kok, Schaalma, and Parcel, 1995).

Communities. Community-based health education draws on social relationships and organizations to reach large populations with media and interpersonal strategies. Models of community organization enable program planners both to gain support for and to design suitable health messages and delivery mechanisms (see Chapter Thirteen). Community interventions in churches, clubs, recreation centers, and neighborhoods have been used to encourage healthful nutrition, reduce risk of cardiovascular disease, and use peer influence to promote breast cancer detection among minority women (see Chapters Nine and Ten).

Worksites. Since its emergence in the mid-1970s, worksite health promotion has grown and spawned new tools for health educators. Because people spend so much time at work, the workplace is both a source of stress and a source of social support (Israel and Schurman, 1990). Effective worksite programs can harness social support as a buffer to stress, with the goal of improving worker health and health practices. Today many businesses, particularly large corporations, provide health promotion programs for their employees (National Center for Health Statistics, 2001). Both high-risk and populationwide strategies have been used in programs to reduce the risk of cancer (Tilley, Glanz, and others, 1999; Tilley, Vernon, and others, 1999; Sorenson and others, 1996) and cardiovascular disease (Glasgow and others, 1995).

Health Care Sites. Health education for high-risk persons, patients, their families, and the surrounding community and inservice training for health care providers are all part of health care today. The changing nature of health service delivery has stimulated greater emphasis on health education in physicians' offices, health maintenance organizations, public health clinics, and hospitals (Walsh and McPhee, 1992; King and others, 1993). Primary care settings, in particular, provide an opportunity to reach a substantial number of people (Campbell and others, 1993; Glanz and others, 1990). Health education in these settings focuses on preventing and detecting disease, helping people make decisions about genetic testing, and managing acute and chronic illnesses.

Homes. Health behavior change interventions are delivered to people in their homes, both through traditional public health means—home visits—and through a variety of communication channels and media such as the Internet, telephone, and mail (Science Panel on Interactive Communication and Health, 1999; McBride and Rimer, 1999). The use of strategies such as mailed tailored messages (Skinner, Campbell, Rimer, Curry, and Prochaska, 1999) and motivational interviewing by telephone (Emmons and Rollnick, 2001) makes it possible to reach larger groups and high-risk groups in a convenient way that reduces barriers to their receiving motivational messages.

The Consumer Marketplace. The advent of home health and self-care products, as well as the use of "health" appeals to sell consumer goods, has created new opportunities both for health education and for misleading consumers about the potential health effects of items they can purchase (Glanz and others, 1995). Social marketing, with its roots in consumer behavior theory, is used increasingly by health educators to enhance the salience of health messages and to improve their persuasive impact (see Chapter Nineteen). Theories of Consumer Information Processing (CIP) provide a framework for understanding why people do or do not pay attention to, understand, and make use of consumer health information such as nutrient labels on packaged food products (Rudd and Glanz, 1990).

Audiences: Who Are the Recipients of Health Education?

For health education to be effective, it should be designed with an understanding of the recipients, or target audiences, and their health and social characteristics as well as their beliefs, attitudes, values, skills, and past behaviors. These audiences consist of people who may be reached as individuals, in groups, through organizations, as communities or sociopolitical entities, or through some combination of these. They may be health professionals, clients, people at risk for disease, or patients. This section discusses four dimensions in which the potential audiences can be characterized: sociodemographic characteristics, ethnic or racial background, life cycle stage, and disease or at-risk status.

Sociodemographic Characteristics and Ethnic or Racial Background. Socio-economic status has been linked with both health status and health behavior, with less affluent persons consistently experiencing higher morbidity and mortality (Adler and others, 1994). The recognition of differences in disease and mortality rates across socioeconomic and ethnic or racial groups has led to increasing efforts to reduce or eliminate such health disparities (U.S. Department of Health and Human Services, 2000). For example, it has long been known that African Americans die at earlier ages than do whites. As of 1998, life expectancy for African American males was 67.6 years compared to 74.5 years for white males. The difference is slightly less for African American women, 74.8 versus 80 for white women, but still alarmingly discrepant (National Center for Health Statistics, 2000).

A variety of sociodemographic characteristics such as gender, age, race, marital status, place of residence, and employment characterize health education audiences. These factors, while generally not *modifiable* within the bounds of health education programs, are useful in guiding the tailoring of strategies and educational material and identifying channels through which to reach consumers. Printed educational materials should be appropriate to, and, ideally, tailored to the educational and reading levels of particular target audiences and be consistent with their ethnic and cultural backgrounds. Chapter Twenty-One examines the role of culturally diverse and other unique populations in health behavior theory, research, and practice.

Life Cycle Stage. Health education is provided for people at every stage of the life cycle, from childbirth education, the beneficiaries of which are not yet born, to self-care education and rehabilitation for the very old. Developmental perspectives help guide the choice of intervention and research methods. Children may have misperceptions about health and illness, such as that illnesses are a punishment for bad behavior (Armsden and Lewis, 1993). Knowledge of children's cognitive development helps provide a framework for understanding these beliefs and ways to respond to them. Adolescents may feel invulnerable to accidents and chronic diseases. The Health Belief Model (see Chapter Three) is a useful framework for understanding the factors that may predispose youth to engage in unsafe sexual practices. Older adults may attribute symptoms of cancer to the inexorable process of aging. Beliefs such as this must be considered in designing, implementing, and evaluating health education programs (Rimer and others 1983; Keintz, Rimer, Fleisher, and Engstrom, 1988).

Disease and At-Risk Status. People who are diagnosed with specific diseases often experience not only symptoms but also the distress associated with their prognosis and with having to make decisions about medical care (see Chapter Ten, on stress and coping). Thus, while they may benefit from receiving health education, their ability to attend to new information may be compromised at critical points due to their illness. Because of this, the timing, channels, and audiences for patient education need to be carefully considered. Successful patient education depends on a sound understanding of the patient's view of the world (Glanz and Oldenburg, 2001). For individuals at high risk due to family history or identified risk factors, health behavior change interventions may have heightened salience when linked to strategies for reducing individual risk (see Chapter Six, on the Precaution Adoption Process Model). Even so, strategies used to enable initial changes in behavior, such as quitting smoking, may be insufficient for maintaining behavior change over the long term even in these persons. Models and theories of health behavior can suggest strategies for relapse prevention for high-risk individuals (Glanz and Oldenburg, 2001).

Progress in Health Promotion and Health Behavior Research

Over the past two decades, research programs have been established to identify and test the most effective methods for achieving health behavior change. More precise quantification of personal health behaviors and improved health outcomes has grown from partnerships between behavioral health scientists and biomedical experts. During this period, findings from some major health behavior intervention studies have become available and have provided important insights for the field.

In the late 1970s and early 1980s, three large community cardiovascular disease intervention studies were begun in California, Minnesota, and Rhode Island (Winkleby, 1994). Each study addressed smoking, hypertension, high-fat diets, obesity, and physical inactivity—all widespread risk factors that many practitioners were tackling. The multicomponent risk reduction programs in these trials used mass media, interpersonal education programs for the public, professionals, and those at high risk. Community organization strategies were used to create institutional and environmental support for the programs, and theory-derived program planning strategies emphasized community participation (Winkleby, 1994). In the 1990s, all three studies reported their findings for risk factor changes. They each found favorable secular trends in control sites and modest or nonsignificant intervention effects on risk factor reduction (Farquhar and others, 1990; Luepker and others, 1994; Carleton and others, 1995). Two large worksite trials of multicomponent nutrition and smoking interventions yielded similar findings (Glasgow and others, 1995; Sorensen and others, 1996).

These studies produced a wealth of knowledge about health behavior, and many of the short-term targeted interventions within the larger studies were found to be effective (Winkleby, 1994). Nonetheless, the results cast doubt on the presumed effectiveness of population-based intervention strategies over the long term, especially against the backdrop of a dynamic, changing environment. Still, the lack of significant communitywide impacts in these studies should not be assumed to "disprove" the conceptual foundations of the intervention methods. An alternative view is to regard the interventions used in these studies as contributors to the substantial secular trend in chronic disease prevention (Winkleby, 1994). Also, more attention must be paid to how to reach the people who have resisted previous messages and programs.

While randomized, controlled trials provide the most rigorous test of health behavior interventions, the past decade has been marked by an increase in carefully designed evaluation research in health education that combines quantitative and qualitative methods. Recently published evaluations of community-based AIDS prevention projects (Janz and others, 1996) and coalitions for prevention of alcohol, tobacco, and other drug abuse (Butterfoss, Goodman and Wandersman, 1996) exemplify new applications of community research methodologies that offer in-depth process information across multiple programs in diverse settings.

Overall, there has been a growing trend toward evidence-based health education and health behavior as the findings of numerous large health behavior intervention studies have been published (Rimer, Glanz, and Rasband, 2001). As the research literature grows, it is increasingly important that the evidence base become accessible to both researchers and practitioners.

Evidence reviews have come to be defined as reviews using a formalized method of assembling and weighing the findings of intervention research. Important progress has been made over the past decade to improve the process of systematic reviews and meta-analysis (Mulrow, Cook, and Davidoff, 1997). However, in reality, literature reviews cut across a continuum of scientific rigor in their methodologies for selecting, evaluating, and reporting the evidence. They may exclude all but the most rigorous studies or be all-inclusive, may provide detailed information on methodology or only report on findings, and may be highly quantitative in drawing conclusions or rely heavily on an expert judgment base (Rimer, Glanz, and Rasband, 2001). An important effort under way in the United States promises to significantly advance the evidence base in HEHB in the next few years. The U.S. Task Force on Community Preventive Services aims to define, categorize, summarize, and rate the quality of evidence on the effectiveness of population-based interventions for disease prevention and control; to provide recommendations on these interventions and methods for their delivery based on the evidence; and to identify and summarize research gaps (Briss and others, 2000; www.thecommunityguide.org).

The challenge of understanding and improving health behavior is a central challenge for health policy today, and is "one of the most complex tasks yet confronted by science. To competently address that challenge, the . . . research community must simply do more and do it better" in certain key areas of behavioral research (McGinnis, 1994). A coordinated and focused effort will be essential to resolving many of the most vexing health issues facing our society (Smedley and Syme, 2000). The integration of the best available knowledge from theory, research, and health promotion and education practice can help advance that agenda in the next decade.

Health Behavior and Health Education Foundations and the Importance of Theory, Research, and Practice

This chapter has discussed the dynamic nature of health education and health behavior today in the context of changing patterns of disease and trends in health care, health education, and disease prevention. It has provided definitions of health education, health promotion, and health behavior and has described the broad and diverse parameters of this maturing field. Health behavior research has experienced great progress, but mixed findings raise new questions and pose methodological, theoretical, and substantive challenges. The interrelationships and importance of theory, research, and practice are set against a backdrop of the important, growing, and complex challenges in health education and health behavior.

References

Adler, N. E., and others. "Socioeconomic Status and Health: The Challenge of the Gradient." *American Psychologist*, 1994, *49*(1), 15–24.

Armsden, G., and Lewis, F. "The Child's Adaptation to Parental Medical Illness: Theory and Clinical Implications." *Patient Education and Counseling*, 1993, *22*, 153–165.

Breckon, D. J., Harvey, J. R., and Lancaster, R. B. *Community Health Education: Settings, Roles and Skills for the 21st Century.* Gaithersburg, Md.: Aspen Publishers, 1994

Briss, P., and others. "Developing an Evidence-Based Guide to Community Preventive Services—Methods." *American Journal of Preventive Medicine*, 2000, *18*(1S), 35–43.

Butterfoss, F. D., Goodman, R., and Wandersman, A. "Community Coalitions for Prevention and Health Promotion: Factors Predicting Satisfaction, Participation, and Planning." *Health Education Quarterly*, 1996, *23*(1), 65–79.

Campbell, M., and others. "The Impact of Message Tailoring on Dietary Behavior Change for Disease Prevention in Primary Care Settings." *American Journal of Public Health*, 1993, *84*(5), 783–787.

Carleton, R., and others. "The Pawtucket Heart Health Program: Community Changes in Cardiovascular Risk Factors and Projected Disease Risk." *American Journal of Public Health*, 1995, *85*(6), 777–785.

Center for the Advancement of Health. *Health Behavior Change in Managed Care: A Status Report.* Washington, D.C.: Center for the Advancement of Health, 2000.

Derryberry, M. "Health Education: Its Objectives and Methods." *Health Education Monographs*, 1960, *8*, 5–11.

Edwards, A., and Elwyn, G. "How Should Effectiveness of Risk Communication to Aid Patients' Decisions Be Judged? A Review of the Literature." *Medical Decision Making*, 1999, *19*, 428–434.

Emmons, K. M., and Rollnick, S. "Motivational Interviewing in Health Care Settings: Opportunities and Limitations." *American Journal of Preventive Medicine*, 2001, *20*, 68–74.

Epp, L. *Achieving Health for All: A Framework for Health Promotion in Canada.* Toronto: Health and Welfare, Canada, 1986.

Farquhar, J. W., and others. "Effect of Communitywide Education on Cardiovascular Disease Risk Factors: The Stanford Five-City Project." *Journal of the American Medical Association*, 1990, *264*, 359–365.

Fotheringham, M. J., Owies, D., Leslie, E., and Owen, N. "Interactive Health Communication in Preventive Medicine: Internet-Based Strategies in Teaching and Research." *American Journal of Preventive Medicine*, 2000, *19*, 113–120.

Frosch, D. L., and Kaplan, R. M. "Shared Decision Making in Clinical Medicine: Past Research and Future Directions." *American Journal of Preventive Medicine*, 1999, *17*, 285–294.

Glanz, K., and Oldenburg, B. "Utilizing Theories and Constructs Across Models of Behavior Change." In R. Patterson (ed.), *Changing Patient Behavior: Improving Outcomes in Health and Disease Management.* San Francisco: Jossey-Bass, 2001.

Glanz, K., and Rimer, B. K. *Theory at a Glance: A Guide to Health Promotion Practice.* Bethesda, Md.: National Cancer Institute, 1995.

Glanz, K., and Yang, H. "Communicating About Risk of Infectious Diseases." *Journal of the American Medical Association*, 1996, *275*(3), 253–256.

Glanz, K., and others. "Patient Reactions to Nutrition Education for Cholesterol Reduction." *American Journal of Preventive Medicine*, 1990, *60*(6), 311–317.

Glanz, K., and others. "Environmental and Policy Approaches to Cardiovascular Disease Prevention Through Nutrition: Opportunities for State and Local Action." *Health Education Quarterly*, 1995, *22(4)*, 512–527.

Glasgow, R., and others. "Take Heart: Results from the Initial Phase of a Work-Site Wellness Program." *American Journal of Public Health*, 1995, *85*(2), 209–216.

Gochman, D. S. "Labels, Systems, and Motives: Some Perspectives on Future Research." *Health Education Quarterly*, 1982, *9*, 167–174.

Gochman, D. S. "Health Behavior Research: Definitions and Diversity." In D. S. Gochman (ed.), *Handbook of Health Behavior Research, Vol. I. Personal and Social Determinants.* New York: Plenum Press, 1997.

Green, L. W., and Kreuter, M. W. *Health Promotion Planning: An Educational and Environmental Approach* (Second Edition). Mountain View, Calif.: Mayfield, 1991.

Green, L. W., Kreuter, M. W., Partridge, K., and Deeds, S. *Health Education Planning: A Diagnostic Approach.* Mountain View, Calif.: Mayfield, 1980.

Griffiths, W. "Health Education Definitions, Problems, and Philosophies." *Health Education Monographs,* 1972, *31,* 12–14.

Hawe, P., Degeling, D., and Hall, J. (1990). *Evaluating Health Promotion: A Health Worker's Guide.* Sydney: MacLennan and Petty.

Hochbaum, G. *Public Participation in Medical Screening Programs: A Sociopsychological Study.* Public Health Service Publication no. 572, 1958.

House, J. S., and Williams, D. R. "Understanding and Reducing Socioeconomic and Racial/Ethnic Disparities in Health." In B. D. Smedley and S. L. Syme (eds.), *Promoting Health: Intervention Strategies from Social and Behavioral Research.* Washington, D.C.: National Academy Press, 2000.

Iglehart, J. "Managed Care and Mental Health." *New England Journal of Medicine,* 1996, *334*(2), 131–135.

Israel, B., and Schurman, S. "Social Support, Control, and the Stress Process." In K. Glanz, F. M. Lewis, and B. K. Rimer (eds.), *Health Behavior and Health Education: Theory, Research, and Practice.* San Francisco: Jossey-Bass, 1990.

Janz, N. K., and others. "Evaluation of 37 AIDS Prevention Projects: Successful Approaches and Barriers to Program Effectiveness." *Health Education Quarterly,* 1996, *23*(1), 80–97.

Kanfer, F. H., and Schefft, B. *Guiding the Process of Therapeutic Change.* Champaign, Ill.: Research Press, 1988.

Kasl, S. V., and Cobb, S. "Health Behavior, Illness Behavior, and Sick-Role Behavior: I. Health and Illness Behavior." *Archives of Environmental Health,* 1966a, *12,* 246–266.

Kasl, S. V., and Cobb, S. "Health Behavior, Illness Behavior, and Sick-Role Behavior: II. Sick-Role Behavior." *Archives of Environmental Health,* 1966b, *12,* 531–541.

Keintz, M., Rimer, B., Fleisher, L., and Engstrom, P. "Educating Older Adults About Their Increased Cancer Risk." *Gerontologist,* 1988, *28,* 487–490.

King, E., and others. "Promoting Mammography Through Progressive Interventions." *American Journal of Public Health,* 1993, *84*(1), 1644–1656.

Kolbe, L. J. "The Application of Health Behavior Research: Health Education and Health Promotion." In D. S. Gochman (ed.), *Health Behavior: Emerging Research Perspectives.* New York: Plenum Press, 1988.

Lalonde, M. *A New Perspective on the Health of Canadians: A Working Document.* Toronto: Health and Welfare Canada, 1974.

Lederberg, J., Shope, R., and Oakes, S. (eds.). *Emerging Infections: Microbial Threats to Health in the United States.* Washington, D.C.: National Academy Press, 1992.

Levinsky, N. "Social, Institutional, and Economic Barriers to the Exercise of Patients' Rights." *New England Journal of Medicine,* 1996, *334*(8), 532–534.

Luepker, R. V., and others. "Community Education for Cardiovascular Disease Prevention: Risk Factor Changes in the Minnesota Heart Health Program." *American Journal of Public Health,* 1994, *84,* 1383–1393.

Luepker, R. V., and others. "Outcomes of a Trial to Improve Children's Dietary Patterns and Physical Activity: The Child and Adolescent Trial for Cardiovascular Health (CATCH)." *Journal of the American Medical Association,* 1996, *275,* 768–776.

Marshall, J. R. "Editorial: Improving Americans' Diet—Setting Public Policy with Limited Knowledge." *American Journal of Public Health,* 1995, *85*(12), 1609–1611.

Matarazzo, J. D., Weiss, S. M., Herd, J. A., Miller, N. E., and Weiss, S. M. (eds.). *Behavioral Health: A Handbook of Health Enhancement and Disease Prevention.* New York: Wiley, 1984.

McBride, C. M., and Rimer, B. K. "Using the Telephone to Improve Health Behavior and Health Service Delivery." *Patient Education and Counseling,* 1999, *37,* 3–18.

McGinnis, J. M. "The Role of Behavioral Research in National Health Policy." In Blumenthal, S., Matthews, K., and Weiss, S. (eds.), *New Research Frontiers in Behavioral Medicine: Proceedings of the National Conference.* Bethesda, Md.: NIH Health and Behavior Coordinating Committee, 1994, 217–222.

McGinnis, J. M., and Foege, W. H. "Actual Causes of Death in the United States." *Journal of the American Medical Association,* 1993, *270*(18), 2207–2212.

McLeroy, K. R., Bibeau, D., Steckler, A., and Glanz, K. "An Ecological Perspective on Health Promotion Programs." *Health Education Quarterly,* 1988, *15,* 351–377.

Minkler, M. "Health Education, Health Promotion, and the Open Society: A Historical Perspective." *Health Education Quarterly,* 1989, *16,* 17–30.

Mullen, P. D., and others. "Settings as an Important Dimension in Health Education/ Promotion Policy, Programs, and Research." *Health Education Quarterly,* 1995, *22,* 329–345.

Mulrow, C. D., Cook, D. J., and Davidoff, F. "Systematic Reviews: Critical Links in the Great Chain of Evidence." *Annals of Internal Medicine,* 1997, *126,* 389–391.

National Center for Health Statistics. *Health, United States, 2000. With Adolescent Chartbook.* Hyattsville, Md.: Public Health Service, 2000.

National Center for Health Statistics. *Healthy People 2000: Final Review.* Hyattsville, Maryland: Public Health Service, 2001. (DHHS Publication No. 01–0256)

National Task Force on the Preparation and Practice of Health Educators. *A Framework for the Development of Competency-Based Curricula.* New York: National Task Force, Inc., 1985.

Noell, J., and Glasgow, R. E. "Interactive Technology Applications for Behavioral Counseling: Issues and Opportunities for Health Care Settings." *American Journal of Preventive Medicine,* 1999, *17,* 269–274.

Nyswander, D. "The Open Society: Its Implications for Health Educators." *Health Education Monographs,* 1966, *1,* 3–13.

O'Donnell, M. P. "Definition of Health Promotion: Part III: Expanding the Definition." *American Journal of Health Promotion,* 1989, *3,* 5.

Parkerson, G., and others. "Disease-Specific Versus Generic Measurement of Health-Related Quality of Life in Insulin-Dependent Diabetic Patients." *Medical Care,* 1993, *31,* 629–637.

Paulussen, T. G., Kok, G., Schaalma, H. P., and Parcel, G. S. "Diffusion of AIDS Curricula Among Dutch Secondary School Teachers." *Health Education Quarterly,* 1995, *22,* 227–243.

Rimer, B., and others. "Planning a Cancer Control Program for Older Citizens." *Gerontologist,* 1983, *23,* 384–389.

Rimer, B. K., Glanz, K., and Rasband, G. "Searching for Evidence About Health Education and Health Behavior Interventions." *Health Education and Behavior,* 2001, *28,* 231–248.

Rudd, J., and Glanz, K. "How Individuals Use Information for Health Action: Consumer Information Processing." In K. Glanz, F. M. Lewis, and B. K. Rimer (eds.), *Health Behavior and Health Education: Theory, Research, and Practice.* San Francisco: Jossey-Bass, 1990.

Science Panel on Interactive Communication and Health. *Wired for Health and Well-Being: The Emergence of Interactive Health Communication.* Washington, D.C.: U.S. Department of Health and Human Services, U.S. Government Printing Office, April 1999.

Simonds, S. "Health Education in the Mid-1970s: State of the Art." In *Preventive Medicine USA.* New York: Prodist, 1976.

Skinner, C. S., Campbell, M. K., Rimer, B. K., Curry, S., and Prochaska, J. O. "How Effective Is Tailored Print Communication?" *Annals of Behavioral Medicine*, 1999, *21*, 290–298.

Smedley, B. D., and Syme, S. L. (eds.). *Promoting Health: Intervention Strategies from Social and Behavioral Research*. Washington, D.C.: National Academy Press, 2000.

Sorensen, G., and others. "Working Well: Results from a Worksite-Based Cancer Prevention Trial." *American Journal of Public Health*, 1996, *86*, 939–947.

Stokols, D. "Establishing and Maintaining Healthy Environments: Toward a Social Ecology of Health Promotion." *American Psychologist*, 1992, *47*, 6–22.

Taubes, G. "Epidemiology Faces Its Limits." *Science*, July 14, 1995, *269*, 164–169.

Tilley, B., Glanz, K., Kristal, A., Hirst, K., Li, S., Vernon, S., and Myers, R. "Nutrition Intervention for High-Risk Auto Workers: Results of the Next Step Trial." *Preventive Medicine*, 1999, *28*, 284–292.

Tilley, B., Vernon, S., Myers, R., Glanz, K., Lu, M., Hirst, K., and Kristal, A. "The Next Step Trial: Impact of a Worksite Colorectal Cancer Screening Promotion Program." *Preventive Medicine*, 1999, *28*, 276–283.

U.S. Department of Health, Education, and Welfare. *Healthy People: The Surgeon General's Report on Health Promotion and Disease Prevention*. Public Health Service Publication No. 79–55071, 1979.

U.S. Department of Health and Human Services. *Promoting Health and Preventing Disease: Health Objectives for the Nation*. Washington, D.C.: U.S. Government Printing Office, 1980.

U.S. Department of Health and Human Services. *Healthy People 2000: National Health Promotion and Disease Prevention Objectives*. Washington, D.C.: U.S. Government Printing Office, 1991. (DHHS Publ. No. PHS 91–50213)

U.S. Department of Health and Human Services. *Healthy People 2010: Understanding and Improving Health*. Washington, D.C.: U.S. Government Printing Office, 2000.

Walsh, J., and McPhee, S. "A Systems Model of Clinical Preventive Care: An Analysis of Factors Influencing Patient and Physician." *Health Education Quarterly*, 1992, *19*, 157–176.

Weston, B., and Lauria, M. "Patient Advocacy in the 1990s." *New England Journal of Medicine*, 1996, *334*(8), 543–544.

Winkleby, M. A. "The Future of Community-Based Cardiovascular Disease Intervention Studies." *American Journal of Public Health*, 1994, *84*, 1369–1372.

www.thecommunityguide.org. Web site for The Guide to Community Preventive Services: Systematic Reviews and Evidence Based Recommendations, 2001.

CHAPTER TWO

THEORY, RESEARCH, AND PRACTICE IN HEALTH BEHAVIOR AND HEALTH EDUCATION

The Editors

Theory, Research, and Practice: Interrelationships

Aristotle distinguished between *theoria* and *praxis*. *Theoria* signifies those sciences and activities that are concerned with knowing for its own sake, whereas *praxis* corresponds to the ways in which we now commonly speak of action or doing. This contrast between theory and practice (Bernstein, 1971) permeates Western philosophical and scientific thought from Aristotle to Marx and on to Dewey and other contemporary twentieth-century philosophers. Dewey attempted to resolve the dichotomy by focusing on the similarities and continuities between theoretical and practical judgments and inquiries. He described "experimental knowing" essentially as an art that involves a conscious, directed manipulation of objects and situations. "The craftsman perfects his art, not by comparing his product to some 'ideal' model, but by the cumulative results of experience—experience which benefits from tried and tested procedures but always involves risk and novelty" (Bernstein, 1971). Dewey thus described empirical investigation, that is, research, as the ground between theory and practice and the testing of theory in action.

Although the perception of theory and practice as a dichotomy has a long tradition in intellectual thought, we follow in Dewey's tradition and focus on the similarities and continuities rather than on the differences. Theory, research, and practice are a continuum along which the skilled professional should move with ease. Not only are they related but they are both essential to health education and health behavior. Theory and research are not solely the province of the academic, just as practice is not solely the field of the practitioner. Researchers and practitioners may differ in their priorities, but the relationship between research and its application can and should move in both directions (D'Onofrio, 1992; Freudenberg and others, 1995). "The search for truth and for an ultimate understanding of the forces that make humans think, feel, and act as they do is the long-term goal" (Kanfer and Schefft, 1988).

The task of health education is both to understand health behavior and to transform knowledge about behavior into effective strategies for health enhancement. Research in health education and health behavior (HEHB) ultimately will be judged by its contributions to improving the health of populations. Although basic behavioral research is important in developing theories, ultimately we must test our theories iteratively in the real world (Rosenstock, 1990). When we do so, theory, research, and practice begin to converge. The authors of this book examine theories in light of their applicability.

However, the relationships between theory, research, and practice are not simple or linear. The larger picture of health improvement and disease reduction is better described as a cycle of interacting types of endeavors, including fundamental research (research into determinants as well as development of methodologies), intervention research (research aimed toward change), surveillance research (tracking populationwide trends including maintenance of change), and application and program delivery (Hiatt and Rimer, 1999; National Center for Chronic Disease Prevention and Health Promotion, 2000; Sallis, Owen, and Fotheringham, 2000). At the heart of this cycle is knowledge synthesis; continually updated critical appraisals of the available literature are central to identifying interventions that should be disseminated in order to reduce the burden of disease (Rimer, Glanz, and Rasband, 2001).

Health Behavior and Health Education aims to help educators, whatever their background or disciplines, understand some of the most important theoretical underpinnings of health education and health behavior and use theory to inform research and practice. "Clearly, application of well-defined and carefully tested theories to the program development process holds tremendous advantages for health educators in terms of coherence, effectiveness, and evaluation of interventions" (van Ryn and Heancy, 1992, p. 328).

The authors of *Health Behavior and Health Education* believe that "there is nothing so useful as a good theory" (Lewin, 1935). Each chapter demonstrates the practical value of theory; each synthesizes what was learned through conceptually sound research and practice; and each draws the linkages between theory, research, and practice.

Professionals charged with responsibility for health education and health behavior are, by and large, interventionists. They are action oriented. They use their knowledge to design and implement programs to improve health. This is true whether they are working to encourage positive changes in individual or in community behavior. It is equally true of most health education and health behavior research. Such research is conducted primarily in the real world, not in isolated laboratories. Usually, in the process of attempting to change behavior or policies, researchers must do precisely what practitioners do—develop and deliver interventions. At some level, both practitioners and researchers are accountable for results, whether these are measured in terms of participants' satisfaction with programs or changes in awareness, knowledge, attitudes, beliefs, health behaviors; improved decision making; institutional norms; community integration; or more distal results including morbidity, mortality, and quality of life. Health educators may assess these results anecdotally, or they may conduct more rigorous evaluations.

The design of interventions that yield desirable changes can best be done with an understanding of theories of behavior change and an ability to use them skillfully in practice. Most health educators work in situations in which resources are limited, which makes judgments about the choice of intervention very important. There may be no second chance to reach a critical target audience.

A synthesis of theory, research, and practice will advance what is known about health behavior. A health educator without a theory is like a mechanic or a mere technician, whereas the professional who understands theory and research comprehends the *why?* and can design and craft well-tailored interventions. He or she does not blindly follow a cookbook recipe but constantly creates the recipe anew, depending on the circumstances. In health education, the circumstances include the nature of the target audience, setting, resources, goals, and constraints (Prochaska, DiClemente, and Norcross, 1992; Green and others, 1994).

An understanding of theory also guides the user to measure more carefully and astutely in order to assess the impact of interventions. Learning from successive interventions and from published evidence strengthens not only the knowledge base of the individual health professional but also, over time, such cumulative learning contributes to the knowledge base of all. Along their continuum, theory, research, and practice nurture and are nurtured by each other.

The health educator in a health maintenance organization who understands the relevance of The Transtheoretical Model (TTM) or Social Cognitive Theory (SCT) may be able to design better interventions to help patients lose weight or stop smoking. The community health educator who understands principles of social marketing and media communication can make far better use of the mass media than one who docs not. The nurse who recognizes that modeling is important to how people learn, as postulated in SCT, may do a better job of teaching diabetics how to administer their injections. A working knowledge of community organization can help the educator identify and mobilize key individuals and groups to develop or maintain a health promotion program. The physician who understands interpersonal influence can communicate more effectively with patients. The health psychologist who understands The Transtheoretical Model of change will know how to design better smoking cessation and exercise interventions and how to tailor them to the needs of his or her patients.

What Is Theory?

A *theory* is a set of interrelated concepts, definitions, and propositions that present a *systematic* view of events or situations by specifying relations among variables in order to *explain* and *predict* the events or situations (Kerlinger, 1986). The notion of *generality*, or broad application, is important, as is *testability* (van Ryn and Heaney, 1992). Theories are by their nature abstract: that is, they do not have a specified content or topic area (Glanz and Rimer, 1995). Like an empty coffee cup, they have a shape and boundaries but nothing concrete inside. They only come alive when they are filled with practical topics, goals, and problems.

A fully developed formal theory—more an ideal than a reality—is a completely closed deductive system of propositions that identifies the interrelationships among the concepts and is a systematic view of the phenomena (Kerlinger, 1986; Blalock, 1969). In reality, there is no such system in the social sciences or health promotion and education; it can only be approximated (Blalock, 1969). Theory has been defined in a variety of ways, each consistent with Kerlinger's definition. Table 2.1 summarizes several definitions of theory. These definitions, put forth in the 1970s and 1980s, have stood the test of time. They have been articulated in more recent works without substantive changes (Isaac and Michael, 1995; Sussman, 2001).

Theories can help us during the various stages of planning, implementing, and evaluating an intervention. Program planners can use theories to shape the pursuit of answers to *why? what?* and *how?* That is, theories can be used to guide the search for *why* people are not following public health and medical advice or not caring for themselves in healthy ways. They can help pinpoint *what* you need to know before developing and organizing an intervention program. They can provide insight into *how* to shape program strategies to reach people and organizations and make an impact on them. They also help to identify *what* should be monitored, measured, or compared in a program evaluation (Glanz, Lewis, and Rimer, 1996; Glanz and Rimer, 1995).

Thus, theories and models *explain* behavior and suggest ways to achieve behavior *change*. Explanatory theories, often called a *theory of the problem*, help describe

TABLE 2.1. DEFINITIONS OF THEORY.

Definition	Source
A set of interrelated constructs (concepts), definitions, and propositions that presents a systematic view of phenomena by specifying relations among variables, with the purpose of explaining and predicting phenomena	Kerlinger, 1986, p. 9
A systematic explanation for the observed facts and laws that relate to a particular aspect of life	Babbie, 1989, p. 46
A formal and abstract statement about a selected aspect of reality	Kar, 1986, pp. 157–158
Knowledge writ large in the form of generalized abstractions applicable to a wide range of experiences	McGuire, 1983, p. 2
A set of relatively abstract and general statements that collectively purport to explain some aspect of the empirical world	Chafetz, 1978, p. 2
An abstract, symbolic representation of what is conceived to be reality—a set of abstract statements designed to "fit" some portion of the real world	Zimbardo, Ebbesen, and Maslach, 1977, p. 53

and identify why a problem exists. These theories guide the search for modifiable factors such as knowledge, attitudes, self-efficacy, social support, lack of resources, and so on. Change theories, or *theories of action,* guide the development of interventions. They also form the basis for evaluation, pushing the evaluator to make explicit her or his assumptions about how a program should work. These two types of theory often have different foci, but are quite complementary.

Even though various theoretical models of health behavior may reflect the same general ideas (Cummings, Becker, and Maile, 1980; Weinstein, 1993; Mullen, Hersey, and Iverson, 1987), each theory employs a unique vocabulary to articulate the specific factors considered to be important. The *why* tells us about the processes by which changes occur in the target variables. Theories vary in the extent to which they have been conceptually developed and empirically tested. Bandura (1986) points out that "theories are interpreted in different ways depending on the stage of development of the field of study. In advanced disciplines, theories integrate laws; in less advanced fields, theories specify the determinants governing the phenomena of interest." The term *theory* must be used in the latter sense in *Health Behavior and Health Education* because the field is still relatively young.

Concepts, Constructs, and Variables

Concepts are the major components of a theory; they are the building blocks or primary elements of a theory. Concepts can vary in the extent to which they have meaning or can be understood outside the context of a specific theory. When concepts have been developed or adopted for use in a particular theory, they are called *constructs* (Kerlinger, 1986). The term *subjective normative belief* is an example of a construct within Ajzen and Fishbein's Theory of Reasoned Action (1980) (also see Chapter Four); the specific construct is understood only within the context of that theory. Another example of a construct is the term *perceived susceptibility* in the Health Belief Model (see Chapter Three).

Variables are the empirical counterparts or operational forms of constructs. They specify how a construct is to be measured in a specific situation. It is important to keep in mind that *variables* should be matched to *constructs* when identifying what should be assessed in the evaluation of a theory-driven program.

Principles

Theories go beyond *principles*. Principles are general guidelines for action. They are broad and nonspecific and may actually distort realities or results based on research. Principles may be based on precedent or history, *or* they may be based on research. At their worst, principles are so broad that they invite multiple interpretations and are therefore unreliable. In their weakest form, principles are like horoscopes: Anyone can derive whatever meaning he or she wants from them. At their best, principles are based on accumulated research. In their best form, principles provide hypotheses and serve as our most informed hunches about how or what we should do to obtain a desired outcome in a target population.

Models

Health behavior and the guiding concepts for influencing it are far too complex to be explained by a single, unified theory. *Models* draw on a number of theories to help understand a specific problem in a particular setting or context. They are often informed by more than one theory as well as by empirical findings (Earp and Ennett, 1991). Several models that support program planning processes are widely used in health promotion and education: Green and Kreuter's PRECEDE-PROCEED model (1999; also see Chapter Eighteen), social marketing (see Chapter Nineteen), and ecological planning approaches (Green and others, 1994; McLeroy, Bibeau, Steckler, and Glanz, 1988; also see Chapter Twenty). New frameworks to integrate various theories and incorporate multilevel influences have also been proposed by Stokols (1992), Winett (1995), and Rothman (2000).

Paradigms for Theory and Research in Health Promotion and Education

A *paradigm* is a basic schema that organizes our broadly based view of something (Babbie, 1989). Paradigms are widely recognized scientific achievements that, for a time, provide model problem-solving approaches to a community of practitioners and scientists. They include theory, application, and instrumentation and comprise models that represent coherent traditions of scientific research (Kuhn, 1962). Paradigms gain status because they are more successful at solving pressing problems than are their competitors (Kuhn, 1962).

Paradigms create boundaries within which the search for answers occurs; they do not answer particular questions, but they do direct the search for answers to questions (Babbie, 1989). Paradigms circumscribe or delimit what is important to examine in a given field of inquiry. The collective judgments of scientists define the dominant paradigm that constitutes the body of science (Wilson, 1952).

In the fields of health education and health behavior (and in this text), the dominant paradigm that supports the largest body of theory and research is that of *logical positivism*, or *logical empiricism*. This basic view, developed in the Vienna Circle from 1924 to 1936, has two central features: (1) an emphasis on the use of induction, or sensory experience, feelings, and personal judgments as the source of knowledge; and (2) the view that deduction is the standard for verification or confirmation of theory so that theory must be tested through empirical methods and systematic observation of phenomena (Runes, 1984). Logical empiricism reconciles the deductive and inductive extremes; it prescribes that the researcher begin with a hypothesis deduced from a theory and then test it, subjecting it to the jeopardy of disconfirmation through empirical test (McGuire, 1983).

An alternative worldview in health promotion and education relies more heavily on induction and is often identified as a predominantly constructivist paradigm. This perspective argues that the organization and explanation of events must be revealed through a process of discovery rather than organized into prescribed conceptual categories before a study begins (Lewis, 1996). As such, data collection methods such as standardized questionnaires and predetermined response categories have a limited place. Ethnography, phenomenology, and grounded theory are examples of approaches using a constructivist paradigm (Strauss, 1987). It has become increasingly common in the field for work to originate within a constructivist paradigm and shift toward a focus on answering specific research questions using methodologies from the logical positivist paradigm.

Lewin's metatheory stipulates the rules to be followed for building good theory; it is consistent with logical positivism but focuses on his view that the function of social psychology is to further understand the interrelationships between the individual and the social environment (Gold, 1992). This "metatheory" is an orientation or approach, distinct from Lewin's specific field theory (Gold, 1992), and has been influential in health behavior theory since the earliest attempts to use social science to solve public health problems (Rosenstock, 1990). Key rules of Lewin's metatheory require analysis that starts with the situation as a whole, contemporaneity, a dynamic approach, constructive method, mathematical representation of constructs and variables, and a psychological approach that explains both inner experiences and overt actions from the actor's perspective (Lewin, [1942] 1951). The latter rule implies a single level of analysis requiring "closed theory" and poses a serious limitation to solving the problems of contemporary health promotion. It raises the issue—one that those concerned with health behavior often grapple with—that we must often trade off theoretical elegance in favor of relevance (Gold, 1992).

While the paradigms described above focus on the basic schema for development and application of knowledge, health education and health behavior are also concerned with approaches to solving social problems; in other words, how to bring about change. Considerable scholarly and practitioner efforts have been devoted to developing techniques that change behavior. While such techniques grew out of a desire to produce a better world, those that "push" people to change were experienced by many as manipulating, reducing freedom of choice, and sustaining a balance of power in favor of the "change agent" (Kipnis, 1994). A paradigm shift has occurred whereby most behavioral techniques today (for example, social support, empowerment, personal growth) are based on *reducing restraints against change* and promoting informed decision making, rather than on pushing people to change. Nevertheless, as Kipnis (1994) notes, even when health education (or social science) uses these techniques for the elimination of injustice, the inherent exercise of power remains a problem.

New paradigms for understanding, studying, and applying knowledge about human behavior continue to arise and may be influential in the future of applied social sciences in health behavior and education. Sperry (1993) suggests that a "cognitive revolution" that explains conscious behavior as based on subjective mental states is increasingly blending free will and determinism and regarding subjective human values as the underlying key to world change. Barton (1994) notes that models based on concepts of chaos, nonlinear dynamics, and self-organization provide a new paradigm for understanding systems and system change. The Institute of Medicine's Committee on Capitalizing on Social Science and Behavioral Research to Improve the Public's Health recommends strongly that "interventions on social and behavioral factors should link multiple levels of influence" rather than focusing on a single or limited number of health determinants (Smedley and Syme, 2000, p. 7).

Trends in the Use of Health Behavior Theories and Models

Theories that gain recognition in a discipline shape the field, help define the scope of practice, and influence the training and socialization of its professionals. No single theory or conceptual framework dominates research or practice in health promotion and education today. Instead, there is a multitude of theories from which to choose. In a review of 116 theory-based articles published between 1986 and 1988 in two major health education journals, conducted during planning for the first edition of this book, we found fifty-one distinct theoretical formulations. At that time, the three most frequently mentioned theories were: Social Learning Theory, the Theory of Reasoned Action, and the Health Belief Model (Glanz, Lewis, and Rimer, 1990).

To plan for the second edition of this book, we reviewed 526 articles from twenty-four journals in health education, medicine, and behavioral sciences, published from mid-1992 to mid-1994. Sixty-six different theories and models were identified, and twenty-one of these were mentioned eight times or more. Two-thirds of the total instances of theory use in the 497 articles using one or more of the twenty-one most common theories or models were accounted for by the first eight: the Health Belief Model, Social Cognitive Theory, Self-Efficacy (Bandura, 1997), the Theory of Reasoned Action and the Theory of Planned Behavior, community organization, The Transtheoretical Model, also known as the Stages of Change model, social marketing, and social support and social networks (Glanz, Lewis, and Rimer, 1996).

Through the mid-1990s, several publications described experts' views of the dominant theoretical models used in health behavior and education today. Among the most frequently mentioned theories and models were the Health Belief Model, Social Cognitive Theory, The Transtheoretical Model or Stages of Change model, the Theory of Reasoned Action, Diffusion Theory, and ecological models (Freudenberg and others, 1995; van Ryn and Heaney, 1992; Earp and Ennett, 1991; Glanz and Rimer, 1995; Weinstein, 1993). Glanz and Oldenburg (2001) identified some key constructs that cut across often-cited models for understanding behavior and behavior change: the importance of the individual's view of the world, multiple levels of influence, behavior change as a process, motivation versus intention, intention versus action, and changing behavior versus maintaining behavior change.

Along with the published observations about *which* theories are being used, concerns have been raised about *how* the theories are used (or not used) in research and practice. A common refrain is that researchers may not understand how to measure and analyze constructs of health behavior theories (Rejeski, Brawley, McAuley, and Rapp, 2000; Marsh, Johnson, and Carey, 2001). Considerable conceptual confusion—among both researchers and practitioners—about interrelationships between related theories and variables has also been observed (Rosenstock, Strecher and Becker, 1988; Weinstein, 1993; Mullen, Hersey, and Iverson, 1987). Clearly, the need for clarification and illustration of applied theory continues to be a priority.

Selection of Theories for This Book

Our selection of theories and models to be included in the third edition of *Health Behavior and Health Education* was based on the published information summarized above, supplemented by an updated analysis of the health behavior literature. We reviewed all issues of twelve journals in health education, health behavior, and preventive medicine published in 1999 and 2000, using a process similar to what we did in the mid-1990s. Ten theories or models clearly emerged as the most often used. The first two, and by far the most dominant, were Social Cognitive Theory (sometimes referred to by the core construct of Self-Efficacy [Bandura, 1997]) and The Transtheoretical Model. The remainder of the top ten theories and models were: the Health Belief Model, social support and social networks, patient-provider communication, the Theory of Reasoned Action and the Theory of Planned Behavior, stress and coping, community organization, ecological models or social ecology, and Diffusion Theory.

An additional source of data regarding frequently used theories of health behavior is a recently released evidence review on dietary behavior change interventions for cancer prevention (Ammerman and others, 2001). In what appears to be an emerging trend, the evidence tables reported on theories and models used in the 104 intervention studies included in the review. While nearly two dozen theories were listed, only three were used in more than three studies: Social Cognitive Theory, The Transtheoretical Model, and the Health Belief Model (Ammerman and others, 2001).

Each of the most often cited theories and models are the focus of chapters in this third edition of *Health Behavior and Health Education*. These theories have been selected to provide readers with a range of theories representing different units of intervention: individual, group, and community. They were also chosen because they represent, as with Social Cognitive Theory, The Transtheoretical Model, and the Health Belief Model, dominant theories of health behavior and health education.

Others, such as social marketing, the PRECEDE/PROCEED Model, and community organization, were chosen for their practical value in applying theoretical formulations in a way that has demonstrated usefulness to professionals concerned with health behavior change.

Our selection of theories resulted from our review and also reflects some difficult editorial decisions. Three criteria that are consistent with and confirmatory of our review also helped to define the content of this book. First, we determined that the theory must meet basic standards of adequacy for research and practice, thus having the potential for effective use by health education practitioners. Second, *current* health behavior and health education research must be using the theory. (That is why, for example, we include the Health Belief Model rather than Lewin's Field Theory.) The third criterion is that there must be at least promising, if not substantial, empirical evidence supporting the theory's validity in predicting or changing health behavior.

In some cases, a purpose rather than the theory is the identifying title for a chapter—as in the case of Chapter Eleven, which describes theories of interpersonal communication and social influence and illustrates their use for health education. Chapter Thirteen, on community organization, is named for the resultant intervention strategies rather than for the convergent theoretical bases that form the foundation for community organization work. Chapters in Part Five present the PRECEDE-PROCEED model for program planning, social marketing, and ecological models, each of which draws on multiple theories to understand health behavior and assist in development of effective intervention programs and strategies.

We recognize the lack of consensus regarding the definition and classification of theories. We have taken a liberal, ecumenical stance toward theory. And we concede that the lowest common denominator of the theoretical models herein might be that they are all conceptual or theoretical frameworks, or broadly conceived perspectives used to organize ideas. Nevertheless, we have not abandoned the term *theory* because it accurately describes the spirit of this book and describes the goal to be attained for developing frameworks and the tools for refining health education research and practice.

Fitting a Theory or Theories to Research and Practice: Building Bridges and Forging Links

Effective health education depends on marshaling the most appropriate theory and practice strategies for a given situation. Different theories are best suited to different units of practice, such as individuals, groups, and organizations. For example, when one is attempting to overcome women's personal barriers to obtaining mammograms, the Health Belief Model may be useful. The Transtheoretical Model may be especially useful in developing smoking cessation interventions. The Precaution Adoption Process Model may be appropriate when trying to explain how people respond to risk communications. When one is trying to change physicians' mammography practices by instituting reminder systems, organizational change theories are more suitable. The choice of a suitable theory or theories should begin with identifying the problem, goal, and units of practice (van Ryn and Heaney, 1992; Sussman and Sussman, 2001), *not* with selecting a theoretical framework because it is intriguing, familiar, or in vogue.

The adequacy of a theory most often is assessed in terms of three criteria: (1) its *logic*, or *internal consistency* in not yielding mutually contradictory derivations, (2) the extent to which it is *parsimonious* or broadly relevant while using a manageable number of concepts, and (3) its *plausibility* in fitting with prevailing theories in the field (McGuire, 1983).

Theories are further judged in the context of activities of practitioners and researchers. Practitioners apply the pragmatic criterion of *usefulness* to a theory and are concerned with whether it is consistent with everyday observations (Burdine and McLeroy, 1992; Glanz and Rimer, 1995). Researchers make scientific judgments of a theory's *ecological validity*, the extent to which it conforms to observable reality when empirically tested (McGuire, 1983). We need to test our theories iteratively in the real world (Rosenstock, 1990). When we do so, theory, research, and practice begin to converge.

Health education and health behavior theory are eclectic and derivative. Adaptations and refinements of theories of health behavior and health education occur in response to the concerns of both scientists and practitioners. A circularity exists between theory and practice. As Roberts (1959) astutely noted more than three decades ago, "The theoretical base of our profession must be augmented and modified by continuing, careful analysis of documented practice and from collaborative action research."

Practitioners of health education at once benefit from and are challenged by the eclectic and derivative nature of their endeavor: a multitude of theoretical frameworks and models from the social sciences are available for their use, but the best choices and direct translations may not be immediately evident. There is an inherent danger in a book like this: one can begin to think that the links between theory, research, and health promotion practice are easily forged. They are not. For the unprepared, the choices can be overwhelming, but for those who understand the commonalities and differences among theories of health behavior and health education, the growing knowledge base can provide a firm foundation upon which to build. We hope that *Health Behavior and Health Education* will provide and strengthen that foundation for readers.

Science is by definition cumulative, and the same applies to the science base that supports long-standing as well as innovative health behavior interventions. More research is needed at all points along the research continuum. We need more basic research to develop and test theories, more intervention research to develop and test evidence-based interventions, and more concerted, focused attention to dissemination of evidence-based interventions (Rimer, Glanz, and Rasband, 2001). Moreover, both the research and practice communities in HEHB are sorely in need of more rigor and precision in theory development and testing—in measures, assessment of mediating variables, and in specification of theoretical elements (Rejeski, Brawley, McAuley, and Rapp, 2000).

The gift of theory is that it provides the conceptual underpinnings to well-crafted research and informed practice. "The scientist values research by the size of its contribution to that huge, logically articulated structure of ideas which is already, though not half built, the most glorious accomplishment of mankind" (Medawar, 1967).

In this book, we aim to demystify theory and to communicate theory and theoretically inspired research alongside their implications for practice. We encourage informed criticism of theories. Only through rigorous scrutiny will our theories improve. The ultimate test of these ideas and this information rests on its use over time. Like any long-term behavior, this will require social support, supportive environments, and periodic reinforcement. The beneficiaries will be practitioners, researchers, and the participants in health education programs.

As this chapter and the preceding one demonstrate, health education and health behavior are concerns of ever-increasing importance to the well-being of humankind worldwide. As scholars, researchers, and practitioners, all of us grapple with the complexities of human beings and society. We press forward within the limits of current methodologies while striving to build a cumulative body of knowledge in a fast-changing world. The results of some of our efforts are disappointing, but this should motivate, not deter us in pursuing high-quality work. Continual dialogue between theory, research, and practice involves compromise, creativity, healthy criticism, appreciation of others' skills, and a willingness to cooperate to learn and to set high standards. "We must learn to honor excellence in every socially accepted human activity, however humble the activity, and to scorn shoddiness, however exalted the activity. An excellent plumber is infinitely more admirable than an incompetent philosopher. The society that scorns excellence in plumbing because plumbing is a humble activity and tolerates shoddiness in philosophy because it is an exalted activity will have neither good plumbing nor good philosophy. Neither its pipes nor its theories will hold water" (Gardner, 1984).

Limitations of This Book

No text can be all-inclusive. This is certainly true of *Health Behavior and Health Education.* Some theories and frameworks presented in previous editions of this book do not appear in this edition: Consumer Information Processing (Rudd and Glanz, 1990), Multiattribute Utility Theory (Carter, 1990), Attribution Theory (Lewis and Daltroy, 1990), and Media Advocacy (Wallack, 1990). These theories and frameworks remain important, but we found them to be less widely used than those included in this edition. Interested readers should refer to the first edition of this book and to other sources (Glanz and Rimer, 1995) for coverage of these frameworks.

There are other important theories and conceptual frameworks that could not be included because of space limitations. These include Self-Regulation Theory (Leventhal, Zimmerman, and Gutmann, 1984), Protection Motivation Theory (Rogers, 1975), and more familiar classical theories such as Field Theory (Lewin, 1935) and Cognitive Consistency (Festinger, 1957). Some of these are described as part of the historical origins of the various theories discussed in this book. Others are discussed in the synthesis and perspectives chapters.

This book is not intended to be a how-to guide or a manual for program planning and development in health education and health behavior. Other books in health education, nursing, medicine, psychology, and nutrition serve that purpose, and readers should seek out key sources in each discipline for more on the "nuts and bolts" of practice. In addition, this volume will be most useful when it is included as part of a problem-oriented learning program, whether in a formal professional education setting or through continuing education venues.

Neither is this volume intended to serve as an in-depth treatise on research methods in health behavior and health education. Instead, it demonstrates by example how theories are operationalized in a modest number of examples. The reader who wishes more guidance regarding applied research for studies of health behavior and education will find ample resources in books on social science research methodology and measurement in health behavior and education.

We hope that readers will emerge with a critical appreciation of theory and with the curiosity to pursue not only the theories presented in *Health Behavior and Health Education* but other promising theories as well. This book should be regarded as a starting point, not the finish.

Theories—or conceptual frameworks—can be, and *are*, useful because they enrich, inform, and complement the practical technologies of health promotion and education. Thus the readers of this book should "pass with relief from the tossing sea of Cause and Theory to the firm ground of Result and Fact" (Churchill, 1898). As the ocean meets the shore, so we hope you will find that theory, research, and practice in health promotion and education stretch out to converge in a single landscape.

References

Ajzen, I., and Fishbein, M. *Understanding Attitudes and Predicting Social Behavior.* Englewood Cliffs, N.J.: Prentice-Hall, 1980.

Ammerman, A., and others. "Efficacy of Interventions to Modify Dietary Behavior Related to Cancer Risk." Evidence Report/Technology Assessment No. 25 (Contract No. 290–97–0011 to the Research Triangle Institute-University of North Carolina at Chapel Hill Evidence-Based Practice Center), AHRQ Publication No. 01-E029, Rockville, Md.: Agency for Healthcare Research and Quality, February 2001.

Babbie, E. *The Practice of Social Research.* (5th ed.) Belmont, Calif.: Wadsworth, 1989.

Bandura, A. *Social Foundations of Thought and Action: A Social Cognitive Theory.* Englewood Cliffs, N.J.: Prentice Hall, 1986.

Bandura, A. *Self-Efficacy: The Exercise of Control.* New York: W.H. Freeman and Company, 1997.

Barton, S. "Chaos, Self-Organization, and Psychology." *American Psychologist,* 1994, *49*(1), 5–14.

Bernstein, R. *Praxis and Action.* Philadelphia: University of Pennsylvania Press, 1971.

Blalock, H. M., Jr. *Theory Construction, from Verbal to Mathematical Constructions.* Englewood Cliffs, N.J.: Prentice Hall, 1969.

Burdine, J. N., and McLeroy, K. R. "Practitioners' Use of Theory: Examples from a Workgroup." *Health Education Quarterly,* 1992, *19*(3), 315–330.

Carter, W. "Health Behavior as a Rational Process: Theory of Reasoned Action and Multiattribute Utility Theory." In K. Glanz, F. M. Lewis, and B. K. Rimer (eds.), *Health Behavior and Health Education: Theory, Research, and Practice.* San Francisco: Jossey-Bass, 1990.

Chafetz, J. *A Primer on the Construction of Theories in Sociology.* Itasca, Ill.: Peacock, 1978.

Churchill, W. *The Malakand Field Force.* 1898.

Cummings, K. M., Becker, M. H., and Maile, M. C. "Bringing the Models Together: An Empirical Approach to Combining Variables Used to Explain Health Actions." *Journal of Behavioral Medicine,* 1980, *3*, 123–145.

D'Onofrio, C. N. "Theory and the Empowerment of Health Education Practitioners." *Health Education Quarterly,* 1992, *19*(3), 385–403.

Earp, J. A., and Ennett, S. T. "Conceptual Models for Health Education Research and Practice." *Health Education Research,* 1991, *6*(2), 163–171.

Festinger, L. *A Theory of Cognitive Dissonance.* Stanford, Calif.: Stanford University Press, 1957.

Freudenberg, N., and others. "Strengthening Individual and Community Capacity to Prevent Disease and Promote Health: In Search of Relevant Theories and Principles." *Health Education Quarterly,* 1995, *22*(3), 290–306.

Gardner, J. *Excellence* (Revised Ed.). New York: W.W. Norton, 1984.

Glanz, K., Lewis, F. M., and Rimer, B. K. (eds.). *Health Behavior and Health Education: Theory, Research, and Practice.* San Francisco: Jossey-Bass, 1990.

Glanz, K., Lewis, F. M., and Rimer, B. K. (eds.). *Health Behavior and Health Education: Theory, Research, and Practice.* (2nd ed.) San Francisco: Jossey-Bass, 1996.

Glanz, K., and Oldenburg, B. "Utilizing Theories and Constructs Across Models of Behavior Change." In R. Patterson (ed.), *Changing Patient Behavior: Improving Outcomes in Health and Disease Management.* San Francisco: Jossey-Bass, 2001.

Glanz, K., and Rimer, B. K. *Theory at a Glance: A Guide for Health Promotion Practice.* (Monograph) Bethesda, Md.: National Cancer Institute, NIH Publication No. 95–3896, 1995.

Gold, M. "Metatheory and Field Theory in Social Psychology: Relevance or Elegance?" *Journal of Social Issues,* 1992, *48*(2), 67–78.

Green, L. W., and Kreuter, M. W. *Health Promotion Planning: An Educational and Ecological Approach.* (3rd ed.) Mountain View, Calif.: Mayfield, 1999.

Green, L. W., and others. "Can We Build On, or Must We Replace, the Theories and Models in Health Education?" *Health Education Research,* 1994, *9*(3), 397–404.

Hiatt, R. A., and Rimer, B. K. "A New Strategy for Cancer Control Research." *Cancer, Epidemiology, Biomarkers and Prevention,* 1999, *8*, 957–964.

Isaac, S., and Michael, W. B. *Handbook of Research and Evaluation.* (3rd ed.) San Diego: Educational and Industrial Testing Services, 1995.

Kanfer, F. H., and Schefft, B. *Guiding the Process of Therapeutic Change.* Champaign, Ill.: Research Press, 1988.

Kar, S. B. "Introduction: Theoretical Foundations of Health Education and Promotion." *Advances in Health Education and Promotion,* 1986, *1*, 157–163.

Kerlinger, F. N. *Foundations of Behavioral Research.* (3rd ed.) New York: Holt, Rinehart and Winston, 1986.

Kipnis, D. "Accounting for the Use of Behavior Technologies in Social Psychology." *American Psychologist,* 1994, *49*(3), 165–172.

Kuhn, T. S. *The Structure of Scientific Revolution.* Chicago: University of Chicago Press, 1962.

Leventhal, H., Zimmerman, R., and Gutmann, M. "Compliance: A Self-Regulation Perspective." In D. Gentry (ed.), *Handbook of Behavioral Medicine.* New York: Guilford Press, 1984.

Lewin, K. *A Dynamic Theory of Personality.* New York: McGraw Hill, 1935.

Lewin, K. "Field Theory and Learning." In D. Cartwright (ed.), *Field Theory in Social Science.* New York: Harper, 1951. (Originally published 1942.)

Lewis, F. "Whom and From What Paradigm Should Health Promotion Serve?" *Health Education Quarterly,* 1996, *23*, 448–452.

Lewis, F. M., and Daltroy, L. "How Causal Explanations Influence Health Behavior: Attribution Theory." In K. Glanz, F. M. Lewis, and B. K. Rimer (eds.), *Health Behavior and Health Education: Theory, Research, and Practice.* San Francisco: Jossey-Bass, 1990.

Marsh, K. L., Johnson, B. T., and Carey, M. P. "Conducting Meta-Analyses of HIV Prevention Literatures from a Theory-Testing Perspective." *Evaluation and the Health Professions,* 2001, *24*, 255–276.

McGuire, W. J. "A Contextualist Theory of Knowledge: Its Implications for Innovation and Reform in Psychological Research." *Advances in Experimental Social Psychology,* 1983, *16*, 1–47.

McLeroy, K. R., Bibeau, D., Steckler, A., and Glanz, K. "An Ecological Perspective on Health Promotion Programs." *Health Education Quarterly,* 1988, *15*, 351–377.

Medawar, P. B. *The Art of the Soluble.* New York: Methuen, 1967.

Mullen, P. D., Hersey, J. C., and Iverson, D. C. "Health Behavior Models Compared." *Social Science and Medicine,* 1987, *24*, 973–981.

National Center for Chronic Disease Prevention and Health Promotion. "Setting the Agenda, CDC Research in Chronic Disease Prevention and Health Promotion." Atlanta: Centers for Disease Control and Prevention, September 2000.

Prochaska, J. O., DiClemente, C. C., and Norcross, J. C. "In Search of How People Change: Applications to Addictive Behaviors." *American Psychologist*, 1992, *47*(9), 1102–1114.

Rejeski, W. J., Brawley, L. R., McAuley, E., and Rapp, S. "An Examination of Theory and Behavior Change in Randomized Clinical Trials." *Controlled Clinical Trials*, 2000, *21*(5 Supplement), 164S-170S.

Rimer, B. K., Glanz, K., and Rasband, G. "Searching for Evidence About Health Education and Health Behavior Interventions." *Health Education and Behavior*, 2001, *28*, 231–248.

Roberts, B. J. "Decision Making: An Illustration of Theory Building." Presidential address, 10th annual meeting of the Society of Public Health Educators, Atlantic City, N.J., Oct. 18, 1959.

Rogers, R. "A Protection Motivation Theory of Fear Appeals and Attitude Change." *Journal of Psychology*, 1975, *91*, 93–114.

Rosenstock, I. M. "The Past, Present, and Future of Health Education." In K. Glanz, F. M. Lewis, and B. K. Rimer, (eds.), *Health Behavior and Health Education: Theory, Research, and Practice*. San Francisco: Jossey-Bass, 1990.

Rosenstock, I. M., Strecher, V. J., and Becker, M. H. "Social Learning Theory and the Health Belief Model." *Health Education Quarterly*, 1988, *15*(2), 175–183.

Rothman, A. J. "Toward a Theory-Based Analysis of Behavioral Maintenance." *Health Psychology*, 2000, *29*(1 Supplement), 64–69.

Rudd, J., and Glanz, K. "How Individuals Use Information for Health Action: Consumer Information Processing." In K. Glanz, F. M. Lewis, and B. K. Rimer, (eds.), *Health Behavior and Health Education: Theory, Research, and Practice*. San Francisco: Jossey-Bass, 1990.

Runes, D. *Dictionary of Philosophy*. Totawa, N.J.: Rowman and Allanheld, 1984.

Sallis, J. F., Owen, N., and Fotheringham, M. J. "Behavioral Epidemiology: A Systematic Framework to Classify Phases of Research on Health Promotion and Disease Prevention." *Annals of Behavioral Medicine*, 2000, *22*, 294–298.

Smedley, B. D., and Syme, S. L. (eds.). *Promoting Health: Intervention Strategies from Social and Behavioral Research*. Washington, D.C.: National Academy Press, 2000.

Sperry, R. W. "The Impact and Promise of the Cognitive Revolution." *American Psychologist*, 1993, *48*(8), 878–885.

Stokols, D. "Establishing and Maintaining Healthy Environments: Toward a Social Ecology of Health Promotion." *American Psychologist*, 1992, *47*(1), 6–22.

Strauss, A. L. *Qualitative Analysis for Social Scientists*. Cambridge, England: Cambridge University Press, 1987.

Sussman, S. (ed.). *Handbook of Program Development for Health Behavior Research and Practice*. Thousand Oaks, Calif.: Sage, 2001.

Sussman, S., and Sussman, A. N. "Praxis in Health Behavior Program Development." In S. Sussman (ed.), *Handbook of Program Development for Health Behavior Research and Practice*. Thousand Oaks, Calif.: Sage, 2001.

van Ryn, M., and Heaney, C. A. "What's the Use of Theory?" *Health Education Quarterly*, 1992, *19*(3), 315–330.

Wallack, L. "Media Advocacy: Promoting Health Through Mass Communication." In K. Glanz, F. M. Lewis, and B. K. Rimer (eds.), *Health Behavior and Health Education: Theory, Research, and Practice*. San Francisco: Jossey-Bass, 1990.

Weinstein, N. D. "Testing Four Competing Theories of Health-Protective Behavior." *Health Psychology,* 1993, *12*(4), 324–333.

Wilson, E. B. *An Introduction to Scientific Research.* New York: McGraw-Hill, 1952.

Winett, R. A. "A Framework for Health Promotion and Disease Prevention Programs." *American Psychologist,* 1995, *50*(5), 341–350.

Zimbardo, P. G., Ebbesen. E. B., and Maslach, C. *Influencing Attitudes and Changing Behavior.* (2nd ed.) Reading, Mass.: Addison-Wesley, 1977.

PART TWO

MODELS OF INDIVIDUAL HEALTH BEHAVIOR

Individuals are one of the essential units of health education and health behavior theory, research, and practice. This does not mean that the individual is the only or necessarily the most important unit of intervention. But all other units, whether they are groups, organizations, worksites, communities, or larger units, are composed of individuals.

A wide range of health professionals, including health educators, physicians, psychologists, dietitians, and nurses, focus all or most of their efforts on changing the health behavior of individuals. To intervene effectively and to make informed judgments about how to measure the success of such interventions, health professionals must understand the role of individuals in health behavior. This section of *Health Behavior and Health Education* helps the reader achieve a greater understanding of theories that focus primarily on individual health behavior.

Lewin's seminal Field Theory (1935) was one of the early and most far-reaching theories of behavior, and most contemporary theories of health behavior owe a major intellectual debt to Lewin. Theories that focus on barriers and facilitators to behavior change and those that posit the existence of stages are rooted in the Lewinian tradition. During the 1940s and 1950s, researchers began to learn how individuals make decisions about health and what determines health behavior. In the 1950s, Rosenstock, Hochbaum, and others, from their vantage point at the U.S. Public Health Service, began their pioneering work to understand why individuals did or did not participate in screening programs for tuberculosis. This and related work led to the development of the Health Belief Model (HBM). In the last twenty years, considerable progress has been made in understanding the determinants of individuals' health-related behaviors and finding ways to stimulate positive behavior changes. Value expectancy theories, which include both the HBM and the Theory of Reasoned Action (TRA) and its companion, the Theory of Planned Behavior (TPB), matured during this time.

The Transtheoretical Model (TTM), also known as the Stages of Change (SOC) model, which developed initially from the work of Prochaska, DiClemente, and colleagues, was developed in the late 1970s and 1980s and matured in the 1990s. For the third edition of this book, we have added discussion about Weinstein's Precaution Adoption Process Model (PAPM) as a separate chapter. The PAPM was identified as an emerging theory for the second edition but is now sufficiently mature to merit its own chapter.

In Chapter Three, Nancy Janz, Victoria Champion, and Victor Strecher review the evolution of the Health Belief Model and the constructs that are part of its current formulation. The authors explain that the HBM is used to understand why people accept preventive health services and why they do or do not adhere to other kinds of health care regimens. The HBM has spawned literally hundreds of health education and health behavior research studies and provided the conceptual basis for many interventions in the years since it was formulated. It has been used across the health continuum, including in disease prevention, early disease detection, and illness and sick-role behavior (Becker and Maiman, 1975; Janz and Becker, 1984). It is among the most widely applied theoretical foundations for the study of health behavior change. The HBM is appealing and useful to a wide range of professionals concerned with behavioral change. Physicians, dentists, nurses, psychologists, and health educators have all used the HBM to design and evaluate interventions to alter health behavior. The HBM also has been used to guide analysis of large data sets to understand health behavior. The chapter authors provide two examples of how the HBM has been used. One focuses on AIDS (prevention) and the other on mammography (early detection of cancer).

In Chapter Four, Daniel Montaño and Danuta Kasprzyk discuss two value expectancy theories, the Theory of Reasoned Action and the Theory of Planned Behavior. This family of theories has had a major influence on both research and practice in health behavior and health education. The TRA, developed by Fishbein and Ajzen (1975), and its extension by Ajzen to the TPB, propose that behavioral intentions and behaviors result from a rational process of decision making. The key constructs are subjective norms and intentions to perform specific actions. The TPB also includes the construct *perceived behavioral control*. These theories have been used to intervene in many health behaviors, including having mammograms, quitting smoking, controlling weight, family planning, and using condoms to prevent AIDS (Jaccard and Davidson, 1972; Ajzen and Fishbein,

1980; McCarty, 1981; Lowe and Frey, 1983). Recently, the theories have been used by AIDS researchers in developing interventions to help people at high risk to lower their risk of infection. Montaño and Kasprzyk show how the TRA was used to understand clinician discussion of HIV prevention, with a special focus on the behavior of white, black, and Hispanic women.

In Chapter Five, James Prochaska, Colleen Redding, and Kerry Evers review The Transtheoretical Model, or Stages of Change model, developed by Prochaska, DiClemente, and colleagues (Prochaska, DiClemente, Velicer, and Rossi, 1993). Over a relatively short time, this theory achieved widespread use and acceptance by researchers and practitioners in health education and health behavior. The authors present the key components of the theory: the concepts of stage and decisional balance, pros and cons, and the processes of change that characterize people in different stages. They discuss the fact that to have a public health impact, it will be necessary for practitioners to use proactive strategies that reach out to people rather than rely on reactive strategies that ultimately reach few individuals. TTM is particularly useful for guiding the development of such proactive interventions. In their examples, Prochaska, Redding, and Evers show how TTM has been used in the development of both smoking cessation interventions and multiple risk factor interventions for minority adolescents.

Chapter Six, on the Precaution Adoption Process Model, is authored by Neil Weinstein, who developed the PAPM, and his colleague, Peter Sandman. Since the second edition of *Health Behavior and Health Education,* the PAPM has received sufficient refinement and use, especially by researchers, to warrant a separate chapter. Like TTM, the PAPM is a stage model. As discussed in the perspectives chapter, there are major differences between the approaches as well. The building blocks of the PAPM are the steps along a path from lack of awareness about a precaution (such as using condoms to protect against AIDS) to decision making and then, in some cases, to adoption of the recommended precaution, initiation, and maintenance. As Weinstein and Sandman discuss, the process is not always quite so neat. They provide an interesting example of the use of the model to assess people's decisions about testing for radon, an environmental health threat.

Taken together, these four chapters provide researchers and practitioners alike with an introduction to widely used theories of health education and health behavior. The different theories are suitable to different problems and populations. Some are more well-developed and easier to use and apply than others. But each has made an important contribution to our understanding of health behavior. Each deserves to be read, studied, and used. Further refinement of the theories will result from their use in research and practice. The distinguished authors have provided chapters that should be accessible to a wide range of health professionals.

Chapter Seven provides a review of the individual chapters, highlights similarities and differences, and identifies some important future challenges.

References

Ajzen, I., and Fishbein, M. *Understanding Attitudes and Predicting Social Behavior.* Englewood Cliffs, N.J.: Prentice Hall, 1980.

Becker, M. H., and Maiman, L. A. "Sociobehavioral Determinants of Compliance with Health and Medical Care Recommendations." *Medical Care,* 1975, *13,* 10–24.

Fishbein, M., and Ajzen, I. *Belief, Attitude, Intention and Behavior: An Introduction to Theory and Research.* Reading, Mass.: Addison-Wesley, 1975.

Jaccard, J. J., and Davidson, A. R. "Toward an Understanding of Family Planning Behaviors: An Initial Investigation." *Journal of Applied Social Psychology,* 1972, *2,* 228–235.

Janz, N. K., and Becker, M. H. "The Health Belief Model: A Decade Later." *Health Education Quarterly,* 1984, *11,* 1–47.

Lewin, K. *A Dynamic Theory of Personality.* New York: McGraw-Hill, 1935.

Lowe, R. H., and Frey, J. D. "Predicting Lamaze Childbirth Intentions and Outcomes: An Extension of the Theory of Reasoned Action to a Joint Outcome." *Basic and Applied Social Psychology,* 1983, *4,* 353–372.

McCarty, D. "Changing Contraceptive Usage Intention: A Test of the Fishbein Model of Intention." *Journal of Applied Social Psychology,* 1981, *11,* 192–211.

Prochaska, J. O., DiClemente, C. C., Velicer, W. F., and Rossi, J. S. "Standardized, Individualized, Interactive, and Personalized Self-Help Programs for Smoking Cessation." *Health Psychology,* 1993, *12,* 399–405.

CHAPTER THREE

THE HEALTH BELIEF MODEL

Nancy K. Janz
Victoria L. Champion
Victor J. Strecher

For five decades, the Health Belief Model (HBM) has been one of the most widely used conceptual frameworks in health behavior. The HBM has been used both to explain change and maintenance of health-related behaviors and as a guiding framework for health behavior interventions. The HBM has been expanded, broken down into components, compared to other frameworks, and analyzed using a wide array of multivariate analytic techniques. Over the past two decades, more research has been conducted to specify measures of health beliefs and relationships between these beliefs.

In this chapter, we review the components of the HBM that remain vital. We also examine other psychosocial constructs that further explain relationships within the HBM. Earlier reviews of HBM research findings provide historical context for this chapter (Becker, 1974; Janz and Becker, 1984). Recent HBM research continues to emphasize individual health beliefs, placing them in multivariate analyses and examining their predictive qualities. This type of analysis does little to further specify measurement of or relationships between health beliefs. While there are certainly new, interesting results to review, a consideration of three aspects of the HBM is most needed: components of the HBM, the relationships between HBM components, and how to use the HBM to understand and change behaviors with public health significance.

We begin by describing the origins of the HBM and its place in psychosocial theory. Issues related to the measurement of and relationships between HBM constructs, areas that have received only minimal attention, are then discussed in some detail. Next, we discuss how the HBM can be used to explain and intervene in cancer-screening behavior and AIDS-related behaviors. These examples are used because they represent two very different, behaviorally based public health problems in our society, but clearly there are many other possible applications of the HBM. We also discuss the use of the HBM in multicultural settings. Finally, we provide some recommendations for further research.

Origins of the Model

The Health Belief Model was developed initially in the 1950s by a group of social psychologists in the U.S. Public Health Service to explain the widespread failure of people to participate in programs to prevent and detect disease (Hochbaum, 1958; Rosenstock, 1960, 1974). Later the model was extended to people's responses to symptoms (Kirscht, 1974) and to their behaviors in response to diagnosed illness, particularly adherence to medical regimens (Becker, 1974). Although the model evolved gradually in response to very practical programmatic concerns, we summarize its basis in psychological theory as an aid to understanding its rationale, as well as its strengths and weaknesses.

During the early 1950s, academic social psychology was engaged in developing an approach to understanding behavior that grew out of a confluence of learning theories derived from two major sources: *Stimulus Response (S-R) Theory* (Thorndike, 1898; Watson, 1925; Hull, 1943) and *Cognitive Theory* (Tolman, 1932; Lewin, 1935, 1951; Lewin, Dembo, Festinger, and Sears, 1944).

In simple terms, S-R theorists believe that learning results from events (termed *reinforcements*) which reduce physiological drives that activate behavior. Skinner (1938) formulated the widely accepted hypothesis that the frequency of a behavior is determined by its consequences (or reinforcements). For Skinner, the mere temporal association between a behavior and an immediately following reward was regarded as sufficient to increase the probability that the behavior will be repeated. Such behaviors are termed operants; they operate on the environment to bring about changes resulting in rewards or reinforcements. In this view, no mentalistic concepts such as *reasoning* or *thinking* are required to explain behavior.

Cognitive theorists, on the other hand, emphasize the role of subjective hypotheses and expectations held by the subject (Lewin, Dembo, Festinger, and Sears, 1944). In this perspective, behavior is a function of the subjective *value* of an outcome and of the subjective probability, or *expectation*, that a particular action will achieve that outcome.

Such formulations are generally termed *value-expectancy* theories. Mental processes such as thinking, reasoning, hypothesizing, or expecting are critical components of all cognitive theories. Cognitive theorists, along with behaviorists, believe that reinforcements, or consequences of behavior, are important. For cognitive theorists, reinforcements operate by influencing expectations (or hypotheses) regarding the situation rather than by influencing behavior directly (Bandura, 1977a).

The HBM is a value-expectancy theory. When value-expectancy concepts were gradually reformulated in the context of health-related behaviors, the interpretations were as follows: (1) the desire to avoid illness or to get well (value) and (2) the belief that a specific health action available to a person would prevent (or ameliorate) illness (expectation). The expectancy was further delineated in terms of the individual's estimate of personal susceptibility to and severity of an illness, and of the likelihood of being able to reduce that threat through personal action.

The development of the HBM grew out of practical concerns with the limited success of various programs of the U.S. Public Health Service in the 1950s. One such early example was the failure of large numbers of eligible adults to participate in tuberculosis screening programs provided at no charge in mobile X-ray units conveniently located in various neighborhoods. The concern of the program operators was with explaining people's behavior by illuminating those factors that facilitated or inhibited positive responses.

Beginning in 1952, Hochbaum (1958) studied probability samples of more than twelve hundred adults to understand their *readiness* to obtain X rays, which included their beliefs that they were susceptible to tuberculosis and their beliefs in the personal benefits of early detection. Among individuals who exhibited both belief in their own susceptibility to tuberculosis and the belief that overall benefits would accrue from early detection, 82 percent had at least one voluntary chest X ray during a specified period preceding the interview. Of the group exhibiting neither of these beliefs, only 21 percent had obtained voluntary X rays during the criterion period.

Components of the HBM

Over the years since Hochbaum's survey, many investigations have helped to expand and clarify the model and to extend it beyond screening behaviors to include preventive actions, illness behaviors, and sick-role behavior (Rosenstock, 1974; Kirscht, 1974; Becker, 1974; Janz and Becker, 1984). In general, it now is believed that people will take action to prevent, to screen for, or to control ill-health conditions if they regard themselves as susceptible to the condition, if they believe it would have potentially serious consequences, if they believe that a course of action available to them would be beneficial in reducing either their susceptibility to or the severity of the condition, and if they believe that the anticipated barriers to (or costs of) taking the action are outweighed by its benefits. Table 3.1 gives definitions and commentary specifying the key variables in greater detail.

Perceived Susceptibility

This construct refers to one's subjective perception of the risk of contracting a health condition. In the case of medically established illness, the dimension has been reformulated to include acceptance of the diagnosis, personal estimates of resusceptibility, and susceptibility to illness in general.

Perceived Severity

Feelings concerning the seriousness of contracting an illness or of leaving it untreated include evaluations of both medical and clinical consequences (for example, death, disability, and pain) and possible social consequences (such as effects of the conditions on work, family life, and social relations). The combination of susceptibility and severity has been labeled the *perceived threat*.

Perceived Benefits

While acceptance of personal susceptibility to a condition also believed to be serious (perceived threat) produces a force leading to behavior, the particular course of action that will be taken depends on beliefs regarding the effectiveness of the various available actions for reducing the disease threat, termed the *perceived benefits* of taking health action. Other factors include nonhealth-related benefits (for example, quitting smoking to save money; getting a mammogram to please a family member). Thus, an individual exhibiting an optimal level of beliefs in susceptibility and severity would not be expected to accept any recommended health action unless that action also was perceived as potentially efficacious.

Perceived Barriers

The potential negative aspects of a particular health action, or perceived barriers, may act as impediments to undertaking the recommended behavior. A kind of nonconscious, cost-benefit analysis occurs, wherein the individual weighs the action's expected effectiveness against perceptions that it may be expensive, dangerous (having negative side effects or iatrogenic outcomes), unpleasant (painful,

TABLE 3.1. KEY CONCEPTS AND DEFINITIONS
OF THE HEALTH BELIEF MODEL.

Concept	Definition	Application
Perceived susceptibility	One's belief regarding the chance of getting a condition	Define population(s) at risk, risk levels
		Personalize risk based on a person's characteristics or behavior
		Make perceived susceptibility more consistent with an individual's actual risk
Perceived severity	One's belief of how serious a condition and its sequelae are	Specify consequences of the risk and the conditions
Perceived benefits	One's belief in the efficacy of the advised action to reduce risk or seriousness of impact	Define action to take: how, where, when; clarify the positive effects to be expected
Perceived barriers	One's belief about the tangible and psychological costs of the advised action	Identify and reduce perceived barriers through reassurance, correction of misinformation, incentives, assistance
Cues to action	Strategies to activate one's "readiness"	Provide how-to information, promote awareness, employ reminder systems
Self-efficacy	One's confidence in one's ability to take action	Provide training, guidance in performing action
		Use progressive goal setting
		Give verbal reinforcement
		Demonstrate desired behaviors
		Reduce anxiety

difficult, upsetting), inconvenient, time-consuming, and so forth. Thus, "the combined levels of susceptibility and severity [provide] the energy or force to act and the perception of benefits (less barriers) provide a preferred path of action" (Rosenstock, 1974, p. 332).

Cues to Action

In various early formulations of the HBM, the concept of cues that trigger action was discussed. Hochbaum (1958), for example, thought that readiness to take action (perceived susceptibility and perceived benefits) could only be potentiated by other factors, particularly by *cues* to instigate action, such as bodily events, or by environmental events, such as media publicity. He did not, however, study the role of cues empirically. Cues to action may ultimately prove to be important, but they have not been systematically studied. Indeed, while the concept of cues as a trigger mechanism is appealing, it has been difficult to study in explanatory surveys; a cue can be as fleeting as a sneeze or the barely conscious perception of a poster.

Other Variables

Diverse demographic, sociopsychological, and structural variables may affect the individual's perceptions and thus indirectly influence health-related behavior. Specifically, sociodemographic factors, particularly educational attainment, are believed to have an indirect effect on behavior by influencing the perception of susceptibility, severity, benefits, and barriers.

Self-Efficacy

Bandura distinguished efficacy expectations from outcome expectations, defined as a person's estimate that a given behavior will lead to certain outcomes. Outcome expectations are similar to but distinct from the HBM concept of *perceived benefits* (Bandura, 1977a; 1977b; 1986). Self-efficacy is defined as "the conviction that one can successfully execute the behavior required to produce the outcomes" (Bandura, 1977b). Rosenstock, Strecher, and Becker (1988) suggested that self-efficacy be added to the HBM as a separate construct from the original concepts of susceptibility, severity, benefits, and barriers.

It is not difficult to see why self-efficacy was never explicitly incorporated into early formulations of the HBM. The original focus of the model was on circumscribed preventive actions, usually of a one-shot nature, such as accepting a screening test or an immunization, actions that generally were simple behaviors for most people to perform. Since it is likely that most prospective members of target groups for the programs had adequate self-efficacy for performing those simple behaviors, that dimension was not even recognized.

The situation is vastly different, however, when the focus is lifestyle behaviors requiring long-term changes. The problems involved in modifying lifelong habits, such as eating high-fat foods, getting no or too little exercise, smoking, and failure to use safe sexual practices, are generally far more difficult to surmount than are those for accepting a one-time immunization or a screening test. It requires a good deal of confidence that one can, in fact, alter such lifestyles before successful change is possible. Thus, for behavior change to succeed, people must (as the original HBM theorizes) feel threatened by their current behavioral patterns (perceived susceptibility and severity) and believe that change of a specific kind will result in a valued outcome at acceptable cost. They also must feel themselves competent (self-efficacious) to overcome perceived barriers to taking action. A growing body of literature supports the importance of self-efficacy in accounting for initiation and maintenance of behavioral change (Bandura, 1995, 1997).

The HBM, originally developed to explain health-related behavior, focused on cognitive variables. Efforts to change cognitions about health matters have often involved attempts to arouse affect—particularly fear through threatening messages (Leventhal, 1970). According to Protection Motivation Theory (Rogers and Prentice-Dunn, 1997), the most persuasive communications are those that arouse fear while enhancing perceptions central to the HBM of the severity of an event, the likelihood of exposure to that event, *and* the efficacy of responses to that threat. Self-efficacy also has been incorporated into Protection Motivation Theory. This view of the joint role of fear and reassurance in persuasive communications is generally accepted.

The Health Belief Model components are summarized in Figure 3.1.

Evidence for and Against the Model

In 1974, *Health Education Monographs* devoted an entire issue to the Health Belief Model and personal health behavior (Becker, 1974). That issue summarized findings from research on the HBM to understand why individuals did or did not engage in a wide variety of health-related actions, and it provided considerable support for the model in explaining behavior pertinent to prevention and behavior in response to symptoms or to diagnosed disease.

During the decade following publication of that issue, the HBM continued to be a major organizing framework for explaining and predicting acceptance of health and medical care recommendations. Accordingly, an updated critical review was made of HBM studies conducted between 1974 and 1984, which also

FIGURE 3.1. HEALTH BELIEF MODEL COMPONENTS AND LINKAGES.

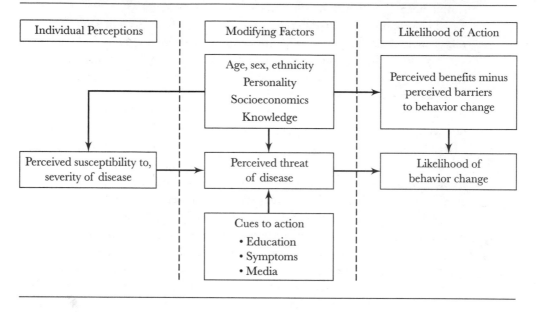

combined the new results with earlier findings to permit an overall assessment of the model's performance (Janz and Becker, 1984).

Summary results provided substantial empirical support for the HBM, with findings from prospective studies at least as favorable as those obtained from retrospective research. Perceived barriers was the most powerful single predictor of the HBM dimensions across all studies and behaviors. While both perceived susceptibility and perceived benefits were important overall, perceived susceptibility was a stronger predictor of preventive health behavior than sick-role behavior; the reverse was true for perceived benefits. Overall, perceived severity was the least powerful predictor; however, this dimension was strongly related to sick-role behavior.

Measuring HBM Constructs

One of the most important deficits in the research on the HBM has been inconsistent measurement of HBM concepts in both descriptive and intervention research. The vast majority of studies using the HBM have failed to establish validity and reliability of measures prior to model testing. Theory testing and development of measures are interdependent. Prior to engaging in instrument development, researchers should search for instruments that have previously been developed and have established validity and reliability. Only when these cannot be found should scale development be undertaken.

When developing new HBM measures, several important principles and procedures should be considered. First, researchers should use construct definitions that are consistent with the HBM theory. Second, construct measurement must be specific to the behavior being addressed. For example, barriers to mammography will be quite different from barriers to colonoscopy. Conducting focus groups with the target population is one strategy to determine barriers that are specific to a behavior. Third, to reduce measurement error, multiple items should be developed for each scale. Finally, validity and reliability of measures must be reexamined with each study. Cultural and population differences make applying scales without such examination risky.

An additional concern for investigators involves addressing the relationship between HBM constructs. Ambiguity about the relationship of theoretical constructs to each other makes tests of construct validity more difficult. Although the HBM clearly identifies the constructs that lead to outcome behaviors, the relationships between concepts are less clear. Whereas many studies have attempted to establish each of the major dimensions as independent, others have tried multiplicative approaches. Investigators have been most successful when looking at models that measure direct as well as conditional effects of variables on behavior (Rosenstock, Strecher, and Becker, 1994). Temporality of relationships also is an issue. When health beliefs and behaviors are measured concurrently, belief-behavior relationships might well turn out to be spurious. Finally, when theoretical concepts (models) are combined, researchers must consider independence of constructs. For example, *outcome expectations* from Bandura's Social Cognitive Theory overlaps with perceived benefits in the HBM.

The past decade has produced several good examples of HBM scale development in the area of cancer screening behaviors (see, for example, Rawl and others, 2000). In relation to breast cancer screening, Champion and colleagues have developed scales to measure constructs of perceived risk, benefits, and barriers to screening (Champion, 1999; Champion and Scott, 1997). Scales were initially developed to address breast self-examination. Further revisions resulted in including mammography benefits and barriers and extending testing to an African American sample. Champion and Scott (1997) found that when scales were developed for African American women, unique issues related to scheduling a mammogram and understanding the procedure surfaced. When revised to be specific to the culture, the scales demonstrated good to excellent reliability and validity similar to those for white samples.

Using the HBM to Address Public Health Concerns

The HBM has been used extensively to determine relationships between constructs and behaviors of public concern as well as to inform interventions. A comprehensive review of all work using the HBM to address health behaviors is beyond the scope of this chapter. In this section, we discuss use of the HBM in two important areas, mammography screening and AIDS-related behaviors, and we show how key HBM components are associated with these behaviors.

The HBM and Mammography Screening Behaviors

Many descriptive studies have reported the predictive ability of the HBM for mammography screening, in particular the constructs of perceived susceptibility to breast cancer and perceived benefits and barriers to action (Champion and Menon, 1997; Friedman, Neff, Webb, and Latham, 1998; Phillips and others, 1998). Determinants of mammography behavior in low-income minority women included perceived susceptibility and barriers related to fear, embarrassment, and costs (Thompson and others, 1997). Research also has addressed differences in perceived susceptibility and barriers by adherent and nonadherent women. Champion and colleagues found that women who were adherent to mammography recommendations had higher perceived susceptibility scores and lower perceived barriers than other groups. Perceived benefits of mammography were lower for women who did not intend to have mammograms (Champion, Skinner, and Foster, 2000).

Several studies have used HBM variables in tailored intervention studies to increase mammography adoption. These are interventions created especially for individual women based on information about the women. Combinations of physician reminder letters and counseling using HBM constructs have shown promise in increasing mammography use. King and colleagues (1994) found that reminder letters and follow-up telephone calls were effective at both steps in increasing adherence. Janz and colleagues (1997) found that a two-step intervention, including a physician letter and peer counseling, resulted in a 38 percent adherence rate compared to 16 percent in the control group for a group of 460 women. The telephone intervention addressed benefits of mammography and barriers identified by respondents.

The most promising strategies for increasing mammography adherence have evolved from individually tailored messages based on HBM beliefs about screening. The constructs of susceptibility, benefits, and barriers have been used for tailoring beliefs. Strecher and Hospers (1994) found that tailored materials increased adherence with women of lower socioeconomic levels. A total of 435 women who had visited family practice groups within the previous two years were selected randomly to receive individually tailored or standardized mammography recommendation letters mailed from physicians' offices. HBM variables of perceived risk and barriers were incorporated into the tailored letters. A significant intervention effect was shown for black and low-income women for movement toward mammography adherence.

An intervention study using the HBM variables of perceived susceptibility, benefits, and barriers was delivered to over three hundred African American women who were at 150 percent of poverty or lower. An in-person counselor addressed each woman's baseline beliefs regarding susceptibility to breast cancer and benefits and barriers to mammography screening. The counselors clarified misconceptions and provided information to change perceptions to be theoretically consistent with obtaining mammography. The most frequently mentioned barriers were fear of finding something wrong, fear of pain, and fear of radiation. For women who had never had a mammogram, adherence was significantly higher in the experimental group (50 percent) than in the control group (18 percent) (Champion, Ray, Heilman, and Springston, 2000).

Mammography intervention trials using the HBM via telephone counseling have shown significant effects. Duan, Fox, Derose, and Carson (2000) assessed the effectiveness of telephone counseling in a church-based mammography promotion intervention trial. Churches were randomized to either telephone counseling or control conditions. A total of 1443 women aged fifty to eighty were recruited as study participants. The intervention was based on the HBM using perceived risk, perceived barriers, and cues to action. Mammography adherence was assessed at one year following the intervention. The HBM-based intervention maintained mammography adherence among baseline-adherent participants and reduced the nonadherence rate from 23 percent to 16 percent.

In a longitudinal intervention study, researchers used the HBM to target mammography screening messages to women receiving care in one of two settings: a health maintenance organization serving insured middle-class women and a general medicine clinic that provided care for underserved women. A randomized six-group design was implemented to test delivery of messages based on HBM constructs by contrasting telephone-delivered messages with in-person counseling. Additionally, a letter encouraging mammography by the woman's personal physician was tested alone and in combination with the targeted counseling. The groups to which women were randomized included (1) standard care, (2) targeted telephone counseling, (3) targeted in-person counseling, (4) physician letter only, (5) targeted telephone counseling plus physician letter, and (6) targeted in-person counseling plus letter. A total of 808 women aged fifty to eighty-five were randomized to one of the six groups. Eligibility requirements specified that women had no previous history of breast cancer and had not undergone a mammogram in the previous fifteen months. At two, four, and six months after the intervention, mammography results were obtained from electronic medical records.

Results indicated significant intervention effects in both HBM beliefs and subsequent behavior. The majority of the women who became adherent did so within two months, after which time the results were linear over time and parallel across groups. All intervention groups except those receiving the physician letter only were significantly different from standard care, with the combination of in-person and physician letter being the most significant. Intervention effects did vary across sites, with the women in the HMO being more affected by the intervention than the women from the general medicine clinic (Champion and others, forthcoming, a).

Most recently, comparing tailored letters with tailored telephone counseling, Champion and colleagues (forthcoming, b) found that telephone counseling plus mailings resulted in the highest adherence (40 percent), but that telephone alone (36 percent) and tailored mailings (37 percent) also were significantly better than standard care. Thus, tailoring messages for breast cancer screening using the HBM constructs of susceptibility, benefits, and barriers has been found to increase mammography adherence.

The HBM and AIDS-Protective Behaviors

The Health Belief Model suggests that for individuals who exhibit high-risk behaviors, perceived susceptibility is necessary before commitment to changing these risky behaviors can occur. In a study of over four hundred young men and women, Steers and others (1996) found that perceived susceptibility to HIV/AIDS was associated with behavior changes, including increased condom use, fewer sex partners, and a decreased number of sexual encounters. Other cross-sectional studies (Ford and Norris, 1995; Liau and Zimet, 2000; Maguen, Armistead, and Kalichman, 2000) also have found significant susceptibility-behavior associations. Countering these findings are several cross-sectional studies that did not find significant susceptibility-behavior associations (Falck, Siegal, Wang, and Carlson, 1995; Lollis, Johnson, Antoni, and Chitwood, 1995; Mahoney, Thombs, and Ford, 1995).

Variations in results are found by the measures used to assess susceptibility. A number of articles we reviewed used a behavioral anchor in their susceptibility measures, for example, asking the question, "If you do not practice safer sex, how likely are you to become infected with the AIDS virus?" as opposed to simply asking, "How likely are you to become infected with the AIDS virus?" Research by

Ronis (1992) suggests that susceptibility questions should be clearly conditional on action or inaction. Unconditional susceptibility measures can lead to a pattern of personalized interpretation—respondents who indicate that their risk of infection is great largely *because* they are not practicing safer sex.

Booth, Zhang, and Kwiatkowski (1999) evaluated a peer-based intervention for runaway and homeless adolescents that was based on principles derived from the HBM. The intervention aimed to first reduce the drug and sex-related HIV-risk behaviors among the peer leaders. The intervention to train peers included discussing individual participants' perceived vulnerability to HIV, identifying skills in negotiating safer sex, avoiding situations where sexual intercourse was likely, and practicing refusal skills when drugs were offered. The authors found that those who perceived they had a great chance of infection were more likely to have used drugs and reported a higher number of sex partners in the previous three months. As described previously, without a behavioral anchor, the authors speculated that the observed relationship may reflect an accurate appraisal of the participants' increased risk. Consistent with the HBM, lower concern with HIV infection was independently associated with the use of heroin and cocaine as well as the overall number of drugs used among the runaway and homeless adolescents. There was not a significant association found between HIV concern and sex risk behavior; however, runaways who used drugs reported nearly twice as many sex partners. HBM-based interventions may need to focus more attention on the interrelationships between concern with HIV infection, drug-risk behaviors, and sex-risk behaviors.

Perceptions of AIDS severity must address the perceived costs of being HIV-positive and of having AIDS. Perceived seriousness, in this case, refers to personal evaluations of the probable biomedical, financial, and social consequences of contracting HIV and having AIDS. Some might argue that asking about AIDS severity would be a waste of respondents' time because it might be assumed that everyone would report AIDS to be an extremely severe disease. Unfortunately, most studies in the research literature do not include measures on the importance of HIV/AIDS severity (Rosenstock, Strecher, and Becker, 1994).

When perception of threat from AIDS is high, the HBM hypothesizes that AIDS-protective behavior decisions become largely a function of perceptions of benefits minus perceived barriers to behavioral change. If the perception of AIDS threat is not high, strong perceived benefits of AIDS-protective behavior may still influence behavioral change. For example, a person who uses condoms because his partner prefers them may adopt and maintain condom-use behavior regardless of his perception of AIDS threat. Although there are perceived benefits in this example, they are not directly related to AIDS-protective behavior, but rather to the benefits of pleasing one's partner. In a similar fashion, reported condom use among Central Harlem youth was motivated by the perceived value of condoms to avoid pregnancy as well as HIV/AIDS, with the strongest motivation being to avoid pregnancy (Laraque and others, 1997). If the perceptions of AIDS threat and benefits are not high, it is not likely that low perceived barriers would necessarily influence AIDS-preventive behavior.

Of the possible perceived benefits, *response efficacy,* or the perception that adopting and maintaining AIDS-preventive behaviors will reduce AIDS risk, is one of the most commonly studied. Perceived benefits also have been found to predict who will participate in HIV testing. In a study by Kalichman, Carey, and Johnson (1996), individuals who received HIV testing were more likely to believe it would help them feel better about their health.

Relationships between perceived barriers and AIDS-preventive behaviors have been mixed across both longitudinal and cross-sectional studies. Often, studies with negative findings have included questionable measures of barriers. Studies using more relevant barriers measures tended to find results in the expected direction. Maguen, Armistead, and Kalichman (2000) found strong associations in the expected direction between an eleven-item barrier scale and being tested for HIV among gay, lesbian, and bisexual youth. In a study of gay men's safer sex behavior, Wulfert, Wan, and Backus (1996) found that most men were convinced about the benefits of using condoms, but these perceived benefits were not associated with behavior. However, perceived barriers representing items about *pleasure reduction* (that is, condoms reduce sensation; condoms interfere with spontaneity) and *partner-related concerns* (that is, condoms create distrust in the relationship; condoms cause embarrassment) were associated with increased risk behavior. The authors found that the more respondents associated sensation and pleasure reduction with condom use, and the more they worried about negative reactions from their partners, the higher the reported risk behavior (that is, unprotected anal intercourse). In a previous study, beliefs that condoms diminish sexual enjoyment were shown to have a strong and consistent relationship with self-efficacy (Wulfert and Wan, 1995).

If perceived HIV/AIDS threat is high, and perceived benefits outweigh perceived barriers, the HBM predicts that a cue to action could prompt an individual to adopt AIDS preventive behaviors. The cue is thought to stimulate the belief-action link. It is best to analyze the cue-to-action dimension in combination with perceived threat. Cues to action should be more strongly associated with AIDS preventive behavior among individuals who have a high perceived AIDS threat. Unfortunately, the cue to action construct has not been examined in recent AIDS-related studies.

Use of the HBM in Multicultural Settings

While it is reasonable to assume that a theory such as the HBM is applicable to different cultures, it also is important to realize that constructs may have to be adapted to make them more relevant to the target culture. Over the past decade, there have been numerous studies examining the utility of the HBM in multicultural settings. Some studies have compared the relative importance of HBM constructs in understanding health behavior across multiple cultures, others have focused on the redefinition and measurement of HBM constructs within certain cultures, and a few have used the HBM to inform interventions in multicultural settings.

A number of studies comparing differences in HBM constructs between white and African American women regarding cancer screening have found that African American women perceive different barriers and experience increased levels of cancer fatalism (Miller and Champion, 1997). Fulton, Rakowski, and Jones (1995) used the HBM to identify predictors of breast cancer screening among Hispanic, nonHispanic black, and nonHispanic white women. Hispanic women were less likely than others to perceive themselves as susceptible and less likely to perceive breast cancer as curable.

Using the HBM to better understand why some Hispanic women begin prenatal care in the later stages of pregnancy, Byrd, Mullen, Selwyn, and Lorimor (1996) identified several barriers that were frequently endorsed by Hispanic women: embarrassment with the physical exam, lack of time spent in the doctor-patient encounter, and long waiting times in clinics. Women in the study who perceived fewer barriers to care were more likely to enter prenatal care earlier. A stronger belief in the benefits of prenatal care to the baby also was associated with earlier initiation to prenatal care. In addition, Lee (2000) found embarrassment about the exam to be a significant barrier among Korean American women seeking cervical cancer screening.

Tang and colleagues (Tang, Solomon, Yeh, and Worden, 1999; Tang, Solomon, and McCracken, 2000) examined the importance of perceived risk and barriers in understanding cancer screening practices among Chinese and Asian American women. The investigators had an interest in developing a *cultural barriers measure*, as distinct from the *common barriers measure*. Across several studies that included such screening behaviors as clinical breast exam, breast self-exam, mammography, cervical cancer screening, and colorectal cancer screening, cultural factors were found to play a role in screening behavior. However, the specific role of cultural issues differed according to age as well as to specific ethnicity within and among cultures.

For example, while barriers to access and familiarity with Western health care were more predictive of screening practices among older women, modesty and health care orientation were more predictive among younger women.

A cervical cancer screening education program for Native American women, guided in part by the HBM, was developed by Dignan and others (1994). Barriers that were endorsed frequently by the target population included reluctance among Native American women to talk openly about their personal health and transportation to health care services. Physician recommendations were not highly valued in Native American culture, so lay health educators, called *project guides,* were chosen to present the screening education program to local women.

In summary, the dimensions of the HBM can be useful in understanding health behaviors in multicultural settings. It is important to consider if the underlying assumptions of the HBM regarding the value placed on health and illness are consistent with the cultural beliefs in the target population. The wording of items should be examined to check for cultural distinctions and understanding. The relative importance of HBM constructs has been found to vary between and within cultures, as well with the health behavior being examined. The reliability and validity of measures must be reexamined when used in a different cultural setting.

Recommendations for Further Research on the Health Belief Model

The following recommendations detail goals and principles for studies using the Health Belief Model.

1. Test the Health Belief Model as a model, or, at minimum, as a combination of constructs—not as a collection of equally weighted variables operating simultaneously. Good examples of more careful examinations of Health Belief Model constructs include the work of Ronis (1992) and of Witte (1994). The following hypotheses serve as a starting point for testing the Health Belief Model as a model:

- Perceived threat is a sequential function of perceived severity and perceived susceptibility. A heightened state of severity is required before perceived susceptibility becomes a powerful predictor. Perceived susceptibility, under the state of high perceived severity, will be a stronger predictor of intention to engage in health-related behaviors than it will be a predictor of actual engagement in health-related behaviors.

- Perceived benefits and barriers will be stronger predictors of behavior change when perceived threat (perceived severity times perceived susceptibility) is high than when it is low. Under conditions of low perceived threat, benefits of and barriers to engaging in health-related behaviors will not be salient. An exception to this may be that when certain benefits of the recommended behavior are perceived to be high (for example, a partner's encouragement for safe sex), perceived threat may not need to be high. Another example of when threat may not need to be high is if perceived barriers are very low (for example, if flu shots are available at very convenient locations like grocery stores).
- Self-efficacy, a factor now included in the Health Belief Model, will be a strong predictor of many health-related behaviors. Self-efficacy will be a particularly strong predictor of behaviors that require significant skills to perform.
- Cues to action will have a greater influence on behavior in situations in which perceived threat is great. We know little about cues to action or their relative impact; more research is needed.

2. Specify in publications the measures used to study belief constructs. An important reason for variance in results between studies is probably due to large variations in the specific measures used. When the actual questions were included in the article or could be uncovered in some manner, a disconcertingly large proportion did not appear to be good indicators of HBM constructs.

3. Researchers should be cautious about aggregating items that measure benefits and barriers into scales. Specifically, barrier items can have low interitem correlations. Barriers should be examined individually both for prediction of the behavior of interest and for identification of the most relevant concerns to address in interventions.

4. Include a behavioral anchor when measuring perceived susceptibility. (See the section on the HBM and AIDS protective behaviors, for example.) The reader is referred to research by Ronis (1992), which finds strong evidence for the importance of asking susceptibility questions that are conditional on action or inaction.

5. A common direction in research involving the HBM is to determine its usefulness in combination with other models and frameworks. Several examples are provided in this chapter. Investigators should recognize that while this approach holds promise in further understanding health-related behaviors, it is important to consider the relationship and independence between constructs and the additional complexity required to evaluate the unique contribution of various model constructs. While differences exist among models of health behavior change, especially with respect to how many different elements (for example, self-efficacy) are combined and used to predict behavioral outcomes, they are largely complementary with significant degrees of overlap (Weinstein, 1993). Therefore,

the central issue is not which model is superior to other models or which variables may be more important, but instead what the relative utility and changes in relative utility with different behaviors and situations are over time (Maddux, Brawley, and Boykin, 1995).

Recommendations for Health Education and Health Promotion Practice

It is timely for professionals who are attempting to influence health-related behaviors to make use of the health belief variables, including self-efficacy, in program planning, both in needs assessment and in program strategies. Programs to deal with a health problem should be based, in part, on knowledge of how many and which members of a target population feel susceptible to a particular health-related outcome, believe the health-related outcome to constitute a serious health problem, and believe that the threat of having the health-related outcome could be reduced by changing their behavior at an acceptable psychological cost. Moreover, health professionals also should assess the extent to which clients possess adequate self-efficacy to carry out the prescribed action(s), sometimes over long periods of time.

The collection of data on health beliefs, along with other data pertinent to the group or community setting, permits the planning of more effective programs than would otherwise be possible. Interventions can then be targeted to the specific needs identified by such an assessment. This is true whether one is dealing with the problems of individual patients, groups of clients, or entire communities. In the planning of programs to influence the behavior of large groups of people for long periods of time, the role of the HBM (including self-efficacy) must be considered in context. Permanent changes in behavior can rarely be wrought solely by direct attacks on belief systems. Even more, when the behavior of large groups is the target, interventions at societal levels (for example, social networks, work organizations, the physical environment, the legislature) along with interventions at the individual level will likely prove more effective than single-level interventions.

Conclusion

This chapter has described both strengths and limitations in the HBM as formulated to date. It is hoped that future theory-building and theory-testing research will direct efforts more toward strengthening the HBM where it is weak than toward repeating what already has been established. More work is needed on experimental interventions to modify health beliefs and health behavior than on surveys to reconfirm already established correlations. More work also is needed to specify and measure factors that should be added to the HBM to increase its predictive power. The addition of self-efficacy to the traditional HBM should improve explanation and prediction, particularly in the area of lifestyle practices.

We should never lose sight of the fact that a crucial way station on the road to improved health is in the beliefs and behavior of each of a series of individuals.

References

Bandura, A. *Social Learning Theory.* Englewood Cliffs, N.J.: Prentice Hall, 1977a.

Bandura, A. "Self-Efficacy: Toward a Unifying Theory of Behavioral Change." *Psychological Review,* 1977b, *84,* 191–215.

Bandura, A. *Social Foundations of Thought and Action.* Englewood Cliffs, N.J.: Prentice Hall, 1986.

Bandura, A. *Self-Efficacy in Changing Societies.* New York: Cambridge University Press, 1995.

Bandura, A. *Self-Efficacy: The Exercise of Control.* New York: W. H. Freeman and Company, 1997.

Becker, M. H. (ed). "The Health Belief Model and Personal Health Behavior." *Health Education Monographs,* 1974, *2,* entire issue.

Booth, R. E., Zhang, Y., and Kwiatkowski, C. F. "The Challenge of Changing Drug and Sex Risk Behaviors of Runaway and Homeless Adolescents." *Child Abuse and Neglect,* 1999, *23*(12), 1295–1306.

Byrd, T. L., Mullen, P. D., Selwyn, B. J., and Lorimor, R. "Initiation of Prenatal Care by Low-Income Hispanic Women in Houston." *Public Health Reports,* 1996, *111*(6), 536–540.

Champion, V., and Menon, U. "Predicting Mammography and Breast Self-Examination in African-American Women." *Cancer Nursing,* 1997, *20*(5), 315–322.

Champion, V. L. "Revised Susceptibility, Benefits, and Barriers Scale for Mammography Screening." *Research in Nursing and Health,* 1999, *22*(4), 341–348.

Champion, V. L., and Scott, C. R. "Reliability and Validity of Breast Cancer Screening Belief Scales in African American Women." *Nursing Research,* 1997, *46*(6), 331–337.

Champion, V. L., Skinner, C., and Foster, J. "The Effects of Standard Care Counseling or Telephone/In-Person Counseling on Beliefs, Knowledge and Behavior related to Mammography Screening." *Oncology Nursing Forum,* 2000, *27*(10), 1565–1571.

Champion, V. L., Ray, D., Heilman, D., and Springston, J. "A Tailored Intervention for Mammography Among Low-Income African-American Women." *Journal of Psychosocial Oncology,* 2000, *18*(4), 1–13.

Champion, V. L., and others. "Comparison of Tailored Interventions to Increase Mammography Screening in Nonadherent Older Women." *Preventive Medicine,* forthcoming (a).

Champion, V. L., and others. "Comparison of Tailored Mammography Interventions at Two Months Post Intervention." *Annals of Behavioral Medicine,* forthcoming (b).

Dignan, M., and others. "Development of a Cervical Cancer Education Program for Native American Women in North Carolina." *Journal of Cancer Education,* 1994, *9*(4), 235–242.

Duan, N., Fox, S. A., Derose, K. P., and Carson, S. "Maintaining Mammography Adherence through Telephone Counseling in a Church-Based Trial." *American Journal of Public Health,* 2000, *90*(9), 1468–1471.

Falck, R. S., Siegal, H. A., Wang, J., and Carlson, R. G. "Usefulness of the Health Belief Model in Predicting HIV Needle Risk Practices Among Injection Drug Users." *AIDS Education and Prevention*, 1995, *7*(6), 523–533.

Ford, K., and Norris, A. E. "Factors Related to Condom Use with Casual Partners Among Urban African-American and Hispanic Males." *AIDS Education and Prevention*, 1995, *7*(6), 494–503.

Friedman, L. C., Neff, N. E., Webb, J. A., and Latham, C. K. "Age-Related Differences in Mammography Use and in Breast Cancer Knowledge, Attitudes, and Behaviors." *Journal of Cancer Education*, 1998, *13*(1), 26–30.

Fulton, J. P., Rakowski, W., and Jones, A. C. "Determinants of Breast Cancer Screening Among Inner-City Hispanic Women in Comparison with Other Inner-City Women." *Public Health Reports*, 1995, *110*(4), 476–482.

Hochbaum, G. M. *Public Participation in Medical Screening Programs: A Sociopsychological Study.* PHS publication no. 572. Washington, D.C.: Government Printing Office, 1958.

Hull, C. L. *Principles of Behavior.* New York: Appleton-Century-Crofts, 1943.

Janz, N. K., and Becker, M. H. "The Health Belief Model: A Decade Later." *Health Education Quarterly*, 1984, *11*(1), 1–47.

Janz, N. K., and others. "A Two-Step Intervention to Increase Mammography Among Women 65 and Older." *American Journal of Public Health*, 1997, *87*(10), 1683–1686.

Kalichman, S. C., Carey, M. P., and Johnson, B. T. "Prevention of Sexually Transmitted HIV Infection: A Meta-Analytic Review of the Behavioral Outcome Literature." *Annals of Behavioral Medicine*, 1996, *18*(1), 6–15.

King, E. S., and others. "Promoting Mammography Use Through Progressive Interventions: Is It Effective?" *American Journal of Public Health*, 1994, *84*(1), 104–106.

Kirscht, J. P. "The Health Belief Model and Illness Behavior." *Health Education Monographs*, 1974, *2*, 2387–2408.

Laraque, D., and others. "Predictors of Reported Condom Use in Central Harlem Youth as Conceptualized by the Health Belief Model." *Journal of Adolescent Health*, 1997, *21*(5), 318–327.

Lee, M. C. "Knowledge, Barriers, and Motivators Related to Cervical Cancer Screening Among Korean-American Women: A Focus Group Approach." *Cancer Nursing*, 2000, *23*(3), 168–175.

Leventhal, H. "Findings and Theory in the Study of Fear Communications." In L. Berkowitz (ed.), *Advances in Experimental Social Psychology.* New York: Academic Press, 1970.

Lewin, K. *A Dynamic Theory of Personality.* New York: McGraw-Hill, 1935.

Lewin, K. "The Nature of Field Theory." In M. H. Marx (ed.), *Psychological Theory.* New York: Macmillan, 1951.

Lewin, K., Dembo, T., Festinger, L., and Sears, P. S. "Level of Aspiration." In J. Hunt (ed.), *Personality and Behavior Disorders.* New York: The Ronald Press, 1944.

Liau, A., and Zimet, G. D. "Undergraduates' Perception of HIV Immunization: Attitudes and Behaviors as Determining Factors." *International Journal of STD and AIDS*, 2000, *11*(7), 445–450.

Lollis, C. M., Johnson, E. H., Antoni, M. H., and Chitwood, D. D. "The Predictive Utility of the Health Belief Model for Explaining Condom Usage and Risky Sexual Behavior in Injection Drug User and University Women." Proceedings of the HIV Infected Women's Conference, February 22–24, 1995, p. P130.

Maddux, J. E., Brawley, L., and Boykin, A. "Self-Efficacy and Health Behavior: Prevention, Promotion and Detection." In J. E. Maddux (ed.), *Self-Efficacy, Adaptation, and Adjustment: Theory, Research, and Application.* New York: Plenum Press, 1995.

Maguen, S., Armistead, L. P., and Kalichman, S. "Predictors of HIV Antibody Testing among Gay, Lesbian, and Bisexual Youth." *Journal of Adolescent Health,* 2000, *26*(4), 252–257.

Mahoney, C. A., Thombs, D. L., and Ford, O. J. "Health Belief and Self-Efficacy Models: Their Utility in Explaining College Student Condom Use." *AIDS Education and Prevention,* 1995, *7*(1), 32–49.

Miller, A. M., and Champion, V. L. "Attitudes About Breast Cancer and Mammography: Racial, Income, and Educational Differences." *Women and Health,* 1997, *26*(1), 41–63.

Phillips, K. A., and others. "Factors Associated with Women's Adherence to Mammography Screening Guidelines." *Health Services Research,* 1998, *33*(1), 29–53.

Rawl, S. M., and others. "Colorectal Cancer Screening Beliefs: Focus Groups with First-Degree Relatives." *Cancer Practice,* 2000, *8*(1), 32–37.

Rogers, R. W., and Prentice-Dunn, S. "Protection Motivation Theory." In D. S. Gochman (ed.), *Handbook of Health Behavior Research I: Personal and Social Determinants.* New York: Plenum Press, 1997.

Ronis, D. L., "Conditional Health Threats: Health Beliefs, Decisions, and Behaviors Among Adults." *Health Psychology,* 1992, *11*(2), 127–134.

Rosenstock, I. M. "What Research in Motivation Suggests for Public Health." *American Journal of Public Health,* 1960, *50,* 295–301.

Rosenstock, I. M. "Historical Origins of the Health Belief Model." *Health Education Monographs,* 1974, *2,* 328–335.

Rosenstock, I. M., Strecher, V. J., and Becker, M. H. "Social Learning Theory and the Health Belief Model." *Health Education Quarterly,* 1988, *15*(2), 175–183.

Rosenstock, I. M., Strecher V. J., and Becker M. H. "The Health Belief Model and HIV Risk Behavior Change." In J. Peterson and R. DiClemente (eds.), *Preventing AIDS: Theory and Practice of Behavioral Interventions.* New York: Plenum Press, 1994.

Skinner, B. F. *The Behavior of Organisms.* Englewood Cliffs, N.J.: Appleton-Century-Crofts, 1938.

Steers, W. N., and others. "Health Beliefs as Predictors of HIV-Preventive Behavior and Ethnic Differences in Prediction." *Journal of Social Psychology,* 1996, *136*(1), 99–110.

Strecher, V. J., and Hospers, H. "Physicians' Recommendations for Mammography: Do Tailored Messages Make a Difference?" *American Journal of Public Health,* 1994, *84*(1), 43–49.

Tang, T. S., Solomon, L. J., and McCracken, L. M. "Cultural Barriers to Mammography, Clinical Breast Exam, and Breast Self-Exam Among Chinese-American Women 60 and Older." *Preventive Medicine,* 2000, *31*(5), 575–583.

Tang, T. S., Solomon, L. J., Yeh, C. J., and Worden, J. K. "The Role of Cultural Variables in Breast Self-Examination and Cervical Cancer Screening Behavior in Young Asian Women Living in the United States." *Journal of Behavioral Medicine,* 1999, *22*(5), 419–436.

Thompson, B., and others. "Attitudes and Beliefs Toward Mammography Among Women Using an Urban Public Hospital." *Journal of Health Care for the Poor and Underserved,* 1997, *8*(2), 186–201.

Thorndike, E. L. "Animal Intelligence: An Experimental Study of the Associative Processes in Animals." *Psychological Monographs,* 1898, *2*(8), entire issue.

Tolman, E. C. *Purposive Behavior in Animals and Men.* New York: Appleton-Century-Crofts, 1932.

Watson, J. B. *Behaviorism.* New York: Norton, 1925.

Weinstein, N. D. "Testing Four Competing Theories of Health-Protective Behavior." *Health Psychology,* 1993, *12*(4), 324–333.

Witte, K. "Fear Control and Danger Control: A Test of the Extended Parallel Process Model (EPPM)." *Communication Monographs,* 1994, *61*(2), 113–134.

Wulfert, E., and Wan, C. K. "Safer Sex Intentions and Condom Use Viewed from a Health Belief, Reasoned Action, and Social Cognitive Perspective." *The Journal of Sex Research,* 1995, *32*(4), 299–311.

Wulfert, E., Wan, C. K., and Backus, C. A. "Gay Men's Safer Sex Behavior: An Integration of Three Models." *Journal of Behavioral Medicine,* 1996, *19*(4), 345–366.

CHAPTER FOUR

THE THEORY OF REASONED ACTION AND THE THEORY OF PLANNED BEHAVIOR

Daniel E. Montaño
Danuta Kasprzyk

This chapter presents the Theory of Reasoned Action (TRA) and the Theory of Planned Behavior (TPB). Both theories focus on theoretical constructs that are concerned with individual motivational factors as determinants of the likelihood of performing a specific behavior. Theory constructs are shown graphically in Figure 4.1, and are defined in Table 4.1. The TRA includes measures of attitude and social normative perceptions that determine behavioral intention. Behavioral intention in turn affects behavior. The TPB is an extension of the TRA rather than an independent theory. The TPB includes an additional construct concerned with perceived control over performance of the behavior. Both theories assume that all other factors including demographics and environment operate through the model constructs and do not independently contribute to explaining the likelihood of performing a behavior.

The TRA, first introduced in 1967, is concerned with the relations between beliefs (behavioral and normative), attitudes, intentions, and behavior. Fishbein (1967) developed the TRA through an effort to understand the relationship between attitudes and behavior. Many previous studies of this relationship found relatively low correspondence between attitudes and behavior, and some theorists proposed eliminating attitude as a factor underlying behavior (Fishbein, 1993; see also Abelson, 1972; Wicker, 1969). In his work that led to development of the TRA, Fishbein distinguished between attitude toward an object and attitude toward a behavior with respect to that object. A health-related example of this is

FIGURE 4.1. THEORY OF REASONED ACTION
AND THEORY OF PLANNED BEHAVIOR.

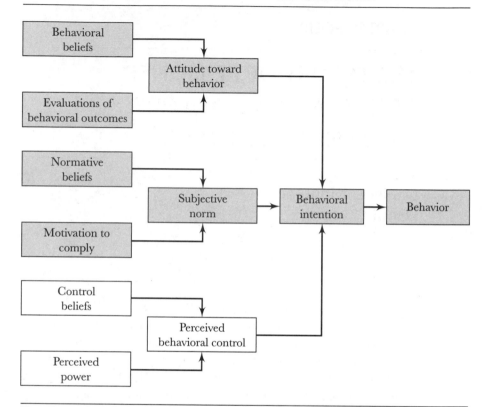

Note: Upper shaded section shows the Theory of Reasoned Action; the entire figure shows the Theory of Planned Behavior.

attitude toward the *object* of breast cancer versus the *behavior* of seeking mammographic screening for breast cancer. Most prior studies attempted to test the correspondence between attitude toward an object (for example, breast cancer) and behavior (for example, mammographic screening) with respect to the object. Fishbein demonstrated that attitude toward a behavior is a much better predictor of that behavior than attitude toward the target at which the behavior is directed (Fishbein and Ajzen, 1975). Thus, in the breast cancer screening example, attitude toward breast cancer is expected to be a poor predictor of mammography screening behavior, whereas attitude toward seeking mammographic screening is expected to be a good predictor.

TABLE 4.1. TRA AND TPB CONSTRUCTS AND DEFINITIONS.

Construct	Definition	Measure
Behavioral Intention	Perceived likelihood of performing the behavior	Bipolar unlikely-likely scale; scored −3 to +3
Attitude		
Direct Measure:	Overall evaluation of the behavior	Semantic differential scales: for example, good-bad
Indirect Measure:		
Behavioral belief	Belief that behavioral performance is associated with certain attributes or outcomes	Bipolar unlikely-likely scale; scored −3 to +3
Evaluation	Value attached to a behavioral outcome or attribute	Bipolar bad-good scale; scored −3 to +3
Subjective Norm		
Direct Measure:	Belief about whether most people approve or disapprove of the behavior	Bipolar disagree-agree scale
Indirect Measure:		
Normative belief	Belief about whether each referent approves or disapproves of the behavior	Bipolar disagree-agree scale; scored −3 to +3
Motivation to comply	Motivation to do what each referent thinks	Unipolar unlikely-likely scale; scored 1 to 7
Perceived Behavioral Control		
Direct Measure:	Overall measure of perceived control over the behavior	Semantic differential scales: for example, up to me– not up to me
Indirect Measure:		
Control belief	Perceived likelihood of occurrence of each facilitating or constraining condition	Unlikely-likely scale; scored −3 to +3 or 1 to 7
Perceived power	Perceived effect of each condition in making behavioral performance difficult or easy	Bipolar difficult-easy scale; scored −3 to +3

Fishbein draws clear distinctions in the definitions and measurement of beliefs, attitudes, intentions, and behavior. He argues that it is critical to have a high degree of correspondence between measures of attitude, intention, and behavior in terms of action, target, context, and time. Operationalization of the TRA constructs was developed from a long history of attitude measurement theory rooted in the concept that an attitude (toward an object or an action) is determined by expectations or beliefs concerning the attributes of the object or action, and by evaluations of those attributes. This expectancy-value conceptualization has been applied extensively in psychology in many areas, including learning theory, attitude theory, and decision making (for example, see Rotter, 1954; Rosenberg, 1956; Edwards, 1954).

The main constructs of these theories are described in more detail in the remainder of this chapter, along with a description of measurement of the constructs and the empirical support for the theories. We also describe the similarity between the key constructs of these theories and constructs from other behavioral theories. Too much attention has been paid to differences between theories, while their similarities have often been ignored (Weinstein, 1993). Finally, we describe two applications of the theories to understand health behaviors.

The Theory of Reasoned Action

The TRA presented in the upper section of Figure 4.1 asserts that the most important determinant of *behavior* is a person's *behavioral intention*. The direct determinants of an individual's behavioral intention are their *attitude* toward performing the behavior and their *subjective norm* associated with the behavior. Attitude is determined by the individual's beliefs about outcomes or attributes of performing the behavior (*behavioral beliefs*) weighted by evaluations of those outcomes or attributes. Thus, a person who holds strong beliefs that positively valued outcomes will result from performing the behavior will have a positive attitude toward the behavior. Conversely, a person who holds strong beliefs that negatively valued outcomes will result from the behavior will have a negative attitude toward the behavior. Similarly, a person's subjective norm is determined by his or her *normative beliefs,* whether important referent individuals approve or disapprove of performing the behavior, weighted by his or her motivation to comply with those referents. Thus, a person who believes that certain referents think he or she should perform a behavior, and is motivated to meet the expectations of those referents, will hold a positive subjective norm. Conversely, a person who believes these referents think he or she should not perform the behavior will have a negative subjective norm, and a person who is less motivated to comply with those referents will have a relatively neutral subjective norm.

The TRA assumes a causal chain that links behavioral beliefs and normative beliefs to behavioral intention and behavior, via attitude and subjective norms. The measurement of model components and causal relationships among the components are clearly specified (Ajzen and Fishbein, 1980). All measures typically use 5- or 7-point scales. In this chapter we mostly show examples using 7-point scales. A person's behavioral beliefs about the likelihood that performance of the behavior will result in certain outcomes are measured on bipolar "unlikely"-"likely" or "disagree"-"agree" scales. Evaluations of each outcome are measured on bipolar "good"-"bad" scales. For example, one outcome of "my quitting smoking" may be that this "will cause me to gain weight." A person's behavioral belief about this outcome is measured by having him or her rate the likelihood that "my quitting smoking will cause me to gain weight." The person's evaluation of this outcome is measured by having him or her rate the degree to which "my gaining weight" is good versus bad. These behavioral belief and evaluation ratings are usually scored from −3 to −3, thus capturing the psychology of double negatives, in which a belief that a behavior will *not* result in a negative outcome contributes positively to the person's attitude. An *indirect measure* of the person's attitude toward performing the behavior is computed by first multiplying his or her behavioral belief concerning each outcome by his or her corresponding outcome evaluation ratings and then summing these product scores across all outcomes of the behavior. In the previous example, a person may believe that "quitting smoking" is very unlikely to result in "gaining weight" (belief scored as −3), and may evaluate gaining weight as very bad (evaluation scored as −3), resulting in a belief-evaluation product score of +9. Thus, the strong belief that performance of the behavior will *not* result in (will avoid) a negatively valued outcome contributes just as positively to the person's attitude as would a strong belief that the action will result (+3) in a positively valued (+3) outcome (product = +9). Conversely, a strong belief that the behavior will *not* result (−3) in a positively valued outcome (+3) contributes negatively (product = −9) to the person's attitude, as performance of the behavior will *not* achieve a highly valued outcome. In the example of "quitting smoking," the beliefs and evaluations of *all* salient outcomes of this behavior will enter into the computation of an indirect measure of the person's attitude.

Similarly, a person's normative beliefs about whether each referent thinks he or she should perform the behavior are measured on bipolar scales scored −3 to +3, while the person's motivation to comply with each referent is measured on unipolar scales scored 1 to 7. For example, one potential referent with regard to "quitting smoking" might be the person's physician. A person's normative belief concerning the physician is measured by asking the person to rate the degree to which he or she believes the physician thinks the person should or should not quit smoking. Motivation to comply is measured by having the person rate his or her agreement versus disagreement with the statement "Generally, I want to do what my physician thinks I should do." An indirect measure of the person's subjective norm is computed by multiplying his or her normative belief about each referent by his or her motivation to comply with that referent, and then summing these product scores across all referents. The measurement and computation of the TRA model components are described in much more detail by Ajzen and Fishbein (1980).

In addition to the indirect measures computed from behavioral and normative beliefs, it is important to obtain a *direct measure* of each model component. Table 4.1 summarizes the direct and indirect measures of attitudes and subjective norms. A direct measure of attitude toward performing the behavior is obtained using semantic differential scale items such as "good" or "bad" and "pleasant" or "unpleasant," and summing them. A direct measure of subjective norm is obtained with a single item asking the person to rate the statement: "Most people important to me think I should" perform the behavior. This rating is made on a bipolar "unlikely"-"likely" or "agree"-"disagree" scale. These direct measures are important for two reasons. First, the direct measures are usually more strongly associated with intention and behavior than are the indirect measures, and it is necessary to demonstrate this association before conducting analyses on the indirect measures. Second, it is necessary to demonstrate that the indirect measures are strongly associated with the direct measures, to have confidence that the appropriate beliefs were measured and that the composite of these beliefs (behavioral and normative) are adequate measures of the respective TRA constructs. Once this is demonstrated, the indirect measures are of most interest, because the behavioral and normative beliefs help us to understand what drives behavior and provide a focus for interventions (von Haeften, Fishbein, Kasprzyk, and Montaño, 2001).

A prospective study design is recommended to discern the relationships between the constructs, with attitude, subjective norm, and intention measured at one time point and behavior measured following a time interval. A cross-sectional study may provide poor prediction and understanding of previous behavior if study respondents' motivations change subsequent to the behavior. Multiple regression is usually used to test the relationships in the TRA, assessing the effects of attitude and subjective norm in explaining intention at that time and in predicting subsequent behavior. The relative weights of attitude and subjective norm depend upon the behavior and the population under investigation. Some behaviors are entirely under attitudinal control, while others are under normative control. The same behavior has been found to be under attitudinal control in one population but under normative control in another population (Fishbein, 1990; Fishbein, von Haeften, and Appleyard, 2001). The relative weights are determined empirically for the particular behavior and population under investigation. This information provides guidance as to whether attitude or subjective norm is the best focus for behavioral change efforts. Correlation and analysis of variance can be used to determine which specific behavioral beliefs or normative beliefs are most strongly associated with intention and behavior, thus providing empirically identified targets for intervention efforts.

The name of this theory has led to the misperception that this is a model of "rational behavior." This is far from correct. The assumption of the TRA is that individuals are "rational actors." That is, all individuals process information and are motivated to act on it. The TRA assumes that there are underlying reasons that determine one's motivation to perform a behavior. These reasons, made up of a person's behavioral and normative beliefs, determine their attitude and subjective norm, regardless of whether those beliefs are rational, logical, or correct by some objective standard. The strength of the TRA is that it provides a framework for discerning those reasons. It offers a framework for deciphering individuals' actions by identifying, measuring, and combining beliefs that are relevant to individuals or groups, allowing us to understand their own reasons that motivate the behavior of interest. The TRA does not specify the particular beliefs about behavioral outcomes or normative referents that should be measured. The relevant behavioral outcomes and referents will be different for different behaviors. Likewise, they may be different for the same behavior but for different populations. For example, the outcomes affecting mammography use appear to be quite different for low-income than for middle-income women (Thompson and others, 1996).

A critical step in applying the TRA involves conducting open-ended elicitation interviews to identify the relevant behavioral outcomes and referents for each particular behavior and population under investigation. Elicitation interviews are conducted with a sample of at least fifteen to twenty individuals from the population under investigation, about half of whom have performed or intend to perform the behavior under investigation and half of whom have not performed the behavior. These individuals are asked to provide two types of information. First, they are asked to describe any positive or negative attributes or outcomes of performing the behavior. Second, they are asked to describe any individuals or groups to whom they might listen, who are either in favor of or opposed to their performing the behavior. These elicitation interviews are then content analyzed to identify the relevant attributes or outcomes of the behavior and the relevant social referents. This information then provides the questionnaire content, and the TRA measures are developed. A poorly conducted elicitation phase will likely result in inadequate identification of the underlying outcomes and referents, resulting in poor TRA measures and behavioral prediction and thus yielding inadequate information for the development of effective interventions.

The TRA provides a framework for identifying key behavioral and normative beliefs affecting behavior. Interventions then can be designed to target and change these beliefs or the value placed upon them, thereby affecting attitude and subjective norm and leading to a change in intention and behavior. The TRA has been used successfully to predict and explain a wide range of health behaviors and intentions, including smoking, drinking, contraceptive use, mammography use, use of health care services, exercise, seat belt use, safety helmet use, sun protection, breast feeding, substance use, and HIV or sexually transmitted disease (STD) prevention behaviors; and findings have been used to develop behavior change interventions (Albarracin, Fishbein, and Goldestein de Muchinik, 1997; Albarracin, Johnson, Fishbein, and Muellerleile, 2001; Bandawe and Foster, 1996; Bogart, Cecil, and Pinkerton, 2000; Bosompra, 2001; Fishbein, 1993; Fisher, Fisher, and Rye, 1995; Gastil, 2000; Jemmott, Jemmott, and Fong, 1992; Montaño and Taplin, 1991; Morrison, Spencer, and Gillmore, 1998; Steen, Peay, and Owen, 1998; Trafimow, 1996).

The Theory of Planned Behavior

Because the TRA assumes that the most important direct determinant of behavior is behavioral intention, the success of the theory in explaining behavior is dependent upon the degree to which the behavior is under volitional control (that is, situations in which individuals can exercise a large degree of control over the behavior). Under conditions of high volitional control, motivation as measured by intention and its attitudinal and normative determinants is expected to be the main determinant of behavior. However, it is not clear that the TRA components are sufficient for predicting behaviors in which volitional control is reduced. For example, a person who has high motivation to perform a behavior may not actually perform that behavior due to environmental conditions that intervene. Thus, Ajzen and colleagues proposed the Theory of Planned Behavior (TPB), summarized in Figure 4.1, to predict behaviors over which people have incomplete volitional control. Ajzen and colleagues (Ajzen, 1991; Ajzen and Driver, 1991; Ajzen and Madden, 1986) added *perceived behavioral control* to the TRA in an effort to account for factors outside of the individual's control that may affect his or her intention and behavior. This extension was based in part on the idea that behavioral performance is determined jointly by motivation (intention) and ability (behavioral control). Ajzen argues that a person will expend more effort to perform a behavior when his or her perception of behavioral control is high. A person's perception of control over behavioral performance, together with intention, is expected to have a direct effect on behavior, particularly when perceived control is an accurate assessment of actual control over the behavior and when volitional control is not high. The effect of perceived control declines and intention is a sufficient behavioral predictor in situations in which volitional control over the behavior is high (Madden, Ellen, and Ajzen, 1992).

In addition, the TPB postulates that perceived control is an independent determinant of behavioral intention along with attitude toward the behavior and subjective norm. With attitude and subjective norm held constant, a person's perception of the ease or difficulty of behavioral performance will affect his or her behavioral intention. The relative weights of these three factors in determining intention are expected to vary for different behaviors and populations.

According to the TPB, perceived control is determined by *control beliefs* concerning the presence or absence of facilitators and barriers to behavioral performance, weighted by the *perceived power* or impact of each factor to facilitate or inhibit the behavior. Thus, a person who holds strong control beliefs about the existence of factors that facilitate the behavior will have high perceived control over the behavior. Conversely, a person who holds strong control beliefs about the existence of factors that impede the behavior will have low perceived control over the behavior. Few studies have operationalized perceived control using the underlying measures of control beliefs and perceived power.

As in the TRA, the particular resources and impediments that are to be measured are not specified by the theory but are identified through elicitation interviews for the particular population and behavior under investigation. Once these factors are identified, a person's control beliefs and perceived power regarding each factor are measured. Although Ajzen has not completely specified how control beliefs are to be measured, applications of the TPB suggest that control beliefs regarding each factor should be measured on a bipolar likelihood-of-occurrence scale scored −3 to +3. Perceived power of each factor is measured on a bipolar "easy-difficult" scale (Terry, Gallois, and McCamish, 1993; Ajzen, 1991). For example, elicitation interviews might identify "restaurant smoking restrictions" as a factor that affects a person's perceived behavioral control over quitting smoking. A person's control belief regarding this factor is measured by having him or her rate the likelihood of encountering "a restaurant smoking restriction," while perceived power is measured by having the person rate his or her perception of the effect of "restaurant smoking restrictions" in making it easier or more difficult to quit smoking. These measures are obtained for all factors identified as facilitating or impeding the behavior. An indirect measure of the person's perceived behavioral control is then computed by multiplying each control belief by the corresponding perceived power (impact) rating and then summing these product scores across all control factors (Ajzen and Driver, 1991). A direct measure of perceived behavioral control should also be obtained as noted previously, to demonstrate that the indirect measure (based on control beliefs) is associated with the direct measure, and that the direct measure is associated with intention and behavior. The direct measure of perceived behavioral control is usually measured using semantic differential scale items such as "up to me" or "not up to me" and "difficult" or "easy." These measures are summarized in Table 4.1.

Ajzen's construct of perceived behavioral control is similar to Bandura's (1991) construct of self-efficacy, which is concerned with an individual's judgments of how well he or she can perform a behavior under various inhibiting conditions. However, operationalization of these constructs is somewhat different in the TPB compared with Bandura's theory. Perceived control is also very similar to Triandis's (1980) conceptualization of *facilitating conditions*, which is concerned with characteristics of an individual (for example, knowledge or ability) or the environment that make it easier or more difficult to perform the behavior, independent of an individual's behavioral intention. Facilitating conditions are considered to moderate the effect of intention on behavior. However, Triandis has not described methods for measuring facilitating conditions as has been done for perceived control. Each of these theorists is describing different dimensions of the same construct, one concerned with the factors that influence whether intention is translated into behavior. Both Triandis and Ajzen view this construct as moderating the effect of intention on behavior. Intention will have a greater effect on behavioral performance if perceived behavioral control is high, and perceived behavioral control will have a greater effect on performance if intention is high. However, this interaction hypothesis has received very little empirical support (Ajzen, 1991).

In recent years, the TPB has been increasingly applied to explain a variety of health behaviors, including exercise behavior, smoking and drug use, HIV/STD prevention behaviors, mammography use, clinician provision of preventive services, and oral hygiene behaviors. These studies have generally found support for perceived control as a direct predictor of both intention and behavior (Ajzen, 1991; Albarracin, Johnson, Fishbein, and Muellerleile, 2001; Blue, 1995; Craig, Goldberg, and Dietz, 1996; Godin and Kok, 1996; Millstein, 1996; Montaño, Phillips, and Kasprzyk, 2000; Montaño, Thompson, Taylor, and Mahloch, 1997). However, most of these studies have used a direct measure of perceived control rather than computing perceived control from measures of control beliefs and perceived power concerning specific facilitators and constraints. The few studies that have measured control beliefs (indirect measure) found them to be important predictors of intention and behavior (Ajzen and Driver, 1991; Kasprzyk, Montaño, and Fishbein, 1998). Clearly, if perceived behavioral control is an important determinant of intention or behavior, knowledge of the effects of control beliefs concerning each facilitator or constraint would be useful in the development of interventions. This can provide a focus in targeting those specific environmental factors in which control beliefs are most strongly associated with intention or behavior.

TRA and TPB Applications

In this section, we provide two examples of research applying the models. The first describes a thorough elicitation phase used to design a questionnaire for investigating primary care clinician behavior (in this case, provision of HIV prevention health services). The second example describes a study conducted to explain condom use behavior among individuals at risk for contracting HIV and analyses to identify foci for behavior change interventions. Together, these examples provide descriptions of the phases involved in the application of the models, including the critical elicitation phase; descriptions of model component measurement; and descriptions of analyses to explain behavior.

Understanding Clinician Provision of HIV Prevention Discussion and Advice

HIV is spreading more quickly in the United States than previous estimates had indicated, and into populations that had not been considered to be high risk. The STD rates in the United States are also some of the highest in the world (Cates and American Social Health Associate Panel, 1999). Catania (1992) reports that between 15 and 31 percent of heterosexuals nationally report at least one STD/HIV risk factor. The vast majority of Americans see a physician for a routine checkup in any year, with over 91 percent doing so within the past five years (Centers for Disease Control and Prevention, 2000). Thus, primary care clinicians are in a unique position to have an impact on STD/HIV transmission by talking to their patients about behavioral risk for acquiring STD/HIV and by providing prevention advice. The U.S. Preventive Services Task Force (1996) recommends that primary care clinicians conduct a complete sexual and drug history on all adolescent and adult patients and provide STD/HIV prevention advice to sexually active patients. There is a dearth of research on STD-control practices in the private medical sector, in which most of the STD detection, treatment, and screening occurs, as most of the research conducted to date regarding STD treatment has been in the public health sector. The data available in this area indicate that primary care clinicians seldom ask patients questions to assess risk for STD/HIV, and HIV prevention advice is given in fewer than 1 percent of patient visits (Makadon and Silin, 1995; Wenrich and others, 1996). Thus, the Institute of Medicine (Ruiz and others, 2001) has identified as a priority the need to integrate

STD/HIV prevention activities into the clinical care setting, including the taking of sexual and drug use histories and provision of prevention counseling to patients.

We conducted a study that applied the TPB in identifying the determinants affecting the provision by primary care clinicians of behavioral STD/HIV risk assessment and prevention counseling to their patients. Below we describe the findings from the elicitation phase of this study, which led to the design of a clinician questionnaire to measure psychosocial factors that may explain clinician provision of these services.

Methods. An open-ended elicitation interview instrument was designed to elicit from primary care clinicians the factors that may affect their provision of two services: (1) asking patients specific questions about their sexual risk for STD/HIV and (2) providing STD/HIV prevention advice to their patients. The TPB was the framework that guided the interview. Discussion about each action was begun by asking clinicians to describe whether, how, and under what circumstances they ask their patients questions about sexual risk for STD/HIV and offer prevention advice to patients. In order to elicit behavioral beliefs about each action, clinicians were first asked to describe any plusses, advantages, or positive outcomes that would result from taking each action. They were asked to consider this from both their own perspective and that of their patients. Next clinicians were asked to describe any minuses, disadvantages, or negative outcomes of taking each action. Normative beliefs for each action were elicited by asking clinicians to describe any people, groups, or organizations that support or discourage their provision of each action. Finally, to elicit control beliefs, clinicians were asked to describe any environmental or other factors and situations that make it easier or harder to provide each action.

The elicitation interview was designed with multiple questions to ask clinicians to think about and discuss each of the just-described factors. Probes and follow-up questions were used throughout the instrument to encourage discussion. Open-ended semistructured elicitation interviews were conducted with fifty-four randomly selected primary care clinicians (thirteen family physicians, twelve general internists, twelve obstetrician-gynecologists, and seventeen nurse practitioners) in Washington State. Interviews were audiotaped and transcribed verbatim. Next, content analysis using a qualitative software package (NUD*IST) was conducted to code and extract all statements that were relevant to each of the TPB components. For each of the two clinical actions, summary analyses were conducted to place these verbatim statements into the following lists: (1) positive and negative behavioral beliefs about outcomes or attributes of the action, (2) people or groups that encourage or discourage the action, and (3) factors or situations that make it easier or more difficult to perform the action. Discussion and consensus among investigators were used to organize the statements in each list into major themes and to design statements of those themes using actual phrases provided by the clinicians (Montaño, Kasprzyk, Phillips, and Fisher-Allison, 1998).

Results. Table 4.2 lists the outcomes or attributes of each action that were identified in the content analysis. Twenty-eight behavioral beliefs about "asking patients specific questions about their sexual history and behavioral risk for STD/HIV" were identified through the content analysis of clinician interviews. Twenty-two of these behavioral beliefs were also identified for "providing advice to patients about STD/HIV prevention" while one additional belief was unique to this action. These beliefs cover a wide range of issues, which are organized in Table 4.2 by six main categories or themes: patient confidence in their clinician, patient discomfort, valuable patient care, impact on time and money, professional protection, and clinician competence.

Content analysis of clinician descriptions of sources of normative influence resulted in twelve categories of normative influence for both clinical actions (see Table 4.3.) These include patients, colleagues, medical practice administration, official health organizations, legislators, and popular and professional media. Eight conditions that make it easier or more difficult to provide each clinical service were identified as important control beliefs (Table 4.3). These include the sex of the patient, the relationship between the patient and clinician, and circumstances during the patient encounter.

A quantitative clinician questionnaire was designed to measure each of the factors or issues that were identified in the content analysis with regard to each of the two clinical actions. To measure behavior, questions were designed to ask the clinician how often he or she takes each clinical action. Behavioral belief measures for each clinical action were designed to have clinicians rate how strongly they agree or disagree that each of the outcomes listed in Table 4.2 would result from the clinical action. Normative beliefs were measured by asking clinicians to rate how strongly each normative referent listed in Table 4.3 encourages or discourages their taking the two clinical actions. Control belief measures were designed to have clinicians rate how often they encounter each control factor listed in Table 4.3. Perceived power of each control factor was measured by having clinicians rate the degree to which each factor makes it easy or hard to provide each clinical action. Since clinician response to surveys can be dependent on survey length, we decided not to ask clinicians to rate their evaluations of each behavioral outcome or their motivation to comply with each normative referent. Instead we assumed equal weight for all behavioral outcomes, with a positive weight assigned to positive outcomes and a negative weight assigned to negative outcomes. Similarly we assumed equal motivation to comply with each normative referent.

TABLE 4.2. RESULTS OF ELICITATION INTERVIEWS PERTAINING TO CLINICIANS' BEHAVIORAL BELIEFS.

My asking patients specific questions about their sexual history and behavioral risk for STD/HIV . . .	r	My providing advice or counseling about STD/HIV prevention . . .	r
Patient Confidence		*Patient Confidence*	
Helps patients address their worries and concerns about possible risk of HIV infection.	.36	Helps patients address their worries and concerns about possible risk of HIV infection.	.31
Helps patients address their worries and concerns about possible risk of STD infections.	.28	Helps patients address their worries and concerns about possible risk of STD infections.	.27
Is an opportunity to provide reliable information and to educate patients.	.33	Lets me serve as a reliable source of information to educate patients.	.32
Provides an opportunity to change patient behavior and reduce their risk of infection.	.28	Is effective in changing patient behavior and reducing their risk of infection.	.21
Would involve dealing with patient concerns and emotions regarding their relationships.	.15	Would involve dealing with patient concerns and emotions regarding their relationships.	.05
Reduces discomfort among patients who would like to raise the issue.	.32		
Lets me serve as a safe person with whom patients can discuss sexual and other concerns.	.38		
Patient Discomfort		*Patient Discomfort*	
Causes my patients to feel embarrassed or uncomfortable.	−.30	Causes my patients to feel embarrassed or uncomfortable.	−.22
Is viewed by patients as intrusive or an invasion of their privacy.	−.27	Is viewed by patients as intrusive or an invasion of their privacy.	−.22
Is a discussion topic that patients do not want to talk about honestly.	−.26	Is a discussion topic that patients do not want to think or hear about.	−.17
Causes patients to feel anxious and worried.	−.17	Causes patients to feel anxious and worried.	−.11
Would alienate patients and discourage them from returning.	−.29	Would alienate patients and discourage them from returning.	−.25
Causes patients to feel singled out, judged, and stigmatized.	−.27	Causes patients to feel singled out, judged, and stigmatized.	−.27
Raises patient concerns about confidentiality (of medical records, insurance, partner).	−.08		

TABLE 4.2. RESULTS OF ELICITATION INTERVIEWS PERTAINING TO CLINICIANS' BEHAVIORAL BELIEFS, Continued.

My asking patients specific questions about their sexual history and behavioral risk for STD/HIV . . .	r	My providing advice or counseling about STD/HIV prevention . . .	r
Valuable Patient Care		*Valuable Patient Care*	
Is a standard of practice in my community.	.41	Is a standard of practice in my community.	.35
Makes me feel that I am providing comprehensive health care.	.48	Makes me feel that I am providing comprehensive health care.	.41
Is viewed by patients as unnecessary because they feel that they are not at risk for STDs or HIV.	−.32	Is viewed by patients as unnecessary because they feel that they are not at risk for STDs or HIV.	−.28
Helps develop rapport with patients and encourages communication about any problem.	.41	Helps develop rapport with patients and encourages communication about any problem.	.35
Protects the health of the public by preventing the spread of STDs.	.29	Protects the health of the public by preventing the spread of STDs.	.29
Helps me identify patients who would benefit from STD or HIV testing.	.30	Is something patients do not want to discuss, because they have heard it all before.	−.19
Time and Money		*Time and Money*	
Takes time and resources away from other patient needs.	−.40	Takes time and resources away from other patient needs.	−.30
Wastes time because I have few at-risk patients in my practice.	−.45	Wastes time because I have few at-risk patients in my practice.	−.40
Is a service that I will not be compensated or reimbursed for.	−.09	Is a service that I will not be compensated or reimbursed for.	−.16
Would lead to my spending more time on HIV testing and discussing test results with distressed patients.	−.08		
Professional Protection		*Professional Protection*	
Protects me from liability.	.21	Protects me from liability.	.20
Protects my staff and me from exposure and infection.	.08		
Competence		*Competence*	
Is something that I feel competent and knowledgeable enough to do.	.42	Is something that I feel competent and knowledgeable enough to cover with patients.	.32
Causes me to feel uncomfortable or awkward.	−.32	Causes me to feel uncomfortable or awkward.	−.21

TABLE 4.3. CLINICIANS' SOURCES OF
NORMATIVE INFLUENCE AND CLINICIANS' CONTROL BELIEFS.

Source of Influence	Behavior Correlation	
	Risk Assessment	Prevention Advice
Patients	.38	.37
Parents of minor patients	.10	.12
My colleagues	.36	.31
My professional medical organization	.32	.32
Professional journals	.29	.27
Health insurance companies	.12	.17
Legislators and government officials	.16	.18
Advocacy groups	.15	.15
The popular media (television, radio, magazines)	.15	.19
The medical director in my practice organization	.12	.10
The administration in my practice organization	.09	.07
National or local health organizations (for example, CDC, NIH, Public Health Departments)	.29	.26
Control Beliefs		
Having an established clinician-patient relationship	.11	.15
The stigma of STDs and HIV	.11	.09
The community in which I practice	.20	.20
If the patient is male	−.03	−.01
If the patient is female	.17	.25
Significant cultural, religious, or linguistic differences between me and my patient	.03	.07
Having the opportunity to see the patient without family or friends present	.15	.16
My knowledge or intuition that a given patient has engaged in risky behavior	.08	−.01

In addition to the clinical actions just described, the elicitation and question design procedures were also used to investigate two additional actions: offering STD/HIV testing, and asking patients questions about drug use. Additionally, a similar questionnaire was designed to measure the determinants of these clinical actions with prenatal patients. The surveys were sent to a random sample of nine hundred primary care clinicians in Washington State, with a response rate of 80 percent. In addition to clinician self-report of behavior, rates of provision of these services are being obtained through patient surveys. The clinician survey data will be analyzed to determine how well the TPB measures predict clinician rates of providing STD/HIV risk assessment and prevention counseling.

Discussion and Implications. In applying the TRA-TPB, a very thorough elicitation phase is crucial to ensure that the behavioral, normative, and control beliefs that are relevant to the population and their behavior are comprehensively identified and measured. If this process is not done well, then it is unlikely that good prediction of behavior will be obtained. In this study, the comments from questionnaire pretest participants indicated that we captured all important issues. Additionally, the 80 percent response rate on a twenty-four-page questionnaire, from busy practicing clinicians, suggests that clinicians felt that the issues covered by the survey were relevant.

At the time of this writing, the patient survey data collection was being completed, and a complete analysis to determine prediction of clinician behavior from TPB components had not yet begun. However, a preliminary analysis was conducted to compute the correlations of behavioral beliefs, normative beliefs, and control beliefs with clinician self-reports of their provision of risk assessment and prevention advice to patients. These correlations are shown in Tables 4.2 and 4.3. All but two behavioral beliefs were significantly correlated with clinician behavior, and nearly all had magnitudes above .20. Similarly, all but one normative belief was significant with most correlations above .15, while fewer control beliefs were significant though half were above .15. These preliminary findings provide support for the view that the elicitation and content analysis were successful in identifying the outcomes, normative referents, and facilitators and barriers that are potentially most relevant to explaining the behaviors.

Prediction of Condom Use Among Black, Hispanic, and White Women

This example describes the analysis of questionnaire data to identify the TRA-TPB measures that best predict behavioral intention. The findings from these analyses can determine which factors are most relevant for the development of intervention messages.

Condom Use Among Individuals at Risk for Sexually Transmitted Infections.
The transmission of sexually transmitted infections (STIs), including HIV, can be prevented through consistent use of latex condoms. Thus, in the past decade there has been a great deal of research designed to understand the factors associated with condom use, and recognition of the need to develop theory-based behavioral interventions to increase condom use among individuals at risk for STIs (National Institutes of Health, 1997).

Epidemiological and sociological approaches focus on macro factors such as age, gender, and socioeconomic factors to describe behavior, and can be useful for identifying groups to target with scarce intervention resources. However, these studies have limited utility in driving the design of intervention messages. To design interventions that are likely to affect behavior, it is important to focus studies on factors underlying behaviors such as attitudes or perceptions of norms that are changeable (Kasprzyk, Montaño, and Fishbein, 1998). These findings can then drive the design of intervention and health education messages. Demographic factors may be useful for segmenting audiences if descriptive analyses indicate that mutable factors are different among different groups.

Most studies that have examined factors affecting condom use among individuals at risk for STIs are either retrospective or cross-sectional. These study designs make it difficult to identify the *predictors* of behavior. Factors predicting future behavior may be different than the factors that are correlates of behavior measured cross-sectionally. Thus, there was a need to conduct a theory-driven, prospective study to identify and understand the factors affecting the likelihood of condom use among people who are at higher risk for contracting or transmitting HIV. We expected that such a study would provide useful insights into the development of more effective HIV prevention intervention programs. Between 1990 and 1994 we conducted such a study, applying an integrative behavioral model that included components from several behavioral theories. That model is described elsewhere (Fishbein and others, 1992; Kasprzyk, Montaño, and Fishbein, 1998; Montaño, Kasprzyk, von Haeften, and Fishbein, 2001), and it demonstrated support for the TPB. It also demonstrated that the relative importance of attitude, norms, and perceived control as determinants of condom use intentions varied with type of sex, partner, and risk group. In this section we describe the findings from the application of the TPB to explain condom use intentions among women and demonstrate that the determinants vary by racial or ethnic group.

Methods. This study was conducted in Seattle and targeted four groups at risk for HIV infection: injecting drug users, men who have sex with men, female commercial sex workers, and multipartnered heterosexuals. Purposive sampling was used to recruit approximately equal numbers of each risk group and to stratify the groups to include about equal numbers of whites, blacks, and Hispanics. The injecting drug user and multipartnered heterosexual groups were also stratified to include equal numbers by gender. Community-based recruitment was conducted by a multiracial, multiethnic team recruiting study participants from locations identified through prior ethnographic research. The recruitment effort included support and coordination from other community-based organizations.

A prospective design was used with participants recruited for two interviews. They were interviewed at baseline with a questionnaire that measured all model components including self-reported condom use. Participants were interviewed three months later, and again all model components and self-reported condom use during the previous three months were measured. A total of 935 participants completed Time 1 interviews and were asked to return for follow-up interviews, with 686 returning for Time 2 interviews (73 percent return).

The questionnaire used in this study was developed through an extensive formative-research phase. Open-ended, semistructured elicitation interviews were conducted with 171 individuals from the four target groups. Participants were asked about their condom use and their beliefs about the consequences of using or not using condoms with different types of partners (regular, casual, customers) and for different types of sex (vaginal, anal, oral). They were asked to describe factors that make it easier or more difficult for them to use condoms and to indicate the individuals or groups that would support or oppose their condom use. Content analysis of responses to these questions was conducted to develop the measures for attitude, subjective norm, and perceived control, respectively. Separate measures of model constructs were developed for condom use with each type of partner for each type of sex. It was clear from the ethnographic interviews that these are distinct behaviors, and participants described different factors affecting each behavior. The questionnaire development has been described in detail elsewhere (Montaño, Kasprzyk, von Haeften, and Fishbein, 2001).

Model component measures and computation were as follows.

Behavior. At Time 2, participants rated on a 10-point scale how often they had each type of sex with each type of partner during the previous three months. For each type of partner and type of sex they engaged in, they rated on a 7-point scale with endpoints "never" and "all the time" how often they used a condom. The validity of this measure was assessed by testing its correlation with rates obtained using a thirty-day calendar recall measure. Correlations were between .81 and .94.

Intention. Intention to use condoms for each type of sex with each type of partner was measured on a 7-point bipolar scale with endpoints "extremely unlikely" and "extremely likely."

Attitude. Direct measures of attitude toward condom use for each type of sex with each type of partner were assessed on nine-item semantic differential 7-point bipolar scales with endpoints including "good"-"bad," "smart"-"dumb," and "healthy"-"unhealthy." The endpoints were identified in the qualitative analysis. The attitude scores were computed as the sum of these nine items, obtaining internal consistency ranging from Cronbach's alpha = .83 to .90.

Indirect measures of attitude (weighted behavioral beliefs) toward condom use for each type of sex with each type of partner were constructed from belief and evaluation items. The elicitation interview content analysis identified between thirty and thirty-two outcomes and attributes of each condom use behavior. Behavioral belief measures were developed for each behavior using 7-point bipolar scales with endpoints "extremely unlikely" and "extremely likely." These measures included items such as "Using a condom every time you have vaginal sex during the next three months with your regular partner will decrease your sexual sensation" or ". . . implies you don't trust your partner." Evaluations of each behavioral outcome were rated on 7-point bipolar scales with endpoints "extremely bad" and "extremely good." Belief and evaluation ratings were coded from −3 to −3 and attitude scores were computed by summing the products of beliefs and evaluations. Internal consistency of these scales ranged from Cronbach's alpha = .83 to .89.

Subjective Norm. Direct measures of subjective norm with respect to each type of partner and each type of sex were assessed by having participants rate whether "Most people important to me think I should use condoms every time I have sex." Ratings were made on a 7-point scale with endpoints "extremely unlikely" and "extremely likely."

Indirect measures of subjective norm scores (weighted normative beliefs) were obtained by having participants rate normative beliefs about whether fifteen different referents think they should use condoms and the participants' motivation to comply with those referents. Referents identified from the elicitation interviews included individuals and groups such as friends, mother, counselor, and sexual partners. Normative beliefs ratings for each source of influence were made on 7-point bipolar scales with endpoints "extremely unlikely" and "extremely likely," and coded −3 to +3. Ratings of motivation to comply with each source of influence were made on 7-point scales with endpoints "disagree" and "agree," coded 1 to 7. Subjective norm scores were calculated by computing the mean of normative belief times motivation to comply products. A mean was used because several influence sources were not applicable to all participants. The internal consistency of these scales ranged from Cronbach's alpha = .90 to .93.

Perceived Behavioral Control. Direct measures of perceived control were obtained by summing two-item semantic differential 7-point bipolar scales with endpoints "up to me"-"not up to me" and "under my control"-"not under my control." Correlations between these items ranged from .67 to .71.

Indirect measures of perceived control (weighted control beliefs) were constructed from control belief and perceived power items. The content analysis of elicitation interviews identified ten circumstances and conditions that facilitate or impede condom use. These include having sex in a usual place, being high on drugs, being in a hurry to have sex, and having a partner who is open to the idea of using condoms. Measures of perceived control were obtained by asking participants to rate how often each of these ten conditions occur when they have sex with each type of partner (control beliefs), and the degree to which each condition makes it easy versus difficult to use a condom (perceived power). Control beliefs were rated on an 11-point scale ranging from "0 of 10 times" to "10 of 10 times." Perceived power of each condition was rated on 7-point bipolar scales with endpoints "difficult" and "easy," coded −3 to +3. Perceived control scores were computed by summing the products of control belief and perceived power ratings. Internal consistency of these scales ranged from Cronbach's alpha = .69 to .71.

Analysis. In this section we present the analyses and results for identifying the determinants of black (N = 168), Hispanic (N = 57), and white (N = 167) women's condom use for vaginal sex with their main partners. The findings from similar analyses for other study participant subgroups have been reported elsewhere (Johnson and others, 2001; Kenski and others, 2001; Levina and others, 2001; von Haeften and Kenski, 2001). The overall correlation between intention to use a condom for vaginal sex with one's main partner during the next three months and self-reported behavior three months later was highly significant (r = .55, p < .001). Thus, changes in intention to always use condoms for vaginal sex with one's main partner should lead to increased condom use behavior. Therefore the analyses focused on identifying the TRA-TPB factors influencing intention to always use condoms with one's main partner.

Consistent with expectations based on the theories, the indirect measure of attitude (weighted behavioral beliefs) toward using condoms for vaginal sex with one's main partner is significantly associated with the direct attitude measure (r = .81), and the indirect measure of subjective norm (weighted normative beliefs) was significantly associated with the direct measure of subjective norm (r = .51). However, the indirect measure of perceived control (weighted control beliefs) is not highly correlated with the direct measure of perceived control, suggesting that these two measures may be assessing different psychological constructs that may independently contribute to the prediction of intention. Additionally, the data from this study as well as prior research suggest that in this behavioral domain, the perceived partner norm contributes to prediction of intention over and above the subjective norm, so prediction may be improved by treating these as separate predictors. Therefore, our analyses treated attitude, subjective norm, perceived control, weighted control beliefs, and partner norm as potential direct predictors of behavioral intention.

The analyses proceeded in two main steps. First, correlation and multiple regression were used to assess the level at which the direct measure of attitude, direct measure of subjective norm, perceived control, partner norm, and weighted control beliefs contributed to predicting intention. Second, correlation and regression were used to determine which behavioral beliefs, normative beliefs, or control beliefs are most strongly associated with intention.

Results. Table 4.4 shows that all five of the direct psychosocial determinants were significantly correlated with black, Hispanic, and white women's intentions to always use condoms for vaginal sex with their main partners. Thus, for black, Hispanic, and white women, intention was regressed on attitude, subjective norm, partner norm, perceived control, and the weighted control beliefs. Stepwise regression indicated that all five psychosocial components independently contributed to predicting condom use intention among Black women. Attitude (beta = .28) and partner norm (beta = .30) were the most important predictors, followed by perceived control (beta = .17), subjective norm (beta = .15), and control beliefs (beta = .12). These predictors explained 59 percent of the variance in intentions ($R = .77$). For Hispanic women, only attitude (beta = .53) and partner norm (beta = .39) independently contributed to predicting condom use intentions. These two psychosocial variables explained 71 percent of the variance in Hispanic women's intentions ($R = .84$). Among white women, attitude (beta = .44) was the most important predictor, followed by partner norm (beta = .30) and perceived behavioral control (beta = .14). These three variables explained 54 percent of the variance in condom use intentions ($R = .74$). Thus, for all three groups of women, the TPB model led to very accurate prediction of condom use intentions. Attitude and partner norm were important predictors for all three groups. Perceived control was also

TABLE 4.4. ASSESSMENT OF ASSOCIATION BETWEEN TPB VARIABLES AND WOMEN'S INTENTIONS TO ALWAYS USE CONDOMS.

	Black		Hispanic		White	
	r	beta	r	beta	r	beta
Model Construct						
Attitude	.67	.28	.79	.53	.69	.44
Subjective norm	.49	.15	.58	n.s.	.51	n.s.
Perceived control	.47	.17	.44	n.s.	.40	.14
Control beliefs	.43	.12	.57	n.s.	.48	n.s.
Partner norm	.64	.30	.75	.39	.62	.30
Multiple R		.77		.84		.74

important for both black and white women. In addition, black women's intentions are affected by subjective norm over and above the partner norm, and by control beliefs over and above perceived behavioral control.

To identify potential targets for an intervention, the weighted beliefs associated with attitude, subjective norm, and perceived control were correlated with intentions (see Table 4.5). Because attitude was an important predictor of intention for all three groups of women, the individual weighted behavioral beliefs underlying attitude were each correlated with intention. Among black and white women, the majority of the weighted behavioral beliefs were significantly correlated with intention. For Hispanic women, only half of the weighted behavioral beliefs were significantly related to intention. Because subjective norm and control beliefs were also significant determinants of intention among black women, the underlying weighted normative beliefs and control beliefs were each correlated with intention. In addition to partner norm, six normative beliefs were significantly related to black women's intentions to use condoms with their main partners. Five weighted control beliefs were also significantly correlated with black women's intentions. Although the weighted normative and control belief correlations with intention are listed in Table 4.5 for Hispanic and white women (and many of these are significant), these measures were excluded from further analyses because the overall subjective norm and control belief measures did not independently contribute to the prediction of intention in the previous regression analyses (Table 4.4).

To identify the weighted beliefs that independently contribute to the prediction of intention, all weighted beliefs underlying the psychosocial variables that were significantly related to intention were entered into a stepwise regression. Thus, for all three groups of women, intention was regressed on the significant weighted behavioral beliefs. In addition, for black women, intention was regressed on the significant weighted normative beliefs and on the significant weighted control beliefs.

Although twenty-four of the black women's weighted behavioral beliefs were significantly related to intentions, the regression analysis found that only five independently contributed to the prediction of intention. These were the beliefs that always using a condom for vaginal sex with a main partner will "make him feel more relaxed" (beta = .23), "feel more clean" (beta = .25), "disrupt his mood" (beta = .21), "make insertion easier" (beta – .17), and "cause him to think you don't trust him" (beta = .17). Among Hispanic women, although fifteen weighted behavioral beliefs were related to intention, only three independently contributed to the prediction of intention: "makes you feel relaxed" (beta = .63), "makes him angry" (beta = .29), and "means he will not come inside you" (beta = .27). Similarly, among white women twenty-nine weighted behavioral beliefs were related

TABLE 4.5. CORRELATION OF BELIEFS
WITH INTENTIONS TO ALWAYS USE CONDOMS.

	Correlations		
Behavioral Beliefs	**Black**	**Hispanic**	**White**
Condom use . . .			
Makes you relaxed	.46	.73*	.71*
Makes partner relaxed	.53*	.58	.56
Decreases your sexual sensation	.21	.38	.37
Decreases partner's sexual sensation	.16	n.s.	.30
Makes sex less intimate	.31	.31	.33
Feels more clean	.44*	.32	.39
Makes sex less messy	n.s.	n.s.	.22
Prevents infection	n.s.	n.s.	.23
Protects partner from AIDS	.17	n.s.	.26
Protects yourself from AIDS	.16	.29	.29
Protects your partner from STDs	n.s.	n.s.	.31
Protects yourself from STDs	.17	.35	.27
Prevents pregnancy	.28	.31	.43
Makes partner angry	.39	.34*	.35
Makes partner think you don't trust him	.32*	.29	.37
Prolongs sex	.24	n.s.	.26
Makes sex less spontaneous	n.s.	n.s.	n.s.
Costs money	n.s.	n.s.	n.s.
Disrupts your mood	.31	n.s.	.36
Disrupts partner's mood	.42*	n.s.	.38
Makes you feel awkward	.26	n.s.	.50*
Shows partner you care	.45	.58	.30
Is the responsible thing to do	.33	.43	.49
Makes insertion easier	.36*	.43	.36
Makes you worry that condom may break	n.s.	n.s.	.24
Makes partner think you have STD	.29	n.s.	.35
Makes partner think you think partner has STD	.36	n.s.	.38
Makes partner lose erection	.19	n.s.	.20
Makes sex physically uncomfortable	.25	n.s.	.30
Makes sex too dry for you	.30	.34	.34
Means he will not come inside you	n.s.	.36*	.31
Normative Beliefs	**Black**	**Hispanic**	**White**
Social worker	n.s.	.33	.33
Mother or grandmother	.20	n.s.	.23
Family	.20	n.s.	.35
Best friend	.30	.38	.41
Other friends	.22	.41	.31
People with HIV	n.s.	n.s.	.25
Doctor or nurse	.16	.30	.31
People like me	.31*	.45	.42
Famous people	n.s.	n.s.	.24
Community	n.s.	n.s.	.23

**TABLE 4.5. CORRELATION OF BELIEFS
WITH INTENTIONS TO ALWAYS USE CONDOMS, Continued.**

	Correlations		
Normative Beliefs	Black	Hispanic	White
Churches	n.s.	n.s.	n.s.
Spiritual healer	n.s.	n.s.	n.s.
Media	n.s.	n.s.	n.s.
Main partner	.62*	.73*	.61*
Control Beliefs	**Black**	**Hispanic**	**White**
Using alcohol	n.s.	n.s.	n.s.
High on drugs	n.s.	n.s.	n.s.
Condoms available	.38*	.45	.36
Partner open to idea	.59*	.58	.60
In hurry to have sex	.18	n.s.	.16
Other birth control	.22	n.s.	.25
Partner suggests	.61	.64	.49
Sex in usual place	n.s.	n.s.	.29

* = Beliefs with significant regression weights in predicting Intention

to intention, but only two of these weighted beliefs independently contributed to the prediction of those intentions: "makes you feel relaxed" (beta = .61) and "makes you feel awkward" (beta = .23).

Among black women, although seven weighted normative beliefs were related to intention, only two—"my main partner thinks I should" (beta = .56) and "people like me think I should" (beta = .16)—independently contributed to the prediction of intention. Similarly, five weighted control beliefs were significantly related to black women's intentions, but only two of these control beliefs independently contributed to prediction of intentions: "partner open to the idea of using condoms" (beta = .52) and "having condoms with you and available" (beta = .16).

To identify critical targets for possible intervention, the final step in these analyses regressed intention on all the significant multivariate predictors identified in the above analyses. Thus, for black women five weighted behavioral beliefs, one weighted normative belief, two weighted control beliefs, the partner norm, and perceived behavioral control were used to predict intention. The variables that independently contributed to prediction of intention were the partner norm (beta = .36), the weighted control belief concerning the "partner open to the idea of using condoms" (beta = .30), perceived behavioral control (beta = .23), and the weighted behavioral belief that using condoms would "feel more clean" (beta = .19). These four variables explained 59 percent of the variance in intentions (R = .77). For Hispanic women, three weighted behavioral beliefs and partner norm were entered as predictors in the stepwise regression. The partner norm (beta = .46) and the weighted behavioral belief that using condoms "makes you feel relaxed" (beta = .42) independently contributed to predicting intention and explained 64 percent of the variance (R =.81). For white women, two weighted behavioral beliefs, the partner norm and perceived behavioral control, were entered in the stepwise regression. Both weighted behavioral beliefs ("makes you feel relaxed" and "feels awkward") (beta = .45 and .18, respectively), the partner norm (beta = .17), and perceived behavioral control (beta = .17) independently contributed to prediction of intention and explained 64 percent of the variance (R = .80).

Discussion and Implications. The TPB provided an organizing framework for studying and explaining condom use. This framework provided a structure for elicitation interviews that identified behavioral, normative, and control beliefs relevant to the population and behaviors under investigation. Findings from the overall sample suggested a benefit to including partner norm and weighted control beliefs as separate components in addition to the three TPB components. Analysis of the data from the women in the sample provided strong support for the TPB. All three TPB components as well as partner norm and weighted control beliefs were significantly associated with black, Hispanic, and white women's intentions to always use condoms for vaginal sex with their main partners. All five components independently contributed to predicting black women's intentions. Only attitude and partner norm were necessary to predict Hispanic women's intentions, while attitude, partner norm, and perceived behavioral control independently contributed to explaining white women's intentions. Attitude and partner norm were consistently the strongest predictors of intention for all three groups of women. Overall, the TPB components explained a very high proportion of the variance in women's condom use intentions (54 percent to 71 percent).

Further regression analyses of the beliefs underlying attitude, subjective norm, and perceived control found a small number of very specific critical targets for interventions for each group of women. An effective intervention for black women would (1) increase their normative beliefs that their main partners think they should use condoms, (2) increase their control belief that their partner is open to the idea, (3) increase their perceived behavioral control by increasing their beliefs that condom use is "under their control" and "up to them," and (4) increase their behavioral beliefs that condom use will make them feel more clean. For Hispanic women, an effective intervention would (1) increase their normative beliefs that their main partners think they should use condoms and (2) increase their behavioral beliefs that using condoms will make them feel more relaxed. For white women, an effective intervention would (1) increase their normative beliefs that their main partners think they should use condoms, (2) increase their perceived behavioral control by increasing their beliefs that condom use is "under their control" and "up to them," (3) increase their behavioral beliefs that using condoms will make them feel relaxed, and (4) decrease their behavioral beliefs that using condoms would make them feel awkward.

Clearly, it will be easier to develop intervention messages to influence some of these critical targets than others. Thus, as described by von Haeften, Fishbein, Kasprzyk, and Montaño (2001), one can target related beliefs or underlying themes. These can be identified by a review of the beliefs that are significantly related to intention (Table 4.4) and by determining which of these are strongly associated with the critical targets that were identified in the analyses above. A more comprehensive description of TPB analyses to identify predictors of condom use intentions among other subgroups and implications for intervention message development has been published in *Psychology, Health & Medicine*, Special Section on Project SAFER (von Haeften, Fishbein, Kasprzyk, and Montaño, 2001; Fishbein, von Haeften, and Appleyard, 2001). Because so many of the psychosocial measures were associated with intention, different critical predictors of intention were found for blacks, Hispanics, and whites, and a high percentage of variance was accounted for, the results suggest that the elicitation phase of this study was effective in identifying relevant measures for all three ethnic or racial groups. These findings indicate that separate behavioral models are not necessary to explain behavior across different ethnicities, races, or cultures.

Conclusion

Theoretical frameworks organize thought and planning of research, intervention, and analysis. The Theory of Reasoned Action and the Theory of Planned Behavior provide excellent frameworks for conceptualizing, measuring, and identifying factors that determine behavior. The TRA focuses on cognitive factors (beliefs and values) that determine motivation (behavioral intention), and the theory has been very useful in explaining behavior, particularly behavior under volitional control. The TRA provides a very precise rationale for identifying and measuring behavioral and normative beliefs and for testing their association with intentions and behaviors. In applying behavioral theories, it is important to continually reassess them and to consider other theory-driven constructs that may add to the explanatory power. The TPB extends the TRA by adding perceived behavioral control concerned with facilitating or constraining conditions that affect intention and behavior. This is particularly important for behaviors over which a person has less volitional control. This component has not been as extensively tested, and Ajzen only recently specified control beliefs as the underlying determinants of behavioral control. Our study of condom use found strong support for perceived behavioral control as a behavioral determinant.

We cannot stress enough the importance of conducting in-depth, open-ended elicitation interviews to identify the behavioral, normative, and control beliefs that are relevant to the particular behavior and population under investigation and that are to be measured. This process allows one to ground the measures empirically as well as identify information that can later be used in the process of designing specific intervention messages.

For theory to help drive interventions, it must focus attention on how to select the important factors we can influence from among many factors associated with behavior. The TRA and its extension in the TPB seem particularly useful in this regard. Application of these models to understand a particular behavior will identify underlying beliefs that determine one's attitude, subjective norm, and perceived behavioral control, and thereby affect the likelihood of performing the behavior. Often, the important beliefs affecting behavior are different for different related behaviors and for different populations. We found this to be the case in our condom use study.

The TRA and TPB provide a framework for empirically identifying factors on which intervention efforts should focus. However, selection of the specific beliefs to change through health education interventions must be done carefully. Targeting a few beliefs may not be effective if they are a small proportion of the total set of beliefs affecting intention. Similarly, targeting beliefs that constitute a model component that does not have a strong regression coefficient may be ineffective. It is also important to consider the effect of intervention messages on the entire set of beliefs underlying behavior. An intervention communication may change one targeted belief in the desired direction, but could adversely affect other important beliefs, thus negating the effect of the targeted belief. Further, intervention development must pay attention to all model components simultaneously. For example, attempting to modify control beliefs concerning factors that facilitate carrying out one's intention will not be effective if a person is not motivated to perform the behavior in the first place. Conversely, changing attitude and intention may not result in behavior change if the person holds strong control beliefs about conditions that constrain the behavior.

It is therefore critical to assess the effect of interventions on the beliefs targeted and on other components of the model. The TRA and TPB provide a basis for evaluating behavior change interventions because they provide hypotheses about how the intervention targeting a set of beliefs will affect the model component that those items compose (for example, attitude) and thereby affect intention and behavior. It is important to use an evaluation design that includes the measurement of the TRA and TPB components as intermediate outcomes, both at baseline and after the intervention has been implemented, to assess how they are affected by the intervention. It is also important to note that the TRA and TPB can be applied in conjunction with other theories to design and deliver behavioral change interventions. For example, we are currently applying the TPB along with Diffusion Theory to design and implement an HIV-prevention intervention in Zimbabwe. The TPB is being applied to identify the intervention messages, while Diffusion Theory is used to design the intervention delivery methods via local community opinion leaders. Evaluation instruments will assess delivery of the intervention messages, whether the beliefs (behavioral, normative, and control) targeted by the messages change over time, and whether this leads to behavioral change. In this way the TRA and TPB can complement the use of other theories of change and thereby improve behavioral change research and practice.

References

Abelson, R. P. "Are Attitudes Necessary?" In B. T. King and E. McGinnies (eds.), *Attitudes, Conflict, and Social Change.* New York: Academic Press, 1972.

Ajzen, I. "The Theory of Planned Behavior." *Organizational Behavior and Human Decision Processes,* 1991, *50,* 179–211.

Ajzen, I., and Driver, B. L. "Prediction of Leisure Participation from Behavioral, Normative, and Control Beliefs: An Application of the Theory of Planned Behavior." *Leisure Sciences,* 1991, *13,* 185–204.

Ajzen, I., and Fishbein, M. *Understanding Attitudes and Predicting Social Behavior.* Englewood Cliffs, N.J.: Prentice Hall, 1980.

Ajzen I., and Madden, T. J. "Prediction of Goal-Directed Behavior: Attitudes, Intentions, and Perceived Behavioral Control." *Journal of Experimental Social Psychology,* 1986, *22,* 453–474.

Albarracin, D., Fishbein, M., and Goldestein de Muchinik, E. "Seeking Social Support in Old Age as Reasoned Action: Structural and Volitional Determinants in a Middle-aged Sample of Argentinean women." *Journal of Applied Social Psychology,* 1997, *27*(6), 463–476.

Albarracin, D., Johnson, B. T., Fishbein, M., and Muellerleile, P. A. "Theories of Reasoned Action and Planned Behavior as Models of Condom Use: A Meta-analysis." *Psychological Bulletin,* 2001, *127*(1), 142–161.

Bandawe, C. R., and Foster, D. "AIDS-Related Beliefs, Attitudes and Intentions Among Malawian Students in Three Secondary Schools." *AIDS Care,* 1996, *8*(2), 223–232.

Bandura, A. "Social Cognitive Theory of Self Regulation." *Organizational Behavior and Human Decision Processes,* 1991, *50,* 248–285.

Blue, C. L. "The Predictive Capacity of the Theory of Reasoned Action and the Theory of Planned Behavior in Exercise Research: An Integrated Literature Review." *Research in Nursing and Health,* 1995, *18*(2), 105–121.

Bogart, L. M., Cecil, H., and Pinkerton, S. D. "Intentions to Use the Female Condom Among African American Adults." *Journal of Applied Social Psychology*, 2000, *30*(9), 1923–1953.

Bosompra, K. "Determinants of Condom Use Intentions of University Students in Ghana: An Application of the Theory of Reasoned Action." *Social Science and Medicine*, 2001, *52*, 1057–1069.

Catania, J. A., and others. "Prevalence of AIDS-Related Risk Factors and Condom Use in the United States." *Science*, 1992, *258*, 1101–1106.

Cates, W., and the American Social Health Associate Panel. "Estimates of the Incidence and Prevalence of Sexually Transmitted Diseases in the United States." *Sexually Transmitted Diseases*, 1999, *26*(Supplement), S2–S7.

Centers for Disease Control and Prevention. "Behavioral Risk Factor Surveillance System." [http://apps.nccd.cdc.gov/brfss]. 2000.

Craig, S., Goldberg, J., and Dietz, W. H. "Psychosocial Correlates of Physical Activity Among Fifth and Eighth Graders." *Preventive Medicine*, 1996, *25*(5), 506–513.

Edwards, W. "The Theory of Decision Making." *Psychological Bulletin*, 1954, *51*, 380–417.

Fishbein, M. (ed.). *Readings in Attitude Theory and Measurement.* New York: Wiley, 1967.

Fishbein, M. "AIDS and Behavior Change: An Analysis Based on the Theory of Reasoned Action." *Interamerican Journal of Psychology*, 1990, *24*, 37–56.

Fishbein, M. "Introduction." In D. J. Terry, C. Gallois, and M. McCamish (eds.), *The Theory of Reasoned Action: Its Application to AIDS Preventive Behaviour.* Oxford, U.K.: Pergamon Press, 1993.

Fishbein, M., and Ajzen I. *Belief, Attitude, Intention, and Behavior: An Introduction to Theory and Research.* Reading, Mass.: Addison-Wesley, 1975.

Fishbein, M., von Haeften, I., and Appleyard, J. "The Role of Theory in Developing Effective Interventions: Implications from Project SAFER." *Psychology, Health & Medicine*, 2001, *6*(2), 223–238.

Fishbein, M., and others. *Factors Influencing Behavior and Behavior Change.* Final Report, Theorists Workshop. Bethesda, Md.: National Institute of Mental Health, 1992.

Fisher, W. A., Fisher, J. D., and Rye, B. J. "Understanding and Promoting AIDS Preventive Behavior: Insights from the Theory of Reasoned Action." *Health Psychology*, 1995, *14*, 255–264.

Gastil, J. "Thinking, Drinking, and Driving: Application of the Theory of Reasoned Action to DWI Prevention." *Journal of Applied Social Psychology*, 2000, *30*(11), 2217–2232.

Gerbert, B., MaGuire, B. T., and Coates, T. J. "Are Patients Talking to Their Physicians About AIDS?" *American Journal of Public Health*, 1990, *80*, 467–468.

Godin, G., and Kok, G. "The Theory of Planned Behavior: A Review of Its Applications to Health-Related Behaviors." *American Journal of Public Health*, 1996, *11*(2), 87–98.

Jemmott, J. B., Jemmott, L. S., and Fong, G. T. "Reductions in HIV Risk—Associated Sexual Behaviors Among Black Male Adolescents: Effects of an AIDS Prevention Intervention." *American Journal of Public Health*, 1992, *82*(3), 372–377.

Johnson, B. L., and others. "Factors Influencing IDU and Non-IDU Female Commercial Sex Workers' Intentions to Always Use Condoms for Vaginal Sex With Their Regular Partner." *Psychology, Health & Medicine*, 2001, *6*(2), 207–222.

Kasprzyk, D., Montaño, D. E., and Fishbein, M. "Application of an Integrated Behavioral Model to Predict Condom Use: A Prospective Study Among High HIV Risk Groups." *Journal of Applied Social Psychology*, 1998, *28*(17), 1557–1583.

Kenski, K., and others. "Theoretical Determinants of Condom Use Intentions for Vaginal Sex With a Regular Partner Among Male and Female Injecting Drug Users." *Psychology, Health & Medicine,* 2001, *6*(2), 179–190.

Levina, M., and others. "Factors Influencing MSM's Intentions to Always Use Condoms for Vaginal, Anal and Oral Sex with Their Regular Partners." *Psychology, Health & Medicine,* 2001, *6*(2), 191–206.

Madden, T. J., Ellen, P. S., and Ajzen, I. "A Comparison of the Theory of Planned Behavior and the Theory of Reasoned Action." *Personality and Social Psychology Bulletin,* 1992, *18*, 3–9.

Makadon, H. J., and Silin, J. G. "Prevention of HIV Infection in Primary Care: Current Practices, Future Possibilities." *Annals of Internal Medicine,* 1995, *123*, 715–719.

Millstein, S. G. "Utility of the Theories of Reasoned Action and Planned Behavior for Predicting Physician Behavior: A Prospective Analysis." *Health Psychology,* 1996, *15*(5), 398–402.

Montaño, D., Kasprzyk, D., Phillips, W., and Fisher-Allison, N. "Factors Affecting Provision of Sexual Risk Assessment and HIV/STD Preventive Counseling by Primary Care Clinicians." Paper presented at the 12th World AIDS Conference, Geneva, Switzerland, June 1998.

Montaño, D., Kasprzyk, D., von Haeften, I., and Fishbein, M. "Toward an Understanding of Condom Use Behaviors: A Theoretical and Methodological Overview of Project SAFER." *Psychology, Health & Medicine,* 2001, *6*(2), 139–150.

Montaño, D., Phillips, W., and Kasprzyk, D. "Explaining Physician Rates of Providing Flexible Sigmoidoscopy." *Cancer Epidemiology, Biomarkers & Prevention,* 2000, *9*, 665–669.

Montaño, D., and Taplin, S. "A Test of an Expanded Theory of Reasoned Action to Predict Mammography Participation." *Social Science and Medicine,* 1991, *32*, 733–741.

Montaño, D., Thompson, B., Taylor, V. M., and Mahloch, J. "Understanding Mammography Intention and Utilization among Women in an Inner City Public Hospital Clinic." *Preventive Medicine,* 1997, *26*, 817–824.

Morrison, D. M., Spencer, M. S., and Gillmore, M. R. "Beliefs about Substance Use Among Pregnant and Parenting Adolescents." *Journal of Research on Adolescence,* 1998, *8*, 69–95.

National Institutes of Health. *Consensus Development Conference Statement. Interventions to Prevent HIV Risk Behavior.* Bethesda, Md.: National Institutes of Health, 1997.

Rosenberg, M. J. "Cognitive Structure and Attitudinal Affect." *Journal of Abnormal and Social Psychology,* 1956, *53*, 367–372.

Rotter, J. B. *Social Learning and Clinical Psychology.* Englewood Cliffs, N.J.: Prentice Hall, 1954.

Ruiz, M. S., and others (eds.). *No Time to Lose: Getting More from HIV Prevention.* Committee on HIV Prevention Strategies in the United States, Division of Health Promotion and Disease Prevention, Institute of Medicine. Washington, D.C.: National Academy Press, 2001.

Steen, D. M., Peay, M. Y., and Owen, N. "Predicting Australian Adolescents' Intentions to Minimize Sun Exposure." *Psychology and Health,* 1998, *13*(1), 111–119.

Terry, D., Gallois, C., and McCamish, M. "The Theory of Reasoned Action and Health Care Behaviour." In D. J. Terry, C. Gallois, and M. McCamish (eds.), *The Theory of Reasoned Action: Its Application to AIDS Preventive Behaviour.* Oxford, U.K.: Pergamon Press, 1993.

Thompson, B., and others. "The Use of Qualitative Methodology to Identify Attitudes and Beliefs Toward Mammography Among Women Utilizing an Urban Public Hospital." *Journal of Health Care for the Poor and Underserved,* 1996, *8*, 186–201.

Trafimow, D. "The Importance of Attitudes in the Prediction of College Students' Intentions to Drink." *Journal of Applied Social Psychology,* 1996, *26*(24), 2167–2188.

Triandis, H. C. "Values, Attitudes and Interpersonal Behavior." In H. E. Howe Jr. (ed.), *Nebraska Symposium on Motivation*, 1980, *27*, 195–259.

U.S. Preventive Services Task Force. *Guide to Clinical Preventive Services*. (2nd ed.) Baltimore, Md.: Williams & Wilkins, 1996.

von Haeften, I., Fishbein, M., Kasprzyk, D., and Montaño, D. "Analyzing Data to Obtain Information to Design Targeted Interventions." *Psychology, Health & Medicine*, 2001, *6*(2), 151–164.

von Haeften, I., and Kenski, K. "Multi-Partnered Heterosexual's Condom Use for Vaginal Sex with Their Main Partner as a Function of Attitude, Subjective Norm, Partner Norm, Perceived Behavioural Control, and Weighted Control Beliefs." *Psychology, Health & Medicine*, 2001, *6*(2), 165–178.

Weinstein, N. D. "Testing Four Competing Theories of Health-Protective Behavior." *Health Psychology*, 1993, *12*(4), 324–333.

Wenrich, M. D., and others. "Patient Report of HIV Risk Screening by Primary Care Physicians." *American Journal of Preventive Medicine*, 1996, *12*(2), 116–122.

Wicker, A. W. "Attitudes Vs. Actions: the Relationship of Verbal and Overt Behavioral Responses to Attitude Objects." *Journal of Social Issues*, 1969, *25*, 41–78.

CHAPTER FIVE

THE TRANSTHEORETICAL MODEL AND STAGES OF CHANGE

James O. Prochaska
Colleen A. Redding
Kerry E. Evers

The Transtheoretical Model (TTM) uses stages of change to integrate processes and principles of change from across major theories of intervention; hence, the name *trans*theoretical. This model emerged from a comparative analysis of leading theories of psychotherapy and behavior change. The goal was systematic integration of a field that had fragmented into more than three hundred theories of psychotherapy (Prochaska, 1979). During the developmental phase, comparative analyses identified ten processes of change, such as consciousness raising from the Freudian tradition, contingency management from the Skinnerian tradition, and helping relationships from the Rogerian tradition, that characterized people in various stages of change.

We assessed how frequently each group used each of the ten processes in an empirical analysis of self-changers compared to smokers in professional treatments (DiClemente and Prochaska, 1982). Research participants said that they used different processes at different times in their struggles with smoking. These naive subjects taught professionals about a phenomenon that was not explicitly included in any of the multitude of therapy theories—that behavior change unfolds through a series of stages (Prochaska and DiClemente, 1983).

From the initial studies of smoking, the stage model rapidly expanded in scope to include investigations and applications with a broad range of health and mental health behaviors. These include alcohol and substance abuse, anxiety and panic disorders, delinquency, eating disorders and obesity, high-fat diets, HIV/AIDS prevention, mammography screening, medication compliance, unplanned pregnancy prevention, pregnancy and smoking, sedentary lifestyles, sun exposure, and physicians practicing preventive medicine. Over time, these studies have expanded, validated, applied, and challenged the core constructs of the Transtheoretical Model.

Core Constructs

Table 5.1 briefly describes the core constructs of The Transtheoretical Model.

Stages of Change

The *stage construct* is important because it represents a temporal dimension. Change implies phenomena occurring over time. Surprisingly, none of the leading theories of psychotherapy contained a core construct representing time. In the past, behavior change often was construed as a finite event, such as quitting smoking, drinking, or overeating. The Transtheoretical Model construes change as a process-involving progress through a series of six stages.

Precontemplation is the stage in which people do not intend to take action in the foreseeable future, usually measured as the next six months. People may be in this stage because they are uninformed or underinformed about the consequences of their behavior, or they may have tried to change a number of times and became demoralized about their abilities to change. Both groups tend to avoid reading, talking, or thinking about their high-risk behaviors. In other theories, they often are characterized as resistant or unmotivated clients or as not ready for therapy or health promotion programs. Such people are often labeled the "hard to reach."

Contemplation is the stage in which people intend to change within the next six months. They are more aware of the pros of changing but also acutely aware of the cons. The difficult balance between the costs and benefits of changing can produce profound ambivalence that can keep people stuck in this stage for long periods of time. This phenomenon is often characterized as chronic contemplation or behavioral procrastination. These people are not ready for traditional action-oriented programs that expect participants to take immediate action.

Preparation is the stage in which people intend to take action in the immediate future, usually measured as the next month. They have typically taken some significant action in the past year. These individuals have a plan of action such as joining a health education class, consulting a counselor, talking to their physician, buying a self-help book, or relying on a self-change approach. These are the people who should be recruited for such action-oriented programs as traditional smoking cessation or weight loss clinics.

TABLE 5.1. TRANSTHEORETICAL MODEL CONSTRUCTS.

Constructs	Description
Stages of change	
Precontemplation	Has no intention to take action within the next six months
Contemplation	Intends to take action within the next six months
Preparation	Intends to take action within the next thirty days and has taken some behavioral steps in this direction
Action	Has changed overt behavior for less than six months
Maintenance	Has changed overt behavior for more than six months
Decisional balance	
Pros	The benefits of changing
Cons	The costs of changing
Self-efficacy	
Confidence	Confidence that one can engage in the healthy behavior across different challenging situations
Temptation	Temptation to engage in the unhealthy behavior across different challenging situations
Processes of change	
Consciousness raising	Finding and learning new facts, ideas, and tips that support the healthy behavior change
Dramatic relief	Experiencing the negative emotions (fear, anxiety, worry) that go along with unhealthy behavioral risks
Self-reevaluation	Realizing that the behavior change is an important part of one's identity as a person
Environmental reevaluation	Realizing the negative impact of the unhealthy behavior or the positive impact of the healthy behavior on one's proximal social and physical environment
Self-liberation	Making a firm commitment to change
Helping relationships	Seeking and using social support for the healthy behavior change
Counterconditioning	Substituting healthier alternative behaviors and cognitions for the unhealthy behavior
Reinforcement management	Increasing the rewards for the positive behavior change and decreasing the rewards of the unhealthy behavior
Stimulus control	Removing reminders or cues to engage in the unhealthy behavior and adding cues or reminders to engage in the healthy behavior
Social liberation	Realizing that the social norms are changing in the direction of supporting the healthy behavior change

Action is the stage in which people have made specific overt modifications in their lifestyles within the past six months. Since action is observable, behavior change often has been equated with action. But in The Transtheoretical Model, action is only one of six stages. Not all modifications of behavior count as action in this model. People must attain a criterion that scientists and professionals agree is sufficient to reduce risks for disease, for example, abstinence among smokers who have participated in a self-change program.

Maintenance is the stage in which people strive to prevent relapse but do not apply change processes as frequently as do people in action. They are less tempted to relapse and increasingly more confident that they can continue their changes. Based on temptation and self-efficacy data, maintenance of abstinence from smoking lasts from six months to about five years. While this estimate may seem somewhat pessimistic, longitudinal data from the 1990 Surgeon General's report supported this temporal estimate (U.S. Department of Health and Human Services, 1990). After twelve months of continuous abstinence, the percentage of individuals who returned to regular smoking was 43 percent. It was not until five years of continuous abstinence that the risk for relapse dropped to 7 percent.

Termination is the stage in which individuals no longer succumb to temptation and have total self-efficacy. No matter whether they are depressed, anxious, bored, lonely, angry, or stressed, they are sure they will not return to their old unhealthy habit as a way of coping. It is as if they never acquired the habit in the first place. In a study of former smokers and alcoholics, less than 20 percent of each group had reached the criteria of zero temptation and total self-efficacy (Snow, Prochaska, and Rossi, 1992). The criteria may be too strict or it may be that this stage is an idealized goal for the majority of people. In other areas, such as exercise, consistent condom use, and weight control, the realistic goal may be a lifetime of maintenance, with the recognition that no one is perfect. Since termination may not be a practical reality for a majority of people, it has not been given as much emphasis in TTM research.

Decisional Balance

Decisional balance reflects the individual's relative weighing of the pros and cons of changing. Originally, TTM relied on Janis and Mann's (1977) model of decision making that included four categories of pros (instrumental gains for self and for others and approval from self and from others), and four categories of cons (instrumental costs to self and to others and disapproval from self and from others). In a long series of studies attempting to produce this structure of eight factors, a much simpler structure always was found—just the pros and cons of changing.

Self-efficacy

Self-efficacy is the situation-specific confidence that people have that they can cope with high-risk situations without relapsing to their unhealthy or high-risk behavior. This construct was integrated from Bandura's (1982) self-efficacy theory.

Temptation reflects the intensity of urges to engage in a specific habit when in the midst of difficult situations. Typically, three factors reflect the most common types of tempting situations: negative affect or emotional distress, positive social situations, and craving.

Processes of Change

Processes of change are the covert and overt activities that people use to progress through the stages. Processes of change provide important guides for intervention programs. Ten processes have received the most empirical support.

Consciousness raising involves increased awareness about the causes, consequences, and cures for a particular problem behavior. Interventions that can increase awareness include feedback, confrontations, interpretations, bibliotherapy, and media campaigns.

Dramatic relief initially produces increased emotional experiences followed by reduced affect if appropriate action is taken. Psychodrama, role playing, grieving, personal testimonies, and media campaigns are examples of techniques that can move people emotionally.

Self-reevaluation combines both cognitive and affective assessments of one's self-image with and without a particular unhealthy habit, such as one's image as a couch potato and one's different image as an active person. Value clarification, healthy role models, and imagery are techniques that can move people evaluatively.

Environmental reevaluation combines both affective and cognitive assessments of how the presence or absence of a personal habit effects one's social environment, such as the effect on others of smoking. It also can include the awareness that one can serve as a positive or negative role model for others. Empathy training, documentaries, and family interventions can lead to such reassessments.

Self-liberation is both the belief that one can change and the commitment and recommitment to act on that belief. New Year's resolutions, public testimonies, and multiple rather than single choices can enhance what the public calls willpower.

Helping relationships combine caring, trust, openness, and acceptance as well as support for healthy behavior change. Rapport building, a therapeutic alliance, counselor calls, and buddy systems can be sources of social support.

Counterconditioning requires the learning of healthier behaviors that can substitute for problem behaviors. Relaxation, assertion, desensitization, nicotine replacement, and positive self-statements are strategies for safer substitutes.

Contingency management provides consequences for taking steps in a particular direction. While contingency management can include the use of punishments, we found that self-changers rely on rewards much more than on punishments. Reinforcements are emphasized, because the TTM aims to work in harmony with how people change naturally. Contingency contracts, overt and covert reinforcements, and group recognition are procedures for increasing reinforcement and the probability that healthier responses will be repeated.

Stimulus control removes cues for unhealthy habits and adds prompts for healthier alternatives. Avoidance, environmental reengineering, and self-help groups can provide stimuli that support change and reduce risks for relapse.

Social liberation requires an increase in social opportunities or alternatives, especially for people who are relatively deprived or oppressed. Advocacy, empowerment procedures, and appropriate policies can produce increased opportunities for minority health promotion, gay health promotion, and health promotion for impoverished people. These same procedures also can be used to help people change. Strategies such as smoke-free zones, salad bars in school lunches, and easy access to condoms have been used in the past. The Transtheoretical Model has concentrated on five stages of change, ten processes of change, the pros and cons of changing, self-efficacy, and temptation. The Transtheoretical Model also is based on critical assumptions about the nature of behavior change and interventions that can best facilitate such change.

Critical Assumptions

The following are the assumptions that drive TTM theory, research, and practice.

1. No single theory can account for all of the complexities of behavior change. Therefore, a more comprehensive model will most likely emerge from an integration across major theories.
2. Behavior change is a process that unfolds over time through a sequence of stages.
3. Stages are both stable and open to change just as chronic behavioral risk factors are both stable and open to change.
4. The majority of at-risk populations are not prepared for action and will not be served by traditional action-oriented prevention programs.
5. Specific processes and principles of change should be applied at specific stages if progress through the stages is to occur.

Empirical Support and Challenges

Each of the core constructs have been studied across a broad range of behaviors and populations. Only a sampling of these studies can be reviewed here.

Stage distribution. If interventions are to match the needs of entire populations, there is a need to know the stage distributions for specific high-risk behaviors. A series of studies on smoking in the United States demonstrated that less than 20 percent of smokers are in the preparation stage in most populations (see for example, Velicer and others, 1995). Approximately 40 percent of smokers are in the contemplation stage, and another 40 percent are in precontemplation. Action-oriented cessation programs will not match the needs of the vast majority of smokers. Within a sample of twenty-thousand members of an HMO across fifteen health-risk behaviors, only a small minority were ready for action (Rossi, March 1992). The distribution varies for different types of health-related behaviors.

Pros and Cons Structure Across Twelve Behaviors. Across studies of twelve different behaviors (smoking cessation, quitting cocaine, weight control, dietary fat reduction, safer sex, condom use, exercise acquisition, sunscreen use, radon testing, delinquency reduction, mammography screening, and physicians practicing preventive medicine), the two-factor structure of pros and cons was remarkably stable.

Integration of Pros and Cons and Stages of Change Across Twelve Behaviors. Stage is not a theory; it is a construct. A theory requires systematic relationships between a set of constructs, ideally culminating in mathematical relationships. Systematic relationships have been found between stages of change and pros and cons of changing for the twelve health behaviors listed previously.

In all twelve studies, the cons of changing were higher than the pros for people in precontemplation (Prochaska and others, 1994). Likewise, the pros increased between precontemplation and contemplation. From contemplation to action, across all twelve behaviors, the cons of changing were lower in action than in contemplation. In eleven of the twelve studies, the pros of changing were higher than the cons for people in action. These relationships suggest that to progress from precontemplation, the pros of changing must increase; to progress from contemplation, the cons must decrease; to progress to action, the pros must be higher than the cons.

Strong and Weak Principles of Progress. Across these same twelve studies, mathematical relationships were found between the pros and cons of changing and progress across the stages (Prochaska, 1994).

The Strong Principle is

$$PC \rightarrow A \cong 1 \ SD \uparrow PROS$$

Progress from precontemplation to action involves approximately one standard deviation increase in the pros of changing. On intelligence tests, a one SD increase would be fifteen points, a substantial increase.

The Weak Principle is

$$PC \rightarrow A \cong 0.5 \text{ SD} \downarrow \text{CONS}$$

Progress from precontemplation to action involves approximately .5 SD decrease in the cons of changing.

Practical implications of these principles are that the pros of changing must increase twice as much as the cons must decrease. Perhaps twice as much emphasis should be placed on raising the benefits as on reducing the costs or barriers. For example, if couch potatoes in precontemplation can only list five pros of exercise, then being too busy will be a big barrier to change. But if program participants come to appreciate that there can be more than fifty benefits for sixty minutes a week, being too busy becomes a relatively smaller barrier.

Processes of Change Across Behaviors. One of the assumptions of The Transtheoretical Model is that there is a common set of change processes that people can apply across a broad range of behaviors. The higher order structure of the processes (experiential and behavioral) has been replicated across problem behaviors better than have specific processes (Rossi, August 1992). Typically, support has been found for the standard set of ten processes across such behaviors as smoking, diet, cocaine use, exercise, condom use, and sun exposure. But the structure of the processes across studies has not been as consistent as the structure of the stages and the pros and cons of changing. In some studies, fewer processes are found, and occasionally evidence for one or two additional processes are found. For some behaviors, fewer change processes may be used. With an infrequent behavior such as a yearly mammogram, for example, fewer processes may be required to progress to long-term maintenance (Rakowski and others, 1996; 1998).

Relationship Between Stages and Processes of Change. One of the earliest empirical integrations was the discovery of systematic relationships between the stages people were in and the processes they were applying. This discovery allowed an integration of processes from theories that were typically seen as incompatible and in conflict. For example, Freudian theory that relied almost entirely on consciousness raising for producing change was viewed as incompatible with Skinnerian theory that relied entirely on contingency management for modifying behavior. But self-changers did not know that these processes were theoretically incompatible, and they showed that processes from very different theories were emphasized at different stages of change. Table 5.2 presents the current empirical integration (Prochaska, DiClemente, and Norcross, 1992). This integration suggests that in early stages people apply cognitive, affective, and evaluative

TABLE 5.2. PROCESSES OF CHANGE THAT MEDIATE PROGRESSION BETWEEN THE STAGES OF CHANGE.

	Stages of Change				
	Precontemplation	Contemplation	Preparation	Action	Maintenance
Processes	Consciousness raising Dramatic relief Environmental reevaluation				
		Self-reevaluation			
			Self-liberation		
				Counterconditioning Helping relationships Reinforcement management Stimulus control	

Note: Social liberation was omitted due to its unclear relationship to the stages.

processes to progress. In later stages, people rely more on commitments, conditioning, contingencies, environmental controls, and support for progressing toward maintenance or termination.

To help people progress from precontemplation to contemplation, such processes as consciousness raising and dramatic relief should be applied (see Table 5.2). Encouraging processes such as contingency management, counterconditioning, and stimulus control to people in precontemplation could be a theoretical, empirical, and practical mistake. But for people in action, such strategies would represent optimal matching.

As with the structure of the processes, the integration of the processes and stages has not been as consistent as the integration of the stages and pros and cons. While part of the problem may be due to the greater complexity of integrating ten processes across five stages, the processes of change need more basic research.

Studies That Challenge TTM. As with any model, not all of the research is supportive. Farkas and others (1996) and later Abrams, Herzog, Emmons, and Linnan (2000) compared addiction variables to TTM variables as predictors of cessation over twelve to twenty-four months. Addiction variables, such as number of cigarettes smoked and duration of prior quits (for example, more than one hundred days), out-predicted TTM variables, suggesting that addiction models were preferable to TTM. Responses to these comparative studies included the observation that Farkas and colleagues compared fourteen addiction type variables to just the single stage variable from TTM (Prochaska and Velicer, 1996). The Abrams and colleagues study included self-efficacy and the contemplation ladder measure of stage as part of their addiction model, although these are part of TTM.

In the first of a series of studies, Herzog and others (1999) found that six processes of change were not adequate predictors of stage progress over a twelve-month period. In a second report, the processes predicted stage progress but only when the contemplation ladder was used (Herzog, Abrams, Emmons, and Linnan, 2000). In the third report, TTM measures predicted twelve-month outcomes, but self-efficacy and the contemplation ladder were not counted as TTM variables (Abrams, Herzog, Emmons, and Linnan, 2000). Other research has found that change processes and other TTM variables predict stage progress (for example, Prochaska and others, 1985, 1991; DiClemente and others, 1991; Johnson and others, 2000). Johnson and others (2000) sought to explain some of the inconsistencies in previous research, such as predictions over six months versus twelve months and using all ten processes of change instead of a subset.

Applied Studies. Within a large and diverse body of applied TTM studies, there are several trends. The most common application involves tailored communications, which match intervention messages to an individual's particular needs (for example, Kreuter, Strecher, and Glassman, 1999; Skinner and others, 1999). For example, individuals in precontemplation could receive feedback designed to increase their pros of changing to help them progress to contemplation.

The largest number of TTM-related intervention studies have been for smoking (Aveyard and others, 1999; Curry and others, 1995; Dijkstra, DeVries, and Roijackers, 1999; O'Neill, Gillespie, and Slobin, 2000; Pallonen and others, 1994, 1998; Prochaska, DiClemente, Velicer, and Rossi, 1993; Prochaska and others, 2001a, 2001b; Strecher and others, 1994; Velicer and others, 1999); diet (Beresford and others, 1997; Brug and others, 1998; Campbell and others, 1994; Glanz and others, 1998; Horwath, 1999); and exercise (Cardinal and Sachs, 1996; Marcus and others, 1998). There are a growing range of applications, including mammography (Rakowski and others, 1998); alcohol abuse (Project Match Research Group, 1997; Carbonari and DiClemente, 2000); condom use (CDC AIDS Community Demonstration Projects Research Group, 1999; Schneider Jamner, Wolitski, and Corby, 1997); organ donation (Robbins and others, 2001); and multiple behavior changes (Gold, Anderson, and Serxner, 2000; Kreuter and Strecher, 1996; Steptoe, Kerry, Rink, and Hilton, 2001). There also are an increasing number of settings in which TTM is being applied, including primary care (Goldstein and others, 1999) at home (Curry and others, 1995; Gold, Anderson, and Serxner, 2000); in churches (Voorhees and others, 1996); schools (Aveyard and others,

1999); and communities (CDC AIDS Community Demonstration Projects Research Group, 1999). While many of these applications have been effective, some have not (see for example, Aveyard and others, 1999). Future applied research should determine which types of TTM interventions are effective for which behaviors and populations and in which intervention settings.

Application: Population-Based Approaches to Smoking Cessation

Smoking is costly to individual smokers and to society. In the United States, approximately forty-four million Americans continued to smoke in 2000 (National Cancer Institute, 2000). Over four hundred thousand preventable deaths per year are attributable to smoking. Globally, the problem is catastrophic. Of the people alive in the world today, five hundred million are expected to die from this single behavior, a loss of approximately five billion years of life to tobacco use (Peto and Lopez, 1990). Providing effective smoking cessation to entire populations could prevent millions of premature deaths and help preserve billions of years of life.

Recruitment and Retention

Population cessation requires interventions that reach or recruit high percentages of smokers. In two home-based programs with approximately five thousand smokers in each study, we reached out either by telephone alone or by personal letters followed by telephone calls if needed and recruited smokers to stage-matched interventions. For each of five stages, these interventions included self-help manuals, individualized computer feedback reports based on assessments of the pros and cons, processes, self-efficacy and temptations, and counselor protocols based on the computer reports. Using these proactive recruitment methods and stage-matched interventions, we obtained participation rates of 80 to 85 percent, respectively (Prochaska and others, 2001a; 2001b). Such recruitment rates provide the potential to generate unprecedented results with entire populations of smokers.

Impact on population equals participation rate times the rate of efficacy or action (Velicer and DiClemente, 1993; see also Chapter Twenty-Four). If a program produced 30 percent efficacy (such as long-term abstinence), historically it was judged to be better than a program that produced 25 percent abstinence. But a program that generates 30 percent efficacy but only 5 percent participation has an impact of only 1.5 percent (30 percent × 5 percent). A program that produces only 25 percent efficacy but 60 percent participation has an impact of 15 percent. For health promotion programs, this would mean a ten-fold greater population impact.

TTM programs shift outcomes from efficacy alone to impact. To achieve such high impact, we must shift from reactive recruitment, in which we advertise or announce programs and react when people reach us (for example, Lichtenstein and Hollis, 1992), to proactive recruitments, in which we reach out to interact with all potential participants. In addition, programs should match people's stages.

The best strategy to promote retention is matching interventions to stage of change. In three smoking cessation studies using such matching strategies, smokers in the precontemplation stage were retained at the same high levels as were those who started in the preparation stage (Prochaska, DiClemente, Velicer, and Rossi, 1993; Prochaska and others, 2001a, 2001b).

Progress

The amount of progress participants make following health promotion programs directly relates to the stage they were in at the start of the interventions. Across sixty-six different predictions of progress, smokers starting in contemplation were about two-thirds more successful than those in precontemplation at six-, twelve-, and eighteen-month follow-ups. Similarly, those in preparation were about two-thirds more successful than those in contemplation at the same follow-ups (Prochaska and others, 2001b).

These results can be used clinically. A reasonable goal for each therapeutic intervention with smokers is to help them progress one stage. If over the course of brief therapy they progress two stages, they will be about 2.66 times more successful at longer-term follow-ups (Prochaska and others, 2001b).

This strategy has been taught to more than six thousand primary-care physicians, nurses, and physicians' assistants in Britain's National Health System. With stage-matched counseling, the strategic goal is to help each patient progress one stage following one brief intervention. One of the first reports describes a marked improvement in the morale of such health promoters intervening with all patients who smoke, abuse substances, and have unhealthy diets. These professionals now have strategies that match the needs of all of their patients, not just the minority prepared to take action. Furthermore, these professionals can assess progress across stages for the majority of these patients, where previously they experienced mostly failure when taking action was their only measure of movement (Steptoe, Kerry, Rink, and Hilton, 2001).

Process

One of the fundamental principles for progress in behavior change is that different processes of change need to be applied at different stages of change. Classic conditioning processes such as counterconditioning, stimulus control, and contingency control can be highly successful for participants taking action but can produce resistance with individuals in precontemplation. With these individuals, more experiential processes, such as consciousness raising and dramatic relief, can move people cognitively and affectively, and can help them shift to contemplation (Prochaska, Norcross, and DiClemente, 1994).

After fifteen years of research, fourteen variables have been identified on which to intervene to accelerate progress across the first five stages of change (Prochaska, Norcross, and DiClemente, 1994). At any particular stage, a maximum of six variables are intervened upon. To help guide individuals at each stage of change, computer-based expert systems have been developed to deliver individualized and interactive tailored interventions to entire populations (Velicer and others, 1993; Redding and others, 1999). These computer programs can be used alone or in conjunction with counselors.

Outcomes

In our first large-scale clinical trial, we compared four treatments: (1) one of the best home-based action-oriented cessation programs (standardized), (2) stage-matched manuals (individualized), (3) expert system computer reports plus manuals (interactive), and (4) counselors plus computers and manuals (personalized). We randomly assigned by stage 739 smokers to one of the four treatments (Prochaska, DiClemente, Velicer, and Rossi, 1993).

In the computer condition, participants answered by mail or telephone forty questions that were used to generate feedback reports. These reports informed participants about their stage of change, their pros and cons of changing, and their use of change processes appropriate to their stages. At baseline, participants were given positive feedback on what they were doing correctly and guidance on which principles and processes they needed to apply more to progress. In two progress reports delivered over the next six months, participants also received positive feedback on any improvements they made on any of the variables relevant to progressing. Demoralized and defensive smokers could begin progressing without having to quit and without having to work too hard. Smokers in the contemplation stage could begin taking small steps, such as delaying their first cigarette in the morning for an extra thirty minutes. They could choose small steps that would increase their self-efficacy and help them become better prepared for quitting. In the personalized condition, smokers received four proactive counselor calls over the six-month intervention period.

Outcomes for the two self-help manual conditions paralleled each other for twelve months. At eighteen months, the stage-matched manual participants moved ahead. This is an example of a *delayed action effect,* which is often observed with stage-matched programs specifically and self-help programs more generally

(Glynn, Anderson, and Schwarz, 1992). It takes time for participants in early stages to progress to action.

The computer alone and computer plus counselor conditions paralleled each other for twelve months. Then the effects of the counselor condition flattened out while the computer condition effects continued to increase. Participants in the personalized condition may have become somewhat dependent on the social support and social control of the counselor. The last call was after the six months assessment, and benefits would be observed at twelve months. Termination of the counselors could result in no further progress because of the loss of social support and control. The classic pattern in smoking cessation clinics is rapid relapse beginning as soon as the treatment is terminated. Some of this rapid relapse could well be due to the sudden loss of social support or social control provided by the counselors and other participants in the clinic.

In this clinical trial, smokers were recruited reactively in response to advertisements, announcements, and articles. How would their results compare to the smokers proactively recruited to programs? Most people would predict that smokers who call for help would succeed more than smokers who were called to have help offered.

Figure 5.1 shows the impressive results of comparing smokers in a study who called (reactive) (Prochaska, DiClemente, Velicer, and Rossi, 1993) to those in a study who were called (proactive) (Prochaska and others, 2001a). Both groups received the same home-based expert system computer reports delivered over a six-month period. While the reactively recruited subjects were slightly more successful at each follow-up, the results are similar. The replication and dissemination of

FIGURE 5.1. ABSTINENCE RATES FOR SMOKERS RECRUITED BY REACTIVE AND PROACTIVE STRATEGIES.

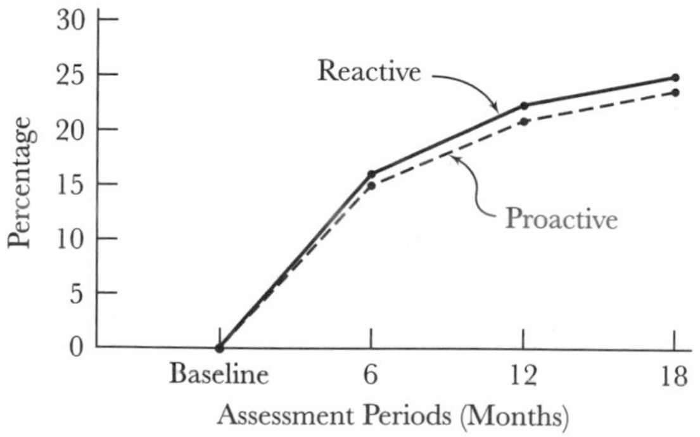

such programs could produce substantial impacts on entire populations. However, scientific and professional shifts will be required:

1. From an action paradigm to a stage paradigm
2. From reactive to proactive recruitment
3. From expecting participants to match the needs of programs to programs that match their needs
4. From clinic-based to community-based behavioral health programs that apply the field's most powerful individualized and interactive intervention strategies

Application: Mammography Screening

Every year, about one hundred and eighty thousand women in the United States are diagnosed with breast cancer, and deaths from breast cancer exceed forty-three thousand yearly (Parker, Tong, Bolden, and Wingo, 1997). Breast cancer is the second leading cause of cancer deaths among women. The most effective method of detecting and reducing mortality from breast cancer is screening mammography. Although the number of women having a mammogram has increased since the mid-1980s, there is still much room for improvement. Several studies have applied The Transtheoretical Model to increase women's participation in mammography screening within a variety of populations, including a worksite sample (Rakowski and others, 1992), women chosen from selected census tracts (Rakowski, Fulton, and Feldman, 1993), random samples of women from an HMO in southeastern New England (Rakowski and others, 1996), and studies from across the United States (Rakowski and others, 1997a).

The majority of this research has focused on the stages of change and decisional balance measures (Rakowski, Fulton, and Feldman, 1993; Rakowski and others, 1996). Studies have examined the application of the Stages of Change construct to this behavior, exploring alternative ways of assessing an individuals' stage of adoption (Rakowski and others, 1996). Definitions of the traditional TTM stages of precontemplation, contemplation, action, and maintenance have been refined and findings have identified additional stages. Precontemplation has been defined as never having had a mammogram and not planning to have one within the next two years. Women in contemplation are those who never had a mammogram, but plan to have one in the coming two years, or are off schedule after having a prior mammogram but intend to have one in the next two years. The action stage has been defined as having had one mammogram on schedule, and intending to have another on schedule, or already having one scheduled. Finally, the maintenance stage includes women who have had at least two mammograms on schedule and intend to have another on time. Two other stages also have been incorporated: *relapse*, defined as having had a mammogram but not intending to have another in the next two years, and *risk for relapse*, defined as having had regular mammograms but not planning to have another within a scheduled time frame. Because women in these two other stages have no intention to have a mammogram in the next two years, they could be viewed as comparable to precontemplation.

Several studies have focused on the development and validation of the decisional balance measures for mammography use. These studies found that decisional balance scores did vary predictably with stage of mammography adoption (Rakowski and others, 1992, 1997b).

Rakowski and colleagues examined whether women who received a mailed, stage-matched, tailored intervention received more mammography screening than did women who received either no materials or standard materials (Rakowski and others, 1998). Women involved in this study participated in four telephone surveys over twenty-one months (baseline, three to five months, twelve months, and nineteen to twenty-one months). Women randomized to the no materials group participated in the telephone surveys and did not receive any mailed interventions. Individuals in the standard materials group received a mailed intervention packet following the baseline and first follow-up timepoints, which included a question-and-answer sheet, a breast health guide, a tip sheet, and a breast self-examination shower card. Women randomized into the stage-matched materials group also received mailed intervention packets following the baseline and first follow-up timepoints, which included an expert system computer-generated letter tailored to the individual's responses on stage of adoption, decisional balance, and processes of change. In addition to the expert system letter, women in this group also received a packet of information matched to their stage of adoption that included versions of a question-and-answer sheet about mammography, a tumor-size sheet that was tailored to specific stages, and a tip sheet and breast self-exam shower card. Finally, a provider-training component was included across all three groups that incorporated an introduction to the study for health care providers and a training session to increase mammography screening.

Women between the ages of forty and seventy-four were recruited into the intervention study through a staff-model HMO, with a response rate of 73.5 percent. Outcome analyses on a total of 1,397 women found that 64 percent of the women who received the stage-matched materials obtained mammograms compared to 55 percent of women who received no intervention materials and 59 percent of those who received standard materials (OR = 1.43) (Rakowski and others, 1998). These findings demonstrate the ability to intervene effectively on this important health behavior with minimal stage-matched materials mailed to participants.

Conclusion

Increasing impact on population health should be one of the top priorities for health behavior research. One promising approach is to intervene on multiple behaviors. Using the same type of stage-matched and tailored interventions as those proven to be effective for smoking and other single behaviors, a growing number of projects are treating multiple behaviors. In parallel projects, adolescents at school and their parents at home received expert system interventions to change smoking, high-fat diets, and sun exposure. The results of these population trials were very encouraging, though they have not yet been published (Prochaska and others, 2001c).

These population studies have been extended to include alcohol abuse, exercise, and stress management. Innovative approaches also include intervening at both the family and individual level with parents. An integrative approach is being developed to teach teens the principles and processes across stages for multiple behaviors. The goal should be for self change management to become more of a core competency so that young people can apply these principles to whatever behaviors they choose.

The action paradigm suggested that treating multiple behaviors at once would overwhelm people with too many demands. From a stage perspective, our unpublished raw data show that in populations with four behavior risk factors (for example, smoking, diet, exercise, and sun exposure), fewer than 10 percent of individuals are prepared to take action on two or more behaviors at the same time. People can take action on one behavior, while progressing toward action on other behaviors. Nevertheless, more research is needed to determine the optimal number of behaviors to treat simultaneously.

While research results to date are encouraging, much still needs to be done to advance The Transtheoretical Model. Basic research should explore relationships of TTM variables with constructs from other established health behavior theories, including perceived risk, subjective norms, and problem severity. The purpose would be to determine if such constructs relate systematically to the stages and if they predict progress across particular stages. More research is needed on the structure or integration of the processes and stages of change across a broad range of behaviors, including acquisition behaviors such as exercise and extinction behaviors such as smoking cessation (Rosen, 2000). One reason would be to determine what modifications are needed for specific types of behaviors, for example, perhaps fewer processes for infrequent behaviors such as mammography screening.

Because tailored communications represent the most promising interventions for applying the TTM to large populations, more research is needed to compare the effectiveness, cost effectiveness, and impacts of alternative technologies. The Internet is excellent for individualized interactions at lower cost but cannot produce the high participation rates generated by person-to-person outreach via telephone or primary care practitioners.

How do diverse populations respond to stage-matched interventions and to high tech systems? How might programs best be tailored to meet the needs of diverse populations? Might menus of alternative intervention modalities (for example, telephone, Internet, neighborhood or church leaders, person-to-person or community programs) empower diverse populations to best match health-enhancing programs to their particular needs?

The Transtheoretical Model is a dynamic theory of change. It must remain open to modifications and enhancements as more students, scientists, and practitioners apply the stage paradigm to a growing number and diversity of theoretical issues, public health problems, and at-risk populations.

References

Abrams, D. B., Herzog, T. A., Emmons, K. M., and Linnan, L. "Stages of Change Versus Addiction: A Replication and Extension." *Nicotine and Tobacco Research*, 2000, *2*, 223–229.

Aveyard, P., and others. "Cluster Randomised Controlled Trial of Expert System Based on the Transtheoretical ("Stages of Change") Model for Smoking Prevention and Cessation in Schools." *British Medical Journal*, 1999, *319*, 948–953.

Bandura, A. "Self-Efficacy Mechanism in Human Agency." *American Psychologist*, 1982, *37*, 122–147.

Beresford, S.A.A., and others. "A Dietary Intervention in Primary Care Practice: The Eating Patterns Study." *American Journal of Public Health*, 1997, *87*, 610–616.

Brug, J., and others. "The Impact of Computer-Tailored Feedback and Iterative Feedback on Fat, Fruit, and Vegetable Intake." *Health Education and Behavior*, 1998, *25*, 517–531.

Campbell, M. K., and others. "Improving Dietary Behavior: The Effectiveness of Tailored Messages in Primary Care Settings." *American Journal of Public Health*, 1994, *84*, 783–787.

Carbonari, J. P., and DiClemente, C. C. "Using Transtheoretical Model Profiles to Differentiate Levels of Alcohol Abstinence Success." *Journal of Consulting and Clinical Psychology*, 2000, *68*, 810–817.

Cardinal, B. J., and Sachs, M. L. "Effects of Mail-Mediated, Stage-Matched Exercise Behavior Change Strategies on Female Adults' Leisure-Time Exercise Behavior." *Journal of Sports Medicine and Physical Fitness*, 1996, *36*, 100–107.

CDC AIDS Community Demonstration Projects Research Group. "Community-Level HIV Intervention in 5 Cities: Final Outcome Data from the CDC AIDS Community Demonstration Projects." *American Journal of Public Health*, 1999, *89*(3), 336–345.

Curry, S. J., and others. "A Randomized Trial of Self-Help Materials, Personalized Feedback, and Telephone Counseling with Nonvolunteer Smokers." *Journal of Consulting and Clinical Psychology*, 1995, *63*, 175–180.

DiClemente, C. C., and Prochaska, J. O. "Self Change and Therapy Change of Smoking Behavior: A Comparison of Processes of Change in Cessation and Maintenance." *Addictive Behavior*, 1982, *7*, 133–142.

DiClemente, C. C., and others. "The Processes of Smoking Cessation: An Analysis of Precontemplation, Contemplation, and Preparation Stages of Change." *Journal of Consulting and Clinical Psychology*, 1991, *59*, 295–304.

Dijkstra, A., DeVries, H., and Roijackers, J. "Targeting Smokers with Low Readiness to Change with Tailored and Non-Tailored Self-Help Materials." *Preventive Medicine*, 1999, *28*, 203–211.

Farkas, A. J., and others. "Addiction Versus Stages of Change Models in Predicting Smoking Cessation." *Addiction*, 1996, *91*, 1271–1280.

Glanz, K., and others. "Impact of Work Site Health Promotion on Stages of Dietary Change: The Working Well Trial." *Health Education and Behavior*, 1998, *25*, 448–463.

Glynn, T. J., Anderson, D. M., and Schwarz, L. "Tobacco Use Reduction Among High Risk Youth: Recommendations of a National Cancer Institute Expert Advisory Panel." *Preventive Medicine*, 1992, *24*, 354–362.

Gold, D. B., Anderson, D. R., and Serxner, S. A. "Impact of Telephone-Based Intervention on the Reduction of Health Risks." *American Journal of Health Promotion*, 2000, *15*(2), 97–106.

Goldstein, M. G., and others. "Physician-Based Physical Activity Counseling for Middle-Aged and Older Adults: A Randomized Trial." *Annals of Behavioral Medicine*, 1999, *21*, 40–47.

Herzog, T. A., Abrams, D. B., Emmons, K. A., and Linnan, L. "Predicting Increases in Readiness to Quit Smoking: A Prospective Analysis Using the Contemplation Ladder." *Psychology and Health*, 2000, *15*, 369–381.

Herzog, T. A., and others. "Do Processes of Change Predict Stage Movements? A Prospective Analysis of the Transtheoretical Model." *Health Psychology*, 1999, *18*, 369–375.

Horwath, C. C. "Applying the Transtheoretical Model to Eating Behaviour Change: Challenges and Opportunities." *Nutrition Research Review*, 1999, *12*, 281–317.

Janis, I. L., and Mann, L. *Decision Making: A Psychological Analysis of Conflict, Chance and Commitment.* London: Cassil and Collier Macmillen, 1977.

Johnson, J. L., and others. "What Predicts Stage of Change for Smoking Cessation?" *Annals of Behavioral Medicine*, 2000, *22*, S173.

Kreuter, M., and Strecher, V. J. "Do Tailored Behavior Change Messages Enhance the Effectiveness of Health Risk Appraisal? Results from a Randomized Trial." *Health Education Research*, 1996, *11*, 97–105.

Kreuter, M. W., Strecher, V. J., and Glassman, B. "One Size Does Not Fit All: The Case for Tailoring Print Materials." *Annals of Behavioral Medicine*, 1999, *21*(4), 276–283.

Lichtenstein, E., and Hollis, J. "Patient Referral to Smoking Cessation Programs: Who Follows Through?" *The Journal of Family Practice*, 1992, *34*, 739–744.

Marcus, B. H., and others. "Efficacy of an Individualized, Motivationally Tailored Physical Activity Intervention." *Annals of Behavioral Medicine*, 1998, *20*, 174–180.

National Cancer Institute. *Population Based Smoking Cessation: Proceedings of a Conference on What Works to Influence Cessation in the General Population.* Smoking and Tobacco Control Monograph

No. 12. Bethesda, Md.: U.S. Department of Health and Human Services, National Institutes of Health, National Cancer Institute, NIH Pub. No. 00–4892, November 2000.

O'Neill, H. K., Gillespie, M. A., and Slobin, K. "Stages of Change and Smoking Cessation: A Computer-Administered Intervention Program for Young Adults." *American Journal of Health Promotion,* 2000, *15*(2), 93–96.

Pallonen, U. E., and others. "A 2-Year Self-Help Smoking Cessation Manual Intervention Among Middle-Aged Finnish Men: An Application of the Transtheoretical Model." *Preventive Medicine,* 1994, *23*, 507–514.

Pallonen, U. E., and others. "Computer-Based Smoking Cessation Interventions in Adolescents: Description, Feasibility, and Six-Month Follow-up Findings." *Substance Use and Misuse,* 1998, *33*, 935–965.

Parker, S. L., Tong, T., Bolden, S., and Wingo, P. A. "Cancer Statistics, 1997." *CA—A Cancer Journal for Clinicians,* 1997, *47*, 5–27.

Peto, R., and Lopez, A. "World-Wide Mortality from Current Smoking Patterns." In B. Durstone and K. Jamrogik (eds.), *The Global War: Proceedings of the Seventh World Conference on Tobacco and Health.* East Perth, Western Australia: Organizing Committee of Seventh World Conference on Tobacco and Health, 1990.

Prochaska, J. O. *Systems of Psychotherapy: A Transtheoretical Analysis.* Pacific Grove, Calif.: Brooks-Cole, 1979.

Prochaska, J. O. "Strong and Weak Principles for Progressing from Precontemplation to Action Based on Twelve Problem Behaviors." *Health Psychology,* 1994, *13*, 47–51.

Prochaska, J. O., and DiClemente, C. C. "Stages and Processes of Self-Change of Smoking: Toward an Integrative Model of Change." *Journal of Consulting and Clinical Psychology,* 1983, *51*, 390–395.

Prochaska, J. O., DiClemente, C. C., and Norcross, J. C. "In Search of How People Change: Applications to the Addictive Behaviors." *American Psychologist,* 1992, *47*, 1102–1114.

Prochaska, J. O., DiClemente, C. C., Velicer, W. F., and Rossi, J. S. "Standardized, Individualized, Interactive, and Personalized Self-Help Programs for Smoking Cessation." *Health Psychology,* 1993, *12*, 399–405.

Prochaska, J. O., Norcross, J. C., and DiClemente, C. C. *Changing for Good.* New York: William Morrow, 1994.

Prochaska, J. O., and Velicer, W. F. "On Models, Methods and Premature Conclusions." *Addictions,* 1996, *91*, 1281–1283.

Prochaska, J. O., and others. "Predicting Change in Smoking Status for Self-Changers." *Addictive Behaviors,* 1985, *10*, 395–406.

Prochaska, J. O., and others. "Patterns of Change: Dynamic Typology Applied to Smoking Cessation." *Multivariate Behavioral Research,* 1991, *26*, 83–107.

Prochaska, J. O., and others. "Stages of Change and Decisional Balance for Twelve Problem Behaviors." *Health Psychology,* 1994, *13*, 39–46.

Prochaska, J. O., and others. "Evaluating a Population-Based Recruitment Approach and a Stage-Based Expert System Intervention for Smoking." *Addictive Behaviors,* 2001a, *26*, 583–602.

Prochaska, J. O., and others. "Counselor and Stimulus Control Enhancements of a Stage-Matched Expert System Intervention for Smokers in a Managed Care Setting." *Preventive Medicine,* 2001b, *32*, 23–32.

Prochaska, J. O., and others. (Unpublished raw data), 2001c.

Project Match Research Group. "Matching Alcoholism Treatments to Client Heterogeneity: Project MATCH Post Treatment Drinking Outcomes." *Journal of Studies on Alcohol,* 1997, *58,* 7–29.

Rakowski, W., Fulton, J. P., and Feldman, J. P. "Women's Decisions About Mammography: A Replication of the Relationship Between Stages of Adoption and Decisional Balance." *Health Psychology,* 1993, *12,* 209–214.

Rakowski, W., and others. "Assessing Elements of Women's Decisions About Mammography." *Health Psychology,* 1992, *11,* 111–118.

Rakowski, W., and others. "Screening Mammography and Constructs from the Transtheoretical Model: Associations Using Two Definitions of the Stages-of-Adoption." *Annals of Behavioral Medicine,* 1996, *18,* 91–100.

Rakowski, W., and others. "Confirmatory Analysis of Opinions Regarding the Pros and Cons of Mammography." *Health Psychology,* 1997a, *16,* 433–441.

Rakowski, W., and others. Integrating Pros and Cons for Mammography and Pap Testing: Extending the Construct of Decisional Balance to Two Behaviors. *Preventive Medicine,* 1997b, *26,* 664–673.

Rakowski, W. R., and others. "Increasing Mammography Among Women Aged 40–74 by Use of a Stage-Matched, Tailored Intervention." *Preventive Medicine,* 1998, *27,* 748–756.

Redding, C. A., and others. "Transtheoretical Individualized Multimedia Expert Systems Targeting Adolescents' Health Behaviors." *Cognitive and Behavioral Practice,* 1999, *6*(2), 144–153.

Robbins, M. L., and others. "Assessing Family Members' Motivational Readiness and Decision Making for Consenting to Cadaveric Organ Donation." *Journal of Health Psychology,* 2001, *6,* 523–536.

Rosen, C. S. "Is the Sequencing of Change Processes by Stage Consistent Across Health Problems? A Meta-Analysis." *Health Psychology,* 2000, *19,* 593–604.

Rossi, J. S. "Stages of Change for 15 Health Risk Behaviors in an HMO Population." Paper presented at the 13th Meeting of the Society for Behavioral Medicine, New York, March 1992.

Rossi, J. S. "Common Processes of Change Across Nine Problem Behaviors." Paper presented at the 100th meeting of the American Psychological Association, Washington, D.C., August 1992.

Schneider Jamner, M., Wolitski, R. J., and Corby, N. H. "Impact of a Longitudinal Community HIV Intervention Targeting Injecting Drug Users' Stage of Change for Condom Use and Bleach Use." *American Journal of Health Promotion,* 1997, *12,* 15–24.

Skinner, C. S., and others. "How Effective Is Tailored Print Communication?" *Annals of Behavioral Medicine,* 1999, *21*(4), 290–298.

Snow, M. G., Prochaska, J. O., and Rossi, J. S. "Stages of Change for Smoking Cessation Among Former Problem Drinkers: A Cross-Sectional Analysis." *Journal of Substance Abuse,* 1992, *4,* 107–116.

Steptoe, A., Kerry, S., Rink, E., and Hilton, S. "The Impact of Behavioral Counseling on Stages of Change in Fat Intake, Physical Activity, and Cigarette Smoking in Adults at Increased Risk of Coronary Heart Disease." *American Journal of Public Health,* 2001, *91*(2), 26.

Strecher, V. J., and others. "The Effects of Computer Tailored Smoking Cessation Messages in Family Practice Settings." *The Journal of Family Practice,* 1994, *39,* 262–270.

U.S. Department of Health and Human Services. *The Health Benefits of Smoking Cessation: A Report of the Surgeon General.* U.S. Department of Health and Human Services Publication no. CDC 90-8416. Washington, D.C.: U.S. Government Printing Office, 1990.

Velicer, W. F., and DiClemente, C. C. "Understanding and Intervening with the Total Population of Smokers." *Tobacco Control,* 1993, *2,* 95–96.

Velicer, W. F., and others. "An Expert System Intervention for Smoking Cessation." *Addictive Behaviors,* 1993, *18,* 269–290.

Velicer, W. F., and others. "Distribution of Smokers by Stage in Three Representative Samples." *Preventive Medicine,* 1995, *24,* 401–411.

Velicer, W. F., and others. "Interactive Versus Noninteractive Interventions and Dose-Response Relationships for Stage-Matched Smoking Cessation Programs in a Managed Care Setting." *Health Psychology,* 1999, *18,* 21–28.

Voorhees, C. C., and others. "Heart, Body, and Soul: Impact of Church-Based Smoking Cessation Interventions on Readiness to Quit." *Preventive Medicine,* 1996, *25,* 277–285.

CHAPTER SIX

THE PRECAUTION ADOPTION
PROCESS MODEL

Neil D. Weinstein
Peter M. Sandman

I magine that you are a health educator trying to understand why young adults
engage in behaviors that put them at risk for AIDS. You develop a questionnaire that asks them about the likelihood that they will come in contact with someone who is HIV positive, the chances of becoming infected by this person, the
effectiveness of various precautions, the social consequences of taking these precautions, what others think about the risk of AIDS and about AIDS precautions,
and other topics like these that are drawn from widely used theories of health behavior. It seems obvious that assessing these beliefs will help you understand why
someone is or is not engaging in risky behavior.

This approach makes sense today, but what if the year of your study were 1987,
when the public was first learning about AIDS? At that time, young adults might
have known that AIDS is a fatal, progressive disease, but little more. Few would have

This chapter is a modification of one that originally appeared in D. Rutter and L. Quine (eds.), *Changing Health Behavior: Intervention and Research with Social Cognition Models*. Buckingham, U.K.: Open University Press, 2001. Used with permission.

The authors are indebted to Alexander Rothman and Stephen Sutton for their assistance in clarifying the characteristics and testing of stage theories and to Cara Cuite, May Lou Klotz, Judith Lyon,
Paul Miller, and Nancy Roberts for their contributions to our radon research. Funding for the radon
research from the New Jersey Department of Environmental Protection, the New Jersey Agricultural
Experiment Station, and the National Cancer Institute is gratefully acknowledged.

any idea how to answer most of your questions. Still, their behaviors would vary a lot. Some would have had many sexual partners; some few or none. Some would use condoms and others would not. Nevertheless, neither their current behaviors nor the likelihood that they would change these behaviors could be explained or predicted by their beliefs about HIV. They had not yet formed such beliefs.

As this example shows, in 1987 one could not explain risk behaviors for HIV in terms of beliefs about AIDS and AIDS transmission. In general, theories that try to explain behavior by focusing on the perceived costs and benefits of action apply only to the period when someone has already been engaged by the threat and has formed beliefs about possible responses. As the preceding example suggests, there are different phases to precaution taking. Consequently, we need different explanations for what goes on in these different phases.

How Stage Theories Approach the Issue of Explaining and Changing Behavior

Most theories of health behavior, such as those based on perceived costs and benefits of action, specify a single equation to predict behavior. They acknowledge *quantitative* differences among people in their likelihood of action and in their position on various influential variables. However, the theories do not acknowledge changes in the barriers that people must overcome to progress toward action. For all these theories, the goal of interventions is to maximize the variables that increase the value of the prediction equation.

Advocates of stage theories such as the Precaution Adoption Process Model (PAPM) question whether changes in health-relevant behaviors can be described by a single prediction equation. In effect, these advocates suggest that we must try to understand a whole series of changes, identifying for each stage transition the relevant variables and the way in which they combine. This is a much more complicated goal than finding a single prediction rule, but it offers the possibility of greater intervention efficiency and effectiveness.

Essential Elements of Stage Theories

Stage theories have four principal elements (Weinstein, Rothman, and Sutton, 1998). The essential elements apply to the PAPM as well as to other stage theories.

1. *A category system to define the stages.* Stages are theoretical constructs. A "prototype" can be defined for each stage, but few people will match this ideal perfectly. The actual boundaries between stages may not be as clear as our theories and measurements suggest.

2. *An ordering of the stages.* Stage theories assume that people generally pass through all the stages to reach the end point of action or maintenance. However, progression is neither inevitable nor irreversible (compare with Bandura, 1995). There is no minimum length of time people must spend in a particular stage. Sometimes they may progress so rapidly (for example, when a doctor recommends an action that someone had never thought about before) that, for practical purposes, people can be said to skip stages. Also, some stages may lie on side paths that are not on the route to action, and people do not need to pass through them.

3. *Common barriers to change that face people in the same stage.* Stage ideas are helpful in designing programs that encourage people to move toward action if people at one stage have to address similar types of issues before they can progress to the next stage.

4. *Different barriers to change that face people in different stages.* If the factors producing movement toward action were the same regardless of a person's stage, the same intervention could be used for all, and the concept of stages would be superfluous.

A completely specified stage theory would include both the criteria that define the stages and the issues that represent barriers between stages. Although the stage definitions apply across behaviors, the barriers to progress between stages may be behavior-specific.

The particular factors that help people make a decision to lose weight may be quite different from the factors that help people make a decision to use condoms, even though the process of reaching a decision is common to both actions. A model that proposes a particular sequence of stages in the change process could be correct about these stages even if it has not identified all the barriers at each stage. Thus, the PAPM changes should be seen as a framework that needs to be filled in for each behavior with an analysis of how each stage transition occurs.

How Stage Theories, Including the PAPM, Can Be Tested

A variety of approaches have been used to determine whether a particular behavior change passes through the sequence of stages proposed by a stage theory (Weinstein, Rothman, and Sutton, 1998). Many of these approaches have limitations. For example, a common but weak strategy is to use cross-sectional data from interviews to look for differences between people thought to be in different stages. A somewhat stronger approach would be prospective, measuring the stages that people are in and following up with measures of whether they took action or not. Still, simply finding differences among stages tells us little, as nonstage processes will also produce such differences. Explanatory and analytical research is limited to learning about the variables that are assessed.

Intervention research provides a much stronger test of theory. Experimental studies using matched and mismatched interventions would be one of the optimal strategies to use in testing stage theories. If it is true that different variables influence movement at different stages, treatments designed to influence these variables should be most effective when applied to people in the appropriate stage. Thus, individuals in a given stage should respond better to an intervention that is *matched* to their stage than to one that is *mismatched* (that is, matched to a different stage).

Stage models predict that the sequencing of treatments is important. For maximum effectiveness, the order of interventions should follow the hypothesized order of stages. Consequently, sequence effects provide further evidence of a stage process. Unfortunately, because testing for sequence effects requires sequential interventions, such tests are quite difficult to carry out.

The Precaution Adoption Process Model

Description of the Model

The adoption of a new precaution or the cessation of a risky behavior requires deliberate action. The Precaution Adoption Process Model applies to these types of actions rather than to the gradual development of habitual patterns of behavior, such as exercise and diet. It can also be used to explain why and how people make deliberate changes in their habitual patterns.

The goal of the PAPM is to explain how a person comes to the decision to take action, and how he or she translates that decision into action. For this reason the Precaution Adoption Process Model focuses on psychological processes within individuals. As a consequence, the stages prior to action are defined in terms of the mental states that appear to be important, rather than in terms of factors external to the person, such as current behavior, past behavior, or some combination of these with the person's mental state. Stages should not be defined in terms of criteria that are salient only to health professionals, such as the percentage of fat in a person's diet, as they are unlikely to explain a layperson's behavior.

Although several aspects of the PAPM were discussed in 1988 (Weinstein, 1988), the present formulation was published in 1992 (Weinstein and Sandman, 1992). The PAPM identifies seven stages along the path from lack of awareness to action (see Figure 6.1). At some initial point in time people are unaware of the health issue (stage 1). When they first learn something about the issue, they are no long unaware, but they are not necessarily engaged by it either (stage 2). People who reach the decision-making stage (stage 3) have become engaged by the issue and are considering their response. This decision-making process can result in one

FIGURE 6.1. STAGES OF THE PRECAUTION ADOPTION PROCESS MODEL.

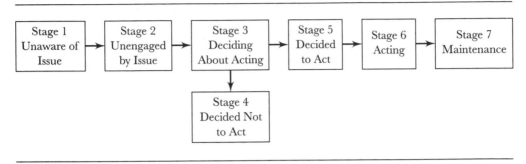

of two outcomes. If the decision is to take no action, the precaution adoption process ends (stage 4), at least for the time being. If people decide to adopt the precaution (stage 5), the next step is to initiate the behavior (stage 6). A seventh stage, if relevant, indicates that the behavior has been maintained over time (stage 7).

Although the stages have been labeled with numbers, there is certainly no implication that these numbers have any more than ordinal value (and they would not even have ordinal value if stage 4 were included, as it is not a step on the path to action). The numbers should never be used to calculate correlation coefficients, nor should one ever calculate the mean stage for a sample. Both of these calculations assume that the stages represent equal-spaced intervals along a single underlying dimension. This assumption violates the basic idea behind a stage model.

The PAPM is relatively new and has been applied to a limited number of health behaviors: osteoporosis prevention, mammography, hepatitis B vaccination, and home testing to detect radioactive radon gas (Blalock and others, 1996; Clemow and others, 2000; Hammer, 1997; Rimer and others, 2001; Weinstein and Sandman, 1992; Weinstein, Lyon, Sandman, and Cuite, 1998). Two concrete examples, the stages relevant to radon testing and to taking calcium for osteoporosis prevention, are shown in Figure 6.2.

The PAPM asserts that people usually pass through the stages in sequence, without skipping any. Although not shown in Figure 6.1, movement backward toward an earlier stage can also occur, without necessarily going back through all the intermediate stages, though obviously it is not possible to go from later stages to stages 1 or 2. The PAPM appears to resemble another stage theory, The Transtheoretical Model developed by Prochaska, DiClemente, Velicer, and their colleagues (described in Chapter Five). However, it is mainly the names that have been given to the stages that are similar. The number of stages is not the same in the two theories, and those stages with similar names are defined quite differently.

FIGURE 6.2. TWO EXAMPLES OF THE STAGES
OF THE PRECAUTION ADOPTION PROCESS MODEL.

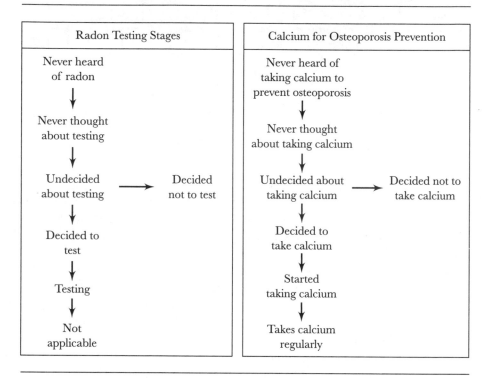

Justification for the PAPM Stages

There should be good reasons for proposing the separate stages in a stage model. What is the justification for the stages in the PAPM?

Stage 1 (Unaware). Much health research deals with well-known hazards, such as smoking, AIDS, and high-fat diets. In such cases, asking someone about his or her beliefs and plans is quite reasonable, because most people have thought about the relevance of these threats to their own lives. But if people have never heard of a hazard, they may not have opinions about it. The reluctance of respondents to answer survey questions about less familiar issues suggests that investigators ought to allow people to say that they "don't know" or have "no opinion" rather than forcing them to state a position. In many studies, participants in health behavior research are not given this opportunity. Even when they are, the "don't know"-"no opinion" responses are typically not used or are collapsed into another category. More importantly, "don't know"-"no opinion" responses indicate something substantive—real data that shouldn't be discarded. In terms of the PAPM, generally, the media have major influence in getting people from stage 1 to stage 2 and from stage 2 to stage 3 and much less influence thereafter.

Stage 2 (Unengaged) Versus Stage 3 (Deciding About Acting). Once people have heard about a hazard and have begun to form opinions about it, they are no longer in stage 1. However, so many issues compete for their limited time and attention that people can know a moderate amount about a hazard without ever having considered whether they need to do anything about it. This idea parallels a well-established finding with respect to mass media effects: that the media are better at "agenda-setting"—persuading people that they ought to consider an issue and have an opinion about it—than they are at influencing the opinion itself, which tends to require more individual sorts of influence (see also Chapter Sixteen, on communication theory).

We believe that this condition of awareness without personal engagement is quite common. In a 1986 survey of radon testing (Weinstein, Sandman, and Klotz, 1987), for example, 50 percent of respondents in a high-risk region said that they had never thought about testing their own homes; all had previously indicated that they knew what radon was and most had correctly answered more than half of the questions on a knowledge test.

The PAPM suggests further that it is important to distinguish between the people who have never thought about an action and those who have given the action some consideration but are undecided. There are several reasons for making this distinction. First, people who have thought about acting are likely to be more knowledgeable. Furthermore, attitudes based on experience with an issue are more predictive of future behavior than attitudes generated on the spot without such experience (Fazio and Zanna, 1981). Also, getting people to think about an issue may require different sorts of communication (and overcoming different sorts of obstacles) than getting them to adopt a particular conclusion. Thus, whether a person has or has not thought about taking action appears to be an important distinction.

Stage 3 (Deciding About Acting) Versus Stage 4 (Decided Not to Act) and Stage 5 (Decided to Act). Research reveals important differences between people who have not yet formed opinions and those who have made decisions. People who have come to a definite position on an issue—especially an issue regarding their own behavior—have different responses to information and are more resistant to persuasion than people who have not formed opinions (Anderson, 1983;

Brockner and Rubin, 1985; Cialdini, 1988; Ditto and Lopez, 1992; Jelalian and Miller, 1984; Nisbett and Ross, 1980, Chapter Eight). This tendency to adhere to one's own position has been termed "confirmation bias," "perseverance of beliefs," and "hypothesis preservation." It manifests itself in a variety of ways. According to Klayman (1995), these include overconfidence in one's beliefs, searches for new evidence that are biased to favor one's beliefs, biased interpretations of new data, and insufficient adjustment of one's beliefs in light of new evidence. For these reasons, the PAPM holds that it is significant when people say that they have decided to act or have decided not to act, and that the implications of someone saying that they have decided to act are not the same as saying it is "very likely" they will act.

We believe that cost-benefit theories of health behavior, such as the Health Belief Model, the Theory of Reasoned Action, the Theory of Planned Behavior, Protection Motivation Theory, and Subjective Expected Utility Theory, are dealing mainly with the factors that govern how people who get to stage 3 decide what to do. The issues these theories have identified are important, but they relate mainly to this one portion of the precaution adoption process.

Perceived susceptibility (or, equivalently, perceived personal likelihood) is one factor that frequently influences what people decide. Most theories of health behavior include this factor (Connor and Norman, 1995). Because people are reluctant to acknowledge personal susceptibility to harm even when they acknowledge the risk faced by others (Weinstein, 1987), it appears that overcoming this reluctance is a major barrier to getting people to decide to act.

Stage 5 (Decided to Act) Versus Stage 6 (Acting). The distinction between decision and action is not a new idea. For example, Ajzen's (Ajzen, 1985; Ajzen and Madden, 1986) Theory of Planned Behavior distinguishes between intentions and action. Similarly, Schwarzer's Health Action Process Approach (Schwarzer, 1992; Schwarzer and Fuchs, 1996) distinguishes between two phases. During the initial, motivation phase, people develop an intention to act, based on beliefs about risk, outcomes, and self-efficacy. After a goal has been established within this motivation phase, people enter the volition phase in which they plan the details of action, initiate action, and deal with the difficulties of carrying out that action successfully.

Protection Motivation Theory is not a stage theory, but its developers implicitly recognize the need for sequencing interventions. According to Rogers and Prentice-Dunn, "PMT experiments always present information in the same order, i.e., threatening information followed by coping information" (Rogers and Prentice-Dunn, 1997, p. 116). These researchers also talk in terms of developing motivation first and then coping skills.

A growing body of research (Gollwitzer, 1999) suggests that there are important gaps between intending to act and carrying out this intention, and that helping people develop specific implementation plans can reduce these barriers. The PAPM suggests that detailed implementation information that would be uninteresting to people in early stages, and even to those who are trying to decide what to do, is often essential to aid the transition from decision to action. For problems with many possible solutions, the decision to take action is distinct from the decision about which action to take.

Stage 6 (Acting) Versus Stage 7 (Maintenance). For any health behavior that is more than a one-time action, the process of adopting the behavior for the first time is different from that involved in repeating the behavior at intervals or continuing a habitual behavior over time. Thus, a person who gets a mammogram or colon cancer screening for the first time will have more information and past experience (perhaps positive as well as negative) that play a part in the decision to be rescreened at recommended intervals. Similarly, someone who stops smoking or loses weight must deal with the acute withdrawal experience and the glow of success in the early stage of taking action but shifts to addressing different challenges in the maintenance stage. The distinction between action and maintenance is widely recognized (for example, Dishman, 1988; Marlatt and Gordon, 1985; Meichenbaum and Turk, 1987).

Stages of Inaction. One value of the PAPM is its recognition of important differences among people who are not acting and not even thinking about acting. People in stage 1 (unaware), stage 2 (unengaged), and stage 4 (decided not to act) all fit in this broad category. Those in stage 1 obviously need basic information about the hazard and the recommended precaution. People in stage 2 need something that makes the threat and action seem personally relevant. Individualized messages and contact with friends and neighbors who have considered action should help these individuals move to the next stage. Another powerful influence on the transition from stage 2 to stage 3 is probably the awareness that others are making up their minds, that one is obliged to have some opinion on this current issue of the day.

As stated earlier, people who have thought about and rejected action, those in stage 4, are a particularly difficult group. Evidence shows that they can be quite well informed (Blalock and others, 1996; Weinstein and Sandman, 1992), and, as noted earlier, they will tend to dispute or ignore information that challenges their decision that action is unnecessary in their case.

Some examples of factors that may be important at different transitions are given in Table 6.1 and in Weinstein (1988).

TABLE 6.1. ISSUES LIKELY TO DETERMINE PROGRESS BETWEEN STAGES.

Stage Transition	Important Issues
Stage 1 to stage 2	Media messages about the hazard and precaution
Stage 2 to stage 3	Communications from significant others Personal experience with hazard
Stage 3 to stage 4 or stage 5	Beliefs about hazard likelihood and severity Beliefs about personal susceptibility Beliefs about precaution effectiveness and difficulty Behaviors and recommendations of others Perceived social norms Fear and worry
Stage 5 to stage 6	Time, effort, and resources needed to act Detailed "how-to" information Reminders and other cues to action Assistance in carrying out action

Application to Home Radon Testing

A field experiment focusing on radon testing (Weinstein, Lyon, Sandman, and Cuite, 1998) was designed to examine several aspects of the PAPM. We describe the experiment here in some detail to show how experiments with stage theories can be constructed and analyzed and to explain what the results of the study tell us about the validity of the model.

Radon is an invisible, odorless, radioactive gas produced by the decay of small amounts of naturally occurring uranium in soil. It enters homes through foundation cracks and other openings. Radiation from the decay of radon can damage cells in the lungs, and radon is the second leading cause of lung cancer after smoking (National Academy of Sciences, 1988; U.S. Environmental Protection Agency, 1992). Radon tests can be carried out by homeowners with a modest degree of effort. A single do-it-yourself test typically costs between $10 and $50. Testing is also provided by private companies at higher costs. If testing reveals a radon problem, mitigation strategies are effective but moderately expensive.

The experiment focused on two stage transitions: from being undecided about testing one's home for radon (stage 3) to deciding to test (stage 5), and from deciding to test (stage 5) to actually ordering a test (stage 6). The study did not look at the transition from being unaware of the radon issue (stage 1) to being aware but not engaged (stage 2), or from being unengaged (stage 2) to thinking about testing (stage 3), because merely agreeing to participate in a radon study and answering questions about testing would probably be sufficient to produce these changes. People who had already decided not to test (stage 4) were excluded, because a brief intervention would probably be unable to reverse that decision. Thus, while this example does not examine all stages of the PAPM, it is a realistic example of how critical stages and stage transitions can be studied.

To determine whether the two transitions studied involve different barriers, as the theory claims, two interventions were used, one matched to each transition. Previous surveys and experiments (Sandman and Weinstein, 1993; Weinstein, Sandman, and Roberts, 1990) gave insights into the potential barriers. They suggested that increasing homeowners' perceptions of their own risk—that is, increasing the perceived likelihood of having unhealthy radon levels in their homes—is important in getting undecided people to decide to test. Thus, information about localized radon risk and rebuttals to myths of invulnerability were chosen as the focus of one intervention. Its goal was to help move people from stage 3 to stage 5.

Interventions focusing mainly on risk had not been effective, however, in getting people to actually order tests (Weinstein, Sandman, and Roberts, 1990, 1991). Instead, several studies had found that test orders could be increased by increasing the ease of testing (Doyle, McClelland, and Schulze, 1991; Weinstein, Sandman, and Roberts, 1990, 1991). Thus, for people who had already decided to test, the second intervention was intended to lower barriers to action by providing information about do-it-yourself test kits and a test order form. Its goal was to move people from stage 5 to stage 6.

Method

Study Design. The study took place in Columbus, Ohio, a city with high radon levels. As the issue had received hardly any local attention for several years, we were concerned that homeowners' thoughts about testing might be weakly held and that any stage assessment would be unstable. Consequently, all participants viewed a general informational video before receiving any experimental treatment. Their stage of testing was assessed after this first video viewing (preintervention measurement).

After the questionnaires had been returned and eligibility to continue had been ascertained, the experimental videos were delivered to participants. One intervention (high-likelihood) focused on increasing the perceived likelihood of having a home radon problem. The second (low-effort) focused on decreasing the perceived and actual effort required to test. These two treatments were combined factorially to create four conditions: control (no intervention), high-likelihood, low-effort, and combination (high-likelihood plus low-effort). Stage of testing was assessed immediately after the experimental treatment (postintervention measurement) and several months later.

Intervention Videos.   Three different videos were developed for the experiment. All participants viewed the six-minute, preintervention tape, titled *Basic Facts About Radon,* that provided an overview of the topic but included only general information about radon risk and testing procedures.

The high-likelihood treatment consisted of a five-minute video, *Radon Risk in Columbus Area Homes,* and an accompanying cover letter. The goal of the video was to convince people that they had a moderate to high chance of finding unhealthy radon levels in their own homes. Results of radon studies indicating high local levels, pictures of actual local homes with high levels, and testimony by a local homeowner and a city health official all presented evidence of the problem. Myths about radon levels that had been identified in past research were presented and refuted. The cover letter mentioned that test kits could be ordered from the American Lung Association (ALA), but did not include an order form.

Participants in the low-effort condition received a five-minute video, *How to Test Your Home for Radon,* an accompanying cover letter, and a form to order test kits through the ALA. The video described how to select a kit type (making an explicit recommendation in order to reduce uncertainty), locate and purchase a kit, and conduct a test. The process was represented as simple and inexpensive.

Participants in the combination condition received a ten-minute video that simply combined the two separate treatments. They received the same letter and order form as did people in the low-effort condition. Participants in the control condition received a letter stating that their assistance in viewing a second video was not needed (they had already screened *Basic Facts About Radon*).

Procedure and Stage Assessment.   Study participants were contacted by telephone. Those homeowners who had at least heard of radon, who had not tested, and who agreed to take part ($N = 4,706$) were mailed the video *Basic Facts About Radon* and a questionnaire assessing their reactions. The particular question designed to assess stage of testing asked, "What are your thoughts about testing your home for radon?" The choices offered were, "I have already completed a test, have a test in progress, or have purchased a test" (stage 6); "I have never thought about testing my home" (stage 2); "I'm undecided about testing" (stage 3); "I've decided I *don't* want to test" (stage 4); and "I've decided I *do* want to test" (stage 5)." (Stage 1 people, who had never heard about radon testing, had been screened out of the study.)

An algorithm for assessing radon testing stages is shown in Table 6.2. This algorithm could be modified easily for other precautions by replacing the text in curly brackets with corresponding text for the new behavior.

TABLE 6.2. PAPM STAGE CLASSIFICATION ALGORITHM.

1. Have you ever heard about {home radon testing}?

    No   Stage 1

    Yes [go to 2]

2. Have you {tested your own house for radon}?

    Yes   Stage 6

    No [go to 3]

3. Which of the following best describes your thoughts about {testing your home}?

I've never thought about {testing}	Stage 2
I'm undecided about {testing}	Stage 3
I've decided I don't want to {test}	Stage 4
I've decided I do want to {test}	Stage 5

Note: The material in curly brackets could be replaced with other precautions to develop a staging algorithm for these precautions.

Those individuals who were either in the "undecided" stage or "decided to test" stage after watching *Basic Facts About Radon* were assigned at random to one of the four experimental conditions and were mailed the intervention materials appropriate for that condition and a feedback questionnaire. The response rate to the second video was 73 percent, with no significant differences among conditions.

Follow-up telephone interviews (completion rate = 95 percent) were carried out nine to ten weeks after respondents returned the second video questionnaire. These asked whether participants had purchased a radon test kit and, if not, determined their final stage. (Buying a test kit is not equivalent to testing. The full behavior sequence requires using the test kit and sending it to the lab for analysis. Because some test kits remain in place for up to a year before they are returned, we chose to use test kit purchase as the main outcome to avoid lengthening the follow-up period.)

Results

The final sample consisted of 1,897 homeowners. After watching *Basic Facts About Radon,* the division among stages of those retained in the study was 29 percent "undecided" and 71 percent "decided to test."

Predicting Progress Toward Action. Table 6.3 shows the percentage of people from each preintervention stage who progressed *one or more* stages toward testing. This criterion (rather than progress of only a single stage toward testing) was

TABLE 6.3. PARTICIPANTS WHO PROGRESSED ONE OR MORE STAGES TOWARD TESTING (PERCENTAGE).

Preintervention Stage	Condition			
	Control	High-Likelihood	Low-Effort	Combination
Undecided	18.8 (138)	41.7 (144)	36.4 (130)	54.5 (139)
Decided-to-test	8.0 (339)	10.4 (338)	32.5 (329)	35.8 (345)

Note: The group size in each cell is shown in parentheses.

chosen because although people who stopped at one stage were hypothesized to lack the requirements to get to the next stage, there was no a priori reason to assume that they did not already possess the information or skills needed to overcome later barriers. The upper half of the table indicates the percentage of people at follow-up who had moved from the undecided stage to either the decided-to-test or the testing stage. The lower half of the table shows the percentage of decided-to-test people who had moved on to the testing stage.

Statistical analyses showed more people progressed from the undecided stage than from the decided-to-test stage, $F(1, 1886) = 61.6$, $p < .0001$. There also was more progress among those who received the high-likelihood treatment than among those who did not, $F(1, 1886) = 31.5$, $p < .0001$. Most important, there was a significant stage by high-likelihood treatment interaction, $F(1, 1886) = 18.5$, $p < .0001$, indicating that the high-likelihood treatment was much more effective for undecided participants than for decided-to-act participants. This is what would be expected from matched and mismatched interventions. Although the study design did not systematically vary the interventions on whether or not they matched participants' baseline stages, our analysis revealed this important finding.

There was also a large main effect of the low-effort treatment, $F(1, 1886) = 89.4$, $p < .0001$. The stage by low-effort treatment interaction, $F(1, 1886) = 5.9$, $p < .02$, indicated that, as hypothesized, the low-effort treatment in the low-effort and combination conditions had a relatively bigger effect on people already planning to test than on people who were undecided. The high-likelihood by low-effort interaction and the three-way interaction were not significant.

Predicting Test Orders. The follow-up interviews revealed that radon tests were ordered by 342 study participants, or 18 percent of the sample (see Table 6.4). For people initially planning to test, "progress" and testing are the same according to the PAPM, so the data in the lower half of Table 6.4 are identical to those in the lower half of Table 6.3. As expected, there was more testing from the decided-

TABLE 6.4. RADON TEST ORDERS (PERCENTAGE).

Preintervention Stage	Condition			
	Control	High-Likelihood	Low-Effort	Combination
Undecided	(a) 5.1	(b) 3.5	(c) 10.1	(d) 18.7
Decided-to-test	(e) 8.0	(f) 10.4	(g) 32.5	(h) 35.8

to-test stage than from the undecided stage, $F(1, 1887) = 42.3$, $p < .0001$. In addition, there was much more testing among people exposed to a low-effort treatment than by those who did not receive this treatment, $F(1, 1887) = 87.9$, $p < .0001$. The high-likelihood treatment effect and the low-effort by high-likelihood interactions were not significant, p's $> .1$. Most important was the highly significant interaction between stage and low-effort treatment, $F(1, 1887) = 18.2$, $p < .0001$. The other interactions (stage by high-likelihood and stage by low-effort by high-likelihood) were not significant (p's $> .1$).

More specific tests involve predicted cell-by-cell contrasts. In subsequent paragraphs, the predictions are presented in brackets and experimental groups are labeled with letters that refer to the cells in Table 6.4.

Test order rates of both undecided and decided-to-test participants in the control condition were expected to be quite low, because both groups were viewed as lacking information needed to progress to action [(a) ≅ (e), both small]. The main problems facing people who had decided to test were hypothesized to be the difficulties in choosing, purchasing, and using radon test kits. Thus, the low-effort treatment was expected to be much more helpful than the high-risk treatment in getting people in this stage to order tests [(g) > (f)]. In fact, past research (Weinstein, Sandman, and Roberts, 1990, 1991) suggested that the high-likelihood treatment would be ineffective in eliciting testing from people planning to test [(f) ≅ (e)], and, more obviously, unable to elicit test orders from undecided people [(b) ≅ (a)]. Furthermore, because it was anticipated that people in the decided-to-test stage did not need further information about risk, we predicted that testing in the combination condition would not be significantly greater than testing in the low-effort condition [(h) ≅ (g)].

According to the PAPM, people who are undecided have to decide to test before acting. Consequently, a low-effort intervention alone was not expected to produce test orders from this group [(c) ≅ (a)]. However, undecided people in the combination condition received both high-likelihood information (seen as important in deciding to test) and low-effort assistance (seen as important for carrying out action intentions). Some of these people might be able to make two stage transitions [(d) > (c)], but not as many as decided-to-test people in the combination condition who needed to advance only one stage [(d) < (h)].

T-tests comparing the means of the cells mentioned in the preceding eight hypotheses demonstrated that none of the pairs predicted to be approximately the same were significantly different (p's > .3), but all pairs predicted to be different were significantly different (all p's < .0001 except for the hypothesis that (d) > (c), p = .03).

Implications for Theory and Practice

Implications for Theory

The study just discussed has several theoretical implications. First, it provides support for our claim that never having thought about an action, being undecided, and having decided to act represent distinct stages, with different barriers between stages. Second, the data support the suggestion that information about risk is helpful in getting people to decide to act, even though this same information may have little value in producing action among those individuals who have already decided to act. Third, information that increases the perceived and actual ease of action appears to greatly aid people who have decided to act, but it is less important among people who are still undecided. More research is needed to determine whether these same factors are important at the same stages for other health behaviors. Additional research is also needed to discern how these factors operate when interventions are purposively tailored to baseline stage, when they are sequentially introduced, and what happens when participants represent the full continuum of the seven PAPM stages.

Acceptance of the idea that stages exist also has implications for theory development. If the factors that facilitate movement toward action vary from stage to stage, few if any factors will be important at all stages. Thus, the standard approach of comparing people who have acted with everyone who has not will be a poor way to discover variables important for precaution adoption.

For example, if we had compared people who had tested for radon to all those who had not, we would have found many differences in beliefs and experiences, and we might have based our interventions on some group of these. Yet when we compared people who had tested with those hypothesized to be in the previous stage, people who had decided to test but had not yet acted, we found almost no differences on these variables. This finding led us to explore the idea that factors external to the individual—especially matters of opportunity and effort—were responsible for getting people to move from intention to action. Much of our success in generating test purchases came from this idea.

A variable may be a powerful determinant of progress at an early stage, but it may look rather weak if all one does is compare people who have acted to everyone else. In fact, when all who have not acted are simply lumped together in a single category, it may happen that some stage is missing or barely represented. In this case, it would be impossible to discover the role of a variable that might be crucial to people reaching or leaving this stage—and therefore crucial to the precaution process—but not relevant to other transitions. Stage theories suggest that we will be better able to identify important barriers if we compare people who are in adjacent stages.

Implications for Practice

The effects produced by the radon testing experiment are large enough to have practical implications. Viewed in terms of odds ratios, the interventions created a three-fold difference in test orders between the undecided and decided-to-test stages in the low-effort condition and a ten-fold difference between cells with the highest and lowest testing rates.

Stage-targeted communications have never been used in actual radon testing promotions, and until relatively recently, had not been used for any health behaviors. The most widely disseminated radon communications, national television public service advertisements, have focused on persuading viewers that the radon hazard is substantial for people in general. To the extent that a target audience stage can be inferred, these public service advertisements appeared to be aimed primarily at viewers who are unaware of the radon problem (stage 1) or had never thought about their own response (stage 2). This was a defensible choice when the issue was new and the medium used (national television) was scattershot. But fifteen years after radon first received substantial public attention, most radon communication campaigns have retained the same focus, even though there is reason to think that much of the audience is beyond stages 1 and 2.

Criteria for Applying Stage-Based Interventions

As the preceding paragraph implies, a variety of issues need to be considered to determine the practical utility of the Precaution Adoption Process Model or any other stage theory.

Superiority Over Unstaged Messages. The practical utility of a stage model depends on the extent to which it leads to interventions that are more effective than generic messages. For the radon testing study described here, we had to develop two different interventions. The interventions chosen were based on years of research on radon testing, plus a sizable pilot project in the target community. Thus, substantial effort is needed to find the barriers between particular stages. However, this effort can be guided by previous research on other precautions, and even approaches not based on stage ideas need to decide what issues to address and to develop interventions to address them. Nevertheless, the experimental design did not prospectively assign interventions according to participants' preintervention stage.

As predicted, individual vulnerability turned out to be a particularly useful message for people in the Columbus area at the undecided stage of the radon testing decision. We suggest that vulnerability is usually a key issue for transitions from stage 3 to stage 5—as opposed to, say, information about illness severity—but this suggestion requires verification. Ease of testing turned out to be particularly useful to those Columbus residents who had already decided to test but had not yet done so. Detailed instructions for carrying out precautions is key to transitions from stage 5 to stage 6, but this assumption also needs testing.

Because the combination treatment in our experiment produced the greatest progress among both undecided and decided-to-test participants, one might be tempted to conclude that the PAPM did not provide any new treatment ideas. "Just use the combination treatment," someone might say. There are several flaws in this reasoning. First, the combination treatment was approximately twice as long as each of its two components. Media time is expensive, speakers usually have a fixed length of time for their presentations, some people will not attend an educational presentation, and audiences have a limited attention span. Thus, attempting to replace the low-effort or high-likelihood interventions with their combination would involve substantial costs.

Second, although no evidence from studies based on the PAPM is available on this point, people seem likely to be more engaged by a treatment that matches their stage, and a mismatched treatment may deter them from attending to the properly matched treatment to come. For example, unlike people who have agreed to participate in a research study, members of the general public who are undecided about taking a precaution may not pay attention to the detailed procedural information they might need later to carry out that precaution. Worse, among people who had decided to act, risk information was superfluous and might deter attention to the more relevant information about how to test. Nevertheless, if only a single message can be given to a mixed-stage audience, the combination intervention would probably be the most appropriate.

Stage Assessment. A second relevant criterion is the ability to identify stages accurately and efficiently. The PAPM requires only a single question to assess a person's stage, so it can be used easily in individual and small-group settings. Clinicians could ask such a question without disrupting their practices. Even in a large audience, a show of hands might be used to quickly determine the distribution of stages present. However, if the audience is dispersed, the budget is small, or time is tight, efforts to measure stage may be impractical.

Furthermore, a single assessment may be insufficient. As mentioned earlier, stage models predict that the sequencing of treatment is important. Progress toward action needs to be monitored over time so that the interventions or messages can change to match the current stages of the intended audiences. To increase mammography use, for example, Rakowski and others (1998) determined stages from telephone interviews twice during the course of the study and used this information both to tailor the materials women received and to change the materials when women's stages changed. Also, the accuracy and reliability of stage assessments require consideration, as these are most often based on self reports (Kristal, Glanz, Curry, and Patterson, 1999). Furthermore, accuracy and reliability are likely to depend on the frequency and recency with which audience members have considered the health topic. When people are asked about new hazards or new precautions or about old ones that they have not thought about for years, their responses may be unreliable and tell us little about their actions or concerns.

Delivery of Stage-Targeted Messages. The feasibility of delivering stage-targeted messages in different situations varies greatly. If communication is one-on-one, as in a doctor's office or counseling session, delivering the message appropriate for an individual is relatively easy. In group settings, such as public lectures, messages can be chosen to fit the overall audience, though not individual members. In mass communications, a stage approach is more often practical with print than with broadcast media. Within print channels, pamphlets and magazines offer more opportunities for stage targeting than do newspapers; within broadcasting, cable offers more opportunities for stage targeting than do networks. New media channels, such as the Internet, offer new opportunities for message targeting.

The ability to deliver targeted messages to members of a group also depends on the range of stages present in that group. The greater the range of stages present, the more difficult it is to choose a single message. For a mass audience, the most efficient way to encourage a new health-protective action may be with a comprehensive broadcast message that ignores stage or assumes everyone to be at a very early stage. As the issue matures, however, distinctive audiences, separable by stage, merit distinctive messages, and print or "narrowcasting" becomes the medium of choice for mass communications. Thus, stage-based messages are likely to be more important for relatively mature health issues than for emerging ones. The reality is that in the modern world, on almost any issue, audiences will be heterogeneous.

Difficulty of Behavioral Change. A final criterion of importance concerns the difficulty of the action being advocated and the expected resistance of the audience to the behavioral change recommendation. When a behavior is easy and resistance is low, stage may matter little. In such situations, the interventions and messages needed to help people progress from stage to stage can be brief, and several may be combined into a single comprehensive treatment. In contrast, when change is difficult and resistance is high, there is a greater need to have separate messages for each stage.

In our radon testing experiment, the general, preintervention videotape moved many participants through two stages from "never thought about acting" to "decided to act." Similarly, the low-effort intervention persuaded many undecided people to progress two stages and order test kits. In this second case, homeowners who had been reluctant to test might have told themselves, "if it is really that simple and inexpensive, I might as well do it"—in effect skipping the decision-making process on the grounds that such a low-effort behavior would be easier to implement than to evaluate. It is easy to imagine people adopting many other simple precautions—changing to a fluoridated toothpaste, bypassing a brand of food reported to be contaminated, or avoiding a street on which a crime has occurred—on the strength of a single message that informs people about the risk, describes who is susceptible, and recommends a particular response.

Radon testing appears so easy, and radon test kits so accessible, that it comes as a surprise to many professionals that there is any need for an effort-reducing intervention. Even apparently simple actions may raise questions that need to be answered before people feel confident they can carry out the behavior successfully. These actions often seem much more difficult to the public than to professionals. Some types of lifestyle changes—exercise, smoking cessation, dietary change, cancer screening, and others—are difficult or frightening for many people, and it is hard to convince audiences that action is needed. In cases such as these, matching interventions to stage would be expected to matter more.

Stage-based, tailored interventions are more complex, and thus usually more expensive, than standardized, one-size-fits-all interventions or even stage-matched interventions. Thus, it seems certain that there will be situations in which the improvement produced by a stage-based intervention is not large enough to justify its use. Nevertheless, there are numerous health behaviors that have proved resistant to standard health promotion approaches. Examples include automobile seat belt use, weight loss, smoking prevention, adherence to medication programs, and condom use. In such situations, the need to try new approaches seems undeniable, and the higher cost may be more than offset by greater success.

Conclusion and Future Directions

The Precaution Adoption Process Model seeks to identify the different steps or stages people pass through as they progress toward action. Most other (non-stage) theories of individual health behavior see the adoption of new precautions as involving only one step: inaction to action (or, perhaps, inaction to intention), and the variables claimed to produce this step clearly characterize it as a judgment about the relative costs and benefits of action. The PAPM does not reject the variables identified by these theories. Rather, it sees the theories as describing just one stage of the behavioral change process, the stage when people are actively weighing options and deciding what to do. The PAPM points out that other issues important to behavioral change arise before people ever think seriously about action and still different issues arise after people have already decided to act.

As mentioned earlier, the PAPM is relatively new and researchers have used it to examine only a limited number of health behaviors. Because it is not composed of a short list of variables, it does not offer a simple process for designing interventions. Instead, it should be seen as an attempt to describe more accurately how people deal with health hazards, and this insight can help us identify the barriers that prevent movement from one stage to the next. As additional research is conducted, we will learn more about the barriers found at each stage and whether there is enough consistency across behaviors to use information about the stages present in a population (or the stage of an individual) to suggest the specific intervention needed.

References

Ajzen, I. "From Intentions to Actions: A Theory of Planned Behavior." In J. Kuhl and J. Beckmann (eds.), *Action Control: From Cognition to Behavior.* Heidelberg: Springer-Verlag, 1985.

Ajzen, I., and Madden, T. J. "Prediction of Goal-Directed Behavior: Attitudes, Intentions, and Perceived Behavioral Control." *Journal of Experimental Social Psychology,* 1986, *22,* 453–474.

Anderson, C. A. "Abstract and Concrete Data in the Perseverance of Social Theories: When Weak Data Lead to Unshakable Beliefs." *Journal of Experimental Social Psychology,* 1983, *19,* 93–108.

Bandura, A. "Moving into Forward Gear in Health Promotion and Disease Prevention." Address presented at the annual meeting of the Society of Behavioral Medicine, San Diego, Calif., March 1995.

Blalock, S. J., and others. "Osteoporosis Prevention in Premenopausal Women: Using a Stage Model Approach to Examine the Predictors of Behavior." *Health Psychology,* 1996, *15,* 84–93.

Brockner, J., and Rubin, J. Z. *Entrapment in Escalating Conflicts: A Social Psychological Analysis.* New York: Springer-Verlag, 1985.

Cialdini, R. B. *Influence: Theory and Practice.* Glenview, Ill.: Scott, Foresman, 1988.

Clemow, L., and others. "Underutilizers of Mammography Screening Today: Characteristics of Women Planning, Undecided About, and Not Planning a Mammogram." *Annals of Behavioral Medicine,* 2000, *22*(1), 80–88.

Connor, M., and Norman, P. *Predicting Health Behavior.* Philadelphia: Open University Press, 1995.

Dishman, R. K. *Exercise Adherence: Its Impact on Public Health.* Champaign, Ill.: Human Kinetics, 1988.

Ditto, P. H., and Lopez, D. F. "Motivated Skepticism: Use of Differential Decision Criteria for Preferred and Nonpreferred Conclusions." *Journal of Personality and Social Psychology,* 1992, *63*, 568–584.

Doyle, J. K., McClelland, G. H., and Schulze, W. D. "Protective Responses to Household Risk: A Case Study of Radon Mitigation." *Risk Analysis,* 1991, *11*, 121–134.

Fazio, R. H., and Zanna, M. P. "Direct Experience and Attitude-Behavior Consistency." In L. Berkowitz (ed.), *Advances in Experimental Social Psychology.* Vol. 14. New York: Academic Press, 1981.

Gollwitzer, P. "Implementation Intentions: Strong Effects of Simple Plans." *American Psychologist,* 1999, *54*, 493–503.

Hammer, G. P. "Hepatitis B Vaccine Acceptance Among Nursing Home Workers." Unpublished doctoral dissertation, Department of Health Policy and Management, Johns Hopkins University, 1997.

Jelalian, E., and Miller, A. G. "The Perseverance of Beliefs: Conceptual Perspectives and Research Developments." *Journal of Social and Clinical Psychology,* 1984, *2*, 25–56.

Klayman, J. "Varieties of Confirmation Bias." *The Psychology of Learning and Motivation.* Vol. 32. New York: Academic Press, 1995.

Kristal, A. R., Glanz, K., Curry, S. J., and Patterson, R. E. "How Can Stages of Change Be Best Used in Dietary Interventions?" *Journal of the American Dietetic Association,* 1999, *99*, 679–684.

Marlatt, G. A., and Gordon, J. R. *Relapse Prevention: Maintenance Strategies in the Treatment of Addictive Behaviors.* New York: Guilford Press, 1985.

Meichenbaum, D., and Turk, D. C. *Facilitating Treatment Adherence: A Practitioner's Handbook.* New York: Plenum, 1987.

National Academy of Sciences. *Health Effects of Radon and Other Internally Deposited Alpha-Emitters: BEIR IV.* Washington, D.C.: National Academy Press, 1988.

Nisbett, R., and Ross, L. *Human Inference: Strategies and Shortcomings of Social Judgment.* Englewood Cliffs, N.J.: Prentice Hall, 1980.

Rakowski, W., and others. "Increasing Mammography Among Women Aged 40–74 by Use of a Stage-Matched, Tailored Intervention. *Preventive Medicine,* 1998, *27*, 748–756.

Rimer, B. K., and others. "The Short-Term Impact of Tailored Mammography Decision-Making Interventions." *Patient Education and Counseling,* 2001, *43*, 269–285.

Rogers, R. W., and Prentice-Dunn, S. "Protection Motivation Theory." In D. Gochman (ed.), *Handbook of Health Behavior Research.* Vol. 1. *Determinants of Health Behavior: Personal and Social.* New York: Plenum, 1997.

Sandman, P. M., and Weinstein, N. D. "Predictors of Home Radon Testing and Implications for Testing Promotion Programs." *Health Education Quarterly,* 1993, *20*, 1–17.

Schwarzer, R. "Self-Efficacy in the Adoption and Maintenance of Health Behaviors: Theoretical Approaches and a New Model." In R. Schwarzer (ed.), *Self-Efficacy: Thought Control of Action.* Washington, D.C.: Hemisphere, 1992.

Schwarzer, R., and Fuchs, R. "Self-Efficacy and Health Behaviors." In M. Conner and P. Norman (eds.), *Predicting Health Behavior: Research and Practice with Social Cognition Models.* Buckingham, England: Open University Press, 1996.

U.S. Environmental Protection Agency Office of Radiation Programs, and U.S. Department of Health and Human Services Centers for Disease Control. *A Citizen's Guide to Radon.* (2nd ed.) Washington, D.C.: Author, 1992.

Weinstein, N. D. "Unrealistic Optimism About Susceptibility to Health Problems: Conclusions From a Community-Wide Sample." *Journal of Behavioral Medicine,* 1987, *10,* 481–500.

Weinstein, N. D. "The Precaution Adoption Process." *Health Psychology,* 1988, *7,* 355–386.

Weinstein, N. D., Lyon, J. E., Sandman, P. M., and Cuite, C. L. "Experimental Evidence for Stages of Precaution Adoption." *Health Psychology,* 1998, *17,* 445–453.

Weinstein, N. D., Rothman A., and Sutton, S. "Stage Theories of Health Behavior." *Health Psychology,* 1998, *17,* 290–299.

Weinstein, N. D., and Sandman, P. M. "A Model of the Precaution Adoption Process: Evidence from Home Radon Testing." *Health Psychology,* 1992, *11,* 170–180.

Weinstein, N. D., Sandman, P. M., and Klotz, M. L. *Public Response to the Risk from Radon, 1986.* New Brunswick, N.J.: Environmental Communications Research Program, Rutgers University, 1987.

Weinstein, N. D., Sandman, P. M., and Roberts, N. E. "Determinants of Self-Protective Behavior: Home Radon Testing." *Journal of Applied Social Psychology,* 1990, *20,* 783–801.

Weinstein, N. D., Sandman, P. M., and Roberts, N. E. "Perceived Susceptibility and Self-Protective Behavior: A Field Experiment to Encourage Home Radon Testing." *Health Psychology,* 1991, *10,* 25–33.

CHAPTER SEVEN

PERSPECTIVES ON INTRAPERSONAL THEORIES OF HEALTH BEHAVIOR

Barbara K. Rimer

Theories that focus on the behavior of individuals constitute an important part of the intellectual foundation of health education and health behavior. Part Two of this book describes four well-developed theories and models of health behavior: the Health Belief Model (HBM), the Theory of Reasoned Action (TRA) and its companion the Theory of Planned Behavior (TPB), The Transtheoretical Model (TTM), and the newest addition to the book, the Precaution Adoption Process Model (PAPM). The PAPM was described in the last edition of *Health Behavior and Health Education* as a developing model. However, in the interim it has become clear that not only has its development progressed, but more and more researchers are using it as the basis for health intervention research.

The theories and models included in this section were among the most widely cited in a recent literature search to identify applications of theories of health behavior (see Chapter Two). This chapter considers some further perspectives on each of the four theories that have been presented in Part Two and offers some thoughts on new theoretical directions.

The Health Belief Model

The Health Belief Model, developed in the 1950s, is one of the oldest and most resilient models of health behavior. It has remained remarkably useful over time. As Janz, Champion, and Strecher write in Chapter Three, the HBM has been used "both to explain change and maintenance of health behavior and as a guiding framework for health behavior interventions."

The HBM was developed by social psychologists in the U.S. Public Health Service expressly to understand health behavior. It grew out of practical questions about why people did not get screened for tuberculosis. Since those early days, health professionals have gained long experience with the model in a variety of health contexts.

The HBM is a value-expectancy theory. Such theories, as the chapter explains, regard behavior as the subjective value of an outcome and of the subjective probability, or expectation, that a particular action will achieve that outcome. A critical dimension of the HBM, the failure to believe in the possibility of having pathology in the absence of symptoms, is as relevant today in studying cancer, AIDS, Hepatitis C, and other diseases as it was in helping to explain tuberculosis screening behavior in the 1950s. These are all diseases that are best diagnosed before a person is symptomatic. Belief in asymptomatology is probably a critical variable in explaining participation in cancer screening. We have learned, for example, that women are often reluctant to obtain mammograms when they are feeling healthy, even if they "know" that a mammogram can detect something too small to be found by a woman or her physician in any other way. A frequent reason women give for not having mammograms is that they are not necessary in the absence of symptoms (Stoddard and others, 1998). It appears that it may take a belief in asymptomatology, almost an act of faith, to perform the behavior.

One of the most appealing aspects of the HBM is its acceptance not only by health educators and health psychologists but by many other health professionals, including physicians, dentists, nurses, dietitians, and other professionals. It has a sort of intuitive logic, the central tenets are clearly stated, and beliefs can be measured by a variety of techniques ranging from clinical interviews to population-based surveys. Mullen, Hersey, and Iverson (1987) showed that the HBM is an economical model in terms of the number of questions needed to assess key variables.

The HBM has been evaluated and its limitations have been identified. Some critics have argued that according to the strictest definitions of theory, the HBM is not a theory at all. Certainly, it never has had the kind of rigorous quantification that Fishbein and Ajzen (1975) have achieved with the Theory of Reasoned Action. However, as Janz and Becker (1984) and Mullen, Hersey, and Iverson (1987) have shown, most of the concepts in the model have received substantial empirical support.

Some components of the HBM still are not well understood, and others, such as severity, have low predictive value. The concept of cue to action deserves further study and experimental manipulation. Janz, Champion, and Strecher stress that we need to know more about the role of fear and how it may foster cognitive and behavioral changes. Other theoretical models, such as Protection Motivation Theory (Prentice-Dunn and Rogers, 1986), the Precaution Adoption Process Model (Weinstein, 1988), and Self-Regulation Theory (Leventhal and Cameron, 1987), used in combination with the HBM, may be helpful in gaining this knowledge. In addition, more research is needed to determine if self-efficacy should be a formal part of the model. The authors of the HBM note that it is frequently included as a part of the HBM, but they did not add self-efficacy to the model schematic.

In the second edition of *Health Behavior and Health Education,* Strecher and Rosenstock (1996) cautioned researchers and practitioners alike to be mindful of how the HBM is measured and analyzed. That is good advice. It is tempting to choose some components of the HBM on which to focus above others. However, when a theory is taken out of context, the results may be both disappointing and difficult to explain. Moreover, the barriers component should be developed with specificity to the population being studied. Janz, Champion, and Strecher identified topic areas in which significant scale development has occurred, for example, mammography. They also emphasized the need for more attention to measurement issues.

Although mature by the standards of health education and health behavior, the HBM is a thoroughly modern theory. Researchers and practitioners should be challenged to use the theory both to develop interventions and to evaluate them. One of the most significant HBM studies was conducted by Becker and Maiman (1980) to examine potential Tay-Sachs carriers and their interest in genetic testing. It may be especially timely to consider the HBM as a model for studying responses to genetic susceptibility testing in light of recent scientific advances.

The Theory of Reasoned Action and the Theory of Planned Behavior

The Theory of Reasoned Action and its later extension, the Theory of Planned Behavior, also are robust models, used to study a wide range of health behaviors. The TRA and the TPB, discussed in Chapter Four, share with the HBM roots in the tradition of value-expectancy theories. However, the TRA and the TPB are newer theories, dating to the late 1960s. As Montaño and Kasprzyk discuss, these theories grew out of a need to understand the relationship between attitudes and behavior. The TRA and the TPB assume a causal chain that links behavioral beliefs and normative beliefs to behavior through attitudes and subjective norms.

The TPB is a refinement of the TRA and includes perceived behavioral control. This is an improvement and addresses criticisms that the TRA is overly rational. The addition of perceived behavioral control to TPB means that all the theories discussed in Part Two include a variable akin to self-efficacy—a central construct in health education and health behavior research. The most important predictor of behavior is intention. Although the other theories in this section implicitly or explicitly recognize intention, its most central place is in the TRA and the TPB. The TRA and the TPB explain relationships between different types of beliefs, intentions, and behaviors, and can be used in conjunction with other theories described in this book when the goal is to develop interventions.

Fishbein and Ajzen (1975; Ajzen and Fishbein, 1980) have devoted much of their research to specifying the concepts and relationships within the TRA and, more recently, the TPB. The authors of Chapter Four have shown how each of the concepts, such as attitude toward the act, subjective norm, behavioral and normative beliefs, and behavioral intention, can be operationalized. Because their components have been so well codified, the TRA and the TPB come closest of all the theories discussed in this section to meeting Kerlinger's strict definition of theory (Kerlinger, 1986; see Chapter Two).

With increased precision of measurement has come improved potential for prediction. The theories are most predictive when the concepts are defined specifically and are measured in close temporal order. The TRA and the TPB provide a method for systematically identifying those issues that are most important to a person's decisions about performing specific behaviors. The end product of these efforts is to identify important, mutable beliefs and attitudes for subsequent use in behavioral interventions.

Although very appealing, especially from a methodological point of view, the TRA and the TPB have limitations, as do all health behavior theories. Mullen, Hersey, and Iverson (1987) criticized the TRA because it did not recognize emotional, fear-arousal elements such as perceived susceptibility to illnesses. The addition of perceived behavioral control is helpful in this regard but does not address all the concerns. For purposes of intervention development, the TRA and the TPB might need to be supplemented by the HBM or another theory, such as the PAPM, Protection Motivation Theory (Rogers and Mewborn, 1976), Self-Regulation Theory (Leventhal and Cameron, 1987), or one of the theories identified in Chapter Ten, on stress and coping, in Part Three of this book.

The measurements required by the TRA and the TPB, though powerful for prediction, are challenging in practice. They rely on extensive interviewer-administered personal interviews. Although ultimately useful, this can be a demanding, costly process. Collecting more than pilot data may be beyond the resources of many practitioners and can be laborious when programs must be developed quickly. Simplification of the theories and their application for practice would make them more accessible to practitioners, who could then more easily use the constructs of the TRA and the TPB to understand and explain health behaviors, develop interventions, and evaluate them. Nevertheless, the emphasis on specificity of the intended behavior is both central to the TRA and the TPB and one of their most important contributions. Moreover, as Fishbein (2000) has stressed, one must go to members of that population to identify relevant outcome, normative, and efficacy beliefs. Thus, he argued, because each use of the theory is based on specific data relevant to a population, the theory can easily be applied across cultures and population groups.

The Transtheoretical Model

The Transtheoretical Model or Stages of Change Model (in Chapter Five), classified as a developing theory in the first edition of this book and presented as a theory in the second edition (Prochaska, Redding, and Evers, 1996), has matured and been diffused so that it is now one of the most widely used models of health behavior. It has been employed not just by health educators and psychologists, but also by nurses, physicians, dietitians, and other health providers. One reason for its widespread acceptance undoubtedly is its intuitive appeal. Treating people as though they are all the same inevitably dilutes the impact of interventions. The TTM allows practitioners to treat individuals as they are—in different stages of readiness to make health behavior changes. To make greater progress in some areas of behavioral science—for example, finding ways to further reduce the number of smokers and achieve greater public health impact—it will be necessary to reach people in the precontemplation and contemplation stages, that is, people who are not ready for change as well as those who are thinking about change (see Chapter Five). As Prochaska and colleagues (Prochaska and others, 1982; Prochaska, DiClemente, Velicer, and Rossi, 1993); Lerman, Orleans, and Engstrom (1993); and Abrams, Marlatt, and Sobell (1995) explained, the vast majority (75 percent) of smokers are in these early stages.

TTM is one of the most popular health behavior models. It recognizes that people in the process of changing should receive interventions that start at their stage in the behavior change process. For example, if a smoker has not started thinking about what smoking is doing to him or her, there is no point in providing detailed information about behavioral coping processes. It would be far better to raise the smoker's consciousness regarding the harms associated with smoking and the benefits to be achieved from quitting. This is similar to the health education principle that Minkler and Wallerstein discuss in Chapter Thirteen with regard to community organization—start where the people are. Once stage of change has been assessed, people can be provided with therapist-guided, self-initiated, or other interventions that meet their needs.

Some important questions about TTM remain. For example, must the processes of change always be measured? How central are they to the model? It certainly adds to the measurement burden. Are the stages really discrete? How many stages are needed? How behavior-specific are the stages? The authors of Chapter Five discuss changes in the formulation of stages over time. As TTM has been extended to new health care settings and screening behaviors, stage definitions have become more complex. For example, Rakowski and others (1993) found it necessary to add a relapse risk stage for mammography. In addition, the contemplation stage seems to have substages, for example, women who say they would have a mammogram if their physicians told them to do so (sometimes called doctor-dependent contemplation). There also are important questions about the appropriate statistical analyses for assessing stage-related changes (for example, see Hedeker, Mermelstein, and Weeks, 1999).

More attention also should be paid to extending the model to other populations, especially low-income and ethnic minority populations. For example, Tessaro and others (1997) found that Prochaska and others' smoking pros and cons scale (1982) had little relevance to low-income African Americans in Durham, North Carolina. Nevertheless, smoking cessation interventions that used tailored messages that reflected stage as well as other information were highly effective (Lipkus, Lyna, and Rimer, 1999). In contrast, Rimer and others (1996) concluded that mammography pro-con scales developed by Rakowski and others (1993) were very robust when applied to African Americans.

More research also is needed to assess what kinds of interventions are best for people in what stages, and to determine if stage-matched interventions are as effective as, or more effective than, tailored interventions created especially for individuals. Although there has been some work in this area, far too little is known about how much and what kind of stage matching is needed (Marcus, Nigg, Riebe, and Forsyth, 2000; Rakowski and others, 1998). Early results are encouraging (Prochaska, DiClemente, Velicer, and Rossi, 1993). For example, Rakowski and others (1998) showed that stage-matched tailored materials produced significantly higher initial mammography rates than standard materials. Clark and others (forthcoming) found that the effect persisted for repeat mammography.

The TTM has an elegant simplicity, but both researchers and practitioners should use it wisely, carefully, comprehensively, and critically. Readers are encouraged to review a series of editorials about TTM that appeared in the *British Journal of Addictions* (Davidson, 1992) for a discussion of strengths and weaknesses of TTM.

The Precaution Adoption Process Model

The Precaution Adoption Process Model (PAPM) is predicated on the assumption that people may go through seven stages in modifying their behavior: (1) they deny having heard of the hazard in question; (2) they acknowledge that the hazard poses risk to others; (3) they acknowledge that the hazard poses personal risk; (4) they make the decision to act; (5) they adopt the behavioral change; (6) they initiate the behavior; and (7) they maintain the behavior. If a person does not adopt or maintain the behavior, he or she may not go through all the stages. Likewise, he or she may regress. As the authors stress, the PAPM posits that people usually pass through all the stages, although in some cases, transit time may be quite rapid. The major determinants of each stage vary, but there are commonalities across some stages (Weinstein, 1988). For example, across the first three stages, indirect and direct experience with the hazard, and communication of who is at risk, facilitate movement across stages. The stage 3 actions of accepting personal risk (that is, understanding that a serious consequence can occur) and recognizing that a precaution is effective are vital to initiating the decision to act (stage 5).

Unfortunately, individuals typically deny personal risk; that is, they are optimistically biased (Weinstein, 1980, 1984, 1987; Perloff and Fetzer, 1986) and are consequently less likely to seek out or pay attention to communications about hazards (Weinstein, 1988). There also may be cultural determinants of inaccurate risk perceptions. For example, people in the Netherlands frequently underestimate their intake of dietary fat, even when it exceeds recommended levels, whereas Americans more often perceive their diets as high in fat (Glanz, Brug, and van Assema, 1997). Thus, health interventions that prescribe precautionary behaviors should communicate information about risk that is clear, credible, culturally appropriate, salient, and individualized (Lipkus and Hollands, 1999) to overcome the biases that may affect receptivity to risk communications (Weinstein and Klein, 1995).

The PAPM provides a dynamic *cognitive* framework of behavioral change that emphasizes the important role of risk perceptions. The PAPM has this emphasis on perceived risk in common with the Health Belief Model (HBM). It highlights processes overlooked in other frameworks, such as consideration of costs and benefits over time and the competition between precautionary behaviors and other life demands. These considerations also can be found in the HBM, but the PAPM articulates them much more precisely. In addition, the PAPM explicitly recognizes a stage in which people may be unaware of a risk or precaution. The growing awareness of the threat of anthrax during September and October 2001 illustrates how quickly people may go from a state of unawareness to awareness and action (such as people who got tested for anthrax exposure and took Cipro).

The PAPM also provides a heuristic model to categorize people at different stages of behavior change, and it includes mediating variables amenable to assessment in intervention programs. In Chapter Six, Weinstein and Sandman provide an excellent, detailed example of how they used the PAPM to increase use of radon testing in Ohio. In the process, they clearly illustrated how the model was used to construct stage-based interventions and to assess their efficacy.

The PAPM has been studied most comprehensively by Weinstein and his collaborators. Given the importance of risk perception, the PAPM should be used more widely. It shares with TTM a stage focus, but the PAPM has a stronger emphasis on how people process risks and communications related to risks.

Commentary

The theories in this section have much in common. The construct of self-efficacy is embodied in three of the theories (HBM, TTM, and TRA-TPB). The concept of readiness is a central component of both the HBM and TTM. Perceived risk is important in both the HBM and the PAPM. Barriers inhibit behavioral change explicitly in both the HBM and TTM and implicitly in the PAPM.

Two theories, the PAPM and TTM, are stage theories. Weinstein and Sandman provide a useful overview of stage theories early in their chapter. The theories deal with awareness of hazards or risks in different ways. The PAPM is the only one that explicitly recognizes a state in which one is unaware of a risk. In TTM, persons who are unaware generally would be classified as in precontemplation. However, as Rakowski (2001) has noted, this puts very different kinds of people in the same category, for example, those strongly opposed to the recommended behavior and those who simply have not heard of it. These groups are actually quite different.

Bandura (2000) has levied strong criticisms against the Stages of Change and other stage models. He has argued that the stage "view substitutes a categorical approach for a process model of human adaptation" (p. 310). As he noted, and this is a reasonable concern, people fluctuate in their efforts to take personal control over behaviors. Thus, discrete stages may not adequately represent the rich complexity of behavior change.

The theories discussed in this section focus on somewhat different outcomes. For example, the TRA and the TPB emphasize the important role of intentions as predictors of behavior, whereas the PAPM focuses on what people decide to do or not to do.

Each of the theories can be used to design interventions. The chapters on TTM and on the PAPM discuss how information might vary for people in different stages. Weinstein and Sandman also speculate about how the choice of media might vary for people in different stages. Likewise, Montaño and Kasprzyk discussed how use of the TRA and the TPB led to the selection of specific beliefs as a focus for interventions. For each of the theories, the identification of such unique model-specific factors is critical. Each theory recognizes that people in different situations need different information and interventions. For example, HBM interventions should address people's specific barriers and facilitators to a behavior. The TRA and the TPB call for specificity of all constructs. Likewise, in both TTM and the PAPM, people in different stages require not only different information, but often different educational strategies as well.

Stage-based theories have a long tradition in behavioral research. The modern theories owe at least some debt to Lewin's stage model (Lewin, 1935). Although stage-based models are appealing, there is not unequivocal support for stage-matched interventions. In an intriguing study, Quinlan and McCaul (2000) deliberately mismatched interventions for smokers who were not planning to quit. They concluded that smokers who received the action intervention were most likely to quit, regardless of stage. Matching was not effective and did not increase the likelihood of quitting.

Some of the theories are easier to use than others. Sherry Turkle (1995) wrote about the appeal of appropriable theories, those that can be manipulated and played with. Part of the appeal of the HBM, the PAPM, and TTM is undoubtedly that they are appropriable theories. The PAPM, the TRA, and the TPB are perhaps more challenging but worth the effort.

Measurement of the key variables in each of the theories requires the serious attention of those who use these theories to understand behavior and create interventions. More attention is needed not only to the appropriate, consistent measures of independent and dependent variables in these models but also to understanding the mediators of behavior (Baron and Kenny, 1986; Sussman, 2000). As Sussman and Wills (2000) noted, many programs do not act directly on health behaviors, but work by altering mediators such as coping patterns and attitudes. Understanding the mediators of behavior change is an important step in developing more effective interventions (Baranowski, Anderson, and Carmack, 1998; Sallis, 2001). Indeed, there are now a growing number of reports of successful interventions using theories described in this section (Bock, Marcus, Pinto, and Forsyth, 2001; Rimer and others, 2001; Legler and others, forthcoming). However, in many cases, while the interventions changed intermediate variables, such as risk perceptions about breast cancer, such changes were not related to changes in mammography use. In their chapter, Weinstein and Sandman make some useful recommendations about how stage models should be evaluated.

Measurement of the TRA and the TPB is perhaps most complex because of the need to conduct elicitation interviews prior to developing questionnaires. However, the additional level of precision may pay dividends in understanding health behaviors.

All the theories and models in this section should be tested further with diverse populations, such as low-income persons, ethnic or racial minorities, and older persons. One of the important points made in all the chapters is that it is important to collect data specific to the behavioral problem and population of interest for use in program planning. With such data, any of these theories should be appropriate for diverse populations. There is no *a priori* reason that the theories should not be applicable to diverse populations, but more research is indicated.

It is now common for researchers and practitioners to combine or blend theories as discussed earlier in this chapter. Thoughtful combinations could potentially result in more robust interventions. However, there is a potential downside. If the relevant constructs in the models are not measured, it may not be possible to really understand how an intervention exerted its impact. This means that there probably is a practical limit to how many theories can be combined. If our theories are to be refined, it is critical that some researchers continue to focus on careful, methodologically rigorous tests of single theories.

In the past several years, there has been increased attention to the larger environment in which behavior occurs. Some groups have criticized a sole focus on individual health behavior as inappropriate (for example, Smedley and Syme, 2000). Others have suggested a broader focus on ecological models that reflect the multiple levels of determinants of health behavior and thus the multiple levels of intervention required to achieve the desired outcomes (McLeroy, Bibeau, Steckler, and Glanz, 1988; Smedley and Syme, 2000). The decisions about what theories or models to use and with what other theories or models to combine them should emanate from a diagnostic understanding of the behavioral problem, using a planning model such as PRECEDE (see Chapter Eighteen). For behaviors requiring individual action, such as stopping smoking or getting mammograms, individual-focused theories are usually appropriate. But that does not mean program developers should ignore the larger array of influences that affect behavior. Nor does it mean that the focus should be exclusively on individual behavior. For example, Legler and others (forthcoming) found that the combination of access-enhancing and individual-directed interventions were the most effective type of strategy for promoting mammography use, resulting in an estimated 27 percent increase in mammography.

More attention in all the theories should be paid to maintenance of behavior change. TTM and the PAPM are theories that explicitly include maintenance, but the others do not exclude it. However, inclusion of maintenance of behavior change may require refinement of constructs and measures. A recent analysis by Sheeran, Conner, and Norman (2001) found that the TPB was useful in predicting attendance at health screening. However, the theory could not reliably differentiate people who delayed attending or initially attended and then relapsed. These apparent nuances are very important not only in classifying and describing health behavior, but also in developing interventions. Measurement of implementation intentions might help to improve the TPB in this regard (Sheeran, Conner, and Norman, 2001).

Emotions may not be considered adequately in any of these theories or models. Salovey, Rothman, Detweiler, and Steward (2000) and, more recently, Schneider and others (2001) have shown that emotions may affect how women respond to messages about mammography and other topics. Messages that are framed to focus on the benefits (gains) or the losses associated with health behaviors may differentially affect adherence. Because people take cues from their emotional states, emotions can affect behavior by influencing the ease with which information comes to mind (Salovey, Rothman, Detweiler, and Steward, 2000). Moods may influence beliefs, which subsequently affect behavior. As Salovey, Rothman, Detweiler, and Steward (2000) observed, emotions also may influence health practices by promoting resilience. They suggest that a positive state of mind may enable people to consider personally unfavorable information. A question for further study is whether the theories presented here would be strengthened by the inclusion of some constructs related to emotions.

As discussed throughout this section, there are many similarities across the different theories. Recognizing this fact, Fishbein (2000) recommended the use of an integrative model that includes key variables from several of the theories in this section as well as Social Learning Theory (see Figure 7.1). The integrative model is appealing because it reflects the importance of intraindividual factors as well as environmental factors and self-efficacy. More research is needed to determine the viability of this model.

There are many other theories of intrapersonal health behavior in addition to those included in this section. None are as well-developed or as frequently cited as the first three we have featured. However, two additional theories, Prospect Theory and Self-Regulation Theory, are worthy of mention. Both are being used by a variety of researchers studying different health behavior topics, and they provide useful guidance for intervention development.

Prospect Theory, which evolved from research by Kahneman and Tversky (1982), is particularly notable for its contributions to message framing (Salovey, Schneider, and Apanovitch, 1999; Rothman and Salovey, 1997). As Salovey, Roth-

FIGURE 7.1. AN INTEGRATIVE MODEL.

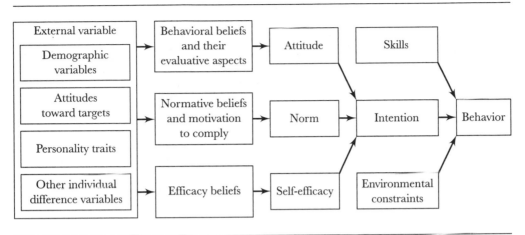

Source: Fishbein, 2000, p. 274.

man, Detweiler, and Steward (2000) explained, message framing refers to the emphasis in a message on the positive or negative consequences. Salovey found that loss-framed messages are more likely to motivate women to get mammograms. Gain-framed messages were more effective in motivating women to use sunscreen.

Self-Regulation Theory was developed over the past three decades by Leventhal and colleagues (Leventhal, Kelly, and Leventhal, 1999). They proposed that self-protective action is the result of the meanings people attach to various appraisals. The belief system underlying motivation, according to Leventhal, Kelly, and Leventhal (1999), has at least four interrelated belief systems: the representation or beliefs about the disease, condition, or recommended action; the timeline, consequences, causes, and beliefs about its susceptibility to control; the representation of the self; and disease-specific and self-relevant beliefs. Action also is affected by representations about available strategies for self-protection.

Both Prospect Theory, and its practical manifestation in message framing, and Self-Regulation Theory complement the theories included in Part Two. With its explicit focus on specific aspects of messages that may enhance persuasion, message framing is a potentially powerful tool. Self-Regulation Theory recognizes the powerful interplay between intra-psychic factors and the broader interpersonal and macro environment. In fact, it provides an excellent bridge to the theories discussed in Part Three.

Conclusion

Although each of the theories reviewed in this section is well developed, there are many important questions about each for researchers to pursue. Researchers and practitioners should be thoughtful and parsimonious when combining constructs from different theories. Bandura (2000) cautioned theory users to beware of the cafeteria approach to theoretical constructs. There are unresolved questions about when and under what conditions constructs from different theories should be combined.

Theory is not theology. Theory needs questioners more than loyal followers. Within this section, some of the chapter authors differ with others about constructs and definitions. This should not be seen as problematic. Healthy debate will strengthen theory development. Considerable debate rages currently about whether some of the stage theories are really theories and how stage theories are best evaluated (Weinstein, Rothman, and Sutton, 1998). When conducted with civility and intellectual rigor, such debates are healthy. The advancement of each of the theories discussed here will come from those who are willing to use the theories, test them, and subject them to rigorous evaluation.

References

Abrams, D. B., Marlatt, G. A., and Sobell, M. G. "Overview of Section II: Treatment, Early Intervention, and Policy." In J. Fertig and R. Allen (eds.), *Alcohol and Tobacco: From Basic Science to Policy.* NIAAA Research Monograph, no. 19. Washington, D.C.: National Institute of Alcoholism and Alcohol Abuse, 1995.

Ajzen, I., and Fishbein, M. *Understanding Attitudes and Predicting Social Behavior.* Englewood Cliffs, N.J.: Prentice Hall, 1980.

Bandura, A. "Health Promotion from the Perspective of Social Cognitive Theory." In P. Norman, C. Abraham, and M. Connor (eds.), *Understanding and Changing Health and Behaviour.* Reading, U.K.: Harwood, 2000.

Baranowski, T., Anderson, C., and Carmack, C. "Mediating Variable Framework in Physical Activity Interventions: How Are We Doing?" *American Journal of Preventive Medicine,* 1998, *15,* 266–297.

Baron, R. M., and Kenny, D. A. "The Moderator-Mediator Variable Distinction in Social Psychological Research: Conceptual, Strategic, and Statistical Considerations." *Journal of Personality and Social Psychology,* 1986, *51,* 1173–1182.

Becker, M. H., and Maiman, L. A. "Strategies for Enhancing Patient Compliance." *Journal of Community Health,* 1980, *6,* 113–135.

Bock, B. C., Marcus, B. H., Pinto, B. M., and Forsyth, L. H. "Maintenance of Physical Activity Following an Individualized Motivationally Tailored Intervention." *Annals of Behavioral Medicine,* 2001, *23,* 79–87.

Clark, M. A., and others. "The Effect of a Stage-Matched and Tailored Intervention on Repeat Mammography." *American Journal of Preventive Medicine,* forthcoming.

Davidson, R. "Prochaska and DiClemente's Model of Change: A Case Study?" *British Journal of Addictions,* 1992, *87,* 821–822.

Fishbein, M. "The Role of Theory in HIV Prevention." *AIDS Care,* 2000, *12*(3), 273–278.

Fishbein, M., and Ajzen, I. *Belief, Attitude, Intention and Behavior: An Introduction to Theory and Research.* Reading, Mass.: Addison-Wesley, 1975.

Glanz, K., Brug, J., and van Assema, P. "Are Awareness of Dietary Fat Intake and Actual Fat Consumption Associated? A Dutch-American Comparison." *European Journal of Clinical Nutrition,* 1997, *51,* 542–547.

Hedeker, D., Mermelstein, R. J., and Weeks, K. "The Thresholds of Change Model: An Approach to Analyzing Stages of Change Data." *Annals of Behavioral Medicine,* 1999, *21,* 61–70.

Janz, N. K., and Becker, M. H. "The Health Belief Model: A Decade Later." *Health Education Quarterly,* 1984, *11,* 1–47.

Kahneman, D., and Tversky, A. "The Psychology of Preferences." *Scientific American,* 1982, *247,* 160–173.

Kerlinger, F. N. *Foundations of Behavioral Research.* (3rd ed.) New York: Holt, Rhinehart and Winston, 1986.

Legler, J., and others. "The Effectiveness of Interventions to Promote Mammography Among Women with Historically Lower Rates of Screening." *Cancer, Epidemiology, Biomarkers, and Prevention,* (forthcoming).

Lerman, C., Orleans, C. T., and Engstrom, P. F. "Biological Markers in Smoking Cessation Treatment." *Seminars in Oncology,* 1993, *20,* 359–367.

Leventhal, H., and Cameron, L. "Behavioral Theories and the Problem of Compliance." *Patient Education and Counseling,* 1987, *10,* 117–138.

Leventhal, H., Kelly, K., and Leventhal, E. A. "Population Risk, Actual Risk, Perceived Risk, and Cancer Control: a Discussion." *Journal of the National Cancer Institute Monograph,* 1999, *25,* 81–85.

Lewin, K. *A Dynamic Theory of Personality.* New York: McGraw Hill, 1935.

Lipkus, I. M., and Hollands, J. G. "The Visual Communication of Risk." *Journal of the National Cancer Institute Monographs,* 1999, *25,* 149–163.

Lipkus, I. M., Lyna, P. R., and Rimer, B. K. "Using Tailored Interventions to Enhance Smoking Cessation Among African-Americans at a Community Health Center." *Nicotine and Tobacco Research,* 1999, *1,* 77–85.

Marcus, B. H., Nigg, C. R., Riebe, D., and Forsyth, L. H. "Interactive Communication Strategies: Implications for Population-Based Physical-Activity Promotion." *American Journal of Preventive Medicine,* 2000, *19,* 121–126.

McLeroy, K. R., Bibeau, D., Steckler, A., and Glanz, K. "An Ecological Perspective on Health Promotion Programs." *Health Education,* 1988, *15,* 351–377.

Mullen, P. D., Hersey, J. C., and Iverson, D. C. "Health Behavior Models Compared." *Social Science and Medicine,* 1987, *24,* 973–981.

Perloff, L., and Fetzer, B. K. "Self-Other Judgments and Perceived Vulnerability to Victimization." *Journal of Personality and Social Psychology,* 1986, *2,* 502–510.

Prentice-Dunn, S., and Rogers, R. W. "Protection Motivation Theory and Preventive Health: Beyond the Health Belief Model." *Health Education Research,* 1986, *1,* 153–161.

Prochaska, J. O., DiClemente, C. C., Velicer, W. F., and Rossi, J. S. "Standardized, Individualized, Interactive, and Personalized Self-Help Programs for Smoking Cessation." *Health Psychology*, 1993, *12*, 399–405.

Prochaska, J. O., Redding, C., and Evers, K. "The Transtheoretical Model and Stages of Change." In K. Glanz, F. M. Lewis, and B. K. Rimer (eds.), *Health Behavior and Health Education*. (2nd ed.) San Francisco: Jossey-Bass, 1996.

Prochaska, J. O., and others. "Self-Change Processes, Self-Efficacy and Self-Concept in Relapse and Maintenance of Cessation of Smoking." *Psychological Reports*, 1982, *51*, 983–990.

Quinlan, K. B., and McCaul, K. D. "Matched and Mismatched Interventions with Young Adult Smokers: Testing a Stage Theory." *Health Psychology*, 2000, *19*, 165–171.

Rakowski, W. "Breast Cancer: Current Behavioral Research." Paper presented at the CDC 2001 Cancer Conference, 2001, Atlanta, Ga.

Rakowski, W., and others. "Women's Decision-Making About Mammography: An Application of the Relationship Between Stages of Adoption and Decisional Balance." *Health Psychology*, 1993, *12*, 209–241.

Rakowski, W., and others. "Increasing Mammography Among Women Aged 40–74 by Use of a Stage-Matched, Tailored Intervention." *Preventive Medicine*, 1998, *27*, 748–756.

Rimer, B. K., and others. "Cancer Screening Practices Among Women in a Community Health Center Population." *American Journal of Preventive Medicine*, 1996, *12*, 351–357.

Rimer, B. K., and others. "The Short-Term Impact of Tailored Mammography Decision-Making Interventions." *Patient Education and Counseling*, 2001, *43*, 271–287.

Rogers, R. W., and Mewborn, C. R. "Fear Appeals and Attitude Change: Effects of a Threat's Noxiousness, Probability of Occurrence, and the Efficacy of Coping Responses." *Journal of Personality and Social Psychology*, 1976, *34*, 54–61.

Rothman, A. J., and Salovey, P. "Shaping Perceptions to Motivate Healthy Behavior: The Role of Message Framing." *Psychology Bulletin*, 1997, *121*, 3–19.

Sallis, J. F. "Progress in Behavioral Research on Physical Activity." *Annals of Behavioral Medicine*, 2001, *23*, 77–78.

Salovey, P., Rothman, A. J., Detweiler, J. B., and Steward, W. T. "Emotional States and Physical Health." *American Psychologist*, 2000, *55*, 110–121.

Salovey, P., Schneider, T. R., and Apanovitch, A. M. "Persuasion for the Purpose of Cancer Risk Reduction: A Discussion." *Journal of the National Cancer Institute. Monographs*, 1999, *25*, 119–122.

Schneider, T. R., and others. "The Effects of Message Framing and Ethnic Targeting on Mammography Use Among Low-Income Women." *Health Psychology*, 2001, *20*, 256–266.

Sheeran, P., Conner, M., and Norman, P. "Can the Theory of Planned Behavior Explain Patterns of Health Behavior Change?" *Health Psychology*, 2001, *20*, 12–19.

Smedley, B. D., and Syme, S. L. (eds.). *Promoting Health: Intervention Strategies from Social and Behavioral Sciences*. Washington, D.C.: National Academy Press, 2000.

Stoddard, A. M., and others. "Underusers of Mammogram Screening: Stage of Adoption in Five Subpopulations." *Preventive Medicine* 1998, *27*, 478–487.

Strecher, V. J., and Rosenstock, I. M. "The Health Belief Model." In K. Glanz, F. M. Lewis, and B. K. Rimer (eds.), *Health Behavior and Health Education: Theory, Research, and Practice*. San Francisco: Jossey-Bass, 1996.

Sussman, S., and Wills, T. A. "Rationale for Program Development Needs." In S. Sussman and T. A. Wills (eds.), *Handbook of Program Development for Health Behavior Research and Practice*. Thousand Oaks, Calif.: Sage, 2000.

Tessaro, I., and others. "Readiness to Change Smoking Behavior in a Community Health Center Population." *Journal of Community Health,* 1997, *22,* 15–31.

Turkle, S. *Life on the Screen.* New York: Simon & Schuster, 1995.

Weinstein, N. D. "Unrealistic Optimism About Future Life Events." *Journal of Personality and Social Change,* 1980, *39,* 806–820.

Weinstein, N. D. "Why It Won't Happen to Me: Perceptions of Risk Factors and Susceptibility." *Health Psychology,* 1984, *3,* 431–457.

Weinstein, N. D. "Unrealistic Optimism About Susceptibility to Health Problems: Conclusions from a Community-Wide Sample." *Journal of Behavioral Medicine,* 1987, *10,* 481–500.

Weinstein, N. D. "The Precaution Adoption Process." *Health Psychology,* 1988, *7,* 355–386.

Weinstein, N. D., and Klein, W. M. "Resistance of Personal Risk Perceptions to Debiasing Interventions." *Health Psychology,* 1995, *14,* 132–140.

Weinstein, N. D., Rothman, A. J., and Sutton, S. R. "Stage Theories of Health Behavior: Conceptual and Methodological Issues." *Health Psychology,* 1998, *17,* 290–299.

PART THREE

MODELS OF INTERPERSONAL HEALTH BEHAVIOR

Humans are social creatures who are sustained and affected by interactions with their environments, including other people. The core assumption in all the chapters in Part Three is that the interpersonal environment is among the most powerful sources of influence on health-related behavior and health status.

The chapters in Part Three analyze one theory and three theoretical frameworks. Chapter Eight analyzes Social Cognitive Theory. Chapter Nine reviews social support and social networks. Chapter Ten addresses stress and coping, and Chapter Eleven examines social influence and interpersonal communication.

Each chapter attempts to answer two questions: What is known about how the interpersonal environment and relationships alter or enhance health behavior and health outcomes? and By what mechanisms is health-related behavior improved? Each chapter offers different and often complementary ways to conceptualize and modify the interpersonal environment in which a person's health-related behavior can be enhanced. As each chapter will illustrate, substantial research links the concepts in the theory or theoretical framework with both health behavior and health outcomes.

In Chapter Eight, on Social Cognitive Theory, Tom Baranowski, Cheryl Perry, and Guy Parcel outline its historical development and emergence from an operant conditioning paradigm to its current form as a fully codified predictive and prescriptive theory of behavior. A recent review of published literature found that Social Cognitive Theory is one of the most frequently applied theories of health behavior (see Chapter Two). Two applications of the theory are analyzed, both involving health behavior with school-age children. The first is Project Northland's program for preventing and reducing alcohol use among adolescents. The second application is "Gimme 5," a dietary intervention for grade school children.

Catherine Heaney and Barbara Israel, in Chapter Nine, outline the history of social networks and social support as health-relevant concepts and describe core characteristics of social networks and social support. The two applications in Chapter Nine are intervention studies. The first application is an evaluation study of the "Big Brothers, Big Sisters" youth mentoring program. The second application is an intervention study that uses lay health advisers to increase mammography screening among African American women.

In Chapter Ten, Lari Wenzel, Karen Glanz, and Caryn Lerman draw on the Transactional Model of Stress to explain the links between stress, coping, and health outcomes. The Transactional Model consists of three primary concepts: primary appraisal, secondary appraisal, and coping behavior. Coping behavior can be either problem-focused or emotion-focused. Both types are designed to regulate the impact of stress on the focal person. The chapter authors summarize an expansive literature linking appraisal with coping behavior and types of coping behavior with health-related outcomes. The chapter concludes with two applications, both of which are intervention studies. The first intervention used the Transactional Model of Stress to design and evaluate a problem-solving training for relatives of breast cancer patients. The second application is an intervention to improve quality of life for persons who are BRCA+ mutation carriers.

Megan Lewis, Brenda DeVellis, and Betsy Sleath focus in Chapter Eleven on social influence and interpersonal communication. Interdependence Theory is identified by the chapter authors as the overall social psychological theory into which social influence processes and other interpersonal models of communication can be efficiently organized. A chapter on social influence and interpersonal communication is new in this edition of *Health Behavior and Health Education*. Previous editions emphasized patient-provider interaction and influence (Joos and Hickam, 1990; Roter and Hall, 1996), but this new chapter conceptualizes social influence and interpersonal communication through the broader lens. Within Interdependence Theory, three concepts are identified as particularly relevant to health behavior: relationship interdependence, interdependence, and correspondence of outcomes. The two applications described in the chapter are intervention studies. The first application involves the use of motivational interviewing to increase fruit and vegetable intake in attendees of African American churches. The second application is an evaluation of "Family Matters," a family-directed program for preventing smoking and alcohol use among teenagers.

Finally, Chapter Twelve offers additional perspectives on each of the four preceding chapters and recommendations for future research.

References

Joos, S. K., and Hickam, D. H. "How Health Professionals Influence Health Behavior: Patient-Provider Interaction and Health Care Outcomes." In K. Glanz, F. M. Lewis, and B. K. Rimer (eds.), *Health Behavior and Health Education: Theory, Research, and Practice.* San Francisco: Jossey-Bass, 1990.

Roter, D. L., and Hall, J. A. "Patient-Provider Communication." In K. Glanz, F. M. Lewis, and B. K. Rimer (eds.), *Health Behavior and Health Education: Theory, Research, and Practice.* (2nd ed.) San Francisco: Jossey-Bass, 1996.

CHAPTER EIGHT

HOW INDIVIDUALS, ENVIRONMENTS, AND HEALTH BEHAVIOR INTERACT

Social Cognitive Theory

Tom Baranowski
Cheryl L. Perry
Guy S. Parcel

Social Cognitive Theory (SCT) addresses both the psychosocial dynamics influencing health behavior and methods for promoting behavioral change. Within SCT, human behavior is explained in terms of a triadic, dynamic, and reciprocal model in which behavior, personal factors (including cognitions), and environmental influences all interact. Among the crucial personal factors are the individual's capabilities to symbolize behavior, to anticipate the outcomes of behavior, to learn by observing others, to have confidence in performing a behavior (including overcoming the problems in performing the behavior), to self-determine or self-regulate behavior, and to reflect on and analyze experience (Bandura, 1997).

Health educators and behavioral scientists have creatively used SCT to develop interventions, procedures, or techniques that influence these underlying cognitive variables, thereby increasing the likelihood of behavioral change. This chapter provides a brief history of the development of Social Cognitive Theory, includes a description of key concepts, and analyzes two recent examples of how the theory was used to design health education programs.

The authors' work on this chapter was supported in part by the following grants: HL 47618, CA 61596, AA 08596, HL 39927, CA 75614, HL 65160, and CA 73503.

A Brief History of Social Cognitive Theory

Table 8.1 summarizes publication milestones of SCT in the areas of understanding and changing health behaviors. This summary of major contributions represents some of the key examples among many.

In 1962, Bandura published an article on social learning and imitation (Bandura, 1962). In contrast to operant learning theory, which maintained that rewards had to be directly applied for learning to occur, Bandura and Walters (1963) proposed that children could observe other children to learn a new behavior and did not need to be rewarded directly. Thus, a child learned by ob-

TABLE 8.1. PUBLICATION MILESTONES IN THE DEVELOPMENT OF SOCIAL COGNITIVE THEORY.

1962	Bandura	"Social Learning Through Imitation," *Nebraska Symposium on Motivation*
1963	Bandura and Walters	*Social Learning and Personality Development*
1969	Bandura	*Principles of Behavior Modification*
1977	Bandura	*Social Learning Theory*
	Bandura	"Self-Efficacy: Toward a Unifying Theory of Behavioral Change," *Psychological Review*
	Farquhar and others	"Community Education for Cardiovascular Health," *Lancet*
1978	Bandura	"The Self System in Reciprocal Determinism," *American Psychologist*
1981	Parcel and Baranowski	"Social Learning Theory and Health Education," *Health Education*
1983	Abrams and Follick	"Behavioral Weight-Loss Intervention at the Worksite: Feasibility and Maintenance," *Journal of Consulting and Clinical Psychology*
1986	Bandura	*Social Foundations of Thought and Action*
	Abrams, Elder, Carleton, Lasater, and Artz	"Social Learning Principles for Organizational Health Promotion: An Integrated Approach," *Health and Industry: A Behavioral Medicine Approach*
1995	Bandura	*Self-Efficacy in Changing Societies*
1997	Bandura	*Self-Efficacy: The Exercise of Control*
2001	Bandura	"Social Cognitive Theory: An Agentic Perspective," *Annual Review of Psychology*

Note: See reference section at the end of the chapter for complete bibliographical references.

serving the behavior of others (modeling) and the rewards others received (vicarious reinforcement). Six years later, Bandura provided a conceptual foundation for behavior modification that heavily emphasized traditional learning theory (Bandura, 1969). But in 1977, Bandura refuted the adequacy of traditional learning theory principles for understanding learning and provided the first theoretical treatment of his cognitive concept of self-efficacy (Bandura, 1977a, 1977b).

Farquhar and others (1977) reported the first communitywide intervention for heart disease prevention based on Social Learning Theory. Bandura (1978) proposed the organizing concept of reciprocal determinism, in which environment, person, and behavior are continually interacting. Parcel and Baranowski (1981) applied SCT to health education and delineated stages in the behavioral change process at which each concept was most relevant. Abrams and Follick (1983) first applied social learning concepts to the design of worksite interventions. In 1986, Bandura published a comprehensive framework for understanding human social behavior and renamed Social Learning Theory as Social Cognitive Theory (Bandura, 1986). Shortly thereafter, Abrams, Elder, Carleton, Lasater, and Artz (1986) used SCT as a framework for understanding and integrating organizational and individual approaches to health behavior change.

Bandura (1995) proposed self-efficacy as the construct undergirding many aspects of social change. Bandura (1997, 2001) moved SCT from the domain of mechanistic theories of human behavior to the views of the person as an agent in control of his or her own life. While many other contributions could be cited, this list reflects our interpretation of the major historical roots and some dominant contributions to the public health literature.

Several things should be learned from this historical review. First, there have been both major changes (for example, from behavioral learning to cognitive learning theory foundations for SCT) and minor changes (such as the addition and refinement of constructs) in the development of SCT. Second, change in theory is necessary as we try to better understand the behaviors of interest. Third, readers of this chapter have ample opportunity to conduct relevant research and contribute to the further development in SCT.

SCT is particularly relevant to health education and health behavior programs for three reasons. First, the theory synthesizes previously disparate cognitive, emotional, and behavioristic understandings of behavioral change. Second, as demonstrated in this chapter, the constructs and processes identified by SCT suggest many important avenues for new behavioral research and practice in health education. Third, SCT permits the application to health behaviors and behavioral change of theoretical ideas developed in other disciplines such as psychology, thereby benefiting from their insights and understanding.

Social Cognitive Theory Constructs

Bandura (1977a, 1986) formulated a number of SCT constructs that are important to understand and intervene in health behavior. Table 8.2 summarizes these constructs as well as their implications for potential intervention strategies.

Reciprocal Determinism

Within SCT, behavior is depicted as dynamic, depending on aspects of the environment and the person, all of which influence each other simultaneously. This continuing interaction among the characteristics of a person, the behavior of that person, and the environment within which the behavior is performed is called *reciprocal determinism*. Behavior is not simply the result of the environment and the person, just as the environment is not simply the result of the person and behavior. Instead, these three components are constantly influencing each other. A change in one component has implications for the others (Bandura, 1978, 1986). Reciprocal determinism is accepted within SCT as a principle or a postulate and has not been submitted to empirical test.

Environments and Situations

The term *environment* refers to the objective factors that can affect a person's behavior but that are physically external to that person. Examples of the social environment include family members, friends, and peers at work or in the classroom. The physical environment might include the size of a room, the ambient temperature, or the availability of certain foods. The term *situation* refers to the cognitive or mental representation of the environment (including real, distorted, or imagined factors) that may affect a person's behavior. The situation is a person's perception of the environment, such as place, time, physical features, activity, participants, and his or her own role in the situation. Environment and situation provide an ecological framework for understanding behavior (Parraga, 1990).

A model of family reciprocal determinism (Taylor, Baranowski, and Sallis, 1994; Baranowski, 1990) has been proposed to capture these complexities. The habitual pattern of interactions between family members constitutes an aspect of the environment: emergent family characteristics (Baranowski, 1996). For example, when habitual family interactions are characterized by conflict, whether and how family members seek information and assistance from one another will consistently vary from those characterized as supportive. Within this model, behavior

TABLE 8.2. MAJOR CONCEPTS IN SOCIAL COGNITIVE THEORY AND IMPLICATIONS FOR INTERVENTION.

Concept	Definition	Implications
Environment	Factors physically external to the person	Provide opportunities and social support
Situation	Person's perception of the environment	Correct misperceptions and promote healthful norms
Behavioral capability	Knowledge and skill to perform a given behavior	Promote mastery learning through skills training
Expectations	Anticipatory outcomes of a behavior	Model positive outcomes of healthful behavior
Expectancies	The values that the person places on a given outcome; incentives	Present outcomes of change that have functional meaning
Self-control	Personal regulation of goal-directed behavior or performance	Provide opportunities for decision making, self-monitoring, goal setting, problem solving, and self-reward
Observational learning	Behavioral acquisition that occurs by watching the actions and outcomes of others' behavior	Include credible role models of the targeted behavior
Reinforcements	Responses to a person's behavior that increase or decrease the likelihood of reoccurrence	Promote self-initiated rewards and incentives
Self-efficacy	The person's confidence in performing a particular behavior and in overcoming barriers to that behavior	Approach behavior change in small steps to ensure success; seek specificity about the change sought
Emotional coping responses	Strategies or tactics that are used by a person to deal with emotional stimuli	Provide training in problem solving and stress management; include opportunities to practice skills in emotionally arousing situations
Reciprocal determinism	The dynamic interaction of the person, behavior, and the environment in which the behavior is performed	Consider multiple avenues to behavioral change including environmental, skill, and personal change

is a function of a shared environment with other family members and their behavior and personal characteristics, all of which function within a larger environment. Thus, the eating of certain foods by a child is in part a result of the child's preferences for those foods (Domel and others, 1993a), what foods are available in the home, certain types of prompts by parents to eat those foods (Iannotti, O'Brien, and Spillman, 1994), and what foods are available by time of the year or region (Sallis, 1986).

The environment has been increasingly recognized as important in health behavior change. State and worksite policies restricting smoking have enhanced smoking prevention and cessation (Biener, Abrams, Follick, and Dean, 1989). The unavailability of certain healthful foods in the home precludes their consumption (Kirby, Baranowski, Reynolds, Taylor, and Binkley, 1995). Modifying the foods served in the school cafeteria has been shown to increase students' consumption of low-fat meals (Simons-Morton, Parcel, Baranowski, Forthofer, and O'Hara, 1991).

Observational Learning

The environment is important in SCT in part because it provides *models* for behavior. A person can learn from other people not only by receiving reinforcements from them but also through observing them. *Observational learning* occurs when a person watches the actions of another person and the reinforcements that the person receives. This process has also been called vicarious reward or vicarious experience (Bandura, 1972, 1986, 1997).

Observational learning is more efficient than operant conditioning for learning complex behaviors. In the operant approach, a person must perform a behavior that is subsequently reinforced. Through a trial-and-error process, the person continues to perform behaviors that come progressively closer to the desired performance. Trial and error is an inefficient process. In observational learning, the observer does not need to engage in this time-consuming, trial-and-error process in uncertain circumstances. Instead, the learner discovers rules that account for the behavior of others by observing the behavior and the reinforcements they receive for their behavior.

Many types of behavior can be learned through observational learning (Bandura and Walters, 1963; Bandura, 1972, 1986). This process accounts for why people in the same family often have common behavioral patterns. Children observe their parents when they eat, smoke, drink, and use seat belts and see the various rewards or penalties the parents receive for these types of behavior. Some children observe other children smoking at school and notice the rewards and punishments that the smokers receive. If the smokers get reinforcements that the observers consider rewarding (acceptance from peers or a desirable image), the observers are more likely to perform that behavior in the future.

Behavioral Capability

Behavior can be viewed at many levels (Frederiksen, Martin, and Webster, 1979), from having a meal to eating a specific food to how many bites it took to chew a mouthful of food. Health educators and others interested in changing health behaviors must clearly specify their targeted behavior. The concept of *behavioral capability* maintains that if a person is to perform a particular behavior, he or she must know what the behavior is (knowledge of the behavior) and how to perform it (skill). The concept of behavioral capability distinguishes between learning and performance because a task can be learned and not performed. Performance presumes learning.

Reinforcement

Reinforcement is the primary construct in the operant form of learning theory. *Positive reinforcement,* or reward, is a response to a person's behavior that increases the likelihood that the behavior will be repeated. In traditional operant theory, the reinforcement works in an unknown mechanistic way to affect behavior. For example, complimenting someone will increase the likelihood that the person repeats the behavior for which the compliment was provided, especially if the person doing the behavior values the opinion of the person making the compliment. Negative reinforcement also increases the likelihood of a behavior but by withdrawal of a negative stimulus when the desired behavior is performed. For example, smoking is negatively reinforcing because the inhaled nicotine removes negative affect (depression, anxiety, anger, for example), withdrawal, and craving. Punishment may simply reduce the likelihood that a particular behavior will be performed in those situations in which a person expects to receive punishment but not in other situations. Exercise among obese children was increased both by reinforcing active behaviors and reinforcing decreased time in sedentary behaviors (Epstein, Saelens, and O'Brien, 1995). However, once the rewards are removed, the behavior may revert to its original form or level.

SCT incorporates three types of reinforcement: direct reinforcement (as in operant conditioning), vicarious reinforcement (as in observational learning), and self-reinforcement (as in self-control). SCT further categorizes these types of reinforcement into external (or extrinsic) and internal (or intrinsic) reinforcement (Lepper and Cordova, 1992). External reinforcement is the occurrence of an event or act that is known to have predictable reinforcement value. Internal reinforcement is a person's own experience or perception that an event had some value. Educational programs that are intrinsically reinforcing result in more learning, retention, and interest in the subject matter (Lepper and Cordova, 1992). Participants who reported higher intrinsic motivation than extrinsic motivation were more likely to achieve abstinence from smoking (Curry, Wagner, and Grothaus, 1990).

Outcome Expectations

Expectations are the anticipatory aspects of behavior that Bandura (1977a, 1986) called antecedent determinants of behavior. A person learns that certain events are likely to occur in response to the person's behavior in a particular situation and then expects them to occur when the situation recurs. For behavior that is not habitual, people anticipate many aspects of the situation in which the behavior might be performed, develop and test strategies for dealing with the situation, and anticipate what will happen as a result of their behavior in this situation. In this way, people develop expectations about a situation and expectations for outcomes of their behavior before they actually encounter the situation. In most cases, this anticipatory behavior reduces their anxiety and increases their ability to handle the situation. Expectations are learned in four ways: (1) from previous experience in similar situations (performance attainment), (2) from observing others in similar situations (vicarious experience), (3) from hearing about these situations from other people or social persuasion, and (4) from emotional or physical responses to behaviors (physiological arousal).

An example of how expectations may develop and be changed is provided in adolescent smoking prevention. Generally, adolescents "learn" to expect, from advertising, older peers, or adult role models, that smoking can be a fun or exciting experience or that they can attain a grown-up or even sexy appearance by smoking. In a health education and health behavior program, peers can be taught to direct discussions on the negative social consequences of smoking and on how to handle pressure to smoke from other adolescents. This approach has been successful in deterring smoking onset (Flay, 1985). In essence, this approach succeeds in part because negative social consequences (negative outcome expectations) for these adolescents have changed.

Outcome Expectancies

Outcome expectancies (called incentives by Bandura [1977a, 1986]) are differentiated from expectations in that expectancies are the *values* that a person places on a particular outcome. Expectancies have magnitude: a quantitative value that can be positive or negative and is usually represented on a continuum from −1 to +1. Expectancies influence behavior according to the hedonic principle: if all other things are equal, a person will choose to perform an activity that maximizes a positive outcome or minimizes a negative outcome. Positive outcome expectancies for smoking predicted the severity of withdrawal symptoms, while both positive and negative outcome expectancies predicted success of attempts at smoking cessation (Wetter and others, 1994). Food preferences and tastes can be considered immediate outcome expectancies of eating. Preference was the only predictor of consumption of fruits and vegetables among children (Domel and others, 1996; Resnicow and others, 1997) and taste was a primary predictor of consumption of beverages among adults (Lewis, Sims, and Shannon, 1989).

A person's positive expectancies should be assessed early in a project that is designed to promote changes in health behavior to identify motivators for that behavior. Many researchers have observed, for example, that people are more likely to engage in physical activity to achieve short-term benefits (to become physically attractive, to feel better, or to compete with friends in tennis) than to achieve long-term gains (for example, to avoid a heart attack in thirty years).

Self-Efficacy

Self-efficacy is the confidence a person feels about performing a particular activity, including confidence in overcoming the barriers to performing that behavior. Bandura and colleagues (Bandura, 1977b, 1978, 1982, 1986, 1997) proposed that self-efficacy is the most important prerequisite for behavior change because it affects how much effort is invested in a given task and what level of performance is attained. Self-efficacy was a primary predictor of intention to engage in eight healthy dietary practices among office staff (Sheeshka, Woolcott, and MacKinnon, 1993) and of healthy food choices among third- and fourth-grade students (Parcel and others, 1995). It also has been a consistent predictor of success in quitting smoking and of maintaining other healthful behavior changes.

Both observational and active (participatory) learning techniques can be used to introduce and promote each sequence of a targeted behavior (Bandura, 1986). Through repeated successful enactment of incremental tasks, the person acquires enhanced expectations that he or she will succeed in the task, which in turn affects task persistence, initiation, and endurance, all of which promote behavioral change. Therefore, health professionals who are training people with diabetes to self-inject insulin may divide the self-injection process into many small steps, each of which individuals can learn through repetition (for example, filling the syringe with the correct amount of insulin, ensuring that all items remain sterilized, seeing that no bubbles get into the syringe, and being sure that the fluid is at the precise marker on the syringe). Simplifying each step and allowing individuals to practice each step in isolation with many repetitions enables them to build self-efficacy about performing each step. When persons are self-confident about each step, they can progressively put the steps together and build self-efficacy about the entire task. Measurement of self-efficacy must be specific to the target behavior, and to the barriers faced by, and the understanding and capabilities of, the target audience (Maibach and Murphy, 1995).

Self-Control of Performance

The term *performance* refers to human behavior focused on achievement of a goal. One of the goals of health education is to bring the performance of health behavior under the control of the individual. Bandura (1991) proposed that the self-control system has several component subfunctions. The subfunctions include monitoring of one's own behavior and its determinants and effects; comparison of behavior and its outcomes to personal standards, especially self-set goals; and self-reward, especially affective self-reaction. Self-efficacy has an important role in self-control in terms of selecting the extent of behavior for change and the practice for building confidence in self-regulation. The setting of a criterion of performance, or goal setting, may be one of the most important factors (Cullen, 2001). Promotion of self-control requires a focus on a specific type of behavior.

Managing Emotional Arousal

Bandura (1977a) recognized that excessive emotional arousal inhibits learning and performance. He proposed that certain stimuli give rise to fearful thoughts (stimulus-outcome expectancies), which in turn produce emotional arousal and trigger defensive behaviors. As the defensive behaviors deal effectively with the stimuli, the fear, anxiety, hostility, and emotional arousal are reduced.

Categories of behavioral management for emotional and physiological arousal were identified by Moos (1976). One category includes psychological defenses (denial, repression, and sublimation). Another category involves cognitive techniques, such as problem restructuring. A third category is stress management techniques (progressive relaxation or exercise) that treat the symptoms of the emotional distress. Finally, the fourth category is methods for solving problems effectively (clarifying a problem and identifying, selecting, and implementing solutions for the causes of the emotional arousal). SCT constructs and methods are usually employed to learn these behavioral management skills.

Reciprocal Determinism Revisited

It is instructive to return to the concept of reciprocal determinism and examine it in light of the component SCT constructs just discussed. If a characteristic of the person, environment, or behavior changes, the situation changes, and the behavior, situation, and person are reevaluated. For example, a man may be so opposed to exercise that his friends come to expect him to maintain a sedentary lifestyle. The man has strengthened this expectation about his exercise by avoiding any physical or social environments in which he might be expected to exercise (for example, gyms or playing fields). At some point, however, a dramatic event may occur in his life (for example, the death of a close family member from a heart attack and exposure to information that heart attacks may in part be caused by a sedentary lifestyle) that causes him to decide to start exercising. The man will now encounter the expectations of his sedentary friends, who may pressure him not to exercise. To avoid these negative pressures, he may seek new friends (a new social environment) who value exercise and support his new behavior (reciprocal effect). This change, in turn, may motivate a sedentary friend to begin to exercise as well (a reciprocal effect to that friend), and the friend will then either change the exercise habits of other sedentary friends, or acquire new friends who are interested in exercise.

This kind of behavior change underscores the importance of professionals avoiding the simplicity of "single direction of change" thinking. Reciprocal determinism may be used to advantage in developing programs that do not focus on behavior in isolation but focus instead on changes in the environment and in the individual as well. A recent health promotion program based on Social Cognitive Theory that included environmental and individual changes is the Child and Adolescent Trial for Cardiovascular Health (CATCH), which was designed to improve nutrition and physical activity behavior. In this multicenter trial, interventions for third- through fifth-grade students were tested. The interventions attempted to influence changes in cognitive factors through classroom instruction and through environmental changes by modifying the food service program and the physical education program. The interventions were predicated on reciprocal determinism by addressing behavioral capability, self-efficacy, and perceived norms in the classroom; providing an opportunity for children to practice the new behaviors in the school cafeteria and in physical education; and providing reinforcement from important others in the child's environment (teachers and parents). The evaluations indicated significant changes in cognitive variables, environmental conditions, and nutrition and physical activity behavior (Luepker and others, 1996; Edmundson and others, 1996).

To provide more examples of the use of these SCT concepts, the following sections describe how SCT was used in the design of two health education interventions. The first application of SCT, Project Northland, addresses alcohol use among adolescents. The second application, Gimme 5, deals with fruit and vegetable consumption among school-age children.

Case Study: Project Northland's Programs for Eleventh-Grade Students

Project Northland, a communitywide program, was designed to prevent and reduce alcohol use among adolescents in grades six through twelve (ages eleven through eighteen). SCT concepts were creatively translated into developmentally appropriate educational and environmental programs that would deter high school students from drinking alcohol. Project Northland involved twenty-four school districts and surrounding communities in northeastern Minnesota, an area with high levels of alcohol-related problems (Perry and others, 1993). The project focused on the Class of 1998, that is, students who graduated from high school in 1998. In the intervention communities, Class of 1998 students participated in three years of school-based behavioral health curricula, parental involvement programs, peer leadership opportunities, and communitywide task force activities while in the sixth through eighth grades (Perry and others, 1996). They also took part in an additional short curriculum in the ninth grade, but no other program activities during the tenth grade. At the end of the eighth grade, students in the intervention communities were significantly less likely to say they drank alcohol than those in the delayed-program communities (Perry and others, 1996). The mediating variables for the first phase of Project Northland, at the end of eighth grade, included less observational learning from peers, more negative expectancies around alcohol use, and increased behavioral capability to communicate with parents, as demonstrated by mediation analyses (Komro and others, 2001). By the end of the tenth grade (1996), the differences between treatment conditions were no longer significant.

The goals of the eleventh-grade program were to reduce access to alcohol and to change community norms concerning the acceptability of alcohol use for high school–age students (Perry and others, 2000). To meet the goals, the eleventh-grade intervention consisted of (1) direct-action community organizing with adult action teams to address policies and practices related to teen alcohol use; (2) parental education, including a postcard campaign and a contest (Sound OFF!) to encourage parent-adolescent communication about alcohol; (3) youth-development activities with youth-action teams formed in each school to instigate alcohol-free events such as proms and homecoming, creation of videos of the alcohol environment in each community, mentoring of younger students, and policy projects; (4) media projects including a campaign (Don't Provide!) aimed at young adults, calendars for alcohol merchants, messages in church bulletins, and a celebration poster in 1998; and (5) a classroom-based curriculum that involved six sessions based on a mock trial program, in which students acted as counsel, concerning cases involving teen alcohol use (Perry and others, 2000). SCT guided the development of these eleventh-grade program components as summarized in Table 8.3.

After a year of Phase 2 intervention activities, students in the intervention group drank less, but the difference was not statistically significant. At the end of twelfth grade, however, significant differences between conditions in the rate of increase in alcohol use and heavy drinking over the course of Phase 2, using growth-curve analyses, demonstrated the longer-term effectiveness of this approach. In addition, access to alcohol was reduced and parental norms were less accepting of teen alcohol use at the end of the study. These outcomes suggest that the application of SCT at the community level appears to have yielded results in changing the environment and expectancies related to alcohol use by reducing teen access to alcohol, changing norms, and reducing alcohol use among high school students. Thus, actions at the community level to change these constructs resulted in less drinking among teens.

Case Study: Gimme 5!— Fruit and Vegetables for Fun and Health

SCT was used to define the reasons why (McLeroy and others, 1994) fourth- and fifth-grade children were not eating sufficient servings of fruit, 100 percent juice, and vegetables (FJV) (Baranowski, and others, 1993; Kirby, Baranowski, Reynolds, Taylor, and Binkley, 1995) and then creatively used to design an intervention to remedy those factors (Domel and others, 1993b).

While several dietary guidelines for the United States recommend that everyone should eat five to nine servings of fruit and vegetables every day (Domel and others, 1993c), recent data revealed that children eat somewhere between 1.8 and 2.5 servings per day (Domel and others, 1994). Focus group discussions predicated on SCT (Baranowski and others, 1993; Kirby, Baranowski, Reynolds, Taylor, and Binkley, 1995) revealed that children were not eating fruit, juice, and vegetables (FJV) due to environmental, personal, and behavioral factors. Regarding the environment, FJV were not available in the homes of lower-income families and not accessible in all homes. Regarding personal factors, children did not have positive outcome expectancies, especially preference or taste, for eating vegetables.

TABLE 8.3. EXAMPLES OF SOCIAL COGNITIVE CONSTRUCTS IN PROJECT NORTHLAND'S ELEVENTH-GRADE INTERVENTION.

SCT Constructs	Examples of Construct Use
Environment	Commercial access to alcohol was a primary target of the adult action teams.
	Students planned alcohol-free prom and homecoming parties.
	The "Don't Provide" print media campaign discouraged provision to minors.
	The parent postcards targeted norms at home concerning teen alcohol use.
Situation	Student videos of their communities were played to Class of 1998 students and community members to invoke community concern.
Behavioral capabilities	Students developed skills to assess personal and community responsibility for teen alcohol use.
Expectations	Students learned the legal outcomes of underage alcohol use and abuse.
Expectancies	Prom and homecoming were portrayed as fun and cool when alcohol free.
Self-control	Students taught younger students the skills to remain alcohol free.
Observational learning	Videotaped lawyers provided arguments in Class Action.
	Peer action teams developed engaging alcohol-free activities.
	Alcohol beverage server training was publicized in all communities.
Reinforcement	Students received stipends for involvement in youth-development activities.
	Students received Project Northland certificate at graduation.
Self-efficacy	Group presentations argued their "case" in front of class juries.
Reciprocal determinism	The commercial environment changed, so there was reduced access to alcohol for high school students.
	Parents were aware of the changes via the parent postcards and reinforced normative changes at home.
	Students in intervention communities began to drink less, which provided fewer social opportunities for peers to drink.

And regarding behavioral factors, children were responsible for making their own snacks and some of their own meals but did not have a repertoire of recipes for making their favorite FJV dishes. The primary predictor of FJV consumption was preference for FJV (Domel and others, 1993a; Resnicow and others, 1997).

A school curriculum called Gimme 5! was designed to help remedy these influencing factors and thereby increase FJV consumption (Domel and others, 1993b). The intervention attempted to increase availability and accessibility of FJV through "asking skills." That is, skills-training activities including role-playing were designed to have children go home and ask to purchase their favorite FJV at the grocery store, to have their favorite FJV available at meals and snacks, and to select fast-food eateries that offer a variety of FJV. Gimme 5! attempted to increase preference for FJV by developing and pretasting FaSST (fast, simple, safe, and tasty) recipes that children were likely to enjoy, by increasing exposures to FJV through taste testings of these recipes in the classroom (Birch, 1987), and by associating fun participative activities with FJV (for example, a rap song, role-playing). The children's ability to prepare FJV dishes was addressed by preparing FaSST recipes in the classroom and sending the recipes home through newsletters to the family with homework assignments to prepare them at home. Self-regulation skills were promoted by having students monitor their FJV consumption, set goals for eating more FJV at specific meals or snacks, problem solve when goals were not achieved, and be rewarded when goals were achieved. Rewards came in the form of congratulations and applause from the teacher and students and in the form of small toys to those children who achieved all their goals. The pilot test of the curriculum revealed that children experienced a 50 percent increase in their fruit consumption and changed their most frequently consumed vegetable from french fries (undesired because they are high in fat) to green salad (Baranowski and others, 2000). Further analyses revealed that all these changes occurred at school; in other words, children took more advantage of the FJV offered in school lunch than at home. Examples of the use of SCT constructs in Gimme 5! are found in Table 8.4.

The ensuing implementation of the Gimme 5! curriculum attempted to more effectively target home availability, accessibility, and consumption of FJV (Havas and others, 1995), a home environment variable. The same conceptual analysis was employed, but attempts to reach parents included an expanded weekly newsletter with many tips for helping children eat more FJV recipes and three fifteen-minute videotapes per year with an MTV format, including a local professional basketball player as the VJ and children and parents from the local schools as actors, modeling many of the desired behaviors. Point-of-purchase education at the local grocery stores was also added, addressing parental concerns about how to select low-cost and unlikely-to-perish FJV, offering taste testings, and dispensing free samples through coupons and prizes as incentives to attend the evening sessions in the stores.

TABLE 8.4. EXAMPLES OF SOCIAL COGNITIVE CONSTRUCTS IN GIMME 5!

SCT Constructs	Examples of How Constructs Were Used
Environment	Availability and accessibility of fruit, juice, and vegetables (FJV) at home
Behavioral capability	Skills development to make FaSST recipes
	Skills development to "ask for" more FJV at home and at fast-food eateries
Outcome expectancies	Eating more FJV will enhance students' school performance but will not impair their acceptance by their peers.
Self-control	Setting goals to eat more FJV at targeted meals and snacks
Observational learning	Observing the teacher setting goals for her own dietary change
Reinforcement	Receiving congratulations for attaining all dietary change goals
	Receiving small prizes (neon shoelaces, FJV refrigerator magnets) for completing all homework assignments
Self-efficacy	Enhancing the student's confidence to ask for FJV through role-playing such situations in school
Reciprocal determinism	Children ask for more of their favorite FJV to be available and accessible at home; as the FJV become more available and accessible, children eat more of them because their preferences for FJV have increased; the increased exposure to FJV further increases the preferences for FJV

Outcome analyses of Gimme 5! revealed a 0.2 vegetable serving increase at the end of the fourth grade (right after activities emphasizing vegetable intake) but no difference in FJV at the end of the fifth grade (Baranowski and others, 2000). Change was induced in only a subset of the mediating variables. Process evaluation using observations in the classroom revealed that the classroom teachers implemented only about 50 percent of the Gimme 5! curriculum tasks and only 22 percent of the curriculum tasks most likely to result in behavior change (Davis and others, 2000). Thus, it appears that low implementation of the curriculum impaired the program's ability to influence mediating variables and produce behavior change.

Limitations of Social Cognitive Theory

Some health educators and behavioral scientists have complained that Social Cognitive Theory is too comprehensive in its formulation. There are so many constructs that some authors have found a way to explain almost any phenomenon using one or more of the constructs. Therefore, both practitioners and investigators using SCT must specify the range of phenomena to which it applies, examine the situations in which the theory does not apply, and limit their claims about the utility of SCT to those that are supported by empirical evidence.

Measurement of some of the SCT constructs has been subjected to theoretical criticism (Maibach and Murphy, 1995), and many have modest reliability coefficients. Error in measurement reduces the correlations with other variables, both in predictive models and in mediating variable analyses (Traub, 1994). Thus, improvement in measurement procedures may improve the ability of SCT constructs to explain behavior and the effects of interventions. More research needs to be conducted to elucidate the extent to which social cognitive theory constructs predict health-related behaviors.

Summary

This chapter has focused on Social Cognitive Theory and its relevance in the design of health education programs. SCT is attractive for health education and health behavior programs because it both addresses the dynamics of individual behavior and gives direction to the design of intervention strategies. By incorporating the environment, people, and behavior, SCT provides a framework for designing, implementing, and evaluating comprehensive behavioral change programs. Intervention designers should clearly specify the desired behavioral outcomes, identify the SCT variables most likely to influence each behavior, and develop and test intervention methods to change the targeted SCT variables. Evaluations of programs based on SCT should use measures of relevance to SCT that have established validity and reliability.

References

Abrams, D. B., Elder, J. P., Carleton, R. A., Lasater, T. M., and Artz, L. M. "Social Learning Principles for Organizational Health Promotion: An Integrated Approach." In M. F. Cataldo and T. J. Coates (eds.), *Health and Industry: A Behavioral Medicine Perspective.* New York: Wiley, 1986.

Abrams, D. B., and Follick, M. J. "Behavioral Weight-Loss Intervention at the Worksite: Feasibility and Maintenance." *Journal of Consulting and Clinical Psychology*, 1983, *51*, 226–233.

Bandura, A. "Social Learning Through Imitation." In M. R. Jones (ed.), *Nebraska Symposium on Motivation*, Vol. 10. Lincoln, Nebr.: University of Nebraska Press, 1962.

Bandura, A. *Principles of Behavior Modification*. New York: Holt, Rinehart & Winston, 1969.

Bandura, A. *Psychological Modeling: Connecting Theories*. Chicago: Aldine/Atherton, 1972.

Bandura, A. *Social Learning Theory*. Englewood Cliffs, N.J.: Prentice Hall, 1977a.

Bandura, A. "Self-Efficacy: Toward a Unifying Theory of Behavioral Change." *Psychological Review*, 1977b, *84*, 191–215.

Bandura, A. "The Self System in Reciprocal Determinism." *American Psychologist*, 1978, *33*, 344–358.

Bandura, A. "Self-Efficacy Mechanism in Human Agency." *American Psychologist*, 1982, *37*, 121–147.

Bandura, A. *Social Foundations of Thought and Action*. Englewood Cliffs, N.J.: Prentice Hall, 1986.

Bandura, A. "Social Cognitive Theory of Self-Regulation." *Organizational Behavior and Human Decision Processes*, 1991, *50*, 248–287.

Bandura, A. *Self-Efficacy in Changing Societies*. New York: Cambridge University Press, 1995.

Bandura, A. *Self-Efficacy, The Exercise of Control*. New York: W. H. Freeman, 1997.

Bandura, A. "Social Cognitive Theory: An Agentic Perspective." *Annual Review of Psychology*, 2001, *52*, 1–26.

Bandura, A., and Walters, R. H. *Social Learning and Personality Development*. New York: Holt, Rinehart & Winston, 1963.

Baranowski, T. "Reciprocal Determinism at the Stages of Behavior Change: An Integration of Community, Personal and Behavioral Perspectives." *International Quarterly of Community Health Education*, 1990, *10*, 297–327.

Baranowski, T. "Families and Health Action." In D. Gochman (ed.), *Handbook of Health Behavior Research*, Vol. I. New York: Plenum, 1996.

Baranowski, T., and others. "Increasing Fruit and Vegetable Consumption Among 4th and 5th Grade Students: Results from Focus Groups Using Reciprocal Determinism." *Journal of Nutrition Education*, 1993, *25*, 114–120.

Baranowski, T., and others. "Gimme 5 Fruit, Juice and Vegetables for Fun and Health: Outcome Evaluation." *Health Education & Behavior*, 2000, *27*, 96–111.

Biener, L., Abrams, A. B., Follick, M. J., and Dean, L. A. "Comparative Evaluation of a Restrictive Smoking Policy in a General Hospital." *American Journal of Public Health*, 1989, *79*, 192–195.

Birch, L. L. "Children's Food Preferences: Developmental Patterns and Environmental Influences." *Annals of Child Development*, 1987, *4*, 171–208.

Cullen, K. W., Baranowski, T., and Smith, S. P. "Goal Setting for Dietary Behavior Change." *Journal of the American Dietetic Association*, 2001, *101*, 562–566.

Curry, S., Wagner, E. H., and Grothaus, L. C. "Intrinsic and Extrinsic Motivation for Smoking Cessation." *Journal of Consulting and Clinical Psychology*, 1990, *58*, 310–316.

Davis, M., and others. "Gimme 5 Fruit and Vegetables for Fun and Health: Process Evaluation." *Health Education and Behavior*, 2000, *27*, 167–176.

Domel, S., and others. "Measuring Fruit and Vegetable Preferences Among Fourth and Fifth Grade Students." *Preventive Medicine*, 1993a, *22*, 866–879.

Domel, S., and others. "Development and Evaluation of a School Intervention to Increase Fruit and Vegetable Consumption Among 4th and 5th Grade Students." *Journal of Nutrition Education*, 1993b, *25*, 345–9.

Domel, S., and others. "To Be or Not To Be . . . Fruits and Vegetables." *Journal of Nutrition Education*, 1993c, *25*(6), 352–358.

Domel, S., and others. "Fruit and Vegetable Food Frequencies by Fourth and Fifth Grade Students: Validity and Reliability." *Journal of the American College of Nutrition*, 1994, *13*(1), 1–7.

Domel, S., and others. "Psychosocial Predictors of Fruit and Vegetable Consumption Among Elementary-School Children." *Health Education Research: Theory & Practice*, 1996, *11*, 299–308.

Edmundson, E., and others. "The Effects of Child and Adolescent Trial for Cardiovascular Health upon Psychosocial Determinants of Diet and Physical Activity Behavior. *Preventive Medicine*, 1996, *25*, 442–454.

Epstein, L. H., Saelens, B. E., and O'Brien, J. G. "Effects of Reinforcing Increases in Active Behavior Versus Decreases in Sedentary Behavior for Obese Children." *International Journal of Behavioral Medicine*, 1995, *2*, 41–50.

Farquhar, J. W., and others. "Community Education for Cardiovascular Health." *Lancet*, 1977, *1*, 1192–1195.

Flay, B. R. "What We Know About the Social Influences Approach to Smoking Prevention: Review and Recommendations." In C. S. Bell and R. J. Battles (eds.), *Prevention Research: Deterring Drug Abuse Among Children and Adolescents*. National Institute for Drug Abuse Research Monograph no. 63, 1985.

Frederiksen, L. W., Martin, J. E., and Webster, J. S. "Assessment of Smoking Behavior." *Journal of Applied Behavior Analysis*, 1979, *12*, 653–664.

Havas, S., and others. "5-A-Day for Better Health." *Public Health Reports*, 1995, *110*(1), 68–79.

Iannotti, R. J., O'Brien, R. W., and Spillman, D. M. "Parental and Peer Influences on Food Consumption of Preschool African-American Children." *Perceptual and Motor Skills*, 1994, *79*, 747–752.

Kirby, S., Baranowski, T., Reynolds, K., Taylor, G., and Binkley, D. "Children's Fruit and Vegetable Intake: Socioeconomic, Adult Regional, and Urban-Rural Influences." *Journal of Nutrition Education*, 1995, *27*, 261–271.

Komro, K. A., and others. "How Did Project Northland Reduce Alcohol Use Among Young Adolescents? Analysis of Mediating Variables. *Health Education Research: Theory & Practice*, 2001, *16*, 59–70.

Lepper, M. R., and Cordova, D. I. "A Desire to Be Taught: Instructional Consequences of Intrinsic Motivation." *Motivation and Emotion*, 1992, *16*, 187–208.

Lewis, C. J., Sims, L. S., and Shannon, B. "Examination of Specific Nutrition/Health Behaviors Using a Social Cognitive Model." *Journal of the American Dietetic Association*, 1989, *89*, 194–202.

Luepker, R. V., and others. "Outcomes of a Trial to Improve Children's Dietary Patterns and Physical Activity: The Child and Adolescent Trial for Cardiovascular Health (CATCH)." *Journal of the American Medical Association*, 1996, *275*, 768–776.

Maibach, E., and Murphy, D. A. "Self-Efficacy in Health Promotion Research and Practice: Conceptualization and Measurement." *Health Education Research*, 1995, *10*, 37–50.

McLeroy, K. R., and others. "Social Science Theory in Health Education: Time for a New Model?" *Health Education Research*, 1994, *9*, 305–312.

Moos, R. H. *The Human Context: Environmental Determinants of Behavior*. New York: Wiley, 1976.

Parcel, G., and Baranowski, T. "Social Learning Theory and Health Education." *Health Education*, 1981, *12*, 14–18.

Parcel, G. S., and others. "Measurement of Self-Efficacy for Diet-Related Behaviors Among Elementary-School Children." *Journal of School Health*, 1995, *65*, 23–27.

Parraga, I. M. "Determinants of Food Consumption." *Journal of the American Dietetic Association*, 1990, *90*, 661–663.

Perry, C. L., and others. "Background, Conceptualization, and Design of a Community-Wide Research Program on Adolescent Alcohol Use: Project Northland." *Health Education Research*, 1993, *8*, 125–136.

Perry, C. L., and others. "Project Northland: Outcomes of a Community-Wide Alcohol Use Prevention Program During Early Adolescence." *American Journal of Public Health*, 1996, *86*, 956–965.

Perry, C. L., and others. "Project Northland High School Interventions: Community Action to Reduce Adolescent Alcohol Use." *Health Education & Behavior*, 2000, *27*, 29–49.

Resnicow, K., and others. "Psychosocial Correlates of Fruit and Vegetable Consumption." *Health Psychology*, 1997, *16*, 272–276.

Sallis, J. F., Nader, P. R., Rupp, J. W., Atkins, C. J., and Wilson, W. C. "San Diego Surveyed for Heart-Healthy Foods and Exercise Facilities." *Public Health Reports*, 1986, *101*, 216–219.

Sheeshka, J. D., Woolcott, J. D., and MacKinnon, N. J. "Social Cognitive Theory as a Framework to Explain Intentions to Practice Healthy Eating Behaviors." *Journal of Applied Social Psychology*, 1993, *23*, 1547–1573.

Simons-Morton, B. G., Parcel, G., Baranowski, T., Forthofer, R., and O'Hara, N. "Promoting Diet and Physical Activity Among Children: Results of a School-Based Intervention Study." *American Journal of Public Health*, 1991, *81*, 986–991.

Taylor, W., Baranowski, T., and Sallis, J. "Family Determinants of Childhood Physical Activity: A Social Cognitive Model." In R. K. Dishman (ed.), *Exercise Adherence: Its Impact on Public Health*. Champaign, Ill.: Human Kinetics Publishers, 1994.

Traub, R. E. *Reliability for the Social Sciences, Theory and Applications*. Thousand Oaks, Calif.: Sage, 1994.

Wetter, D. W., and others. "Smoking Outcome Expectancies: Factor Structure, Predictive Validity, and Discriminant Validity." *Journal of Abnormal Psychology*, 1994, *103*, 801–811.

CHAPTER NINE

SOCIAL NETWORKS AND SOCIAL SUPPORT

Catherine A. Heaney
Barbara A. Israel

The powerful influence that social relationships have on health has garnered great interest among health education and health behavior researchers and practitioners. An understanding of the impact of social relationships on health status, health behaviors, and health decision making contributes to the design of effective interventions for promoting health. Although there is no one theory that adequately explicates the link between social relationships and health, various conceptual models and theories have guided research in this area. This chapter provides a conceptual overview of and briefly reviews the empirical support for the link between social relationships and health, discusses implications for intervention, and presents two intervention examples to illustrate how the health-enhancing potential of social relationships has been used in health behavior and health education research and practice.

Definitions and Terminology

Several key terms have been used in studies of the health-enhancing components of social relationships (Berkman, Glass, Brissette, and Seeman, 2000). The term *social integration* has been used to refer to the existence of social ties. The term *social network* refers to the web of social relationships that surround individuals. The provision of *social support* is one of the important functions of social relationships.

Social networks are linkages between people that may (or may not) provide social support and that may serve functions other than providing support.

The structure of social networks can be described in terms of dyadic characteristics (in other words, characteristics of specific relationships between the focal individual and other people in the network) and in terms of characteristics of the network as a whole (Israel, 1982; House, Umberson, and Landis, 1988). Examples of dyadic characteristics include the extent to which resources and support are both given and received in a relationship (reciprocity), the extent to which a relationship is characterized by emotional closeness (intensity), and the extent to which a relationship serves a variety of functions (complexity). Examples of characteristics that describe a whole network include the extent to which network members are similar in terms of demographic characteristics such as age, race, and socioeconomic status (homogeneity); the extent to which network members live in close proximity to the focal person (geographic dispersion); and the extent to which network members know and interact with each other (density).

Social support has been defined and measured in numerous ways. According to House (1981), social support is the functional content of relationships that can be categorized into the following four broad types of supportive behaviors or acts:

- *Emotional support* involves the provision of empathy, love, trust, and caring.
- *Instrumental support* involves the provision of tangible aid and services that directly assist a person in need.
- *Informational support* involves the provision of advice, suggestions, and information that a person can use to address problems.
- *Appraisal support* involves the provision of information that is useful for self-evaluation purposes, in other words, constructive feedback, affirmation, and social comparison.

While these four types of support can be differentiated conceptually, relationships that provide one type often also provide other types, thus making it difficult to empirically study them as separate constructs. (For a comprehensive review of measurement and methodological issues, see Barrera, 2000; Cohen, Underwood, and Gottlieb, 2000). Table 9.1 summarizes the key concepts and their definitions.

Social support can be distinguished from other functions of social relationships (Burg and Seeman, 1994). Social support is always intended (by the sender) to be helpful, thus distinguishing it from intentional negative interactions (for example, angry criticism, hassling, undermining). Whether or not the intended support is perceived or experienced as helpful by the receiver is an empirical question, and indeed, negative perceptions and consequences of well-intended interper-

TABLE 9.1. TYPES AND CHARACTERISTICS OF SOCIAL NETWORKS AND SOCIAL SUPPORT.

Concepts	Definitions
Social network	A person-centered web of social relationships
Selected social network characteristics:	
Reciprocity	Extent to which resources and support are both given and received in a relationship
Intensity	Extent to which social relationships offer emotional closeness
Complexity	Extent to which social relationships serve many functions
Density	Extent to which network members know and interact with each other
Homogeneity	Extent to which network members are demographically similar
Geographic dispersion	Extent to which network members live in close proximity to focal person
Social support	Aid and assistance exchanged through social relationships and interpersonal transactions
Types of social support:	
Emotional support	Expressions of empathy, love, trust, and caring
Instrumental support	Tangible aid and service
Informational support	Advice, suggestions, and information
Appraisal support	Information that is useful for self-evaluation

Source: Based on Israel, 1982; House, 1981.

sonal exchanges have been identified (for example, Wortman and Lehman, 1985). In addition, social support is consciously provided by the sender, which sets it apart from the social influence exerted through simple observation of the behavior of others (Bandura, 1986) or from receiver-initiated social comparison processes (Taylor, Buunk, and Aspinwall, 1990). Finally, although the provision of social support, particularly informational support, can attempt to influence the thoughts and behaviors of the receiver, such informational support is provided in an interpersonal context of caring, trust, and respect for each person's right to make his or her own choices. This quality distinguishes social support from some other types of social influence that derive from the ability to provide or withhold desired resources or approval. See Chapter Eleven for a fuller treatment of social influence processes.

Although many investigations of the effects of social relationships on health have narrowly focused on the provision of social support, a broader social network approach has several advantages. First, a social network approach can incorporate functions or characteristics of social relationships other than social support (Israel, 1982; Berkman and Glass, 2000). For example, there is increasing evidence that negative interpersonal interactions, such as those characterized by mistrust, hassles, criticism, too many demands, and domination, are more strongly related to such factors as negative mood (Fleishman and others, 2000), unhappiness (Antonucci, Akiyama, and Lansford, 1998), risky health behaviors such as cigarette smoking (Burg and Seeman, 1994), and susceptibility to infectious disease (Cohen, Doyle, Skoner, Rabin, and Gwaltney, 1997) than is a lack of social support. Second, whereas a social support approach usually focuses on one relationship at a time, a social network approach allows for the study of how changes in one social relationship affect other relationships. Third, a social network approach facilitates the investigation of how structural and interactional network characteristics influence the quantity and quality of social support that are exchanged (McLeroy, Gottlieb, and Heaney, 2001). This information can be important for the development of effective support-enhancing interventions.

Background of the Concepts

Barnes's (1954) pioneering work in a Norwegian village first presented the concept of a social network to describe patterns of social relationships that were not easily explained by more traditional social units such as extended families or work groups. Much of the early work on social networks was exploratory and descriptive. The findings from these studies provided a knowledge base that helped identify network characteristics. In general, it was found that close-knit networks exchange more affective and instrumental support, and also exert more social influence on members to conform to network norms. Homogenous networks, networks with more reciprocal linkages, and networks with closer geographic proximity were also more effective in providing affective and instrumental support (see Israel, 1982; Berkman and Glass, 2000, for reviews).

The study of social support owes much to the work of social epidemiologist John Cassel (1976). Drawing from numerous animal and human studies, Cassel posited that social support served as a key psychosocial "protective" factor that reduced individuals' vulnerability to the deleterious effects of stress on health. He also specified that psychosocial factors such as social support were likely to play a nonspecific role in the etiology of disease. Thus, social support may influence the incidence and prevalence of a wide array of health outcomes.

From the previous analysis, it is clear that the terms *social network* and *social support* do not connote theories per se. Rather, they are concepts that describe the structure, processes, and functions of social relationships. Various sociological and social psychological theories (such as exchange theory, attachment theory, and symbolic interactionism) have been used to explain the basic interpersonal processes that underlie the association between social relationships and health (Berkman, Glass, Brissette, and Seeman, 2000; Israel and Rounds, 1987).

Conceptual Model of the Relationship of Social Networks and Social Support to Health

The mechanisms through which social networks and social support may have positive effects on physical, mental, and social health are summarized in Figure 9.1. The model depicts social networks and social support as the starting point or initiator of a causal flow toward health outcomes. In actuality, many of the relationships in Figure 9.1 entail reciprocal influence; for example, health status will influence the extent to which one is able to maintain and mobilize a social network.

In Figure 9.1, pathway 1 represents a hypothesized direct effect of social networks and social support on health. By meeting basic human needs for companionship, intimacy, a sense of belonging, and reassurance of one's worth as a person, supportive ties may enhance well-being and health regardless of stress levels (Berkman and Glass, 2000). Pathways 2 and 4 represent a hypothesized effect of social networks and social support on individual coping resources and community resources, respectively. For example, social networks and social support can enhance an individual's ability to access new contacts and information and to identify and solve problems. If the support provided helps to reduce uncertainty and unpredictability or helps to produce desired outcomes, then a sense of personal control over specific situations and life domains will be enhanced. In addition, the theory of symbolic interactionism suggests that human behavior is based on the meaning that people assign to events. This meaning is derived, in large part, from their social interactions (Israel, 1982; Berkman, Glass, Brissette, and Seeman, 2000). Thus, people's social network linkages may help them reinterpret events or problems in a more positive and constructive light (Thoits, 1995).

The potential effects of social networks and social support on organizational and community competence are less well studied. However, strengthening social networks and enhancing the exchange of social support may increase a community's ability to garner its resources and solve problems. Several community-level interventions have shown how intentional network building and the strengthening

FIGURE 9.1. THE RELATIONSHIP OF SOCIAL NETWORKS
AND SOCIAL SUPPORT TO HEALTH.

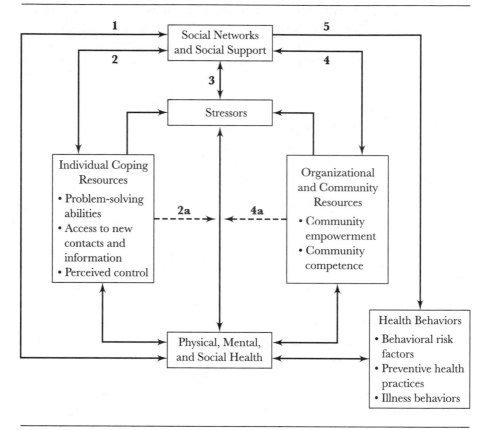

of social support within communities are associated with enhanced community capacity and control (Minkler, 2001; Eng and Parker, 1994).

Resources at both the individual and community levels may have direct health-enhancing effects and may also diminish the negative effects on health due to exposure to stressors. When people experience stressors, having enhanced individual or community resources increases the likelihood that stressors will be handled or coped with in a way that reduces both short-term and long-term adverse health consequences. This effect is called a "buffering effect" and is reflected in pathways 2a and 4a. Research involving people going through major life transitions (such as the loss of a spouse or the birth of a child) has shown how social networks and social support influence the coping process and buffer the effects of the stressor on health (Rhodes, Contreras, and Mangelsdorf, 1994; Hirsch and DuBois, 1992).

Pathway 3 suggests that social networks and social support may influence the frequency and duration of exposure to stressors. For example, a supportive supervisor may ensure that an employee is not given more work to do than time allows for it to be completed. Similarly, having a social network that is able to provide information about new jobs may reduce the likelihood that a person will suffer from long-term unemployment. Reduced exposure to stressors is then, in turn, associated with enhanced mental and physical health.

Pathway 5 reflects the potential effects of social networks and social support on health behaviors. Through the interpersonal exchanges within a social network, individuals are influenced and supported in such health behaviors as adherence to medical regimens (Catz, Kelly, Bogart, Benotsch, and McAuliffe, 2000), help-seeking behavior (McKinlay, 1980; Starrett, Bresler, Decker, Walters, and Rogers, 1990), smoking cessation (Palmer, Baucom, and McBride, 2000), and weight loss (Wing and Jeffery, 1999). Through influences on preventive health behavior, illness behavior, and sick-role behavior, pathway 5 makes explicit that social networks and social support may affect the incidence of and recovery from disease.

Empirical Evidence on the Influence of Social Relationships

Numerous reviews of the empirical studies address the influence of social relationships on health (see for example Barrera, 2000; Berkman and Glass, 2000; Thoits, 1995). Although there are some inconsistencies in this body of research, few today would disagree with House's summary statement made over a decade ago: "Although the results of individual studies are usually open to alternative interpretations, the patterns of results across the full range of studies strongly suggests that what are variously termed social relationships, social networks, and social support have important causal effects on health, exposure to stress, and the relationship between stress and health" (House, 1987, p. 136).

Prospective epidemiological studies, most often using measures of social integration, consistently find a relationship between a lack of social relationships and all-cause mortality (Berkman and Glass, 2000). More recently, a number of studies documented that intimate ties and the emotional support provided by them increase survival rates among people with severe cardiovascular disease (Berkman and Glass, 2000). Evidence for buffering effects is less conclusive, but studies do suggest that social support mobilized to help a person cope with a stressor reduces the negative effects of the stressor on health (Cohen and Wills, 1985; Thoits, 1995). Although the direct effects and the buffering effects of social networks and social support were initially investigated as either-or relationships, evidence suggests that social support and social networks have both types of effects, and that the predominance of one effect over the other depends on the target population, the situation being studied, and the ways in which the social relationship concept is measured (Cohen and Wills, 1985; House, Umberson, and Landis, 1988; Krause, 1995; Thoits, 1995).

The effect of social relationships on all-cause mortality supports the hypothesis, first put forth by Cassel (1976), that the effect of social relationships on health is not specific to any one disease process. This nonspecific role may explain why studies of the effect of social relationships on specific morbidities have not been conclusive (House, Umberson, and Landis, 1988; Berkman and Glass, 2000). Although evidence for a link between social networks and social support and the incidence of particular diseases is inconsistent (Vogt, Mullooly, Ernst, Pope, and Hollis, 1992), a positive role for affective support in the processes of coping with and recovering from serious illness has been consistently documented (Holahan, Moos, Holahan, and Brennan, 1997; Spiegel and Diamond, 2001).

The association between social relationships and health does not follow a linear dose-response curve. Rather, very low levels of social integration are most deleterious, with higher levels being less advantageous once a threshold level has been reached (House, 1981). Having at least one strong intimate relationship is an important predictor of good health (Michael, Colditz, Coakley, and Kawachi, 1999). For example, in a study of African American elderly women, severe social isolation (in other words, living alone and not having had contact with family or friends during the previous two weeks) was associated with a three-fold increase in mortality during a five-year follow-up period (LaVeist, Sellers, Elliott Brown, and Nickerson, 1997).

Of the several types of support that can be exchanged among network members, emotional support is known to be the most strongly and consistently associated with good health and well-being (see Israel and Rounds, 1987 for a review). However, studies also found that low instrumental support is independently and significantly associated with high blood pressure (Strogatz and others, 1997) and depressive symptoms (Israel, Farquahar, Schulz, James, and Parker, forthcoming), particularly within low-income communities of color.

The influence of social network characteristics on social support, health behavior, and health status has been less thoroughly examined than has the relationship between social support and health (Berkman and Glass, 2000). However, the results of earlier reviews of the literature suggest that the social network's reciprocity and intensity were somewhat consistently linked to positive mental health (Israel, 1982; House, Umberson, and Landis, 1988). In addition, networks that were characterized by few ties, high-intensity relationships, high density, and close geographic proximity maintained social identity and the exchange of affective support. Thus, these networks were most health-enhancing when these social network functions were needed. However, during times of transition and change, networks that are larger, more diffuse, and composed of less intense ties may be more adaptive because they are better at facilitating social outreach and the exchange of informational support. Furthermore, more recent studies provide evidence that the size and density of social networks that endorse risk-taking norms are associated with higher levels of risk-taking behaviors such as injection drug use (Berkman and Glass, 2000).

Demographically defined subgroups maintain qualitatively different social networks and experience health benefits from those networks (House, Umberson, and Landis, 1988). Shumaker and Hill (1991) reviewed gender differences in the link between social support and physical health. They suggested that the prospective epidemiological studies investigating the effect of social relationships on mortality found a weaker health-protective effect for women than for men. In addition, women of a particular age group (usually over fifty years of age) experienced a positive association between high levels of social support and mortality. Noting that women tend to cast a "wider net of concern" (that is, maintain more strong ties), are more likely to be both the providers and recipients of social support, and are more responsive to the life events of others than are men, the authors suggest that further study is needed to explore the impact of these differences on the health-protective potential of women's social networks.

Translating Theory and Research into Practice

Results from the literature suggest that any support-enhancing intervention needs to begin with an assessment of the social networks that are maintained by the study population. Such assessments can diagnose aspects of existing social networks that are not meeting the needs of the focal individuals, as well as point out the strengths of the networks. Several network mapping and assessment tools are available (see Barrera, 2000; Berkman and Glass, 2000, for reviews; and Norbeck, Lindsey, and Carrieri, 1983). The evidence for the health-enhancing effects of affective support suggests that interactions with potential helpers should facilitate expressions of trust, closeness, and caring. In addition, the importance of reciprocity for well-being suggests that helping relationships should be founded on a basis of mutual interdependence and exchange.

Although the literature provides clear implications for practice, health education and health behavior researchers who implement social network enhancement interventions face several decision points. House (1981) summarized these decision points in a single question: In order to effectively enhance the health-protective functions of social networks, *who* should provide *what* to *whom* (and *when*)? The issues of *who, what,* and *when* are next discussed.

Who

Social support can be provided by many types of people both in a natural or informal network (for example, family, friends, coworkers, supervisors) and in more formal helping networks (for example, health care professionals, human service workers). Different network members are likely to provide differing amounts and types of support (McLeroy, Gottlieb, and Heaney, 2001). In addition, the effectiveness of the support provided may depend on the source of the support (House, 1981). For example, long-term assistance is most often provided by family members; neighbors and friends more likely provide short-term aid (McLeroy, Gottlieb, and Heaney, 2001). In medical care settings, patients often need emotional support from family and friends and informational support from health care professionals (Blanchard and others, 1995).

Thoits offered a more comprehensive approach to defining an effective source of support. The effective provision of support is likely to stem from people who are socially similar to the support recipients and who have experienced similar stressors or situations (Thoits, 1995). These characteristics enhance the "empathic understanding" of the support provider, making it more likely that the support proffered is in concert with the needs and values of the recipient. In addition, the person who desires the support is more likely to overcome the stigma attached to needing help and to seek or mobilize support when the social network member is perceived to be empathic and understanding. Empathic understanding is particularly relevant to the exchange of emotional support, but it also applies to instrumental and informational support.

Long-standing, intimate social network ties have unique capabilities to provide social support (Gottlieb and Wagner, 1991). However, there can be a downside to depending on these types of relationships for support, particularly informational support. Gottlieb and Wagner (1991) noted that people in close relationships are often distressed by the same stressor and that the nature and quality of the support provided is affected by the distress levels of the helper. Also, because the support providers are very interested in the well-being of the support recipients, when support attempts are not well-received or do not result in positive changes in the receiver, the helpers can react negatively. This is most likely to occur when information or advice are provided. Intimate ties may be best used for emotional support, but other relationships may be better suited for informational support (Gottlieb, 2000).

Considerable debate exists on whether professional helpers are effective sources of social support. Health education interventions may attempt to enhance the social support available to participants by linking them with professional helpers. Professional helpers often have access to information and resources that are not otherwise available in the social network. However, when mapping their social networks, few people include professional helpers as members of their networks (Veroff, Douvan, and Kulka, 1981), and professional helpers are rarely available to provide social support over long periods of time. Additionally, professional-lay relationships are not typically reciprocal and may involve large power differentials or lack of the empathic understanding just described. Thus, a combination of formal and informal helpers may be most effective in situations in which both informational and emotional support are needed.

What

The *perceptions* of support recipients, rather than the *objective* behaviors involved in interactions, are most strongly linked to recipients' health and well-being (Wethington and Kessler, 1986). To design interventions to enhance social support, it is necessary to identify factors that may influence whether behaviors are perceived as supportive. These factors include previous experiences of the support recipient with the helper, the social context of the relationship (for example, are the two people in competition for resources? Does one have the power to reward or punish the other?), role expectations, and individual preferences for types and amounts of social support.

Given the multiple factors that affect how social interactions are perceived, a priori assumptions about which specific behaviors increase perceived social support may be ill-advised. Ways in which social network members can be more supportive can be best identified through participation of the target population. Discussion among the interested parties could include previous successful support efforts and support efforts that have gone awry; such discussion could also generate a set of desired social behaviors and skills specific to the population and problem being addressed. For example, a program designed to enhance coworker and supervisor support used a group format in which employees gleaned suggestions on ways to modify their behavior from the stories of other employees' effective, supportive social interactions (Heaney, 1991). Similar strategies have been used in smoking cessation interventions that attempted to enhance the support for cessation provided by significant others (Palmer, Baucom, and McBride, 2000).

When

Research has suggested that the types of social networks and social support that effectively enhance well-being and health differ according to the age or developmental stage of the support recipient (Kahn and Antonucci, 1980). In addition, people who are experiencing a major life transition or stressor benefit from different types of support during the various stages of coping with the stressor (Thoits, 1995). For example, people whose spouses have just died may benefit from a close-knit, dense social network that is able to provide strong affective support to the bereaved. However, as the widowed individuals modify their lives to adapt to their losses, more diffuse networks that offer access to new social ties and diverse informational support may be most helpful.

Social Network and Social Support Interventions

Several typologies of social network and social support interventions have been suggested (Israel, 1982; McLeroy, Gottlieb, and Heaney, 2001; Gottlieb, 2000). Table 9.2 presents a typology that has four categories of interventions: enhancing existing social network linkages, developing new social network linkages, enhancing networks through the use of indigenous natural helpers, and enhancing networks at the community level through participatory community capacity building and problem-solving processes. A fifth category is composed of interventions that use a combination of these types of interventions. Interventions in these five categories are next briefly described, highlighting the challenges and potential benefits of each type. The quantity and quality of the research investigating the effectiveness of social network interventions differs across the types of intervention. Further research is needed to assess the efficacy of the various interventions and the conditions under which each of the types of interventions are most likely effective.

Enhancing existing network ties. Existing network ties often offer much untapped potential. Interventions aimed at enhancing existing ties attempt to change the attitudes and behaviors of the support recipient, the support provider, or both. The transactional nature of social exchanges suggests that the latter may be most effective, and some research is consistent with this suggestion (Heaney, 1991).

Interventions to enhance existing relationships often include activities to build skills for effective support mobilization, provision, and receipt. They may focus on enhancing the quality of social ties to address specific health issues or to provide support across many different situations. For example, family members were used to provide instrumental aid (monitoring blood pressure) and affective support to those with hypertension (Morisky, DeMuth, Field-Fass, Green, and Levine, 1985). Similarly, partners or significant others were incorporated into smoking cessation programs (Palmer, Baucom, and McBride, 2000) and weight loss programs (Wing and Jeffery, 1999).

Some of the challenges with this type of intervention include identifying existing network members who are committed to providing support and have the resources to sustain the commitment, identifying the changes in attitudes and behaviors that will result in increased perceived support on the part of the support

TABLE 9.2. TYPOLOGY OF SOCIAL NETWORK INTERVENTIONS.

Intervention Type	Examples of Intervention Activities	Selected References
Enhancing existing social network linkages	• Training of network members in skills for providing support • Training of focal individual in mobilizing and maintaining social networks • Systems approach (for example, marital counseling or family therapy	Heaney, 1991 Sandler and others, 1992 Wing and Jeffery, 1999
Developing new social network linkages	• Creating linkages to mentors • Developing buddy systems • Coordinating self-help groups	Heller and others, 1991 Helgeson and Gottlieb, 2000 Chesler and Chesney, 1995
Enhancing networks through the use of indigenous natural helpers	• Identification of natural helpers in the community • Analysis of natural helpers' existing social networks • Training of natural helpers in health topics and community problem-solving strategies	Eng and Hatch, 1991 Earp and others, 1997
Enhancing networks through community capacity building and problem solving	• Identification of overlapping networks within the community • Examination of social network characteristics of members of the selected need or target area • Facilitation of ongoing community problem identification and problem solving	Minkler, 2001 Boutilier, Cleverly, and LaBonte, 2000

recipient, and intervening in ways that are consistent with established norms and styles of interaction.

Developing new social network linkages. Interventions that are designed to develop new social network linkages are most useful when the existing network is small, overburdened, or unable to provide effective support. Sometimes new ties are introduced to alleviate chronic social isolation such as that experienced by the elderly (Heller, Thompson, Trueba, Hogg, and Vlachos-Weber, 1991). Most often new ties are introduced in response to a major life transition or specific stressor.

In such cases, the existing network may lack the requisite experiential or specialized knowledge about the specific stressor.

Some interventions introduce *mentors* or *advisers* who are people who have already coped with the situation being experienced by the focal individual (Eckenrode and Hamilton, 2000). Other interventions introduce *buddies* who are experiencing the stressor or life transition at the same time as the focal person. For example, in some smoking cessation programs and weight-control programs, participants are encouraged to "buddy up" with another participant so the two of them can provide support and encouragement to each other (Palmer, Baucom, and McBride, 2000).

Self-help or mutual aid groups provide a new *set* of network ties. Usually, people come together in self-help groups because they are facing a common stressor or because they want to bring about similar changes, either at the individual level (for example, individual weight loss) or at a community level (for example, increased access to health care in one's community). In self-help or mutual aid groups, the roles of support provider and support recipient are mutually shared among the members. Thus, the ties often entail high levels of reciprocity. Such groups can be particularly effective for participants who cannot mobilize social support from their other social relationships. Although a full description of self-help groups is beyond the scope of this chapter, several good reviews and descriptions exist; for example, see Chesler and Chesney (1995) and Helgeson and Gottlieb (2000).

The use of indigenous natural helpers. Natural helpers are members of social networks to whom other network members naturally turn for advice, support, and other types of aid (Israel, 1985). They are usually respected and trusted network members who are responsive to the needs of others. In addition to providing support directly to network members, natural helpers can link social network members to each other and to resources outside of the network.

One of the first tasks in natural helper interventions is to identify the people who currently fill these helping roles. Although various strategies have been used to do this (Eng and Young, 1992), they commonly ask people in the community for the names of people who demonstrate the characteristics of natural helpers. The participation of community members in the identification process is critical. Those people whose names are repeatedly mentioned can be contacted and recruited. Once the natural helpers are recruited, the health professional can provide the needed information on specific health topics, on health and human service resources available in the community, and on community problem-solving strategies, and can engage in a consultative relationship with the natural helpers.

Natural helper interventions have been conducted in a number of different communities, including urban neighborhoods, rural counties, residential institutions for the elderly, migrant farmworker streams, and church congregations (Israel, 1985; Eng and Hatch, 1991). For example, the Black Churches Project (Eng and Hatch, 1991) identified natural helpers within congregations of black churches in North Carolina and provided training in health promotion concepts and skills to the identified helpers. The goals of the project were to enhance the health behaviors of members of the congregations by having the natural helpers provide information, advice, emotional support, and access to resources.

Enhancing networks through community capacity building and problem solving. Interventions that involve community members in identifying and resolving community problems may indirectly strengthen the social networks that exist in the community. Such interventions (see, for example, Boutilier, Cleverly, and Labonte, 2000; Rothman, Erlich and Tropman, 2001) use community organizing techniques with the goals of (1) enhancing the capacity of a community to resolve its problems, (2) increasing the community's role in making decisions that have important implications for community life, and (3) resolving specific problems. Through participation in collective problem-solving processes, community members forge new network ties and strengthen existing ones. For example, in the Tenderloin Senior Outreach Project, elderly residents in the Tenderloin district of San Francisco formed groups and coalitions to address safety and health concerns. Through participation in these groups, the residents became less socially isolated and began to turn to each other for information, advice, and support (Minkler, 2001). See Chapter Thirteen for an extended analysis of community organizing and capacity development.

Although community problem-solving interventions indirectly affect social networks, social network strategies could be incorporated into both the assessment and implementation stages of these interventions (Israel, 1985). The community assessment could determine how people gain information, resources, and support as well as identify potential problem areas. Examining the extent to which people's networks overlap may aid in the diffusion of new information throughout the community.

Combining strategies. Some programs have combined the intervention strategies described above to maximize the impact of the program. For example, a program that enhances existing network ties and also forges new ties can benefit from well-established social relationships and the infusion of new social resources. In the Family Bereavement Program (Sandler and others, 1992), members of families that experienced a loss attended workshops during which they explored ways family members could provide support to each other. During the workshops, the participants also engaged in supportive interactions with other bereaved families. After participating in the workshops, each family was matched with a family adviser. This adviser then provided ongoing emotional and informational support, shoring up overburdened family sources of support.

Combining natural helper interventions with community problem-solving is another potentially effective strategy (Eng and Hatch, 1991; Schulz and others, forthcoming). Although natural helpers can address the needs of the individual network members, the community-level strategy can address some of the broader social, legal, and economic problems facing the community. This results in a more comprehensive ecological approach to enhancing the health of the community. Lay health advisers may be able to enhance the effectiveness of community-level problem solving by integrating community residents more fully into the life of the community, and, more specifically, into cooperative problem-solving efforts. Future research is needed to evaluate the efficacy of combining these social network strategies.

Health Education and Health Behavior Applications

The following section describes two interventions that illustrate how social network and social support concepts were applied to practice. The first intervention develops new social network linkages by matching youth with adult mentors. The second example involves social network intervention with natural helpers.

Big Brothers Big Sisters

In April 1997, the President's Summit for America's Future highly touted the potential of mentoring programs for reducing the risks faced by American youth. Research documents that social connectedness is a major factor in protecting youths from engaging in behaviors detrimental to their health (see for example Resnick and others, 1997). Because demographic trends such as an increase in single-parent households and longer work hours for many Americans may be limiting adolescents' opportunities to interact with caring adults, programmatic attempts to increase these opportunities have been recommended (Resnick and others, 1997).

One well-known youth-mentoring program in the United States is Big Brothers Big Sisters (BBBS) (Furano, Roak, Styles, and Branch, 1993). BBBS programs have provided mentors to youths living in single-parent households for more than ninety years. The BBBS national office provides program standards and guidelines to its local affiliates. The affiliates then apply these standards and tailor them to the needs and resources of the local community. BBBS recruits adult volunteers who are interested in serving as mentors and matches them with youths who have requested a mentor. Volunteers must commit to spending approximately twelve hours a month with their mentees for at least one year. Program staff match mentors and youths based on gender, geographic proximity, and availability. Some programs also consider the matching preferences of both volunteers and youths in terms of age, race, religion, and interests. Once matches are made, BBBS staff members initiate monthly contact with both the mentor and the youth or the youth's parent. BBBS agencies provide an orientation for volunteers during which program procedures are described. Further training on topics such as child development and relationship building is sometimes offered, but not required (Furano, Roak, Styles, and Branch, 1993).

The impact of the BBBS mentoring program has been evaluated using a randomized controlled trial (Tierney and Grossman, with Resch, 1995). The evaluation study enrolled 959 youths who requested BBBS mentors in eight cities around the country. The youths ranged in age from ten to sixteen years old; 60 percent were boys; more than 50 percent were minorities. The youths were randomly assigned to be matched with a mentor according to usual BBBS procedures or to be waitlisted for the eighteen months of the study. Of the 487 youths who were assigned to the usual intervention group, 378 (78 percent) were matched with mentors.

After eighteen months, comparisons of intervention group youths (including those who had not been matched with a mentor) with those in the control group demonstrated various positive benefits of the program. Intervention group youths had statistically significant better attitudes toward school and better school attendance, improved relationships with their parents and peers, less likelihood of antisocial behavior such as hitting someone, and less likelihood of initiating drug and alcohol use. The intervention group was 46 percent less likely to begin using drugs and 27 percent less likely to begin using alcohol than the control group. The benefits were even more marked among the minority youths. Minority youths in the intervention group were 70 percent less likely to engage in drug use than were their control group counterparts. There was no significant impact of the program on tobacco use (Tierney and Grossman, with Resch, 1995). The impact of the program not only included reducing specific risk behaviors such as substance use, it also improved the mentees' abilities to maintain supportive social relationships. For example, boys in the intervention group experienced a greater exchange of emotional support through their peer relationships and increased trust and communication with their parents.

Although the results of this evaluation study are quite positive, they need to be interpreted cautiously. Results should not be generalized to mentor programs that do not provide careful attention to the selection and training of volunteers and to the monitoring of the mentoring relationship (Tierney and Grossman, with Resch, 1995). Other mentor programs have not been as successful as the BBBS programs in terms of establishing long-lasting mentoring relationships (Mecartney, Styles, and Morrow, 1994). In addition, the BBBS evaluation study provides little guidance on the qualities of the mentoring relationship that were most likely to lead to beneficial outcomes for the youths. To date, there is little empirical evidence available to help mentors establish and maintain effective mentoring relationships. A qualitative study of eighty-two BBBS mentoring relationships (Styles and Morrow, 1992) concluded that mentors who believed that their major role was to support the growth and development of their mentees were more successful than mentors who believed that their major role was to "reform" or change their mentees. The results of this study have been used to inform the development of guidelines for successful mentoring relationships (Jucovy, 2001).

The evaluation of the BBBS program provides rigorous empirical support for the potential benefits of youth-mentoring programs. However, much remains to be learned about how best to implement such programs. Recent reviews of mentoring programs (Barrera and Prelow, 2000; Eckenrode and Hamilton, 2000) suggest that further research is needed to describe the optimal procedures for identifying, recruiting, and orienting both mentors and mentees. The advantages and disadvantages of various procedures for matching mentors with youths are also not yet well understood and require further study. In addition, the effects of such programs on the mentors themselves deserves careful consideration. Knowledge of the benefits and challenges experienced by mentors might aid in future recruitment and training efforts. Last, further examination is needed on whether such programs strengthen aspects of social networks and social support.

North Carolina Breast Cancer Screening Program

Although the incidence of breast cancer is no higher among African American women than among white women in the United States, the five-year survival rates for African American women are lower than they are for whites (Hunter, 2000). Differences in survival are due in part to African American women being diagnosed at a later stage of the disease; an ethnic gap in the use of mammography screening explains some of these differences (McCarthy and others, 1998). In an effort to reduce this ethnic disparity among older African American women, the North Carolina Breast Cancer Screening Program (NC-BCSP) used a natural helper intervention for increasing mammography screening.

The NC-BCSP is an outgrowth of the Save Our Sisters (SOS) Project, which was conducted in one rural county of North Carolina (Eng, 1993). As an initial qualitative investigation of the mammography use behavior of African American women in the county, fourteen focus groups were conducted. Two major themes relevant to the social networks of this population were identified from the focus group data: the women tended to seek support from other women in the community when dealing with matters of women's health, and many of the women belonged to social groups that were an important aspect of the community's vitality (Tessaro, Eng, and Smith, 1994). These themes suggested that building on the strengths of these social networks through the use of natural helpers to serve as "lay health advisers" (LHAs) might be an effective strategy for exchanging informational, emotional, and instrumental support for mammography screening (Eng and Young, 1992). Specifically, those best positioned in African American communities to assist older women in overcoming prevailing fears and reticence about breast cancer were likely to be other women who were slightly younger; active members of community organizations that put them in contact with women from all income groups; and known for their good judgment, discretion, and willingness to help others. The SOS Project then created a structure and context within which LHAs could effectively support women in the community in learning about and gaining access to mammography screening (Eng, 1993).

The NC-BCSP built on the lessons learned through the SOS Project and extended the use of LHAs to five poor, rural counties in North Carolina (Earp and others, 1997; Earp and others, forthcoming). The project included the following components: identification and recruitment of LHAs, provision of training to the LHAs to increase their knowledge of breast cancer and mammography and to enhance their interpersonal and group process skills, ongoing consultation with the LHAs for exchanging informational and emotional support through community projects, and evaluation. All of these components were implemented within a community partnership framework.

Five community outreach specialists were hired to recruit, train, and support the LHAs. These specialists were African American women who were long-time residents of the target counties. They were based in the local health departments and organized Community Advisory Groups (CAGs) in each of the counties. CAG members were African American men and women who were the "movers and shakers" in their communities. Each CAG developed a list of potential LHAs who were contacted by the specialists. In addition to identifying and recruiting LHAs, the CAGs assisted with the logistics of LHA training sessions, helped make links between health care providers and LHAs, and participated in the development of county-specific educational materials and events.

The women who were interested in participating as LHAs completed ten to twelve hours of training. This training provided information about breast cancer, mammography, and the health care system; addressed the potential roles of lay health advisers; and provided opportunities to build skills in interpersonal counseling and small group facilitation. A total of 148 LHAs participated in the training, and approximately 75 percent remained active over the three years of the project. Once training was completed, LHAs met regularly as a group with the community outreach specialists in each county to plan future activities and provide support and encouragement to each other.

Both process and outcome data were collected as part of the evaluation of the NC-BCSP. LHAs were encouraged to submit "activity reports" to the specialists. Although not all LHAs completed these reports on a regular basis, results suggested that LHAs conducted an average of one group presentation every three months and made one to three individual contacts per week (Earp and Flax, 1999). Interviews with women who had had some contact with an LHA suggested that LHAs were perceived as approachable and credible sources of information about mammography (Flax and Earp, 1999). Both LHAs and the women they contacted reported that almost all of the contacts provided informational support, with instrumental and emotional support exchanged in a smaller proportion of the LHA interactions (Flax and Earp, 1999).

For the outcome evaluation, a representative sample of African American women in the five intervention counties and five comparison counties was surveyed both before the intervention began and then three years later. The primary outcome measure was self-reported mammography use during the last two years. Although direct contact with the LHAs was restricted to a relatively small proportion (15 percent) of the women in the survey sample from the intervention counties, the women in the intervention counties reported a marginally statistically significant 6 percent greater increase in communitywide mammography use than did the women in the comparison counties (Earp and others, forthcoming). In addition, the intervention reduced the disparity in use of screening mammography between African Americans and whites, particularly among lower-income women. Among women with family incomes below $12,000 a year, African American women's mammography use increased from 37 percent to 59 percent compared with an increase from 54 percent to 60 percent for white women (Earp, Rauscher, and O'Malley, 2000).

A notable limitation of LHA interventions was that they did not equally benefit all members of the community. Those who were socially isolated and were not already embedded in the social networks of the LHAs were unlikely to benefit. In the NC-BCSP intervention counties, women with higher incomes reported more contact with the LHAs (who tended to have higher incomes themselves) than did lower income women (Earp and others, forthcoming). LHA activity reports indicated that more than two thirds of their direct contacts were with friends and family with whom they interacted regularly (Earp and Flax, 1999). These results underscore the importance of LHAs being recruited from diverse existing social networks.

Future Directions for Research and Practice

Evaluation of carefully designed and meticulously implemented theory-informed social network interventions will help advance our ability to answer the question posed earlier: To effectively enhance the health-protective functions of social networks, *who* should provide *what* to *whom* (and *when*)? There is unlikely to be a generic social network intervention that is effective for everyone. Instead, social network programs need to be tailored to the needs and resources of the participants. Thus, establishing participatory assessment processes during which participants describe the strengths and weaknesses of their social networks will help structure programs to be optimally effective.

Social network interventions are most likely to be effective if developed and implemented within an ecological framework that considers multiple levels of influence. For example, interventions that enhance individuals' motivation and skills for performing healthy behaviors while also enhancing the health-promotive qualities of social networks have great potential. In addition, given our growing understanding of the extent to which broad social forces (for example, crime rates and income disparities) influence the structure and function of social networks (Berkman, Glass, Brissette, and Seeman, 2000), interventions that attempt to enhance social networks within the context of community-based problem-solving efforts hold promise. Thus, an important direction for future research is to develop and evaluate social network interventions that include strategies across multiple units of practice (for example, individual, family, and community).

It is important to evaluate both intervention processes and outcomes (Israel and others, 1995). As the two applications illustrate, effective social network interventions will be advanced through (1) careful description of the intervention activities; (2) monitoring of the effects of these activities on the amount and quality of social support that is both delivered and received; and (3) assessment of changes in knowledge, health behaviors, community capacity, or health status. Rigorous and comprehensive evaluation studies will improve our ability to consistently translate the health protective effects of social networks and social support into effective interventions.

References

Antonucci, T. C., Akiyama, H., and Lansford, J. E. "Negative Effects of Close Social Relations." *Family Relations,* 1998, *47,* 379–384.

Bandura, A. *Social Foundations of Thought and Action.* Englewood Cliffs, N.J.: Prentice Hall, 1986.

Barnes, J. A. "Class and Committees in a Norwegian Island Parish." *Human Relations,* 1954, *7,* 39–58.

Barrera, M. "Social Support Research in Community Psychology." In J. Rappaport and E. Seidman (eds.), *Handbook of Community Psychology.* New York: Kluwer Academic/Plenum, 2000.

Barrera, M., and Prelow, H. "Interventions to Promote Social Support in Children and Adolescents." In D. Cicchetti, J. Rappaport, I. Sandler, and R. P. Weissberg (eds.), *The Promotion of Wellness in Children and Adolescents.* Washington, D.C.: CWLA Press, 2000.

Berkman, L. F., and Glass, T. "Social Integration, Social Networks, Social Support, and Health." In L. F. Berkman and I. Kawachi (eds.), *Social Epidemiology.* New York: Oxford Press, 2000.

Berkman, L. F., Glass, T., Brissette, I., and Seeman, T. E. "From Social Integration to Health: Durkheim in the New Millenium." *Social Science and Medicine,* 2000, *51,* 843–857.

Blanchard, C. G., and others. "The Role of Social Support in Adaptation to Cancer and to Survival." *Journal of Psychosocial Oncology,* 1995, *13,* 75–95.

Boutilier, M., Cleverly, S., and Labonte, R. "Community as a Setting for Health Promotion." In B. D. Poland, L. W. Green, and I. Rootman (eds.), *Settings for Health Promotion: Linking Theory and Practice.* Thousand Oaks, Calif.: Sage, 2000.

Burg, M. M., and Seeman, T. E. "Families and Health: The Negative Side of Social Ties." *Annals of Behavioral Medicine,* 1994, *16,* 109–115.

Cassel, J. "The Contribution of the Social Environment to Host Resistance." *American Journal of Epidemiology,* 1976, *104,* 107–123.

Catz, S. L., Kelly, J. A., Bogart, L. M., Benotsch, E. G., and McAuliffe, T. L. "Patterns, Correlates, and Barriers to Medication Adherence Among Persons Prescribed New Treatments for HIV Disease." *Health Psychology,* 2000, *19,* 124–133.

Chesler, M. A., and Chesney, B. K. *Cancer and Self-Help: Bridging the Troubled Waters of Childhood Illness.* Madison, Wis.: University of Wisconsin Press, 1995.

Cohen, S., Doyle, W. J., Skoner, D. P., Rabin, B. S., and Gwaltney, J. M. "Social Ties and Susceptibility to the Common Cold." *Journal of the American Medical Association,* 1997, *277,* 1940–1944.

Cohen, S., Underwood, L. G., and Gottlieb, B. H. (eds.). *Social Support Measurement and Intervention.* New York: Oxford University Press, 2000.

Cohen, S., and Wills, T. "Stress, Social Support, and the Buffering Hypothesis." *Psychological Bulletin,* 1985, *98,* 310–357.

Earp, J. L., and Flax, V. "What Lay Health Advisors Do." *Cancer Practice,* 1999, *7,* 16–21.

Earp, J. L., Rauscher, G., and O'Malley, M. S. "Closing the Black-White Gap in Mammography Use." Paper presented at the 128th annual meeting of the American Public Health Association. Boston, 2000.

Earp, J. L., and others. "Lay Health Advisors: A Strategy for Getting the Word Out About Breast Cancer." *Health Education & Behavior,* 1997, *24,* 432–451.

Earp, J. L., and others. "Increasing Use of Mammography Among Older Rural African American Women: Initial Results from a Controlled Trial." *American Journal of Public Health,* forthcoming.

Eckenrode, J., and Hamilton, S. "One-to-One Support Interventions: Home Visitation and Mentoring." In S. Cohen, L. G. Underwood, and B. H. Gottlieb (eds.), *Social Support Measurement and Intervention.* New York: Oxford University Press, 2000.

Eng, E. "The Save Our Sisters Project: A Social Network Strategy for Reaching Rural Black Women." *Cancer,* 1993, *72,* 1071–1077.

Eng, E., and Hatch, J. W. "Networking Between Agencies and Black Churches: The Lay Health Advisor Model." *Prevention in Human Services,* 1991, *10,* 123–146.

Eng, E., and Parker, E. "Measuring Community Competence in the Mississippi Delta: The Interface between Program Evaluation and Empowerment." *Health Education Quarterly,* 1994, *21,* 199–220.

Eng, E., and Young, R. "Lay Health Advisors as Community Change Agents." *Family and Community Health,* 1992, *15,* 24–40.

Flax, V. L., and Earp, J. L. "Counseled Women's Perspectives on Their Interactions with Lay Health Advisors: A Feasibility Study." *Health Education Research,* 1999, *14,* 15–24.

Fleishman, J. A., and others. "Coping, Conflictual Social Interactions, Social Support, and Mood Among HIV-Infected Persons." *American Journal of Community Psychology,* 2000, *28*(4), 421–430.

Furano, K., Roak, P. A., Styles, M. B., and Branch, A. Y. *Big Brothers/Big Sisters: A Study of Program Practices.* Philadelphia: Public/Private Ventures, 1993.

Gottlieb, B. H. "Selecting and Planning Support Interventions." In S. Cohen, L. G. Underwood, and B. H. Gottlieb (eds.), *Social Support Measurement and Intervention.* New York: Oxford University Press, 2000.

Gottlieb, B. H., and Wagner, F. "Stress and Support Processes in Close Relationships." In J. Eckenrode (ed.), *The Social Context of Coping.* New York: Plenum Press, 1991.

Heaney, C. A. "Enhancing Social Support at the Workplace: Assessing the Effects of the Caregiver Support Program." *Health Education Quarterly,* 1991, *18,* 477–494.

Helgeson, V. S., and Gottlieb, B. H. "Support Groups." In S. Cohen, L. G. Underwood, and B. H. Gottlieb (eds.), *Social Support Measurement and Intervention.* New York: Oxford University Press, 2000.

Heller, K., Thompson, M. G., Trueba, P. E., Hogg, J. R., and Vlachos-Weber, I. "Peer Support Telephone Dyads for Elderly Women: Was This the Wrong Intervention?" *American Journal of Community Psychology,* 1991, *19,* 53–74.

Hirsch, B. J., and DuBois, D. L. "The Relation of Peer Social Support and Psychological Symptomatology During the Transition to Junior High School: A Two-Year Longitudinal Analysis." *American Journal of Community Psychology,* 1992, *20,* 333–347.

Holahan, C. J., Moos, R. H., Holahan, C. K., and Brennan, P. L. "Social Context, Coping Strategies, and Depressive Symptoms: An Expanded Model with Cardiac Patients." *Journal of Personality and Social Psychology,* 1997, *72,* 918–928.

House, J. S. *Work Stress and Social Support.* Reading, Mass.: Addison-Wesley, 1981.

House, J. S. "Social Support and Social Structure." *Sociological Forum,* 1987, *2,* 135–146.

House, J. S., Umberson, D., and Landis, K. R. "Structures and Processes of Social Support." *Annual Review of Sociology,* 1988, *14,* 293–318.

Hunter, C. P. "Epidemiology, Stage at Diagnosis, and Tumor Biology of Breast Carcinoma in Multiracial and Multiethnic Populations." *Cancer,* 2000, *88,* 1193–1202.

Israel, B. A. "Social Networks and Health Status: Linking Theory, Research, and Practice." *Patient Counseling and Health Education,* 1982, *4,* 65–79.

Israel, B. A. "Social Networks and Social Support: Implications for Natural Helper and Community Level Interventions." *Health Education Quarterly,* 1985, *12,* 65–80.

Israel, B. A., Farquahar, S., Schulz, A., James, S., and Parker, E. "The Relationship Between Social Support, Stress and Health Among Women on Detroit's East Side." *Health Education and Behavior,* forthcoming.

Israel, B. A., and Rounds, K. A. "Social Networks and Social Support: A Synthesis for Health Educators." *Advances in Health Education and Promotion,* 1987, *2,* 311–351.

Israel, B. A., and others. "Evaluation of Health Education Programs: Current Assessment and Future Directions." *Health Education Quarterly,* 1995, *22,* 364–389.

Jucovy, L. *Building Relationships: A Guide for New Mentors.* Portland, Oreg.: Northwest Regional Educational Laboratory, 2001.

Kahn, R. L., and Antonucci, T. C. "Convoys Over the Life Course: Attachments, Roles and Social Support." In P. B. Baltes and O. Brim (eds.), *Life Span Development and Behavior.* (Vol. 3) New York: Academic Press, 1980.

Krause, N. "Assessing Stress-Buffering Effects: A Cautionary Note." *Psychology and Aging,* 1995, *10,* 518–526.

La Veist, T. A., Sellers, R. M., Elliott Brown, K. A., Nickerson, K. J. "Extreme Social Isolation, Use of Community-Based Senior Support Services, and Mortality Among African American Women." *American Journal of Community Psychology,* 1997, *25,* 721–732.

McCarthy, E. P., and others. "Mammography Use Helps Explain Differences in Breast Cancer Stage at Diagnosis Between Older Black and White Women." *Annals of Internal Medicine,* 1998, *128,* 729–36.

McKinlay, J. B. "Social Network Influences on Morbid Episodes and the Career of Help Seeking." In L. Eisenberg and A. Kleinman (eds.), *The Relevance of Social Science for Medicine,* 1980, 77–107.

McLeroy, K. R., Gottlieb, N. H., and Heaney, C. A. "Social Health." In M. P. O'Donnell and J. S. Harris (eds.), *Health Promotion in the Workplace.* (3rd ed.) Albany, N.Y.: Delmar, 2001.

Mecartney, C. A., Styles, M. B., and Morrow, K. V. *Mentoring in the Juvenile Justice System: Findings from Two Pilot Programs.* Philadelphia: Public/Private Ventures, 1994.

Michael, Y. L., Colditz, G. A., Coakley, E., and Kawachi, I. "Health Behaviors, Social Networks, and Healthy Aging: Cross-Sectional Evidence from the Nurses' Health Study." *Quality of Life Research,* 1999, *8,* 711–722.

Minkler, M. "Community Organizing Among the Elderly Poor in San Francisco's Tenderloin District." In J. Rothman, J. L. Erlich, and J. E. Tropman (eds.), *Strategies of Community Intervention.* Itasca, Ill.: Peacock Publishers, 2001.

Morisky, D. E., DeMuth, N. M., Field-Fass, M., Green, L. W., and Levine, D. M. "Evaluation of Family Health Education to Build Social Support for Long-Term Control of High Blood Pressure." *Health Education Quarterly,* 1985, *12,* 35–50.

Norbeck, J., Lindsey, A., and Carrieri, V. "Further Development of the Norbeck Social Support Questionnaire: Normative Data and Validity Testing." *Nursing Research,* 1983, *32,* 4–9.

Palmer, C. A., Baucom, D. H., and McBride, C. M. "Couple Approaches to Smoking Cessation." In K. B. Schmaling and T. G. Sher (eds.), *The Psychology of Couples and Illness: Theory, Research, and Practice.* Washington D.C.: APA, 2000, 311–336.

Resnick, M. D., and others. "Protecting Adolescents from Harm: Findings from the National Longitudinal Study on Adolescent Health." *Journal of the American Medical Association,* 1997, *278,* 823–832.

Rhodes, J. E., Contreras, J. M., and Mangelsdorf, S. C. "Natural Mentor Relationships Among Latina Adolescent Mothers: Psychological Adjustment, Moderating Processes, and the Role of Early Parental Acceptance." *American Journal of Community Psychology,* 1994, *22,* 211–227.

Rothman, J., Erlich, J. L., and Tropman, J. E. *Strategies of Community Intervention.* Itasca, Ill.: Peacock Publishers, 2001.

Sandler, I. N., and others. "Linking Empirically Based Theory and Evaluation: The Family Bereavement Program." *American Journal of Community Psychology,* 1992, *20,* 491–521.

Schulz, A. J., and others. "Addressing Social Determinants of Health Through Community-Based Participatory Research: The East Side Village Health Worker Partnership." *Health Education and Behavior,* forthcoming.

Shumaker, S. A., and Hill, D. R. "Gender Differences in Social Support and Physical Health." *Health Psychology,* 1991, *10,* 102–111.

Spiegel, D., and Diamond, S. "Psychosocial Interventions in Cancer Group Therapy Techniques." In A. Baum and B. L. Andersen (eds.), *Psychosocial Interventions for Cancer.* Washington, D.C.: American Psychological Association, 2001.

Starrett, R. A., Bresler, C., Decker, J. T., Walters, G. T., and Rogers, D. "The Role of Environmental Awareness and Support Networks in Hispanic Elderly Persons' Use of Formal Social Services." *Journal of Community Psychology,* 1990, *18,* 218–227.

Strogatz, D. S., and others. "Social Support, Stress, and Blood Pressure in Black Adults." *Epidemiology,* 1997, *8,* 482–487.

Styles, M., and Morrow, K. *Building Relationships with Youth in Program Settings: A Study of Big Brothers/Big Sisters.* Philadelphia: Public/Private Ventures, 1992.

Taylor, S. E., Buunk, B. P., and Aspinwall, L. G. "Social Comparison, Stress, and Coping." *Personality and Social Psychology Bulletin,* 1990, *16,* 74–89.

Tessaro, I., Eng, E., and Smith, J. "Breast Cancer Screening in Older African-American Women: Qualitative Research Findings." *American Journal of Health Promotion,* 1994, *8,* 286–293.

Thoits, P. A. "Stress, Coping, and Social Support Processes: Where Are We? What Next?" *Journal of Health and Social Behavior,* 1995 (Supplement 1), 53–79.

Tierney, J. P., and Grossman, J. B., with Resch, N. L. *Making a Difference: An Impact Study of Big Brothers Big Sisters.* Philadelphia: Public/Private Ventures, 1995.

Veroff, J., Douvan, E., and Kulka, R. A. *The Inner American: A Self-Portrait from 1957 to 1976.* New York: Basic Books, 1981.

Vogt, T. M., Mullooly, J. P., Ernst, D., Pope, C. R., and Hollis, J. F. "Social Networks as Predictors of Ischemic Heart Disease, Cancer, Stroke, Hypertension—Incidence, Survival, and Mortality." *Journal of Clinical Epidemiology,* 1992, *45,* 659–666.

Wethington, E., and Kessler, R. C. "Perceived Support, Received Support, and Adjustment to Stressful Life Events." *Journal of Health and Social Behavior,* 1986, *27,* 78–89.

Wing, R. R., and Jeffery, R. W. "Benefits of Recruiting Participants with Friends and Increasing Social Support for Weight Loss and Maintenance." *Journal of Consulting and Clinical Psychology,* 1999, *67,* 132–138.

Wortman, C. B., and Lehman, D. R. "Reactions to Victims of Life Crises: Support Attempts that Fail." In I. G. Sarason and B. R. Sarason (eds.), *Social Support: Theory, Research, and Applications.* Dordrecht, The Netherlands: Martinus Nijhoff, 1985.

CHAPTER TEN

STRESS, COPING, AND HEALTH BEHAVIOR

Lari Wenzel
Karen Glanz
Caryn Lerman

An understanding of stress and coping is essential to health education, health promotion, and disease prevention. Stress can contribute to illness directly through physiological effects or indirectly via maladaptive health behaviors (for example, smoking, poor eating habits). However, stress does not affect all people equally; some people live through terribly threatening experiences yet manage to cope well and do not get ill. Moreover, some people experience growth and find positive lessons from negative experiences. Among individuals who are ill or at-risk for illness, their ways of coping can have important influences on psychological and physical health outcomes. The influence of friends, family, and health care providers in the face of stress can have profound effects on these outcomes as well.

The illness experience, medical treatment, a diagnosis of illness, or the fear of developing an illness all can provoke stressful reactions. The way individuals experience and cope with stress affects whether and how they seek medical care and social support and how well they adhere to health professionals' advice. Reactions to stressors can promote or inhibit healthful practices and can influence an individual's motivation to practice positive health habits. The psychosocial aspects of a situation affect the determinants and consequences of health behaviors. A better understanding of theory and the empirical literature on stress and coping is thus essential to develop effective strategies and programs for improving coping and enhancing psychological and physical well-being.

The purpose of this chapter is to review major theories, research, and applications related to stress, coping, and health. We first provide a brief summary of historical concepts of health, stress, and coping. The next section describes an overview of an influential cognitive-behavioral theoretical framework, the Transactional Model of Stress and Coping. We present key variables, definitions, relationships among concepts, and a summary of findings relevant to health behavior. The chapter then describes applications of the model to the design of health behavior interventions.

Historical Concepts of Health, Stress, and Coping

Conceptualizations of health, stress, and coping are derived from numerous branches of research, with the earliest work conducted by scientists in the fields of biology and psychophysiology (for example, Cannon, 1932). In addition, diverse health and behavioral science disciplines have influenced our understanding of stress and health, including epidemiology, personality psychology, and cognitive and social psychology.

Stressors are demands made by the internal or external environment that upset balance or homeostasis, thus affecting physical and psychological well-being and requiring action to restore balance or equilibrium (Lazarus and Cohen, 1977). Early work on stress focused on physiological reactions to stressful stimuli. Cannon (1932) is credited with first describing the "fight or flight" reaction to stress. Hans Selye, the father of modern stress research, extended Cannon's studies with clinical observations and laboratory research. He hypothesized that living organisms (rats and people) exhibited nonspecific changes in response to stressors, labeled as a three-stage General Adaptation Syndrome (GAS). This syndrome consists of an alarm reaction, resistance, and exhaustion (Selye, 1956). Each stage evokes both physiological and behavioral responses, and without curative measures, physical and psychological deterioration will occur.

Another major stream of stress research in the 1960s and 1970s focused on identifying and quantifying potential stressors, or *stressful life events*. Holmes and Rahe (1967) developed the Social Readjustment Rating Scale (SRRS), a tool to measure stressful life events. Studies showed that people with high scores on the SRRS had more illness episodes than did those with low scores. This scale stimulated a substantial body of research (for example, Dohrenwend and Dohrenwend, 1981), despite numerous methodological limitations.

Beginning in the 1960s and 1970s, stress was considered to be a transactional phenomenon dependent on the meaning of the stimulus to the perceiver (Lazarus, 1966; Antonovsky, 1979). The central concept in models developed during this time is that a given event or situation is perceived in different ways by various individuals. Moreover, these perceptions—rather than the objective stressors—are the main determinants of effects on subsequent behaviors and on health status. Some researchers in the field of occupational stress and health used this concept as a foundation for a model that viewed occupational stress as a result of the interaction between individual workers' characteristics and the work environment, or the "person-environment fit" (French and Kahn, 1962; House, 1974). These lines of theory led to an examination of possible buffering, or moderating factors, and in particular to a focus on the role of social support (Cohen and Wills, 1985).

Parallel research in biology and epidemiology indicates that some personality dispositions and psychological states (for example, fatalism, hostility, and emotional suppression) are linked to disease endpoints (Scheier and Bridges, 1995). Chronic stressors and responses to them affect the sympathetic nervous system and endocrine functions, thus influencing the occurrence and progression of health problems including cancer, infectious diseases, and HIV/AIDS (Kiecolt-Glaser and Glaser, 1995). The difficulty of separating psychological and biological causal factors in health status and health behavior is underscored by the apparent complexity of mechanisms proposed for these associations (Borysenko, 1984).

Clearly, there are numerous and important areas of research and theory on stress and health. In this chapter, we emphasize cognitive-behavioral theory and research because of the direct relevance to health education and health behavior change.

The Transactional Model of Stress and Coping: Overview, Key Constructs, and Empirical Support

The Transactional Model of Stress and Coping is a framework for evaluating the processes of coping with stressful events. Stressful experiences are construed as person-environment *transactions,* in which the impact of an external stressor, or demand, is mediated by the person's appraisal of the stressor and the psychological, social, and cultural resources at his or her disposal (Lazarus and Cohen, 1977; Antonovsky and Kats, 1967; Cohen, 1984). When faced with a stressor, a person evaluates the potential threat *(primary appraisal)* as well as his or her ability to alter the situation and manage negative emotional reactions *(secondary appraisal).* Actual *coping efforts,* aimed at problem management and emotional regulation, give rise to the *outcomes* of the coping process (for example, psychological well-being, functional status, adherence).

Recent extensions of coping theory suggest that positive psychological states should also be taken into account. Thus, during a stressful period, numerous affect-inducing events take place that may allow for a cooccurrence of negative and positive affect during the same period of time (Folkman and Moskowitz, 2000). For example, positive affect may facilitate the processing of self-relevant information, serve as a buffer against adverse physiological consequences of stress, and protect against clinical depression (Moskowitz, Folkman, Collette, and Vittinghoff, 1996). Accordingly, Folkman proposed that a cognitive theory of stress and coping should accommodate positive psychological states (Folkman, 1997).

Table 10.1 summarizes the key concepts, definitions, and applications of the Transactional Model of Stress and Coping. Figure 10.1 illustrates the interrelationships among these concepts. As shown in the figure, positive psychological states may be the result of meaning-based coping processes, and they can also lead back to appraisal and coping. For more extensive discussions of theoretical underpinnings of the Transactional Model of Stress and Coping, readers should refer to the work of Lazarus, Folkman, and Moskowitz (Lazarus and Folkman, 1984; Lazarus, 1991a; Folkman, 1997; Folkman and Moskowitz, 2000).

Primary Appraisal

Primary appraisal is a person's judgment about the significance of an event as stressful, positive, controllable, challenging, benign, or irrelevant. Health problems are usually evaluated initially as threatening or as negative stressors. Two basic primary appraisals are perceptions of *susceptibility* to the threat and perceptions of *severity* of the threat. According to the Transactional Model of Stress and Coping, appraisals of personal risk and threat severity prompt efforts to cope with the stressor. For example, a woman who perceives herself at risk for breast cancer may be motivated to obtain mammograms (problem-focused coping) and may seek social support to cope with her concerns about the threat (emotion-focused coping). However, heightened perceptions of risk can also generate distress. Among women with a family history of ovarian cancer, those who perceive themselves as highly susceptible are more prone to experience intrusive ideation and psychological distress (Schwartz, Lerman, Miller, Daly, and Masny, 1995). Appraisals of high threat can also prompt escape-avoidance behaviors (Folkman, Lazarus, Dunkel-Schetter, Delongis, and Gruen, 1986), which can have the paradoxical effect of reducing adherence to health-promoting practices (Lerman and Schwartz, 1993). For example, heightened distress about personal risk of breast cancer has been associated with decreased adherence to recommended breast cancer screening guidelines (Lerman and others, 1993; Kash, Holland, Halper, and Miller, 1992).

Primary appraisals can also serve to minimize the significance of the threat, particularly when a health threat is ambiguous or uncertain. This *appraisal bias*

TABLE 10.1. THE TRANSACTIONAL MODEL OF STRESS AND COPING.

Concept	Definition	Application
Primary appraisal	Evaluation of the significance of a stressor or threatening event	Perceptions of an event as threatening can cause distress. If an event is perceived as positive, benign, or irrelevant, little negative threat is felt.
Secondary appraisal	Evaluation of the controllability of the stressor and a person's coping resources	Perception of one's ability to change the situation, manage one's emotional reaction, or cope effectively can lead to successful coping and adaptation.
Coping efforts	Actual strategies used to mediate primary and secondary appraisals	
Problem management	Strategies directed at changing a stressful situation	Active coping, problem solving, and information seeking can be used.
Emotional regulation	Strategies aimed at changing the way one thinks or feels about a stressful situation	Venting feelings, avoidance, denial, and seeking social support may be used.
Meaning-based coping	Coping processes that induce positive emotion, which in turn sustains the coping process by allowing reenactment of problem- or emotion-focused coping	Positive reappraisal, revised goals, and spiritual beliefs are experienced, and positive events occur.
Outcomes of coping (adaptation)	Emotional well-being, functional status, health behaviors	Coping strategies may result in short- and long-term positive or negative adaptation.
Dispositional coping styles	Generalized ways of behaving that can affect a person's emotional or functional reaction to a stressor; relatively stable across time and situations	
Optimism	Tendency to have generalized positive expectancies for outcomes	Optimists may experience fewer symptoms or faster recovery from illness.
Information seeking	Attentional styles that are vigilant (monitoring) versus those that involve avoidance (blunting)	Monitoring may increase distress and arousal; it may also increase active coping. Blunting may mute excessive worry but may reduce adherence.

FIGURE 10.1. DIAGRAM OF THE TRANSACTIONAL MODEL OF STRESS AND COPING.

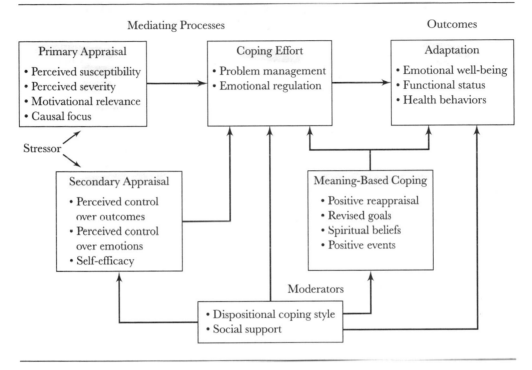

was demonstrated in a series of well-designed studies by Croyle and colleagues (Ditto and Croyle, 1995; Croyle and Sandman, 1988). Employing a test for a fictitious enzyme disorder, they showed that persons who were informed of abnormal test results rated the disorder as less serious and the test itself as less valid than did those who received "normal" test results. Such minimizing appraisals have also been shown to reduce distress associated with real health threats. For example, breast cancer patients who perceived themselves as "invulnerable" to a recurrence experienced less distress and had better overall adjustment than did other patients (Timko and Janoff-Bulman, 1985). Among HIV-positive men, beliefs of invulnerability enhanced perceived control and active coping and reduced distress without compromising performance of safe sexual behaviors (Taylor and others, 1992). However, other studies suggest that minimizing appraisals may also diminish motivation to adopt recommended preventive health behaviors such as cholesterol screening and dietary restriction (Croyle, 1992; Weinstein, 1989). This minimization effect may be particularly pronounced among smokers. Chapman, Wong, and Smith (1993) found that smokers were significantly more likely than nonsmokers to perceive themselves as less personally susceptible to the health effects of smoking.

Other primary appraisals involve the *motivational relevance* and *causal focus* of the stressor. When a stressor is appraised as having a major impact on a person's goals or concerns (high motivational relevance), that person is likely to experience anxiety and situation-specific distress (Smith and Lazarus, 1993). This may be especially true when the relevance is to one's own physical health or well-being (Folkman, Lazarus, Dunkel-Schetter, Delongis, and Gruen, 1986). Perceiving oneself as responsible for the stressor (self-causal focus) may more likely generate guilt and depression than anxiety (Smith, Haynes, Lazarus, and Pope, 1993; Lewis and Daltroy, 1990). When coping with illness, the congruence of the appraisal with the appraisal of a significant other may be more important than the individual's focus of causality (Manne and Taylor, 1993). Alternatively, the most important aspect of causal appraisals of illness may be whether or nor they are generated at all (Lowery, Jacobsen, and DuCette, 1993).

Secondary Appraisal

Secondary appraisal is an assessment of a person's coping resources and options (Cohen, 1984). In contrast to primary appraisals that focus on the features of the stressful situation, secondary appraisals address what one can do about the situation. Key examples of secondary appraisals are *perceived ability to change the situation* (for example, perceived control over the threat), *perceived ability to manage one's emotional reactions* to the threat (for example, perceived control over feelings), and *expectations about the effectiveness of one's coping resources* (for example, coping self-efficacy).

Positive associations between perceptions of control over illness and psychological adjustment have been observed across a wide variety of diseases. These include cancer (Marks, Richardson, Graham, and Levine, 1986), heart disease (Taylor, Helgeson, Reed, and Skokan, 1991), and HIV/AIDS (Taylor and others, 1992). Moreover, perceived control over illness may improve physical well-being by increasing the likelihood that a person will adopt recommended health behaviors (Thompson and Spacapan, 1991). For example, perceived control over health outcomes has been shown to relate positively to safe sexual behavior (Taylor and others, 1992). However, in situations that cannot be altered (such as severe or fatal disease), high levels of perceived control actually may increase distress and dysfunction (Lowery, Jacobsen, and DuCette, 1993; Affleck, Tennen, Pfeiffer, and Fifield, 1987; Thompson, Sobolew-Shubin, Galbraith, Schwankousky, and Cruzen, 1993). Thus, beliefs about personal control are likely to be adaptive only to the extent that they fit with reality (Brownell, 1991).

Beliefs about one's ability to perform the behaviors necessary to exert control (that is, self-efficacy) have been shown to play a central role in the performance of a variety of health behaviors (Strecher, DeVellis, Becker, and Rosenstock, 1986). For example, self-efficacy beliefs predict success with smoking cessation attempts (Strecher, DeVellis, Becker, and Rosenstock, 1986), as well as maintenance of exercise and diet regimens (Ewart, Taylor, Reese, and Debusk, 1984; Jeffrey and others, 1984). Self-efficacy, a central construct of Social Cognitive Theory (Bandura 1989; see Chapter Eight), is specific to a given behavior and is not a global personality trait. For example, a sedentary nonsmoker may have high self-efficacy for avoiding tobacco use but low self-efficacy for exercising regularly.

Coping Efforts

According to the Transactional Model, the emotional and functional effects of primary and secondary appraisals are mediated by actual *coping strategies* (Lazarus and Folkman, 1984; Lazarus, 1991a). Original formulations of the model conceptualized coping efforts along two dimensions: problem management and emotional regulation. Also referred to as problem-focused coping, problem-management strategies are directed at changing the stressful situation. Examples of problem-focused coping include active coping, problem solving, and information seeking. By contrast, emotion-focused coping efforts are directed at changing the way one thinks or feels about a stressful situation. These strategies include the seeking of social support, venting of feelings, avoidance, and denial. The model predicts that problem-focused coping strategies will be most adaptive for stressors that are changeable, whereas emotion-focused strategies are most adaptive when the stressor is unchangeable or when all problem-focused coping attempts have been made.

Empirical studies of coping have focused on the extent to which an individual engages or disengages with the stressor (Carver and others, 1993). When a stressor is perceived as highly threatening and uncontrollable, a person may be more likely to use disengaging coping strategies (Taylor and others, 1992). Examples of disengaging coping strategies include distancing, cognitive avoidance, behavioral avoidance, distraction, and denial. Each of these strategies shifts attention away from the stressor. This attentional shift may allow individuals to minimize their initial distress by avoiding thoughts and feelings about the stressor (Suls and Fletcher, 1985). Ultimately, however, avoidance or denial may lead to intrusive thoughts that can generate increased distress over time (Carver and others, 1993; Schwartz, Lerman, Miller, Daly, and Masny, 1995). For that reason, avoidance and denial are often considered maladaptive; research literature on the usefulness of strategies such as avoidance and denial suggests that they are controversial.

By contrast, when a stressor is appraised as controllable and a person has favorable beliefs about self-efficacy, he or she is more likely to use engaging coping strategies (Aspinwall and Taylor, 1992). Examples of engaging coping strategies include active coping, planning problem solving, information seeking, and use of social support.

Other common coping responses to health threats use meaning-based coping, which can induce positive emotion (Folkman, 1997). These include positive reinterpretation, acceptance, and use of religion and spirituality (Carver and others, 1993; Reed, Kemeny, Taylor, Wang, and Visscher, 1994). These processes involve interpretation of a stressful situation in a personally meaningful way.

There are some interesting parallels between the coping strategies in the Transactional Model and the change processes in the Transtheoretical Model, also known as the Stages of Change model (Prochaska, DiClemente, and Norcross, 1992; see Chapter Five). For example, self-reevaluation is a change process that can facilitate progression from the contemplation stage of behavior change to the preparation stage. Similar to emotion-focused coping strategies such as reappraisal, self-reevaluation involves assessing and, in some cases, altering how one feels about a problem. Likewise, change processes such as stimulus control and counter-conditioning (or substitution of alternatives for problem behaviors) could be considered problem-focused coping strategies.

Several theoretically driven scales have been developed to assess coping efforts. Typically, respondents are asked to describe a stressful situation they have experienced and to answer questions about how they would evaluate and respond to the situation. The most widely used subscales address problem-focused coping and emotion-focused coping (Stone, Greenberg, Kennedy-Moore, and Newman, 1991). Examples of available tools include the Ways of Coping Inventory (WOC) (Folkman and Lazarus, 1980; Mishel and Sorenson, l993), the Multidimensional Coping Inventory (Endler and Parker, 1990), and the Coping Orientations to Problems Experienced (COPE) scale (Carver, Scheier, and Weintraub, 1989). The COPE questionnaire, one of the more recent inventories, uses twelve subscales to measure types of coping strategies, including active coping, suppression of competing activities, planning, restraint, social support, positive reframing, religion, acceptance, denial, disengagement, use of humor, and self-distraction (Carver and others, 1993). There are also scales to measure daily use of coping strategies (Stone and Neale, 1984), which may provide more precise assessments of coping transactions (Stone, Kennedy-Moore, and Neale, 1995). The Cancer Behavior Inventory (CBI) (Merluzzi, Nairn, Hegde, Martinez-Sanchez, and Dunn, 2001) is a new measure of self-efficacy for coping with cancer. The CBI includes eight subscales: maintaining activity and independence, seeking and understanding medical information, managing stress, coping with treatment-related side-effects, accepting cancer or maintaining a positive attitude, affective regulating, and seeking support. This measure of self-efficacy for coping with cancer provides a refined tool to assess secondary appraisal.

The Transactional Model has generated an extensive body of literature on coping strategies, adjustment to illness, and health behavior. In general, these studies provide evidence for the psychological benefits of active coping strategies and acceptance or reappraisal over avoidant or disengaging strategies (for example, Fawzy and others, 1990; Carver and others, 1993; Taylor and others, 1992). More recent studies have reinforced the significant association between use of avoidant coping (for example, avoiding others, hiding feelings, and refusing to think about the illness) and higher levels of psychological distress (Baider and others, 1997; Dunkel-Schetter, Feinstein, Taylor, and Falke, 1992), as well as poorer quality of life (Trask and others, 2001). In addition to adverse effects on psychological well-being, avoidant coping may increase the likelihood of negative health behaviors such as IV drug use in people with AIDS (Fleishman and Vogel, 1994).

By contrast, benefits of more "healthy" or adaptive coping strategies are increasingly evident in the literature. For example, breast cancer patients scoring lowest in avoidant coping were more likely to be actively involved in treatment decision making (Hack and Degner, 1999). In addition, emotionally expressive coping predicted both psychological and physical adjustment to breast cancer (Stanton and others, 2000). The use of spirituality and seeking of social support may reduce the chances that a person will engage in risky behaviors such as unprotected sexual intercourse (Folkman, Chesney, Pollack, and Phillips, 1992). The use of spirituality has also been associated with growth and the capacity to derive a positive meaning from being an ovarian cancer survivor (Wenzel and others, forthcoming). These examples represent a growing body of literature describing the physical and mental health benefits of active coping efforts, including both problem-focused and emotion-focused efforts.

The extent to which specific coping strategies result in desirable or undesirable outcomes, however, may depend on whether short- or long-term outcomes are considered more important (Cohen, 1984). In addition, coping flexibility (the ability to use a variety of different strategies) has been found to be important in health promotion, particularly in prevention of relapse in smokers (Bliss, Garvey, and Heinold, 1989). Moreover, cognitive-behavioral interventions that enhance coping flexibility can improve maintenance of health behavior changes such as smoking cessation (Brandon, Copeland, and Saper, 1995).

Most research on coping strategies evaluates efforts to cope with a particular situation as distinct from generalized coping styles (Stone and Porter, 1995). However, as discussed in the following section, the effects of specific coping strategies on the emotional and functional outcomes of a health threat and the accompanying stress may depend on a person's dispositional coping style and his or her perceptions of support in their environment.

Coping Outcomes

Coping outcomes represent a person's adaptation to a stressor, following from their appraisal of the situation (primary appraisal) and resources (secondary appraisal) and influenced by coping efforts. Because a problem or stressor may change over time, outcomes may occur in differing time frames. Three main categories of outcomes are emotional well-being, functional status (or health status, disease progression, and so forth), and health behaviors. These outcomes may also interact with one another. For example, clinically meaningful links have been made between endocrine function and cancer. Recent studies have demonstrated an association between loss of diurnal variation in cortisol and shorter survival time from breast cancer (Stephton, Sapolsky, Kraemer, and Spiegel, 2000). There are also indications that breast cancer patients' assessment of support from their social environment is associated with lower morning cortisol levels (Turner-Cobb, Stephton, Koopman, Blake-Mortimer, and Spiegel, 2000). This link between social support and cortisol in breast cancer has been confirmed in a clinical trial demonstrating that group support for breast cancer patients reduces mean cortisol levels (Creuss and others, 2000). These recent studies provide support for the premise that reactions to stress may affect health status through physiological processes of the endocrine, immune, and nervous systems (Kiecolt-Glaser and Glaser, 1995; Scheier and Bridges, 1995). However, caution should be used when interpreting relationships between psychological factors and disease progression. Tross and others (1996) examined the contribution of potential psychological predictors to length of disease-free and overall survival over a fifteen-year period. This study, which was conducted within a randomized clinical trial, found no significant predictive effect of the level of distress on disease outcomes.

Health behaviors such as seeking care, communicating with health providers, and adhering to treatment recommendations may be influenced by physical limitations (functional status) and by emotional reactions (worry, depression, denial). Similarly, desirable health behaviors may be influenced by meaning-based processes such as positive reappraisal, which may decrease worry and enhance positive affect.

Theoretical Extensions

Dispositional Coping Styles

In contrast to coping efforts, coping styles are conceptualized as dispositional or stable characteristics of the individual. Another important distinction between coping efforts and coping styles is that the former are situation-specific while the latter are generalized (Lazarus, 1993). Coping efforts change as a function of primary and secondary appraisals, and these processes influence how a person will react emotionally and functionally to the stressor. Thus, coping efforts can be considered *mediators* of the effects of stress and appraisals on emotional and functional outcomes—in other words, the mechanism by which these effects are exerted (Baron and Kenny, 1986). By contrast, coping styles are enduring traits that are believed to drive appraisal and coping efforts (Lazarus, 1993). Individual differences in coping styles can be considered *moderators* of the impact of stress on coping processes and outcomes (Baron and Kenny, 1986). That is, the specific effect of a stressful event or a specific coping behavior on adjustment may depend, in part, on the person's coping style, which may produce a modifying interaction. Coping styles can also have direct effects on the emotional and physical outcomes of stressful events.

Early conceptualizations and research on dispositional coping styles focused on characterizing persons who remained relatively healthy while undergoing stressful life experiences. Hinkle (1974) observed that such people tended to be emotionally insulated and less involved with other people. In contrast, Antonovsky (1979) and Kobasa (1979) suggested that people who exhibited healthful adaptation to internal and environmental stressors had strong resistance resources and a sense of meaningfulness in their lives. Antonovsky (1979) described a "sense of coherence" that involves a strong sense of confidence that the world is predictable and that things will work out "as well as reasonably can be expected" (p. 123). He further proposed that sense of coherence could be found not only in well-adapted individuals but in groups and cultures as well. Kobasa identified a constellation of features she called "hardiness," marked by a strong sense of meaningfulness and commitment to self, a vigorous attitude toward life, and an internal locus of control (Kobasa, 1979; Kobasa, Maddi, and Kahn, 1982). This work was a forerunner of more recent research on purpose and dispositional optimism, which can be considered aspects of "positive" psychology.

"Positive" psychology examines how people develop and sustain characteristics such as hope, wisdom, future mindedness, courage, spirituality, and perseverance in the face of significant stress (Seligman and Csikszentmihalyi, 2000). Several studies have found positive associations between a sense of purpose in life and life satisfaction, positive mood states, and happiness (Ryff, 1989; Ryff and Keyes, 1995; Ryff, Lee, Essex, and Schmutte, 1994). This research also suggests that purpose in life is negatively associated with depression. Lewis (1989) found that purpose in life among a group of late-stage cancer patients was strongly associated with lower self-reported anxiety. In general, these studies suggest that people who endorse a strong purpose in life are likely to experience better emotional well-being.

Optimism. Perhaps the most widely researched coping style is dispositional optimism—the tendency to have positive (optimistic) rather than negative (pessimistic) generalized expectancies for outcomes. Positive expectancies have been shown to be relatively stable over time and across situations (Scheier and Carver, 1992). The direct beneficial effects of optimism on psychological adjustment have been demonstrated in prospective studies of cancer patients (Carver and others, 1993; Epping-Jordan and others, 1999), coronary patients (Scheier and others, 1989), and HIV-positive men (Taylor and others, 1992). Optimists also have been shown to experience fewer physical symptoms during life stresses (Scheier and Carver, 1985) and faster recovery after a myocardial infarction (Scheier and others, 1989).

Studies exploring the effects of optimism on coping responses and adaptation to illness are relevant to the Transactional Model. For example, Carver and others (1993) conducted a one-year prospective study of the effects of optimism and coping strategies on psychological well-being among early-stage breast cancer patients. Dispositional optimism was found to predict psychological adjustment at each timepoint. Moreover, this beneficial effect of optimism was mediated by the use of active coping, planning, problem solving, and acceptance. Optimism was related inversely to avoidance, a coping strategy that generated distress in this sample. Among gay men at risk for AIDS, dispositional optimism was associated with perceived lower risk of AIDS (primary appraisal), higher perceived control over AIDS (secondary appraisal), more active coping strategies, less distress, and more risk-reducing health behaviors in men at risk for AIDS (Taylor and others, 1992). Thus, dispositional optimism appears to exert effects on each of the key processes of the Transactional Model. These effects, in turn, influence how optimists and pessimists respond emotionally and physically to health threats and illness.

Information Seeking. In addition to optimism, there is support for the influence of attentional styles *monitoring*, or seeking information, and *blunting*, or avoiding information (Miller, 1987). Several studies have shown that the vigilant style of *monitors* contributes to heightened perceived risk and excessive worry about health threats (Phipps and Zinn, 1986; Wardle and others, 1993). In a study of women at increased risk for ovarian cancer, monitoring was associated with heightened perceived risk of disease, intrusive thoughts, and distress (Schwartz, Lerman, Miller, Daly, and Masny, 1995). In the same study, perceived risk, an appraisal variable, acted as a mediator of the effects of monitoring on psychological distress.

Effects of monitoring on physical outcomes of stressful events have also been demonstrated. For example, among cancer patients undergoing chemotherapy, monitoring has been associated with more severe nausea and vomiting (Lerman and others, 1990). Monitors have also been shown to experience more physical distress and arousal during an invasive medical procedure than blunters (Miller and Mangan, 1983). In a randomized trial comparing alternate methods of cancer risk counseling in women at high risk for breast cancer, monitors showed increases in distress in both counseling conditions (Lerman and others, 1996b). However, when stressors are short-term and when monitors' needs for information are satisfied (for example, by preparation for stressful medical procedures), active coping is enhanced and emotional and physical distress is minimized (Miller and Mangan, 1983).

Although the foregoing studies suggest that monitoring may be a less adaptive coping style than blunting, there are situations where this may not be the case. For example, monitors may be more inclined to seek health-related information that could have significant medical benefits, as was shown in a study of genetic testing for cancer susceptibility (Lerman, Daly, Masny, and Balshem, 1994). In addition, because monitors are more attentive to health threats, they may also adhere better to recommended health practices than blunters (Steptoe and O'Sullivan, 1986).

Recent research has also shown that patients benefit differentially from how information is framed, depending on their dispositional style. In a study to enhance cervical dysplasia screening follow-up, recommendations were either loss framed (emphasizing cost), or positively framed (emphasizing benefit), or neutrally framed (no emphasis). The results showed that monitors fared worse at the affective level when the message was presented in a loss frame, because the sense of risk was heightened. Blunters, on the other hand, fared better when the information was presented in a loss-framed manner (Miller and others, 1999). The interaction of attentional style with message framing may motivate health actions in addition to its impact on affect.

Social Support

Social support has been conceptualized in a variety of ways (Heaney and Israel, 1997). Some definitions focus on the quantitative and tangible dimensions (for example, number of friendships), while others focus on nontangible aspects such as feelings of interconnectedness or qualitative aspects involving subjective appraisals of adequacy of support networks (Heitzmann and Kaplan, 1988). Although conceptualizations and forms of measurement may vary, there is substantial evidence that social support has beneficial effects on psychological and physical well-being (Heaney and Israel, 1997).

Social support appears to have both direct effects and "stress-buffering" effects on well-being (Cohen and Wills, 1985). The stress-buffering hypothesis predicts that social support will have stronger positive effects on adjustment and physical well-being when a stressor becomes more intense or persistent. Evidence for the buffering model has been found in studies that measure the perceived availability of social support (Cohen and Hoberman, 1983; Littlefield, Rodin, Murray, and Craven, 1990). The direct effects of social support have been observed primarily in studies assessing the extent of social support networks (see Chapter Nine).

By influencing the key processes posited in the Transactional Model, social support can influence how people adapt psychologically to a stressful event such as a significant health threat or illness. For example, the availability of friends with whom to talk could affect a person's perceptions of personal risk or the severity of illness (primary appraisal). These interactions could also bolster beliefs about one's ability to cope with the situation and manage difficult emotions (secondary appraisal) (Cohen and McKay, 1984). Social support can also serve as a mechanism for downward comparison—that is, to compare oneself to someone who is worse off (Cohen and Wills, 1985). Resultant increases in self-esteem and self-efficacy, in turn, could increase the likelihood of active coping strategies rather than avoidance (Holahan and Moos, 1986). A supportive environment can also protect against stress by providing opportunities to explore different coping options and to evaluate their effectiveness (Holahan and Moos, 1986). In addition, disclosure of feelings has been shown to decrease avoidant coping and minimize negative emotional reactions to a stressor (Pennebaker and O'Heeron, 1984).

Social support also can influence health outcomes (Reifman, 1995). In a study of men with coronary artery disease, both quantitative and qualitative dimensions of social support predicted survival, even after controlling for medical variables (Williams and others, 1992). Although the results of studies of social support and cancer outcomes have been mixed (Reifman, 1995), the results of some intervention studies are encouraging. If coping strategies facilitate adjustment to a cancer diagnosis, then psychosocial support should be a potent factor in mediating emotional distress and improving outcome. Two key studies have reported that support group interventions for cancer patients improved emotional adjustment and influenced survival (Fawzy and others, 1993; Spiegel, Bloom, Kraemer, and Gottheil, 1989). A mechanism by which social support may benefit physical well-being is the promotion of active coping behaviors such as adherence to recommended health behaviors (Heitzmann and Kaplan, 1988). Alternatively, by enhancing the expression of negative feelings, social support may have direct physiological and immunological benefits (Pennebaker, 1990). The supportive-expressive group therapy approach (Spiegel, Bloom, Kraemer, and Gottheil, 1989) emphasizes providing support in helping patients face and deal with their disease-related stress and is thought to achieve these positive outcomes. This approach also has recently been shown to reduce distress in patients with metastatic breast cancer (Classen and others, 2001).

Stress Management Interventions

A variety of techniques to manage stress, improve coping, and reduce the deleterious effects of stressors on physical and psychological health have been developed and tested in recent years. Techniques such as biofeedback, relaxation training, and visual imagery can be conceptualized as coping efforts directed at emotional regulation, which is consistent with the original formulation of the Transactional Model (Lazarus and Folkman, 1984). These efforts in turn lead to outcomes of coping efforts (for example, decreased pain or decreased anxiety).

Biofeedback and deep relaxation strategies focus on the interplay between biological and psychological responses to stressors (Critchley, Melmed, Featherstone, Mathias, and Dolan, 2001; Kaplan, Sallis, and Patterson, 1993). Biofeedback systems aim to develop awareness and control of maladaptive responses to stressors and to reduce stress and tension in response to everyday situations. This technique has proven useful in reducing symptoms associated with multiple physical illnesses, including fibromyalgia (Buckelew and others, 1998) and pediatric headache (Kroener-Herwig, Mohn, and Pothmann, 1998).

Use of relaxation techniques assumes that individuals possess alternative responses to fight-or-flight, responses that counteract the effects of stress. The basic elements of the relaxation response, which can be achieved through progressive relaxation training, hypnosis, yoga, and other techniques, are use of a constant mental stimulus, passive attitude, decreased muscle tone, and a quiet environment (Benson, 1984). Research on the effects of relaxation combined with guided imagery (visualizing host defenses destroying tumor cells) on quality of life and response to chemotherapy has shown that in combination, relaxation and imagery improved mood and quality of life, with imagery correlated with clinical response (Walker and others, 1999). As an intervention for breast cancer patients, imagery, when compared with standard care, has also been shown to improve coping skills and social support and to enhance meaning in life (Richardson and others, 1997). In addition, relaxation training has been shown to reduce side effects of cancer chemotherapy (Burish and Jenkins, 1992).

Cognitive-behavioral approaches to improve coping with stress are usually based on five key modes of coping: information seeking, direct action, inhibition of action, intrapsychic processes, and turning to others for support (Cohen and Lazarus, 1979). These approaches, closely derived from the Transactional Model, focus on teaching individuals to evaluate their primary appraisals of stressful situations, to achieve accurate (rather than distorted) primary appraisals, and to evaluate their coping resources and enhance them as necessary (Kaplan, Sallis, and Patterson, 1993). In a study that examined the impact of cognitive-behavioral stress management on personal growth, results indicated that positive contributions were achieved and maintained three months after intervention (Antoni and others, 1999). A cognitive-behavioral approach has also been shown to produce greater short-term and sustained change in anxiety, adjustment to cancer, and use of coping strategies than a nondirective, supportive intervention (Moorey, Greer, Bliss, and Law, 1998).

Applications to Specific Health Behavior Research Areas

Examples of cognitive-behavioral intervention strategies to improve coping and adaptation are given in two applications that follow. These applications relate to family members of breast cancer patients and to persons who receive positive results of genetic tests for cancer.

Application: Problem-Solving Training for Relatives of Breast Cancer Patients

Women with a first-degree relative with breast cancer have a two- to fourfold increased risk of developing this disease (Claus, Risch, and Thompson, 1990). Yet research shows that many high-risk women do not adhere to breast cancer screening (Vogel and others, 1990). In addition, a substantial proportion of these women experience problems in psychological adjustment (Kash, Holland, Halper, and Miller, 1992; Lerman and Schwartz, 1993). Anxiety and distress in high-risk women can interfere with adherence to recommended breast cancer screening (Lerman and others, 1993). For first-degree relatives of newly diagnosed breast cancer patients, psychological adjustment and adherence may be affected by concerns about both their own breast cancer risk and the welfare of loved ones.

The Transactional Model of Stress and Coping was used as the theoretical foundation for the development and evaluation of a cognitive-behavioral intervention to promote adjustment and adherence among first-degree relatives of newly diagnosed breast cancer patients (Schwartz and others, 1998). The intervention used a Problem-Solving Training (PST) approach (D'Zurilla, 1986; Haaga and Davison, 1991) to facilitate adaptive appraisals and to promote effective problem-focused and emotion-focused coping with stressors resulting from the relative's breast cancer diagnosis.

The PST intervention was delivered to the relatives of newly diagnosed breast cancer patients during an extended individual visit with a health educator or nurse. The approach has five steps. The first step is to assess the participant's appraisal of the situation, focusing on her attributions, perceptions of control, and perceived coping resources. Attention is paid to attributions of causality and control, as these beliefs are key determinants of adjustment (Taylor, Lichtman, and Wood, 1984). An adaptive appraisal is fostered by emphasizing that a relative's breast cancer diagnosis can be viewed as an opportunity to protect one's own health and that negative emotions can be used as a "cue" for problem-solving activity. In addition, participants are presented with an overview of the stress and coping model and the problem-solving techniques. Second, specific problem statements are generated; for example, "What can I do to minimize my anxiety about my risk?" and "What can I do to help my sister adjust better to her treatment?" The objective of this stage is to set realistic and attainable short-term goals. The third step is to generate alternative solutions to the problem, focusing on both problem-focused coping strategies and emotion-focused coping strategies. Participants are taught a brainstorming approach to generate a wide range of strategies. The fourth step is to examine the value of these solutions by considering the impact on the participant's well-being, the well-being of the affected relative, the time and effort required, and the potential for problem resolution. Standardized prompts are used to elicit the participant's expectations about the consequences and to apply a cost-benefit strategy to select the best alternative. Finally, evaluation of the success of the specific coping strategies is performed during follow-up telephone booster sessions.

The PST intervention was evaluated in a randomized trial conducted at six cancer centers across the United States. The evaluation focused on the impact of PST, relative to general health counseling (control), on the following elements of the Transactional Model: (1) primary appraisals, including perceptions of risk and perceived threat to oneself and to the affected relative; (2) secondary appraisals, including perceived ability to control the situation and manage negative mood reactions and perceived coping resources; (3) coping behaviors, including active coping, avoidant coping, and spiritual acceptance of coping; (4) quality of life outcomes, including cancer worries, mood, stress impact, and functional health status; and (5) adherence behaviors, including use of mammography, clinical breast examination, and breast self-examination.

Participants included 144 women in the PST group and 197 in the general health counseling (GHC) control group, and the groups did not differ at baseline on any sociodemographic, risk, or psychological distress variables. Study participants in both groups had significant decreases in distress at the three-month follow-up, and the magnitude of the decreases did not differ. However, PST participants who regularly practiced the PST techniques had greater decreases in cancer-specific distress than infrequent practicers or GHC participants (Schwartz and others, 1998). Also, among the women who received the PST, those with higher levels of cancer-specific distress were twice as likely to improve their adherence to breast-self-examination recommendations as were women low in cancer-specific distress (Audrain and others, 1999).

The findings are similar to those of previous research that found that effective problem solvers report greater self-efficacy, exhibit fewer dysfunctional coping efforts, experience less anxiety, and have better physical health than do ineffective problem solvers (Heppner, Reeder, and Larson, 1983). In other randomized trials, PST has had beneficial effects on psychological well-being and adherence (D'Zurilla, 1986). Interventions that include problem-solving skills have also been shown to improve adjustment and adherence to self-care regimens in cancer patients (Glanz and Lerman, 1992; Fawzy and others, 1990; Andersen, 1992).

Application: Intervention to Improve Quality of Life for BRCA+ Mutation Carriers

It is estimated that between 7 and 10 percent of breast and ovarian cancers are attributable to an inherited susceptibility (Claus, Schildkraut, Thompson, and Risch, 1996). Mutations in the BRCA1 and BRCA2 genes are implicated in the majority of high-risk families (Ford and others, 1998). Therefore, genetic testing for inherited BRCA+ mutations is rapidly being integrated into the clinical management of women who have a strong family history of breast or ovarian cancer, and counseling is an important component of the genetic testing process. Genetic counseling includes standardized pretest education and counseling to facilitate informed decision making about whether or not to undergo genetic testing, and postdisclosure counseling to provide information about the results, recommendations for cancer surveillance, and options for breast and ovarian cancer prevention (Biesecker and others, 1993). The genetic counseling process provides a forum to address concerns before testing and to enhance coping and adjustment among individuals who undergo testing. However, women may need more support than they receive in standard genetic counseling.

An intervention based on the Transactional Model of Stress and Coping was developed to augment standard genetic counseling and address medical decision making, emotional reactions, and familial concerns that BRCA+ mutation carriers may experience after test result disclosure. As shown in Figure 10.2, the model addresses these composite concerns in a seamless manner, moving from primary appraisal based on primary stressor disaggregation to secondary appraisal, in which coping is directed toward either problem-focused or emotion-focused coping efforts. The stressor is then reappraised as either resolved or not. Those unresolved stressors can be revisited within the same session to examine other approaches via secondary appraisal, or homework assignments can be generated for the subsequent session.

FIGURE 10.2. TRANSACTIONAL
MODEL APPLIED TO THE BRCA+ EXPERIENCE.

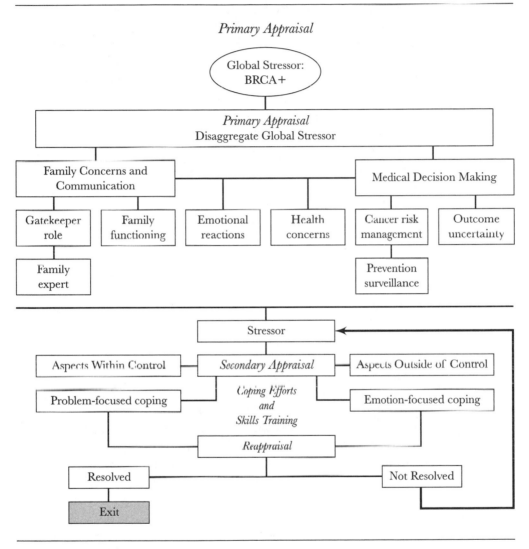

This program is being evaluated in a randomized, controlled trial of the effect of psychosocial telephone counseling (PTC) on quality of life in women who have received a positive BRCA+ genetic test result (Comparing Models of Counseling for BRCA+ Testing; Lerman C, PI). Participants are recruited from genetic testing research programs in Washington, D.C., and Toronto, Ontario, Canada.

The intervention is intended to foster an accurate understanding of personal risk in several ways (primary appraisal). For example, if an unaffected carrier underestimates her cancer risk, she may not initiate coping efforts and may be less motivated to obtain recommended screening tests. If she overestimates her risk, this could lead to increased distress and decreased adherence. Both of these examples imply that the person's appraisal of threat in this situation is likely to have an impact on her cancer risk management and prevention surveillance (see Figure 10.2). Second, the intervention targets a carrier's appraisal of her ability to reduce her risk of developing and dying from cancer and her ability to manage her distress (secondary appraisal). A carrier who does not feel equipped to deal with her risk status or her feelings about it is more likely to experience distress and difficulty when communicating with family members and making decisions regarding cancer screening and prevention. To address this, PTC enhances the participant's confidence in her decisions and actions and increases her ability to manage distress through the use of problem-focused or emotion-focused coping skills training. The coping efforts learned within the PTC intervention are then reinforced to minimize long-term distress and maximize satisfaction with medical decision making and family concerns.

Using the Transactional Model as a foundation for the intervention promotes a consistent process across clients, while still allowing for flexibility to meet a client's unique needs, resources, and circumstances. The intervention consists of five weekly telephone counseling sessions and mailed print materials (CARE Kit) that augment the counseling intervention. Several of the coping strategies were chosen from the Coping Effectiveness Training program (Chesney, Folkman, and Chambers, 1996) and adapted to fit the needs and resources of this audience. The coping strategies include identifying the stressor, which aids in the primary appraisal process; identifying changeable and unchangeable aspects of the stressor, which aids in the secondary appraisal process; and problem-solving, communication, decision making, enhancing social support, and thought changing, which promote healthy or adaptive coping skills. During each counseling session, one coping strategy is applied to the relevant thematic domain. The strategies used in each session provide realistic application and practice. Before and after each session, stress and confidence ratings are taken to help evaluate the success of the strategy as it was applied within the session. Each session includes stressor identification, disaggregation, and application of a suitable coping strategy. The counseling process remains the same across the domains covered in different sessions. This process enables the counselor to be responsive to the participant's needs while maintaining the consistency and structure critical to intervention research.

As this trial is still ongoing, results are not yet available. At present, several important contributions related to genetic testing stressors, and coping associated with these stressors, can be highlighted. As part of this study, data are being collected to determine the prevalence of adverse psychological consequences among genetic testing participants and to identify subgroups of women who may be more psychologically vulnerable. The study will also evaluate genetic counseling methods in terms of how well participants' psychosocial concerns are addressed. However, there is no available measure for assessing the kind of situation-specific psychosocial and clinical concerns that have been noted anecdotally and empirically among mutation-positive women (Dorval and others, 2000). As a result, a brief questionnaire was developed to assess concerns that are very specific to the high-risk cancer clinical setting (Cella and others, forthcoming). This new questionnaire, the Multidimensional Impact of Cancer Risk Assessment (MICRA), taps negative and positive responses to the testing experience as well as concerns about personal and family vulnerability. The MICRA better differentiates participants who were BRCA+ positive from the three BRCA+ negative groups ($p < .01$ in all comparisons) than does a general distress questionnaire. Preliminary results also suggest that genetic testing distress is associated with cognitive appraisal and coping efforts (Hughes, 2001). Findings from this trial of PTC will increase our understanding of whether an assessment and intervention process, based on the Transactional Model, can promote adaptive coping to the specific stressors that may arise over time for this high risk group.

Conclusion

The theory and research presented in this chapter illustrate the complexities of stress and coping and their effects on psychological well-being, health behavior, and health. This work suggests that the outcomes of the stress and coping process are determined by an interplay of situational factors, individual appraisals of the situation, and coping strategies. No particular pattern of relationships among these factors has been related consistently to positive outcomes of the coping process. Rather, the effects of stress and coping processes depend on context (for example, controllability of the stressor), timing (short- versus long-term adaptation), and individual characteristics (for example, information processing styles and meaning-based coping processes).

Although it is difficult to offer simple generalizations about the adaptability of specific coping processes or the efficacy of interventions, the extensive research conducted in this area has several implications for the practice of health promotion and health education. First, because individuals' emotional and health behavior responses to health threats are influenced to a large degree by their subjective interpretations, these appraisals must be assessed. For example, to better understand the determinants of lifestyle practices of cancer patients following treatment, one should assess primary appraisals (such as perceptions of risk of recurrence), secondary appraisals (such as self-efficacy in adopting health behavior recommendations), and specific coping strategies (such as problem-focused coping, emotion-focused coping, and meaning-based coping). These assessments could provide useful information about appraisals that facilitate or hinder lifestyle practices. Such information would be useful for designing motivational messages and coping skills training techniques to be incorporated into standardized interventions.

A second implication of research on stress and coping relates to dispositional coping styles. As described in this chapter, coping strategies are likely to be beneficial to the extent that they fit with the features of the stressful situation and with the individual's own needs for information, control, and level of optimism versus pessimism. Incorporation of coping styles assessments into health promotion and psychoeducational interventions will facilitate the tailoring of these strategies to individual needs. Research on stress, coping, and health behavior suggests that interventions that are tailored to individual appraisals and coping behaviors are likely to be most effective in terms of enhancing coping, reducing stress, and improving health behavior and physical well-being.

References

Affleck, G., Tennen, H., Pfeiffer, C., and Fifield, H. "Appraisals of Control and Predictability in Adapting to a Chronic Stress." *Journal of Personality and Social Psychology,* 1987, *53,* 273–279.

Andersen, B. L. "Psychological Interventions for Cancer Patients to Enhance the Quality of Life." *Journal of Consulting and Clinical Psychology,* 1992, *60,* 552–568.

Antoni, M. H., and others. "Cognitive-Behavioral Stress Management Intervention Decreases the Prevalence of Depression and Enhances Benefit Finding Among Women Under Treatment for Early-Stage Breast Cancer." *Health Psychology,* 1999, *20,* 20–32.

Antonovsky, A. *Health, Stress, and Coping.* San Francisco: Jossey-Bass, 1979. (reprinted 1991).

Antonovsky, A., and Kats, R. "The Life Crisis History as a Tool in Epidemiologic Research." *Journal of Health and Social Behavior,* 1967, *8,* 15–20.

Aspinwall, L. G., and Taylor, S. E. "Modeling Cognitive Adaptation: A Longitudinal Investigation of the Impact of Individual Differences and Coping on College Adjustment and Performance." *Journal of Personality and Social Psychology,* 1992, *63,* 989–1003.

Audrain, J., and others. "The Impact of a Brief Coping Skills Intervention on Adherence to Breast Self-Examination Among First-Degree Relatives of Newly Diagnosed Breast Cancer Patients." *Psycho-Oncology,* 1999, *8,* 220–229.

Baider, L., and others. " The Role of Psychological Variables in a Group of Melanoma Patients: An Israeli Sample." *Psychosomatics,* 1997, *38,* 45–53.

Bandura, A. "Human Agency in Social Cognitive Theory." *American Psychologist,* 1989, *44,* 1175–1184.

Baron, R. M., and Kenny, D. A. "The Moderator-Mediator Variable Distinction in Social Psychological Research: Conceptual, Strategic, and Statistical Considerations." *Journal of Personality and Social Psychology,* 1986, *51*(6), 1173–1182.

Benson, H. "The Relaxation Response and Stress." In J. D. Matarazzo, S. M. Weiss, J. A. Herd, N. E. Miller, and S. M. Weiss (eds.), *Behavioral Health: A Handbook of Health Enhancement and Disease Prevention.* New York: Wiley, 1984.

Biesecker, B. B., and others. "Genetic Counseling for Families with Inherited Susceptibility to Breast and Ovarian Cancer." *Journal of the American Medical Association,* 1993, *269,* 1970–1974.

Bliss, R. E., Garvey, A. J., and Heinold, J. W. "The Influence of Situation and Coping on Relapse Crisis Outcomes After Smoking Cessation." *Journal of Consulting and Clinical Psychology,* 1989, *57,* 443–449.

Borysenko, J. "Stress, Coping, and the Immune System." In J. D. Matarazzo, S. M. Weiss, J. A. Herd, N. E. Miller, and S. M. Weiss (eds.), *Behavioral Health: A Handbook of Health Enhancement and Disease Prevention.* New York: Wiley, 1984.

Brandon, T. H., Copeland, A. L., and Saper, Z. L. "Programmed Therapeutic Messages as a Smoking Treatment Adjunct: Reducing the Impact of Negative Affect." *Health Psychology,* 1995, *14,* 41–47.

Brownell, K. D. "Personal Responsibility and Control over Our Bodies: When Expectation Exceeds Reality." *Health Psychology,* 1991, *10,* 303–310.

Buckelew, S. P., and others. "Biofeedback/Relaxation Training and Exercise Interventions for Fibromyalgia: A Prospective Trial." *Arthritis Care & Research,* 1998, *11,* 196–209.

Burish, T. G., and Jenkins, R. S. "Effectiveness of Biofeedback and Relaxation Training in Reducing the Side-Effects of Cancer Chemotherapy." *Health Psychology,* 1992, *11,* 17–23.

Cannon, W. B. *The Wisdom of the Body.* New York: Norton, 1932.

Carver, C. S., Scheier, M. F., and Weintraub, J. K. "Assessing Coping Strategies: A Theoretically Based Approach." *Journal of Personality and Social Psychology,* 1989, *56,* 267–283.

Carver, C. S., and others. "How Coping Mediates the Effect of Optimism on Distress: A Study of Women with Early Stage Breast Cancer." *Journal of Personality and Social Psychology,* 1993, *65*(2), 375–390.

Cella, D., and others. "A Brief Assessment of Concerns Associated with Genetic Testing for Cancer: The Multidimensional Impact of Cancer Risk Assessment (MICRA) Questionnaire." *Health Psychology,* forthcoming.

Chapman, S., Wong, W. L., and Smith, W. "Self-Exempting Beliefs About Smoking and Health: Differences Between Smokers and Ex-Smokers." *American Journal of Public Health,* 1993, *83,* 215–219.

Chesney, M. A., Folkman, S., and Chambers, D. "Coping Effectiveness Training for Men Living with HIV: Preliminary Findings." *International Journal of Studies on AIDS,* 1996, *7,* 75–82.

Classen C., and others. "Supportive-Expressive Group Therapy and Distress in Patients with Metastatic Breast Cancer: A Randomized Clinical Intervention Trial." *Archives of General Psychiatry,* 2001, *58*(5), 494–501.

Claus, E. B., Risch, N. J., and Thompson, W. D. "Age at Onset as an Indicator of Familial Risk of Breast Cancer." *American Journal of Epidemiology,* 1990, *131*(6), 961–972.

Claus, E. B., Schildkraut, J. M., Thompson, W. D., and Risch, N. J. " The Genetic Attributable Risk of Breast and Ovarian Cancer." *Cancer,* 1996, *77*, 2318–2324.

Cohen, F. "Coping." In J. D. Matarazzo, S. M. Weiss, J. A. Herd, N. E. Miller, and S. M. Weiss (eds.), *Behavioral Health: A Handbook of Health Enhancement and Disease Prevention.* New York: Wiley, 1984.

Cohen, F., and Lazarus, R. S. "Coping with the Stress of Illness." In G. C. Stone, F. Cohen, and N. E. Adler (eds.), *Health Psychology.* San Francisco: Jossey-Bass, 1979.

Cohen, S., and Hoberman, H. M. "Positive Events and Social Supports as Buffers of Life Change Stress." *Journal of Applied Social Psychology,* 1983, *13*(2), 99–125.

Cohen, S., and McKay, G. "Social Support, Stress and the Buffering Hypothesis: A Theoretical Analysis." In A. Baum, J. E. Singer, and S. E. Taylor (eds.), *Handbook of Psychology and Health* (Vol. 4). Mahwah, N.J.: Erlbaum, 1984.

Cohen, S., and Wills, T. A. "Stress, Social Support, and the Buffering Hypothesis." *Psychological Bulletin,* 1985, *98*(2), 310–357.

Creuss, D. G., and others. "Cognitive Behavioral Stress Management Reduces Serum Cortisol by Enhancing Benefit Finding Among Women Being Treated for Early Stage Breast Cancer." *Psychosomatic Medicine,* 2000, *62*, 304–308.

Critchley, H. D., Melmed, R. N., Featherstone, E., Mathias, C. J., and Dolan, R. J. "Brain Activity During Biofeedback Relaxation: A Functional Neuroimaging Investigation." *Brain,* 2001, *124*(5), 1003–1012.

Croyle, R. T. "Appraisal of Health Threats: Cognition, Motivation, and Social Comparison." *Cognitive Therapy and Research,* 1992, *16*(2), 165–182.

Croyle, R. T., and Sandman, G. N. "Denial and Confirmatory Search: Paradoxical Consequences of Medical Diagnosis." *Journal of Applied Social Psychology,* 1988, *18,* 473–490.

Ditto, P. H., and Croyle, R. T. "Understanding the Impact of Risk Factor Test Results: Insights from a Basic Research Program." In R. T. Croyle (ed.), *Psychosocial Effects of Screening for Disease Prevention and Detection.* New York: Oxford University Press, 1995.

Dohrenwend, B. S., and Dohrenwend, B. P. *Stressful Life Events and Their Contexts.* New York: Prodist, 1981.

Dorval, M., and others. "Anticipated Versus Actual Emotional Reactions to Disclosure of Results of Genetic Tests for Cancer Susceptibility: Findings from p53 and BRCA1 Testing Programs." *Journal of Clinical Oncology,* 2000, *18*(10), 2135–2142.

Dunkel-Schetter, C., Feinstein, L., Taylor, S., and Falke, R. "Patterns of Coping with Cancer." *Health Psychology,* 1992, *11*(2), 79–87.

D'Zurilla, T. J. *Problem-Solving Therapy: A Social Competence Approach to Clinical Intervention.* New York: Springer, 1986.

Endler, N., and Parker, J. "Multidimensional Assessment of Coping: A Critical Evaluation." *Journal of Personality and Social Psychology,* 1990, *58*, 844–854.

Epping-Jordan, J. E., and others. "Psychological Adjustment in Breast Cancer: Processes of Emotional Distress." *Health Psychology,* 1999, *18*(4), 315–326.

Ewart, C. K., Taylor, C. B., Reese, L. B., and Debusk, R. F. "Effects of Early Postmyocardial Infarction Exercise Testing on Self-Perception and Subsequent Physical Activity." *American Journal of Cardiology*, 1984, *41*, 1076–1080.

Fawzy, F. I., and others. "A Structured Psychiatric Intervention of Cancer Patients: 1. Changes over Time in Methods of Coping and Affective Disturbance." *Archives of General Psychiatry*, 1990, *47*, 720–725.

Fawzy, F. I., and others. "Malignant Melanoma: Effects of an Early Structured Psychiatric Intervention, Coping, and Affective State on Recurrence and Survival 6 Years Later." *Archives of General Psychiatry*, 1993, *50*, 681–689.

Fleishman, J. A., and Vogel, B. "Coping and Depressive Symptoms Among People with AIDS." *Health Psychology*, 1994, *13*(2), 156–169.

Folkman, S. "Positive Psychological States and Coping with Severe Stress." *Social Science and Medicine*, 1997, *45*, 1207–1221.

Folkman, S., Chesney, M. A., Pollack, L., and Phillips, C. "Stress, Coping, and High-Risk Sexual Behavior." *Health Psychology*, 1992, *11*, 218–222.

Folkman, S., and Lazarus, R. S. "An Analysis of Coping in a Middle-Aged Community Sample." *Journal of Health and Social Behavior*, 1980, *21*, 219–239.

Folkman, S., Lazarus, R. S., Dunkel-Schetter, C., Delongis, A., and Gruen, R. "Dynamics of a Stressful Encounter: Cognitive Appraisal, Coping, and Encounter Outcomes." *Journal of Personality and Social Psychology*, 1986, *50*, 992–1003.

Folkman, S., and Moskowitz, J. "Positive Affect and the Other Side of Coping." *American Psychologist*, 2000, *55*, 647–654.

Ford, D., and others. "Genetic Heterogeneity and Penetrance Analysis of the BRCA1 and BRCA2 Genes in Breast Cancer Families. *American Journal of Human Genetics*, 1998, *62*, 676–689.

French, J.R.P., and Kahn, R. L. "A Programmatic Approach to Studying the Industrial Environment and Mental Health." *Journal of Social Issues*, 1962, *18*, 1–47.

Glanz, K., and Lerman, C. "Psychosocial Impact of Breast Cancer: A Critical Review." *Annals of Behavioral Medicine*, 1992, *14*, 204–212.

Haaga, D. A., and Davison, G. C. "Cognitive Changes Methods." In F. H. Kanfer and A. P. Goldstein (eds.), *Helping People Change*. New York: Pergamon Press, 1991.

Hack, T. F., and Degner, L. F. "Coping with Breast Cancer: A Cluster Analytic Approach." *Breast Cancer Research and Treatment*, 1999, *54*(3), 185–194.

Heaney, C. A., and Israel, B. A. "Social Networks and Social Support." In K. Glanz, F. M. Lewis, and B. K. Rimer (eds.), *Health Behavior and Health Education: Theory, Research, and Practice*. (2nd ed.) San Francisco: Jossey-Bass, 1997.

Heitzmann, C. A., and Kaplan, R. M. "Assessment of Methods for Measuring Social Support." *Health Psychology*, 1988, *7*, 75–109.

Heppner, P. P., Reeder, B. L., and Larson, L. M. "Cognitive Variables Associated with Personal Problem-Solving Appraisal: Implications for Counseling." *Journal of Counseling and Psychology*, 1983, *30*, 537–545.

Hinkle, L. E. "The Effect of Exposure to Cultural Change, Social Change, and Changes in Interpersonal Relationships on Health." In B. S. Dohrenwend and B. P. Dohrenwend (eds.), *Stressful Life Events: Their Nature and Effects*. New York: Wiley, 1974.

Holahan, C. J., and Moos, R. H. "Personality, Coping, and Family Resources in Stress Resistance: A Longitudinal Analysis." *Journal of Personality and Social Psychology*, 1986, *51*, 389–395.

Holmes, T. H., and Rahe, R. H. "The Social Readjustment Rating Scale." *Journal of Psychosomatic Research,* 1967, *11,* 213–218.

House, J. S. "Occupational Stress and Coronary Heart Disease: A Review and Theoretical Integration." *Journal of Health and Social Behavior,* 1974, *15,* 12–27.

Hughes, C. "Cognitive Appraisal and Coping Efforts Following Genetic Testing for BRCA+ Mutations." Personal communication, 2001.

Jeffrey, R. W., and others. "Correlates of Weight Loss and Its Maintenance over Two Years of Follow-Up Among Middle-Aged Men." *Preventive Medicine,* 1984, *13,* 155–168.

Kaplan, R. M., Sallis, J. F., and Patterson, T. L. "Stress and Coping." In *Health and Human Behavior.* New York: McGraw-Hill, 1993.

Kash, K. M., Holland, J. C., Halper, M. S., and Miller, D. G. "Psychological Distress and Surveillance Behaviors of Women with a Family History of Breast Cancer." *Journal of the National Cancer Institute,* 1992, *84,* 24–30.

Kiecolt-Glaser, J. K., and Glaser, R. "Psychoneuroimmunology and Health Consequences: Data and Shared Mechanisms." *Psychosomatic Medicine,* 1995, *57,* 269–274.

Kobasa, S. C. "Stressful Life Events, Personality, and Health: An Inquiry into Hardiness." *Journal of Personality and Social Psychology,* 1979, *37,* 1–11.

Kobasa, S. C., Maddi, S. R., and Kahn, S. "Hardiness and Health: A Prospective Study." *Journal of Personality and Social Psychology,* 1982, *42,* 168–177.

Kroener-Herwig, B., Mohn, U., and Pothmann, R. "Comparison of Biofeedback and Relaxation in the Treatment of Pediatric Headache and the Influence of Parent Involvement on Outcome." *Applied Psychophysiology and Biofeedback,* 1998, *23*(3), 143–157.

Lazarus, R. S. *Psychological Stress and the Coping Process.* New York: McGraw-Hill, 1966.

Lazarus, R. S. *Emotion and Adaptation.* New York: Oxford University Press, 1991a.

Lazarus, R. S. "Progress on a Cognitive-Motivational-Relational Theory of Emotion." *American Psychologist,* 1991b, *46,* 819–834.

Lazarus, R. S. "Coping Theory and Research: Past, Present, and Future." *Psychosomatic Medicine,* 1993, *55,* 234–247.

Lazarus, R. S., and Cohen, J. B. "Environmental Stress." In I. Altman and J. F. Wohlwill (eds.), *Human Behavior and Environment.* (Vol. 2) New York: Plenum, 1977.

Lazarus, R. S., and Folkman, S. *Stress, Appraisal, and Coping.* New York: Springer, 1984.

Lerman, C., Daly, M., Masny, A., and Balshem, A. "Attitudes About Genetic Testing for Breast-Ovarian Cancer Susceptibility." *Journal of Clinical Oncology,* 1994, *12,* 843–850.

Lerman, C., and Schwartz, M. "Adherence and Psychological Adjustment Among Women at High Risk for Breast Cancer." *Breast Cancer Research and Treatment,* 1993, *28,* 145–155.

Lerman, C., and others. "Effects of Coping Style and Relaxation on Cancer Chemotherapy Side-Effects and Emotional Responses." *Cancer Nursing,* 1990, *13,* 308–315.

Lerman, C., and others. "Mammography Adherence and Psychological Distress Among Women at Risk for Breast Cancer." *Journal of the National Cancer Institute,* 1993, *85,* 1074–1080.

Lerman, C., and others. "A Randomized Trial of Breast Cancer Risk Counseling: Interacting Effects of Counseling, Educational Level and Coping Style." *Health Psychology,* 1996, *15,* 75–83.

Lewis, F. M. "Attribution of Control, Experienced Meaning, and Psychosocial Well-Being in Patients with Advanced Cancer." *Journal of Psychosocial Oncology,* 1989, *7,* 105–119.

Lewis, F. M., and Daltroy, L. "How Causal Explanations Influence Health Behavior: Attribution Theory." In K. Glanz, F. M. Lewis, and B. K. Rimer (eds.), *Health Behavior and Health Education: Theory, Research, and Practice.* San Francisco: Jossey-Bass, 1990.

Littlefield, C. H., Rodin, G. M., Murray, M. A., and Craven, J. L. "Influence of Functional Impairment and Social Support on Depressive Symptoms in Persons with Diabetes." *Health Psychology,* 1990, *9,* 737–749.

Lowery, B. J., Jacobsen, B. S., and DuCette, J. "Causal Attribution, Control, and Adjustment to Breast Cancer." *Journal of Psychosocial Oncology,* 1993, *10,* 37–53.

Manne, S., and Taylor, K. Support-Related Interactions Between Women with Cancer and Their Healthy Partners." Presented at the American Psychological Association, Toronto, Canada, 1993.

Marks, G., Richardson, J. L., Graham, J. W., and Levine, A. "Role of Health Locus on Control Beliefs and Expectations of Treatment Efficacy in Adjustment to Cancer." *Journal of Personality and Social Psychology,* 1986, *51,* 443–450.

Merluzzi, T., Nairn, C., Hegde, K., Martinez-Sanchez, M., and Dunn, L. "Self-Efficacy for Coping with Cancer: Revision of the Cancer Behavior Inventory (version 2.0)." *Psycho-Oncology,* 2001, *10*(3), 206–217.

Miller, S. M. "Monitoring and Blunting: Validation of a Questionnaire to Assess Styles of Information-Seeking Under Threat." *Journal of Personality and Social Psychology,,* 1987, *52,* 345–353.

Miller, S. M., and Mangan, C. E. "The Interacting Effects of Information and Coping Style in Adapting to Gynecological Stress: Should the Doctor Tell All?" *Journal of Personality and Social Psychology,* 1983, *45,* 223–236.

Miller, S. M., and others. "Monitoring Styles in Women at Risk for Cervical Cancer: Implications for the Framing of Health-Relevant Messages." *Annals of Behavioral Medicine,* 1999, *21,* 91–99.

Mishel, M., and Sorenson, D. "Revision of the Ways of Coping Checklist for a Clinical Population." *Western Journal of Nursing Research,* 1993, *15*(1), 59–74.

Moorey S., Greer, S., Bliss, J., and Law, M. "A Comparison of Adjuvant Psychological Therapy and Supportive Counselling in Patients with Cancer." *Psycho-Oncology,* 1998, *7*(3), 218–228.

Moskowitz, J. T., Folkman, S., Collette, L., and Vittinghoff, E. "Coping and Mood During AIDS-Related Caregiving and Bereavement." *Annals of Behavioral Medicine,* 1996, *18,* 49–57.

Pennebaker, J. W. *Opening Up: The Healing Power of Confiding in Others.* New York: William Morrow, 1990.

Pennebaker, J. W., and O'Heeron, R. C. "Confiding in Others and Illness Rate Among Spouses of Suicide and Accidental Death Victims." *Journal of Abnormal Psychology,* 1984, *93,* 473–476.

Phipps, S., and Zinn, A. B. "Psychological Response to Amniocentesis: II. Effects of Coping Style." *American Journal of Medical Genetics,* 1986, *25,* 143–148.

Prochaska, J. O., DiClemente, C., and Norcross, J. C. "In Search of How People Change." *American Psychologist,* 1992, *47,* 1102–1114.

Reed, G. M., Kemeny, M. E., Taylor, S. E., Wang, H-Y J., and Visscher, B. R. "Realistic Acceptance as a Predictor of Decreased Survival Time in Gay Men with AIDS." *Health Psychology,* 1994, *13,* 299–307.

Reifman, A. "Social Relationships, Recovery from Illness, and Survival: A Literature Review." *Annals of Behavioral Medicine,* 1995, *17,* 124–131.

Richardson, M. A., and others. "Coping, Life Attitudes, and Immune Responses to Imagery and Group Support After Breast Cancer Treatment." *Alternative Therapy in Health and Medicine,* 1997, *3,* 62–70.

Ryff, C. D. " Happiness Is Everything, or Is It? Explorations on the Meaning of Psychological Well-Being." *Journal of Personality and Social Psychology*, 1989, *57*, 1069–1081.

Ryff, C. D., and Keyes, C. L. " The Structure of Psychological Well-Being Revisited." *Journal of Personality and Social Psychology*, 1995, *69*, 719–727.

Ryff, C. D., Lee, Y. H., Essex, M. J., and Schmutte, P. S. "My Children and Me: Midlife Evaluations of Grown Children and Self." *Psychology and Aging*, 1994, *9*, 195–205.

Scheier, M. F., and Bridges, M. W. "Person Variables and Health: Personality and Predispositions and Acute Psychological States as Shared Determinants for Disease." *Psychosomatic Medicine*, 1995, *57*, 255–268.

Scheier, M. F., and Carver, C. S. "Optimism, Coping, and Health: Assessment and Implications of Generalized Outcome Expectancies." *Health Psychology*, 1985, *4*, 219–247.

Scheier, M. F., and Carver, C. S. "Effects of Optimism on Psychological and Physical Well-Being: Theoretical Overview and Empirical Update." *Cognitive Therapy and Research*, 1992, *16*, 201–228.

Scheier, M. F., and others. "Dispositional Optimism and Recovery from Coronary Artery Bypass Surgery: The Beneficial Effects on Physical and Psychological Well-Being." *Journal of Personality and Social Psychology*, 1989, *57*, 1024–1040.

Schwartz, M., Lerman, C., Miller, S., Daly, M., and Masny, A. "Coping Disposition, Perceived Risk, and Psychological Distress Among Women at Increased Risk for Ovarian Cancer." *Health Psychology*, 1995, *14*, 232–35.

Schwartz, M., and others. "The Impact of a Brief Problem-Solving Training Intervention for Relatives of Recently Diagnosed Breast Cancer Patients." *Annals of Behavioral Medicine*, 1998, *20*, 7–12.

Seligman, M., and Csikszentmihalyi, M. "Positive Psychology: An Introduction." *American Psychologist*, 2000, *55*(1), 5–14.

Selye, H. *The Stress of Life*. New York: McGraw-Hill, 1956.

Smith, C. A., and Lazarus, R. S. "Appraisal Components, Core Relational Themes, and the Emotions." *Cognition and Emotion*, 1993, *7*, 233–269.

Smith, C. A., Haynes, K. N., Lazarus, R. S., and Pope, L. K. "In Search of the 'Hot' Cognitions: Attributions, Appraisals, and Their Relation to Emotion." *Journal of Personality and Social Psychology*, 1993, *65*, 916–929.

Spiegel, D., Bloom, J., Kraemer, H., and Gottheil, E. "Effect of Psychosocial Treatment on Survival of Patients with Metastatic Breast Cancer." *Lancet*, 1989, *2*(8668), 888–891.

Stanton, A. L., and others. "Emotionally Expressive Coping Predicts Psychological and Physical Adjustment to Breast Cancer." *Journal of Consulting and Clinical Psychology*, 2000, *68*(5), 875–882.

Stephton, S. E., Sapolsky, R. M., Kraemer, H. C., and Spiegel, D. "Diurnal Cortisol Rhythm as a Predictor of Breast Cancer Survival." *Journal of the National Cancer Institute*, 2000, *92*, 994–1000.

Steptoe, A., and O'Sullivan, J. "Monitoring and Blunting Coping Styles in Women Prior to Surgery." *British Journal of Clinical Psychology*, 1986, *24*, 143–144.

Stone, A., Greenberg, M., Kennedy-Moore, E., and Newman, M. "Self Report, Situation-Specific Coping Questionnaires: What Are They Measuring?" *Journal of Personality and Social Psychology*, 1991, *61*, 648–658.

Stone, A., Kennedy-Moore, E., and Neale, J. "Coping with Daily Problems." *Health Psychology*, 1995, *14*, 341–349.

Stone, A., and Neale, J. "A New Measure of Daily Coping: Development and Preliminary Results." *Journal of Personality and Social Psychology*, 1984, *46*, 892–906.

Stone, A. A., and Porter, L. S. "Psychological Coping: Its Importance for Treating Medical Problems." *Mind/Body Medicine*, 1995, *1*, 46–54.

Strecher, V. J., DeVellis, B. M., Becker, M. H., and Rosenstock, I. M. "The Role of Self-Efficacy in Achieving Health Behavior Change." *Health Education Quarterly*, 1986, *13*, 73–91.

Suls, J., and Fletcher, B. "The Relative Efficacy of Avoidant and Nonavoidant Coping Strategies: A Meta-Analysis." *Health Psychology*, 1985, *4*, 249–288.

Taylor, S. E., Helgeson, V. S., Reed, G. M., and Skokan, L. A. "Self-Generated Feelings of Control and Adjustment to Physical Illness." *Journal of Social Issues*, 1991, *47*, 91–109.

Taylor, S. E., Lichtman, R. R., and Wood, J. V. "Attributions, Beliefs About Control and Adjustment to Breast Cancer." *Journal of Personality and Social Psychology*, 1984, *46*, 489–502.

Taylor, S. E., and others. "Optimism, Coping, Psychological Distress, and High-Risk Sexual Behavior Among Men at Risk for Acquired Immunodeficiency Syndrome (AIDS)." *Journal of Personality and Social Psychology*, 1992, *63*, 460–473.

Thompson, S. C., Sobolew-Shubin, A., Galbraith, M. E., Schwankousky, L., and Cruzen, D. "Maintaining Perceptions of Control: Finding Perceived Control in Low-Control Circumstances." *Journal of Personality and Social Psychology*, 1993, *64*, 293–304.

Thompson, S. C., and Spacapan, S. "Perceptions of Control in Vulnerable Populations." *Journal of Social Issues*, 1991, *47*(4), 1–21.

Timko, C., and Janoff-Bulman, R. "Attributions, Vulnerability, and Psychological Adjustment: The Case of Breast Cancer." *Health Psychology*, 1985, *4*(6), 521–544.

Trask, P. C., and others. "Psychosocial Characteristics of Individuals with Non-Stage IV Melanoma." *Journal of Clinical Oncology*, 2001, *19*(11), 2844–2850.

Tross, S., and others. "Psychological Symptoms and Disease-Free and Overall Survival in Women with Stage II Breast Cancer: Cancer and Leukemia Group B." *Journal of the National Cancer Institute*, 1996, *88*(10), 629–631.

Turner-Cobb, J. M., Stephton, S., Koopman, C., Blake-Mortimer, J., and Spiegel, D. "Social Support and Salivary Cortisol in Women with Metastatic Breast Cancer." *Psychosomatic Medicine*, 2000, *62*, 337–345.

Vogel, V. G., and others. "Mammographic Screening of Women with Increased Risk of Breast Cancer." *Cancer*, 1990, *66*, 1613–1620.

Walker, L. G., and others. "Psychological, Clinical and Pathological Effects of Relaxation Training and Guided Imagery During Primary Chemotherapy." *British Journal of Cancer*, 1999, *80*, 262–268.

Wardle, F. J., and others. "Psychological Impact of Screening for Familial Ovarian Cancer." *Journal of the National Cancer Institute*, 1993, *85*, 653–657.

Weinstein, N. D. "Optimistic Biases About Personal Risks." *Science*, 1989, *246*, 1232–1233.

Wenzel, L. B., and others. "Ovarian Cancer Survivorship: Resilience, Reflection, and Residual Stress." *Psycho-Oncology*, forthcoming.

Williams, R. B., and others. "Prognostic Importance of Social and Economic Resources Among Medically Treated Patients with Angiographically Documented Coronary Artery Disease." *Journal of the American Medical Association*, 1992, *267*, 520–524.

CHAPTER ELEVEN

SOCIAL INFLUENCE AND INTERPERSONAL COMMUNICATION IN HEALTH BEHAVIOR

Megan A. Lewis
Brenda M. DeVellis
Betsy Sleath

Social influence is a defining feature of many types of relationships (Reis, Collins, and Berscheid, 2000) and a fundamental process used to change health behavior. This influence is often exercised through interpersonal communication. Influence and communication focused on changing health behaviors can occur in both formal and informal relationships, "formal" referring to relationships between physicians and patients or health educators and clients, and "informal" referring to relationships between spouses, friends, or a parent and child.

The study of influence and communication in formal and informal relationships is usually characterized as *goal oriented*. Cialdini and Trost (1999) suggest that most influence attempts are in the service of one or more of three goals: managing self-concept, behaving effectively, and building and maintaining relationships. People's attempts to influence each other can serve any combination of these goals, but this chapter focuses mainly on the second of these goals: how influence and communication affect health behavior.

Because most theories and conceptual models that examine influence and communication focus on dyads, or pairs of people, as the unit of study or practice,

Preparation of this chapter was supported in part by a grant from the NIH (DK56350) to the University of North Carolina, Clinical Nutrition Research Unit, Pilot Feasibility Program. The authors also thank Susan Ennett for comments on this chapter.

most of the concepts and examples in this chapter emphasize dyadic relationships. These models typically consider the target of influence, the agent of influence, and their reciprocal influence on each other's behaviors and outcomes. In spite of this dyadic focus, these models can also be used to understand situations where more than two people are involved, such as a doctor and nurse talking with a patient, or parents having a discussion with their children.

A greater understanding of how influence and communication relate to health behavior is important to health professionals and health educators. First, a better understanding of influence and communication can enhance the effectiveness of health behavior change interventions (van Ryn and Heaney, 1997). Second, core concepts and models of influence and communication can be used to create interventions, programs, and environments that help empower patients in their interactions with health care professionals (McGee and Cegala, 1998; Roter and Hall, 1992). Third, an awareness of influence and communication can be a foundation for more-effective partner-assisted interventions, in which one or more family members or friends are used to leverage or deliver interventions to change health behavior. Finally, distinguishing influence and communication from other interpersonal concepts like social support and social networks leads to greater conceptual clarity in health behavior research and practice (Heller and Rook, 1997; Lewis, Rook, and Schwarzer, 1994; see Chapter Nine for an in-depth discussion of social support).

This chapter introduces Interdependence Theory as a theoretical basis for examining influence and communication in formal and informal interactions. It next presents conceptual models that have been used to describe and understand social influence and interpersonal communication in health-related behavior; these models both share common foundations with and extend the focus of Interdependence Theory. Two interventions that use influence and communication are then described to illustrate strategies for interpersonal influence and communication. One application used motivational interviewing to improve eating patterns and the other addressed family communication about adolescent tobacco and alcohol use. Table 11.1 provides a summary of the concepts on influence and communication that are presented and analyzed in this chapter.

The evidence presented here supports the overarching proposition that influence and communication are most effective in changing health behavior within relationships characterized by mutual trust, respect, and shared power and decision making. Although social influence can be health enhancing or health compromising, depending on the behavior that is the focus of the influence, the relationships among parties, and the intentions of the influencers (House, Umberson, and Landis, 1988), this chapter focuses on how influence and communication, primarily within dyads, can improve health-enhancing behaviors.

TABLE 11.1. KEY CONCEPTS IN
SOCIAL INFLUENCE AND INTERPERSONAL COMMUNICATION.

Concept	Definition	Application
Norm of reciprocity	Norm which states that for rewards and benefits to be received in a relationship, they must also be returned	Provide opportunities to reciprocate, especially when roles or interactions are not clearly defined
Interdependence	Effects that interacting partners exert on each other's motives, preferences, behaviors, and health outcomes	Involve partners in program and target determinants of behavior change that are open to partner or reciprocal influence
Relationship interdependence	Structural relationship characteristics that bring people closer together or drive them apart, such as equality or conflict	Target communication style to bring partners closer together; usually involves going beyond knowledge-based approaches
Correspondence of outcomes	How closely outcomes of communication between persons match	Identify and target values, beliefs, or behaviors that are discrepant between partners
Bases of power	Six sources of power that make people influential in their communication	Combine approaches depending on problem and population; emphasize referent power base
Mutuality	Communication style in which both parties, such as patient and provider, have high control	Educate patients about medical encounters so they have skills and comfort for shared decision making
Motivational interviewing	Client-centered approach to education and behavior change	Use empathic or reflective listening and directive questioning to help clients move toward self-defined behavior-change goals
Authoritative parenting style	Bidirectional communication style that is developmentally appropriate, responsive, and supportive	Teach parents empathic or reflective listening *and* to set rules and standards for behavior
Compliance gaining	Communication tactics and strategies used to influence behavior	Emphasize positive, direct, and bidirectional strategies in communication
Descriptive social norms	Norms that indicate the way most people act	Highlight and correct misperceptions related to acting effectively
Injunctive social norms	Norms that indicate what types of behavior others approve or disapprove of in a given situation	Highlight and correct misperceptions about what is appropriate and acceptable or accepted

Interdependence Theory

Interdependence Theory is a dyad-level social-psychological theory that explains how influence and communication affect behavior by taking into account the outcomes experienced by interacting partners (Kelley and Thibaut, 1978; Rusbult and Van Lange, 1996). Although concepts from Interdependence Theory are not often explicitly referenced in the health education and behavior literature, they underlie many of the research findings. Interacting partners experience outcomes that reflect their own thoughts, emotions, and behaviors related to their interaction; they also experience shared or joint outcomes related to the goals of the interaction (that is, reactions and feelings about the interaction). For example, a doctor and patient may share the joint outcome of treatment success, a health educator and client may share the joint outcome of effectively communicated information, and spouses may share the joint outcome of having a healthy family.

Interdependence Theory is a middle-range theory developed from Social Exchange Theory (Kelley and Thibaut, 1978). Social Exchange Theory focuses on the costs and rewards that interacting partners give and receive from each other. It suggests that we are more likely to continue to interact with people who are best able to provide us with equivalent rewards. A reward is something that a person gains from an interaction. Rewards are subjective and can range from tangible goods such as money or information to intangible states such as satisfaction or positive regard. A central rule in the exchange of rewards in relationships is the *norm of reciprocity* (Goudner, 1960). To *receive* rewards from a relationship, we are usually expected to *give* rewards. Thus, in both formal and informal relationships, influence and communication focused on health behavior change is more likely to be effective when the interactions between that agent and the target of influence are rewarding.

The norm of reciprocity may not apply consistently in two types of circumstances: in formal relationships in which there are well-defined and complementary roles, such as those between a doctor and a patient, and in longer-term, ongoing informal relationships that are emotionally close, such as those between spouses or family members. In the former example, the reciprocity norm does not apply because there are well-defined rules of interaction and obligation. In the latter, the reciprocity norm does not apply because rewards can be exchanged over longer periods of time; in closer relationships, people start to see close others as part of their own identity, and providing rewards to another is like rewarding one's self (Aron, Aron, and Smollen, 1992).

Even so, there are several reasons why the norm of reciprocity may govern influence and communication surrounding health behavior in the previous examples.

Secular trends are leading patients to assume increased responsibility and control for their care. Current empowerment and health education strategies suggest that clients should be more involved in setting the agenda for changes in their health behavior (Emmons and Rollnick, 2001). Also, when interventions use family members or friends as the channel for an intervention, the usual roles and interactions between people are changed. In each of these situations, interactions, roles, and responsibilities in the relationship are different, and the norm of reciprocity becomes increasingly important. What this suggests is that health providers (including counselors and educators) need to be particularly sensitive to the client's needs when roles are uncertain, take more responsibility to make sure the interaction is rewarding, and consider building opportunities for reciprocity into interventions that use influence and communication to change health behaviors.

While Social Exchange Theory examines the exchange of rewards and its consequences, Interdependence Theory emphasizes patterns of outcomes that interacting partners may experience and how these patterns are influenced by the partners' relationship. Key concepts in Interdependence Theory include interdependence, relationship interdependence, and correspondence of outcomes.

Interdependence is the process by which people influence each other's experiences, or the effects an individual exerts on another person's motives, preferences, behavior, and outcomes (Rusbult and Van Lange, 1996). (See Figure 11.1.) Health behavior is partially determined by one's own characteristics, as shown by the parallel lines in Figure 11.1; by the beliefs, values, and behaviors of one's partner, as shown by the crossed lines in the figure; and by the reciprocal or joint influence of both people in an interaction, as shown by the vertical line. In dyads, one person's behavior is never free from the influence of the partner's behavior. In a health care interaction, the relevant dyad can be either a person and his or her family member (for example, a spouse or parent), or a patient and a health professional.

The concept of interdependence is important to health behavior for at least two reasons. Interdependence suggests that interacting partners should be included in interventions that usually target individuals. It also suggests the need to better understand what portion of health behavior is related to the influence of an interacting partner, what portion can be attributed to an individual's own characteristics, and what portion of the health behavior can be attributed to their mutual influence. Using Interdependence Theory to understand adjustment after a heart attack, Coyne and colleagues (Coyne, Ellard, and Smith, 1990) found that the patient's self-efficacy was jointly determined by both patient and spouse variables.

Relationship interdependence refers to the structural characteristics of a relationship that bring people closer together or drive them apart. Just as social networks can have structural properties, such as density or reciprocity (see Chapter Nine), Interdependence Theory suggests that relationship characteristics that bring people closer, such

FIGURE 11.1. INTERDEPENDENCE MODEL OF
SOCIAL INFLUENCE AND INTERPERSONAL COMMUNICATION.

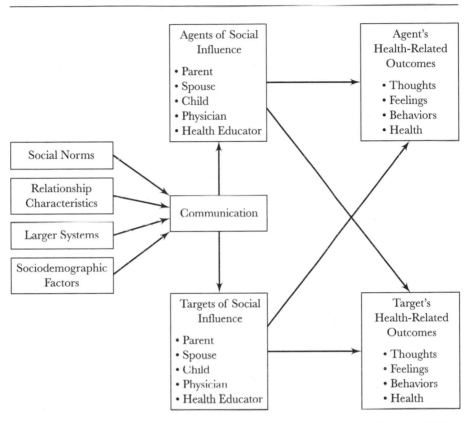

as feelings of attachment or equality, should make influence and communication more effective in changing behavior. Conversely, relationship characteristics that drive people apart, such as conflict or disagreement, impede the effects influence and communication have in changing health behavior (Lewis and Butterfield, 1998b).

Correspondence of outcomes is another concept from Interdependence Theory that has implications in changing health behaviors in relationships. Correspondence of outcomes is the degree to which interacting partners agree about the shared or joint outcomes in the relationship (Rusbult and Van Lange, 1996). Correspondent outcomes occur when partners are fully cooperative with each other in determining the desired behavior (for example, setting goals together); noncorrespondent outcomes occur when partners are completely conflicted in determining behavior.

There are three reasons why the correspondence of outcomes in a dyad is important (Rusbult and Van Lange, 1996). First, the degree of correspondence suggests how much conflict regarding behavioral change may exist in a dyad. For example, a spouse who does not quit smoking after his or her partner quits smoking sets the stage for noncorrespondence in smoking outcomes and for conflict about continued smoking behavior. Likewise, if a physician and patient strongly agree that the best course of action to stem the effects of heart disease is for the patient to change dietary habits, they will have a much easier time working together to achieve this goal. Health educators working with couples in which partners' behaviors are discordant must realize there may be conflict in the relationship over an issue. If conflict exists, then simple knowledge-based approaches to change may not help the couple move toward successful behavioral change.

Second, the degree of correspondence between partners can help focus attention on important values, motivations, and barriers to behavioral change. When potential discrepancies are identified, it may help individuals and couples to reevaluate the barriers to change and the outcomes they value the most. Third, the degree of correspondence is related to how easily interacting partners can make decisions about behavioral change. When there is greater correspondence, decision making should be easier, and the health educator could focus efforts on knowledge, skills building, and maintenance activities to assist couples to change health-related behaviors. Couples' decision making will be most difficult when outcomes are only moderately correspondent (Liebrand, 1992). The opportunity to recognize the interdependence of behavioral change and the goal of making knowledge, values, and behaviors correspond within a family unit may be an advantage of family-focused over individual-focused behavioral change interventions.

Influence and Communication in Formal Dyadic Relationships

This section reviews concepts and literature that relate exchange and interdependence concepts to communication between health care professionals and patients. Most of the literature focuses on physician-patient interaction and on interactions between health educators or counselors and their clients.

Bases of Power and Health Behavior Change

Joos and Hickam (1990) described different types of actual and potential power that have been observed in patient interactions with health providers. The bases of power were first described by French and Raven (1959) and were further elaborated by Raven over thirty years later (Raven, 1993). They were also recently adapted by van Ryn and Heaney (1997) for the specific case of power in health educator–client relationships. This typology identifies six bases of power that make people influential in communication: expert, legitimate, coercive, reward, informational, and referent power.

Expert power involves behavioral change that has as its main basis seeing someone else as more knowledgeable. A related type of power, *legitimate power,* operates when another is viewed has having "the right" to direct a person's behavior and that person feels obligated to comply. This perception of mutual rights and obligations derives from social roles that are imbued with authority and credibility. When people change because they think another can reward or punish them, then *coercive* and *reward powers* are operating. Expert, legitimate, coercive, and reward power are thought to be most useful for achieving short-term influence and less effective in creating long-term behavioral change (Joos and Hickam, 1990). These types of power do not capitalize on reciprocity, which may explain why they are generally less successful than other bases of power (such as informational or referent power) in affecting behavioral change.

Health educators exert *informational power* by providing people with access to information that is conveyed in a clear and persuasive way. As van Ryn and Heaney (1997) observed, the provision of information is a widely used strategy in health education that can lead to health-promoting beliefs and behaviors. However, there may be other persuasive forces such as advertising that interfere with acting on health-promoting information. Also, some health risk behaviors are firmly entrenched and habitual, and provide people with immediate gratification or pleasure. Thus, the exercise of informational power (Raven, 1993) may be a necessary, but not a sufficient, condition for behavioral change.

Referent power, viewed as the most effective source of influence or power in formal dyadic relationships, is based on one's identification with the professional as a person like herself or himself in some respect, and may generate feelings of communality, security, and trust (Joos and Hickam, 1990). Interactions based on referent power begin to approximate a more informal type of relationship. The term *referent* is derived from "the term *reference group,* which is used to describe groups with which we feel psychologically involved. These are the groups to which we refer for our norms and values" (van Ryn and Heaney, 1997, p. 685).

Many recommendations for how health providers should behave are based on referent power. However, the use of referent power is frequently combined with at least one other source of power. For example, the provider may need to provide information about successful strategies others have used to reach a patient's goals (informational power) or may need to gain legitimacy or establish expertise in the eyes of the client (expert power).

One challenge to achieving referent power derives from social status and informational differences between health professionals and their clients or patients. Use of empowerment approaches, however, can help overcome these barriers. For example, with empowerment strategies the health professional would demonstrate respect and empathy, share power with the client, identify and build on the client's strengths, and engage in mutual problem solving. These approaches are more likely to result in successful and longer-term behavioral change because clients are more likely to have their needs and wishes addressed and attribute behavioral change successes to themselves rather than to the health care providers (Rodin and Janis, 1982). Many of the contemporary models for studying influence and communication between physicians and patients are based on the idea of effectively applied referent power.

Influence and Communication Between Health Care Providers and Patients

Health care provider-patient interactions have been studied for over fifty years by medical sociologists and health services researchers (Parsons, 1951; Roter and Hall, 1992). During provider-patient interactions, the level of patient involvement may vary on a continuum from totally passive (Parsons, 1951) to extremely active (Roter and Hall, 1992; Haug and Lavin, 1983). The different types of provider-patient encounters are best illustrated by Roter and Hall's typology of provider-patient relationships. The level of control that the provider and patient possess determines which of the four typologies is operating.

Paternalism is defined as a relationship in which there is high provider control and low patient control over their interaction; it reflects the use of expert and legitimate power. In this type of relationship, the patient is passive and not actively involved during the encounter. Many individuals may prefer this type of relationship and do not want to question their physician (Roter and Hall, 1992).

On the other end of the spectrum is *Consumerism*, defined by low provider control and high patient control (Haug and Lavin, 1983). In this type of relationship, patients actively dominate what occurs during the visit.

Default is characterized by a lack of control by either the patient or the provider (Roter and Hall, 1992). In this type of relationship, a patient may drop out of care because of frustrated goals or failed expectations.

Mutuality is a more balanced type of provider-patient relationship, in which both the patient and provider have high control and are actively involved during the encounter (Roter and Hall, 1992; Sleath, 1996). To have a provider-patient relationship that can be considered mutual, the health care provider would need to use a participatory or patient-centered communication style with the patient. Using this style, he or she would solicit the patient's agenda for the visit and involve the patient in treatment decisions (Kaplan, Greenfield, Gandek, Rogers, and Ware, 1996; Stewart, 2000). The participatory, or shared, decision making involves mutuality and is consistent with referent power.

Participatory patient-centered approaches based on mutuality and referent power are related to better patient outcomes (Adams, Smith, and Ruffin, 2001; Stewart, 2000). These outcomes include better health-related quality of life (Adams, Smith, and Ruffin, 2001), patient recovery, emotional health, and fewer diagnostic tests and referrals (Stewart, 2000). In addition, a participatory decision-making style is related to greater patient satisfaction and loyalty to the physician (Kaplan, Greenfield, Gandek, Rogers, and Ware, 1996). Evidence indicates that a participatory style is also important with children during medical visits (Wissow and others, 1998). These findings are consistent with Interdependence Theory, which suggests that formal relationships that exchange more rewards and acknowledge reciprocity and interdependence will result in improved health behavior. However, it is important to recognize that some patients may prefer a more directive style of health provider communication by virtue of their education, culture, or low tolerance for ambiguity at a given point in the treatment process.

Previous studies have suggested that some patients may be reluctant to ask questions during their visits (Cockburn, Reid, and Sanson-Fisher, 1987). However, Sleath, Roter, Chewning, and Svarstad (1999) found that patients who asked more questions about medications were rated by physicians as more interested and assertive, and that physicians were not irritated or angry by these engaged patients. Thus, patients whose reticence is based on a fear of reprisals can be encouraged to ask questions during their medical visits, as more active involvement by both patients and physicians may result in positive outcomes for both parties.

Health education can play an important role in activating patients in their interactions with health care professionals. Results of randomized trials indicate that patients can be successfully motivated to become more involved during their medical visits by the provision of face-to-face educational sessions conducted by health educators right before their medical visit (Kaplan, Greenfield, and Ware, 1989; Greenfield, Kaplan, Ware, Yano, and Frank, 1988; McGee and Cegala, 1998). Patients who were trained about the purpose of the different phases of the medical encounter and encouraged to ask questions about their conditions asked significantly more questions on medical topics than did untrained patients. The findings also indicate that "trained" active patients have improved health outcomes (Kaplan, Greenfield, and Ware, 1989; Greenfield, Kaplan, Ware, Yano, and Frank, 1988).

Factors That Moderate Patient-Provider Influence and Communication

A variety of background factors are related to more active provider-patient interactions (see left-hand boxes in Figure 11.1). These include the use of similar language (Rivadeneyra, Elderkin-Thompson, Silver, and Waitzkin, 2000), the age of the patient, and higher incomes and educational levels (Lupton, 1997; Haug and Lavin, 1983; Thompson, Pitts, and Schwankovsky, 1993). Other studies found that female patients were more actively involved during medical visits than were male patients (Haug and Lavin, 1983; Thompson, Pitts, and Schwankovsky, 1993; Wallen, Waitzkin, and Stoeckle, 1979; Pendleton and Bochner, 1980).

The health care setting can also influence provider-patient communication. Physicians in higher-volume practices are rated as being less participatory by their patients than those in lower-volume practices. Further, cost-containment strategies, which reduce physicians' time with patients, may decrease physician autonomy and result in lower physician satisfaction and may also negatively affect patient outcomes (Kaplan, Greenfield, Gandek, Rogers, and Ware, 1996).

Secular trends in health care financing, advertising, and use of alternative and complementary medicine can adversely affect physician-patient communication. They may cause patients to be more demanding for potentially inappropriate treatments, make the relationship less rewarding, and heighten conflict over treatment outcomes. Freidson (1989) found that patients who demanded services they felt they had a right to request under prepaid service contracts disturbed many physicians. In addition, the pharmaceutical industry increasingly relies on direct-to-consumer advertising to encourage demand for prescription drugs. Annual expenditures for direct-to-consumer advertising were $1 billion in 1997 and may reach $7.5 billion by 2005 (Burton and Ono, 1997), and research suggests that patients are increasingly more persuasive in their demands for medications (Bell, Wilkes, and Kravitz, 1999). Thus, health care providers may need new skills to effectively communicate and negotiate treatment regimens with patients who demand products they see advertised in magazines or on television.

The increased use of complementary and alternative medicine in the United States is influencing provider-patient communication. The explosion of interest in complementary and alternative medicine is reflected in the fact that 30 to 45 percent of all patients use such alternatives (Eisenberg and others, 1993). Even though many patients use these therapies, few patients commonly discuss them with their physicians (Eisenberg and others, 1993). Part of the problem is that health care providers are not asking patients about their use of alternative treatments. Typically, physicians ask fewer than 5 percent of patients whether they are using any type of alternative therapy (Sleath, Rubin, Campbell, Gwyther, and Clark, 2001).

Influence and Communication in Health Behavior Change Interventions

The emerging attention to patient-centered approaches in clinical and therapeutic interactions has recently been extended to health behavior research and practice. Motivational Interviewing (MI) is a directive but nonconfrontational client-centered communication technique that elicits behavioral change by helping clients explore and work through ambivalence about changing their behavior (Emmons and Rollnick, 2001; Resnicow and others, forthcoming). The technique was originally developed and applied in psychological counseling for addictive behaviors such as alcohol and drug abuse (Miller and Rollnick, 1991). The delivery time of a traditional MI counseling component of a treatment program can range from several to many hours. MI delivered in this context enjoyed successes by advancing clients' readiness to change and also was found to result in actual behavioral change.

Given the success of MI, shortened forms of this approach have been incorporated into strategies for health behavior change (Rollnick, Mason, and Butler, 2000). Health behavior and health education researchers have wondered if this approach could be applied to other health-promoting and disease-preventing behaviors, shortened significantly, and used by practitioners with no training in psychotherapy. There are a number of recently completed health education intervention studies, and many more currently under way, that derive from MI (Miller and Rollnick, 1991; Resnicow and others, forthcoming).

Motivational Interviewing is compatible with referent power and participatory, client-centered approaches to health behavior change advocated almost fifty years ago by Carl Rogers (Rogers, 1957). Practitioners use empathic and reflective listening and directive questioning to help clients focus on their ambivalence about behavioral change. They also focus on the values the clients hold that may be consistent or inconsistent with changing to healthier behavior. Clients are seen as the experts in evaluating their own behavior and generating potential solutions for problem behaviors. The practitioner's role involves offering clients facts and pointing out discrepancies between the clients' goals and behavior. The client is responsible for interpreting the implications of these facts and discrepancies and for generating self-motivating strategies or statements. In this way, the practitioner avoids confrontation and advice giving. From the MI perspective the client, not the practitioner, is viewed as the expert. An example of the application of MI to health behavior change is provided later in this chapter.

Influence and Communication in Informal Relationships

Understanding influence and communication in informal relationships is important for health behavior research and practice. Health behavior interventions have often used informal social network members as the *channel* for delivering health information. This occurs in lay health adviser programs and in family-based prevention programs in which parents act as the channel for health communication messages for children. Other health behavior interventions include the spouse as part of the intervention to change dietary practices, smoking, or medication adherence (Lassner, 1991). For some interventions, social influence and communication are part of a more comprehensive intervention. This contrasts with the research and intervention just presented on formal relationships, in which communication is often the central feature or main intervention component. However, given the increasing use of close social network members to deliver or leverage health behavior interventions, a better understanding of the more successful types of communication is useful.

Influence and Communication Between Parents and Children

Recent research has explored how parenting style affects the health behavior of children and adolescents (Jackson, Henriksen, and Foshee, 1998), and is attempting to elucidate a particular style, termed authoritative parenting (Baumrind, 1978). Studies have found that authoritative parenting is associated with less tobacco and alcohol use in children (Jackson, Henriksen, and Foshee, 1998) and less aggression and drug use among adolescents (Jackson, Henriksen, and Foshee, 1998; Mounts and Steinberg, 1995). Authoritative parenting involves using influence and communication that are bidirectional between the parent and child, setting appropriate standards for a child while also providing developmentally appropriate boundaries for behavior, providing emotional support, and being responsive to a child's concerns (Simons-Morton and Hartos, 2002).

Interventions are currently under way to enhance and teach authoritative parenting to prevent children's early tobacco experimentation (Jackson, 1998) and to prevent problems associated with teen driving (Simons-Morton and Hartos, 2002). Although these interventions involve multiple components that focus on multiple parenting behaviors, the essence of these interventions is to enhance communication and influence between parents and children to prevent children's health-compromising behavior.

These interventions are based on both correlational studies that link authoritative parenting with better behavior and previous interventions that changed parenting style by enhancing communication skills and decreasing conflict between parents and teens. For example, the program Preparing for the Drug Free Years aims to reduce risks, such as family conflict, and improve protective factors, such as parent-child communication, thereby reducing the initiation of early substance use by children. Evaluations of this program based on analyses of videotaped communication between parents and children before and after the intervention indicated that authoritative parenting was successfully increased (Kosterman, Hawkins,

Spoth, Haggerty, and Zhu, 1997). For this program, researchers are currently evaluating how these positive changes in parent-child communication may affect early substance use by children, but results of similar interventions have shown that enhancing communication can lead to reductions in adolescent problem behaviors (Irvine, Biglan, Smolkowski, Metzler, and Ary, 1999).

Influence and Communication in Marital Relationships

A greater understanding of spousal influence and communication is especially important, given the disappointing results from interventions that have used a spouse to help change health behavior. Many behavioral change interventions involving spouses were based on the epidemiological evidence that linked marriage with a lower mortality risk (House, Landis, and Umberson, 1988) and the strong association of spousal support with a variety of health outcomes (Burman and Margolin, 1992). A 1990 meta-analysis of couple interventions that focused on weight loss found that couple interventions were more successful than individual treatment, but the effect was very small and the benefit lasted for no more than two to three months postprogram (Black, Gleser, and Kooyers, 1990). These interventions typically involved a combination of dietary changes, increased physical activity, and medication. There were several limitations to these interventions, including poor assessment of spouses' supportive behaviors during the initiation of behavioral change and the absence of information on actual spouse roles in maintenance of change after the interventions were completed (Kelsey, Earp, and Kirkley, 1997).

Reviews of smoking cessation interventions reached similar conclusions about spousal interventions (Cohen and others, 1988). According to Lichtenstein and Glasgow (1992), intervention efforts that attempted to enhance spousal support yielded uniformly negative results. Although correlational studies reveal positive associations between spousal support and smoking quit rates, the experimental interventions produce negative results (Lichtenstein and Glasgow, 1992). A theoretical analysis of both the weight loss and smoking cessation interventions suggested that when the spouse is involved in a program that is "relationship-based" rather than an adjunct to cognitive-behavioral treatment, spousal support interventions are more successful (Lassner, 1991). Given these findings, a better understanding of spousal influence and communication is needed to develop better partner-assisted interventions.

Influence Strategies Between Spouses

Compliance gaining refers to tactics or strategies a person uses when trying to influence someone else's behavior (Dillard, 1990) and is one type of approach that may help in developing a better understanding of spousal influence and communication.

Recent research suggests ways to link use of compliance-gaining tactics in communication between spouses who are attempting to influence a partner to change his or her health behavior.

Several preliminary conclusions can be drawn from this emerging literature. Qualitative data from focus groups have revealed various health-related influence tactics used by husbands and wives, including modeling the health behavior; making structural changes in the home, workplace, or time management to make it easier for the spouse to engage in healthful behavior; and doing the healthy behavior with the spouse (Lewis, Butterfield, Darbes, and Johnston-Brooks, 1999).

Quantitative analyses of health-related influence and communication between couples indicate that these tactics can be organized into three dimensions, all of which have been related to health behavior change: direct versus indirect, positive versus negative, and bilateral versus unilateral. The use of positive, direct, and bilateral health-related influence tactics by one spouse predicts the partner's health behavior change (Lewis and Butterfield, 1998a). These findings have also been replicated in experimental studies with people in dating relationships (Lewis and Butterfield, forthcoming). Further, a couple's relationship interdependence moderates the association of these influence tactics on behavioral change (Lewis and Butterfield, 1998b). Finally, husbands and wives who are influencing their spouses to initiate a health-enhancing behavior use positive and direct tactics more frequently and negative tactics less frequently (Butterfield and Lewis, forthcoming). While these findings provide some direction for partner-assisted interventions, more research is needed to better understand health-behavior-related influence and communication between spouses.

Factors That Moderate Communication and Influence in Informal Relationships

Social norms regarding health behavior can affect influence and communication in informal relationships. Social norms are expectations held by social groups that dictate appropriate behavior and are thought of as rules or standards that guide behavior (Cialdini and Trost, 1999). Social norms are commonly invoked as an explanation for health behavior, although there is little consensus on how norms should be conceptualized or measured.

Reno and colleagues (Reno, Cialdini, and Kallgren, 1993) attempted to clarify the conceptualization of social norms and distinguished two types of norms—*descriptive norms* and *injunctive norms*. Descriptive norms indicate the way most people act in a given situation and are believed to play a role in motivation by depicting what is considered appropriate or effective behavior in a situation. Descriptive norms have been related to greater intentions to use condoms to prevent HIV transmission (Van den Eijnden, Buunk, Bakker, and Siero, 1998). Injunctive norms indicate what types of behaviors others approve or disapprove of in a given situation and affect motivation by ensuring disapproval or sanctions following undesirable behavior. They tend to be related to the goal of building and maintaining relationships. Foshee and others (1998; 2000) found that injunctive norms about the acceptability of abuse in dating relationships mediated the effects of preventive education on dating violence on abusive behaviors.

Cialdini and Trost (1999) suggested that the salience of either of these norms determines behavior. Whichever norm is made most salient should influence health-related behaviors, especially in three situations: when persons are in uncertain or unfamiliar situations or conditions, when the agent of social influence is similar to the target of social influence, and when the target of social influence is motivated to maintain a relationship with the agent of social influence. Each of these conditions applies when informal relationships are used as a channel for implementing or leveraging health behavior change interventions.

Unequal power and poor relationship quality affects influence and communication in informal relationships, consistent with the findings described earlier for formal relationships. For example, Howard and colleagues (Howard, Blumstein, and Schwartz, 1986) found that spouses in more unequal relationships were more likely to use negative influence tactics such as manipulation. These researchers concluded that positions of weakness or inequality are associated with the increased use of indirect, unilateral, or negative tactics. Along with unequal power, relationship satisfaction affects the tactics people use to influence each other. Those who are satisfied with their relationships are less likely to use tactics that might disrupt relationship functioning (Aida and Falbo, 1991).

Applications of Influence and Communication to Health Behavior Change Interventions

This section describes two applications of social influence and interpersonal communication to health behavior change. The first application involves a test of motivational interviewing to enhance fruit and vegetable consumption among African American churchgoers. The second application describes a family intervention to prevent adolescent smoking and alcohol use.

Using Motivational Interviewing to Increase Fruit and Vegetable Intake

Resnicow and others (2001) evaluated the effectiveness of a Motivational Interviewing intervention to increase fruit and vegetable intake among members of African American churches. Participants were recruited from fourteen churches matched on socioeconomic status and size. Churches were randomly assigned to one of three intervention conditions. Participants who were church members in the first condition served as the comparison group and received standard nutrition education materials. Participants who were church members in the second condition received a multicomponent self-help intervention that included one "cue" telephone call, which prompted participants to read the program materials. Participants in the first two groups also received other culturally sensitive intervention materials.

Participants in the third condition received the same program as did those in the second condition plus three MI telephone calls, each averaging eleven to fifteen minutes. The MI counselors were registered dietitians or dietetic interns who had participated in three two-hour MI training sessions. The MI phone calls, which focused on changing fruit and vegetable intake, were guided by the client-centered, empathic, encouraging, and nonconfrontational methods of MI. More specifically, the counselors began by asking the participants two questions that were then followed by two probes. The first question asked the participants to pick a number from 1 to 10 (with 10 being the highest) that described how motivated or interested they were in eating more fruits and vegetables. The second question asked how confident they were that they could increase the amount of fruits and vegetables they ate. The two follow-up probe questions asked (1) why the participants did not choose a lower number in response to the first question, which would have indicated no-to-low motivation; and (2) why the participants did not choose a higher number in response to the second question. The first probe was designed to elicit positive motivational statements from the participants whereas the second probe was designed to elicit barriers to positive change. The counselor then summarized the participants' reasons for wanting or not wanting to change, prompted the participants to come up with solutions and then, with the participants' permission, added some strategies to the list of solutions "that had worked for others." If the participants wished, the call ended with contracting to try one of the barrier solutions. Of the 1,011 individuals who completed baseline information, 85 percent were assessed at one-year follow-up. Fruit and vegetable intake increases were significantly greater in the MI group than in the other two intervention groups (Resnicow and others, 2001).

Not all intervention studies have been as successful as the one just described. A recent literature review described negative as well as positive findings from other studies (Resnicow and others, forthcoming). It pointed out that applications of MI represents a new field of intervention research when delivered as a relatively brief intervention with professionals who receive systematic but limited training. A key concern about MI interventions like this one relates to its validity: Is the intervention being delivered *really* an MI intervention? Some critics have suggested that health education interventions derived from MI should be called something else, such as "motivational interviewing informed" or "brief negotiation interviewing."

Influence and Communication to Prevent Adolescent Smoking and Alcohol Use

Tobacco and alcohol use by adolescents is a significant and prevalent problem in the United States. In 1997, 43 percent of teens in grades nine through twelve reported using tobacco recently, and 20 percent of those aged twelve to seventeen had used alcohol recently (U.S. Department of Health and Human Services, 2000). Because many school-based programs have small and short-term effects on the use of these substances (for example, Ellickson, Bell, and McGuigan, 1993), some intervention efforts have turned toward family-based programs for preventing substance use.

Family Matters is a family-directed program that focuses on prevention of substance use (smoking and alcohol use) among teens aged twelve to fourteen years. The program is guided by a wide variety of principles from social influence theories, persuasion theories, social learning theory, communication theory, and social developmental theory (Bauman, Foshee, Ennett, Hicks, and Pemberton, 2001). The fundamental assumption of the program is that families can be engaged to influence adolescent substance use through positive family interactions and communication that strengthen family and adolescent norms against substance use. The program involves mailing four consecutive booklets that address topics related to negative consequences of teen substance use (booklet 1); to understanding adolescence, family communication, and family functioning (booklet 2); to how the family can influence substance use (booklet 3); and to how outside influences affect substance use (booklet 4). In addition, each booklet describes activities for both parents and teens. After receiving each booklet, a parent has a discussion with a health educator. The discussions with health educators are meant to serve as an impetus for completing the program as well as a forum for answering questions about the program information or suggested activities. A summary of influence and communication concepts used in Family Matters is shown in Table 11.2. While the program focused heavily on involving *all* family members, the theoretical foundations of the program are consistent with a focus on dyadic communication and influence.

An evaluation of the effectiveness of Family Matters was conducted with a national random sample of teens aged twelve to fourteen and their families. Parent-teen dyads provided baseline data and were then randomly assigned to a control group or to the Family Matters group. Process evaluation indicated the mother (or mother-surrogate) was the primary parent involved in the program (Bauman,

TABLE 11.2. INFLUENCE AND
COMMUNICATION CONCEPTS USED IN FAMILY MATTERS.

Concept	Intervention Activities
Norm of reciprocity	Expect that all family members would participate in intervention activities (general assumption underlying all booklets)
Interdependence	Increase recognition of how adolescent tobacco and alcohol use affects teen *and* family (booklet 1)
Relationship interdependence	Discuss shared experiences, spend time together, reduce conflict (booklet 2)
Correspondence of outcomes	Identify behaviors and characteristics that parent and adolescent share (booklet 1)
Authoritative parenting	Emphasize bidirectional (two-way) communication related to adolescent tobacco and alcohol use *that also* sets developmentally appropriate standards for behavior (booklets 2,3)
Compliance gaining	Emphasize positive, bilateral, and direct communication about expectations regarding adolescent tobacco and alcohol use (all booklets)
Descriptive social norms	Discuss peer influence and resistance to peer influence; watch and discuss television shows that have alcohol and smoking messages to highlight and correct misperceptions (booklet 4)
Injunctive social norms	Agree on rules and sanctions for adolescent alcohol and tobacco use (booklet 3)

Foshee, Ennett, Hicks, and Pemberton, 2001), although by no means the only parent involved. Mothers were the parent involved in the evaluation of the program 96 percent of the time. Telephone interviews to evaluate program effectiveness were made three and twelve months after program completion (Bauman and others, 2001).

Compared with the control condition, Family Matters was successful in reducing smoking initiation by 16.4 percent at the twelve-month follow-up, with an even larger reduction (25 percent) among nonHispanic white teens (Bauman and others, 2001). The program also reduced the overall prevalence of adolescent smoking among nonHispanic whites and the overall prevalence of alcohol use in the entire sample (Ennett and others, 2001). There were no significant effects, however, on onset of alcohol or smokeless tobacco use (Bauman and others, 2001) nor for cigarette or alcohol cessation (Bauman and others, 2000). Bauman and colleagues speculate about a number of methodological and normative factors, which may have accounted for the different program outcomes for smokeless to-bacco, alcohol use, and cessation outcomes, such as the infrequent use of smoke-less tobacco in their sample and the increasing negative publicity about smoking versus alcohol use (Bauman and others, 2001). It is also possible that it was easier for parents to influence initial uptake of smoking behavior than uptake of other substances or of cessation among those who had already tried them. The authors note that the effect of Family Matters on smoking initiation is comparable to that of school-based programs. Programs such as Family Matters, which attempt to capitalize on influence and communication in families, deserve further develop-ment and evaluation.

Conclusion

This chapter focused on influence and communication in informal and formal re-lationships— mainly dyadic ones—with particular emphasis on concepts from In-terdependence Theory. We have highlighted how influence and communication can be effectively applied to health behavior research and practice. In formal health care relationships, there is evidence that influence and communication are more effective when patients and clients are viewed as partners in the behavioral change process and that health educators can gain greater legitimacy by using participatory, client-centered approaches in health education. Although there is less systematic research on what makes influence and communication in informal relationships more successful, communication that is more positive, involves give and take, and directly addresses the issue appears to be more effective.

Several caveats should be noted regarding influence and communication processes in both formal and informal relationships. The act of influence and communication creates a disparity between the target's actual thoughts, feelings, and behaviors and the goal intended by the agent of influence. This disparity can generate feelings of hostility or sadness on the part of the target (Lewis and Rook, 1999). Such findings suggest that when influence and communication are used in interventions, it is important to measure unintended and negative outcomes, such as psychological distress or tension, as well as the intended health behavior change outcomes. It may also be important to perform measurements at different points in time, as the change process may evoke initial negative outcomes that are re-solved with time and successful change among recipients of such communications.

Influence is a characteristic of the social environment, external to the target or recipient, but the goal is behavioral change that is internalized and maintained over time by the client. Long-term maintenance of health-enhancing behavior is only sustained when the target internalizes social influence attempts. Kelman's

(1974) distinction between *compliance, identification,* and *internalization* is helpful in describing the process by which influence and communication result in short-term or long-term behavioral change. Compliance occurs when the target accepts influence attempts to achieve a favorable reaction from the agent, such as approval. Acceptance of influence in this form results in short-term behavioral change. Identification occurs when the target accepts influence attempts to start or maintain a rewarding relationship with the agent. In this case, influence and communication may result in longer-term behavioral change but only when the relationship between the agent and target is maintained. Internalization occurs when the target accepts the agent's influence attempts because the goal advocated by the agent matches his or her own goals and values. Internalized social influence may be the only condition under which long-term behavioral change can be sustained. In this chapter, we have highlighted a number of conditions under which influence and communication are more effective in changing health behaviors. These conditions should also facilitate greater internalization of influence attempts from a health care provider or health educator.

Although influence and communication can lead to the development of more effective intervention research and practice, both processes, if used incorrectly, can be coercive. This chapter has not reviewed what is known about using communication and influence that are intentionally deceptive, manipulative, or coercive. In fact, the theory and evidence presented here clearly argue against the use of these types of interpersonal influence strategies. Such interactions would usually outweigh any positive impact of influence and communication on changing health behavior. Like most health behavior experts, we do not advocate the use of coercive interpersonal communication strategies. Instead, this chapter reflects the contemporary social environment as well as research and theory that support the thoughtful use of interpersonal influence and communication in health behavior research and practice. Using these ideas will advance our understanding of how to maximize the benefits of social influence and interpersonal communication for health improvement.

References

Adams, R. J., Smith, B. J., and Ruffin, R. "Impact of the Physician's Participatory Style in Asthma Outcomes and Patient Satisfaction." *Annals of Allergy, Asthma, and Immunology,* 2001, *86,* 263–271.

Aida, Y., and Falbo, T. "Relationships Between Marital Satisfaction, Resources, and Power Strategies." *Sex Roles,* 1991, *24,* 43–56.

Aron, A., Aron, E. N., and Smollen, D. "Inclusion of Other in the Self Scale and the Structure of Interpersonal Closeness." *Journal of Personality and Social Psychology,* 1992, *63,* 596–612.

Bauman, K. E., Foshee, V. A., Ennett, S. T., Hicks, K., and Pemberton, M. "Family Matters: A Family-Directed Program Designed to Prevent Adolescent Tobacco and Alcohol Use." *Health Promotion Practice,* 2001, *2,* 81–96.

Bauman, K. E., and others. "Influence of a Family-Directed Program on Adolescent Cigarette and Alcohol Cessation." *Prevention Science,* 2000, *1,* 227–237.

Bauman, K. E., and others. "The Influence of a Family Program on Adolescent Tobacco and Alcohol Use." *American Journal of Public Health,* 2001, *91,* 604–610.

Baumrind, D. "Parental Disciplinary Patterns and Social Competence in Children." *Youth & Society,* 1978, *9,* 887–907.

Bell, R. A., Wilkes, M. S., and Kravitz, R. L. "Advertisement-Induced Prescription Drug Requests: Patients' Anticipated Reactions to a Physician Who Refuses." *The Journal of Family Practice,* 1999, *48*(6), 446–452.

Black, D. R., Gleser, L. J., and Kooyers, K. J. "A Meta-Analytic Evaluation of Weight-Loss Programs." *Health Psychology,* 1990, *9,* 330–347.

Burman, B., and Margolin, G. "Analysis of the Association Between Marital Relationships and Health Problems: An Interactional Perspective." *Psychological Bulletin,* 1992, *112,* 39–63.

Burton, T. M., and Ono, Y. "Campaign for Prozac Targets Customers." *Wall Street Journal,* July 1, 1997, pp. B1, B6.

Butterfield, R. M., and Lewis, M. A. "Health-Related Social Influence: A Social Ecological Perspective on Tactic Use." *Journal of Social and Personal Relationships,* forthcoming.

Cialdini, R. B., and Trost, M. B. "Social Influence: Social Norms, Conformity, and Compliance." In D. T. Gilbert, S. T. Fiske, and G. Lindzey (eds.), *Handbook of Social Psychology.* (4th ed.) Boston: McGraw-Hill, 1999, 151–192.

Cockburn, J., Reid, A., and Sanson-Fisher, R. "The Process and Content of General-Practice Consultations That Involve Prescription of Antibiotic Agents." *Medical Journal of Australia,* 1987, *147,* 321–324.

Cohen, S., and others. "Social Support Interventions for Smoking Cessation." In B. H. Gottlieb (ed.), *Marshaling Social Support: Formats, Processes, and Effects.* Thousand Oaks, Calif.: Sage, 1988.

Coyne, J. C., Ellard, J. H., and Smith, D. A. "Social Support, Interdependence, and the Dilemmas of Helping." In B. R. Sarason, I. G. Sarason, and G. R. Pierce (eds.), *Social Support: An Interactional View.* New York: Wiley, 1990.

Dillard, J. P. *Seeking Compliance: The Production of Interpersonal Influence Messages.* Scottsdale, Ariz.: Gorsuch Scarisbrick, 1990.

Eisenberg, D. M., and others. "Unconventional Therapies in the United States: Prevalence, Costs, and Patterns of Use." *New England Journal of Medicine,* 1993, *328,* 246–252.

Ellickson, P. L., Bell, R. M., and McGuigan, K. "Preventing Adolescent Drug Use: Long-Term Results of a Junior High Program." *American Journal of Public Health,* 1993, *83,* 856–861.

Emmons, K. M., and Rollnick, S. "Motivational Interviewing in Health Care Settings: Opportunities and Limitations." *American Journal of Preventive Medicine,* 2001, *20,* 68–74.

Ennett, S. T., and others. "Mediation in a Family-Directed Program for Prevention of Adolescent Tobacco and Alcohol Use." *Preventive Medicine,* 2001, *33,* 333–346.

Foshee, V. A., and others. "An Evaluation of Safe Dates, an Adolescent Dating Violence Prevention Program." *American Journal of Public Health,* 1998, *88,* 45–50.

Foshee, V. A., and others. "The Safe Dates Program: 1-Year Follow-Up Results." *American Journal of Public Health,* 2000, *90,* 1619–1622.

Freidson, E. *Medical Work in America: Essays on Health Care.* New Haven: Yale University Press, 1989.

French, J.R.P., and Raven, B. H. "The Bases of Power." In D. Cartwright (ed.), *Studies in Social Power.* Ann Arbor, Mich.: Institute for Social Research, 1959.

Goudner, A. W. "The Norm of Reciprocity: A Preliminary Statement." *American Sociological Review,* 1960, *25,* 161–178.

Greenfield, S., Kaplan, S. H., Ware, J. E., Yano, E. M., and Frank, H. J. "Patients' Participation in Medical Care: Effects of Blood Sugar Control and Quality of Life in Diabetes." *Journal of General Internal Medicine,* 1988, *3,* 448–457.

Haug, M. R., and Lavin, B. *Consumerism in Medicine: Challenging Physician Authority.* Thousand Oaks, Calif.: Sage, 1983.

Heller, K., and Rook, K. S. "Distinguishing the Theoretical Functions of Social Ties: Implications for Support Interventions." In S. Duck (ed.), *Handbook of Personal Relationships: Theory, Research and Interventions.* (2nd ed.) Chichester, U.K.: Wiley, 1997.

House, J. S., Landis, K. R., and Umberson, D. "Social Relationships and Health." *Science,* 1988, *241,* 540–545.

House, J. S., Umberson, D., and Landis, K. R. "Structures and Process of Social Support." *Annual Review of Sociology,* 1988, *14,* 293–318.

Howard, J. A., Blumstein, P., and Schwartz, P. "Sex, Power, and Influence Tactics in Intimate Relationships." *Journal of Personality and Social Psychology,* 1986, *51,* 102–109.

Irvine, A. B., Biglan, A., Smolkowski, K., Metzler, C. W., and Ary, D. V. "The Effectiveness of a Parenting Skills Program for Parents of Middle School Students in Small Communities." *Journal of Consulting and Clinical Psychology,* 1999, *67,* 811–825.

Jackson, C. "Involving Parents Who Smoke in Smoking Prevention." Paper presented at the Meeting on Youth Smoking Prevention, National Cancer Institute, National Institutes on Health, Rockville, Md., 1998.

Jackson, C., Henriksen, L., and Foshee, V. A. "The Authoritative Parenting Index: Predicting Health Risk Behaviors Among Children and Adolescents." *Health Education & Behavior,* 1998, *25,* 319–337.

Joos, S. K., and Hickam, D. H. "How Health Professionals Influence Health Behavior: Patient-Provider Interaction and Health Care Outcomes." In K. Glanz, F. M. Lewis, and B. K. Rimer (eds.), *Health Behavior and Health Education: Theory, Research, and Practice.* San Francisco: Jossey-Bass, 1990.

Kaplan, S., Greenfield, S., Gandek, B., Rogers, W., and Ware, J. E. "Characteristics of Physicians with Participatory Decision-Making Styles." *Annals of Internal Medicine,* 1996, *124*(5), 497–504.

Kaplan, S., Greenfield, S., and Ware, J. E. "Assessing the Effects of Physician-Patient Interactions on the Outcomes of Chronic Disease." *Medical Care,* 1989, *27,* S110–127.

Kelley, H. H., and Thibaut, J. W. *Interpersonal Relations: A Theory of Interdependence.* New York: Wiley, 1978.

Kelman, H. C. "Further Thoughts on the Process of Compliance, Identification, and Internalization." In J. T. Tedeschi (ed.), *Perspectives on Social Power.* Chicago: Aldine Publishing, 1974.

Kelsey, K., Earp, J. L., and Kirkley, B. G. "Is Social Support Beneficial for Dietary Change? A Review of the Literature." *Family and Community Health,* 1997, *20,* 70–82.

Kosterman, R., Hawkins, J. D., Spoth, R., Haggerty, K. P., and Zhu, K. "Effects of a Preventive Parent Training Intervention on Observed Family Interactions: Proximal Outcomes from Preparing for the Drug-Free Years." *Journal of Community Psychology,* 1997, *25,* 337–352.

Lassner, J. B. "Does Social Support Aid in Weight-Loss and Smoking Interventions? Reply from a Family Systems Perspective." *Annals of Behavioral Medicine,* 1991, *13,* 66–72.

Lewis, M. A., and Butterfield, R. M. "Social Influence Tactics and Health Behavior Change." Paper presented at the annual meeting of the American Psychological Association, San Francisco, 1998a.

Lewis, M. A., and Butterfield, R. M. "Social Control, Relationship Functioning, and Health Behavior Change." Paper presented at the biennial meeting of the International Society for the Study of Personal Relationships, Saratoga Springs, N.Y., 1998b.

Lewis, M. A., and Butterfield, R. M. "Social Control and Health-Related Behavior: Antecedents and Reactions," forthcoming.

Lewis, M. A., Butterfield, R. M., Darbes, L., and Johnston-Brooks, C. "Husbands' and Wives' Use of Health-Related Social Control Tactics." Paper presented at the annual meeting of the Society of Behavioral Medicine, San Diego, 1999.

Lewis, M. A., and Rook, K. S. "Social Control in Personal Relationships: Impact on Health Behaviors and Psychological Distress." *Health Psychology,* 1999, *18,* 63–71.

Lewis, M. A., Rook, K. S., and Schwarzer, R. "Social Support, Social Control, and Health Among the Elderly." In G. N. Penny, P. Bennett, and M. Herbert (eds.), *Health Psychology: A Life Span Perspective.* London: Harwood Academic Publishers, 1994.

Lichtenstein, E., and Glasgow, R. E. "Smoking Cessation: What Have We Learned over the Past Decade?" *Journal of Consulting and Clinical Psychology,* 1992, *60,* 518–527.

Liebrand, W.B.G. "How to Improve Our Understanding of Group Decision Making with the Help of Artificial Intelligence." *Acta Psychologica,* 1992, *80,* 279–295.

Lupton, D. "Consumerism, Reflexivity, and the Medical Encounter." *Social Science and Medicine,* 1997, *45*(3), 373–381.

McGee, D. S., and Cegala, D. J. "Patient Communication Skills Training for Improved Communication Competence in Primary Care Medical Consultation." *Journal of Applied Communication Research,* 1998, *26,* 412–430.

Miller, W. R., and Rollnick, S. *Motivational Interviewing: Preparing People to Change Addictive Behavior.* New York: Guilford Press, 1991.

Mounts, N. S., and Steinberg, L. "An Ecological Analysis of Peer Influence on Adolescent Grade-Point Average and Drug Use." *Developmental Psychology,* 1995, *31,* 915–922.

Parsons, T. *The Social System.* Glencoe, Ill.: Free Press, 1951.

Pendleton, D., and Bochner, S. "The Communication of Medical Information in General Practice Consultations as a Function of Patients' Social Class." *Social Science and Medicine,* 1980, *14A,* 669–673.

Raven, B. H. "The Bases of Power: Origins and Recent Developments." *Journal of Social Issues,* 1993, *49,* 227–251.

Reis, H. T., Collins, W. A., and Berscheid, E. "The Relationship Context of Human Behavior and Development." *Psychological Bulletin,* 2000, *126,* 844–872.

Reno, R. W., Cialdini, R. B., and Kallgren, C. A. "The Trans-Situational Influence of Social Norms." *Journal of Personality and Social Psychology,* 1993, *64,* 104–112.

Resnicow, K., and others. "A Motivation Interviewing Intervention to Increase Fruit and Vegetable Intake Through Black Churches: Results of the Eat for Life Trial." *American Journal of Public Health,* 2001, *91,* 1686–1693.

Resnicow, K., and others. "Motivational Interviewing in Medical and Public Health Settings." In W. Miller and S. Rollnick (eds.), *Motivational Interviewing.* (2nd ed.), forthcoming.

Rivadeneyra, R., Elderkin-Thompson, V., Silver, R., and Waitzkin, H. "Patient-Centeredness in Medical Encounters Requiring an Interpreter." *American Journal of Medicine*, 2000, *108*, 470–474.

Rodin, J., and Janis, I. L. "The Social Influence of Physicians and Other Health Care Practitioners as Agents of Change." In H. S. Friedman and M. R. DiMatteo (eds.), *Interpersonal Issues in Health Care.* Orlando, Fla.: Academic Press, 1982.

Rogers, C. R. "The Necessary and Sufficient Conditions for Therapeutic Personality Change." *Journal of Consulting Psychology,* 1957, *21*, 95–101.

Rollnick, S., Mason, P., and Butler, C. *Health Behavior Change: A Guide for Practitioners.* London: Churchill-Livingstone, 2000.

Roter, D. L., and Hall, J. A. *Doctors Talking with Patients, Patients Talking with Doctors: Improving Communication in Medical Visits.* Westport, Conn.: Auburn House, 1992.

Rusbult, C. E., and Van Lange, P.A.M. "Interdependence Processes." In E. T. Higgins and A. W. Kruglanski (eds.), *Social Psychology: Handbook of Basic Principles.* New York: Guilford Press, 1996, 564–596.

Simons-Morton, B., and Hartos, J. "Application of the Authoritative Parenting Model to Adolescent Health Behavior." In R. DiClemente, R. Crosby, and M. Kegler (eds.), *Emerging Theories and Models in Health Promotion Research and Practice,* San Francisco: Jossey-Bass, 2002.

Sleath, B. "Pharmacist-Patient Interactions: Paternalism, Participatory, or Default?" *Patient Education and Counseling,* 1996, *28*, 253–263.

Sleath, B., Roter, D., Chewning, B., and Svarstad, B. "Question-Asking About Medications: Physician Experiences and Perceptions." *Medical Care,* 1999, *37*(11), 1169–1173.

Sleath, B., Rubin, R., Campbell, W., Gwyther, L., and Clark, T. "Ethnicity and Physician: Older Patient Communication About Alternative Therapies." *Journal of Alternative and Complementary Medicine,* 2001, *7*, 329–335.

Stewart, M. "The Impact of Patient-Centered Care on Outcomes." *The Journal of Family Practice,* 2000, *49*(9), 796–204.

Thompson, S. C., Pitts, J. S., and Schwankovsky, L. "Preferences for Involvement in Medical Decision-Making: Situational and Demographic Influences." *Patient Education and Counseling,* 1993, *22*, 133–140.

U.S. Department of Health and Human Services. *Healthy People 2010: Understanding and Improving Health.* Washington, D.C.: U.S. Government Printing Office, 2000.

Van den Eijnden, R.J.J.M., Buunk, B. P., Bakker, A. B., Siero, F. W. "The Impact of Information About Prevalence of AIDS-Preventive Behavior Among Men and Women: The Mediating Role of Social Norms." *Psychology and Health,* 1998, *13*, 467–478.

van Ryn, M., and Heaney, C. A. "Developing Effective Helping Relationships in Health Education Practice." *Health Education and Behavior,* 1997, *24*, 683–702.

Wallen, J., Waitzkin, H., and Stoeckle, J. "Physician Stereotypes About Female Health and Illness." *Women and Health,* 1979, *4*, 135–146.

Wissow, L., and others. "Patient-Provider Communication During the Emergency Department Care of Children with Asthma." *Medical Care,* 1998, *36*(10), 1439–1450.

CHAPTER TWELVE

PERSPECTIVES ON MODELS OF INTERPERSONAL HEALTH BEHAVIOR

Frances Marcus Lewis

The chapters in Part Three involve interpersonal models of health behavior. The core assumption of these models is that people's interactions with their environments are critical determinants of their health behavior and, in turn, health outcomes. Their environments provide the means, models, reinforcements, resources, and sources of influence from which people gain information, skills, self-confidence, self-management competencies, coping behavior, and support. In the process of interacting with their environments, people are not passive. Instead, the person and the environment operate together, changing each other as they interact. All the models in Part Three aim to enhance health behavior as well as health outcomes.

The chapters in Part Three contain one theory and three theoretical frameworks: Chapter Eight analyzed Social Cognitive Theory, Chapter Nine reviewed social support and social networks, Chapter Ten discussed stress and coping, and Chapter Eleven addressed social influence and interpersonal communication.

This chapter reviews highlights and offers additional perspectives on each of the chapters. It also suggests future directions for research using these models in health behavior and health education.

Social Cognitive Theory

Social Cognitive Theory (SCT) is a theory of skill and competency management and cognitive-behavioral control (Bandura, 1986, 1997, 2001). This theory emphasizes the importance of enhancing a person's behavioral capability (knowledge and skills) and self-confidence (self-efficacy) to engage in a particular health behavior.

Self-efficacy is one of the most essential concepts in this theory. It predicts the initiation of a new health behavior, even under adverse conditions; the continuation of the target health behavior, even under conditions of failure; and the maintenance of complex health behaviors, even under stressful conditions (Bandura, 1997; Parcel and others, 1994; Dougherty, Johnson-Crowley, Lewis, and Thompson, 2001).

SCT is both a predictive and a prescriptive theory: it explains and predicts health-related behavior and it describes methods to enhance health behavior and self-efficacy. Self-efficacy can be altered through four mechanisms: performance enactment, vicarious experience, persuasion, and minimizing emotional arousal.

The most powerful and consistent method of altering self-efficacy is through performance attainment (that is, performance enactment). Successful interventions engage participants in incrementally successful structured experiences in which their own self-monitoring of an enacted target behavior, along with feedback from a valued other, increases their self-view as efficacious over the target behavior. These strategies involve setting achievable goals and providing performance feedback. In SCT, methods for inducting higher levels of behavioral capability and self-efficacy can be structured by the behavioral interventionist or health educator.

The authors of Chapter Eight offer two applications that use SCT in intervention studies with school-age children. However, SCT has wide applicability for different audiences, including healthy adult populations, asymptomatic but at-risk persons, and people with life-threatening or chronic conditions. For example, Social Cognitive Theory has been successfully used in physical activity promotion interventions (Andersen, Bartlett, Moser, Evangelisti, and Verde, 1997; Dunn and others, 1997a, 1997b; Marcus, Owen, Forsyth, Cavill, and Fridinger, 1998). These interventions have documented effectiveness in increasing and maintaining physical activity levels that meet or exceed public health guidelines for previously sedentary adults and obese children (Dunn, Anderson, and Jakicic, 1998). Although the majority of these interventions have been delivered by face-to-face contact in small groups, a small number of studies have demonstrated effectiveness when the intervention is delivered by mail and telephone (Dunn, Anderson, and Jakicic, 1998).

Social Cognitive Theory has been successfully used to structure messages and instructional materials in health education campaigns, including a drowning prevention campaign (Bennett, Cummings, Quan, and Lewis, 1999), and to help family members better manage cystic fibrosis in a child (Parcel and others, 1994). Lorig's SCT-based program of intervention research with persons with arthritis and other chronic medical conditions is particularly noteworthy; it has documented health behavior and health outcome benefits in clinical trials (Lorig, Gonzalez, Laurent, Morgan, and Laris, 1998; Moore, Von Korff, Cherkin, Saunders, and Lorig, 2000). Health maintenance organizations and the National Arthritis Foundation have adopted these SCT-based intervention programs for national dissemination. More tests of applications of this theory are needed across other populations.

In addition to expanding applications of SCT to other populations, future research is needed to test refined methods by which to change self-efficacy and behavioral capability. Interventions that enhance skills, a component of behavioral capability, are not the same as interventions that alter self-efficacy. Operational distinctions need to be made to affect self-efficacy and not merely skills. In addition, it would be useful to know what forms of self-reflection and feedback on performance can alter self-efficacy. In addition, research should explore how we can best use live or symbolic models to affect self-efficacy, including the use of models through media and technological channels.

Social Networks and Social Support

Chapter Nine, on social networks and social support, analyzes both the networks in which the focal person is a member and the support that is available from the network. Social networks are the sets of social relationships to which a person belongs, and social support is the content or types of behavioral acts that members of the network provide to each other.

Heaney and Israel's analysis of social network and social support includes concepts that describe properties of the social network as well as types of supportive behaviors that are hypothesized to affect health outcomes. These acts can include emotional, instrumental, informational, affirmational, or appraisal components.

There is a large descriptive and predictive literature that supports the relationship between network membership, social support, and health. It is now widely recognized that people with close ties, or social support, have a mortality and health advantage over those who are only loosely connected.

Despite the extensive array of correlational and predictive studies using social support or social networks, there is a much more limited literature on intervention studies in which one or more properties of social networks or types of social support have been used to enhance health behavior, health outcomes, or both. We still do not know how best to structure social support in ways that are consistently health-enhancing. Intervention research on suicidal youth by Eggert's team has succeeded in illustrating effective ways to structure the provision of social support to enhance positive health outcomes in high-risk adolescents (Eggert, Thompson, Herting, and Nicholas, 1995; Herting, Eggert, and Thompson, 1996).

Although the chapter authors suggest that there might be optimal combinations of social support under differing situations, there have been only limited tests of such combinations for different problems and for different populations. Further, an explanation of what type of support is best for which situations is not yet well developed or tested. For example, we do not know under what conditions emotional versus instrumental, or affirmational support is health enhancing.

The use of social support is not always normative. Just because social support and social networks exist does not mean people use them. In several studies involving family members experiencing cancer, social support failed to significantly predict any aspect of family member behavior or functioning in either the acute or rehabilitation phases of the illness (Lewis and Hammond, 1992, 1996; Lewis, Zahlis, Shands, Sinsheimer, and Hammond, 1996). Evidence revealed that family members and patients hesitated to burden others by asking for support or, when offered support, did not always know how best to use it. For some family members, the use of support from others outside the household was viewed as a sign of weakness or a failure of their ability to cope.

Over several studies with different populations of cancer patients, the provision of different types of social support from different types of support persons did not consistently predict health behavior or health outcomes. This means that we need to avoid unconditional regard for social support and instead continue to refine and test social support interventions in health behavior and health education research. Evidence from a recently completed clinical trial that offered social support in the form of weekly supportive-expressive groups revealed that such support did not significantly prolong survival for women with metastatic breast cancer, compared with controls. It did, however, improve mood and the perception of pain, particularly for women who were highly distressed when they entered the trial (Goodwin and others, 2001). These results raise caution about thinking that social support is always effective and also raise important methodological questions about the types of outcomes to use to judge the efficacy of social support interventions, especially for people with terminal illnesses.

When interventions with social support are evaluated, it is important to know whether social support was in fact perceived as support. Perceived support often is assumed in an intervention in which objective types of social support are offered. Few health behavior intervention studies have included manipulation checks for perceived support. Social support has its theoretical roots in symbolic interactionism. This means that the meaning and perception of support, not merely its objective properties, are important. Future intervention studies that attempt to modify types of social support need to verify that the intended recipients actually perceived as support the support that was manipulated. It is the perception of support, not merely structural support, that is needed. This suggests that modifications of perceptions of support may require interventions about perceptions, not just interventions about available or proffered support. Attribution theory and cognitive reframing theories, among others, may be useful complements to social support. It is *perceived* support, not merely available support services, that is needed.

Stress, Coping, and Health Behavior

The literature on stress, coping, and health behavior has enjoyed a long history and many applications in both descriptive and intervention research. Its historical roots include research on homeostatic and adaptation processes within animal and human models. Its conceptual articulation with biological processes tightly links it to current research on hormonal and immunological outcomes (Kiecolt-Glaser and Glaser, 1995; Fawzy and others, 1990, 1993).

In the 1960s and 1970s, research documented that stress was a perceptual, specifically transactional, phenomenon. Lazarus, the major author of the Transactional Model of Stress and Coping, suggested that both primary and secondary appraisal interact with coping behavior to result in health-related outcomes. The meaning of the stressor event, not its objective properties, was the main determinant of health behavior and health outcomes. As discussed in Chapter Ten, these theoretical developments led to an elaboration of moderating factors, especially social support, as a buffer for perceived stress.

Research with the Transactional Model of Stress and Coping has led to a large literature on coping and adjustment to illness (for example, Fang, Manne, and Pape, 2001). Many descriptive studies provide evidence of the benefits of coping behavior that attempt to modify the stressor through either behavioral or cognitive strategies. However, despite over thirty years of research, there are still a number of research questions that deserve attention within the Transactional Model of Stress and Coping.

Although the Transactional Model emphasizes the importance of primary and secondary appraisal and coping behavior, more research is needed on ways to modify both appraisals and coping behavior. Much more needs to be learned about operational methods to modify appraisal, especially when the perceived stressor is acute, life-threatening, or chronically unremitting. It may be one thing to modify appraisal when the stressor is delimited and bounded; it may be quite another thing to modify appraisal under life-threatening conditions or when there is a rapid downward trajectory. Issues of controllability, including links with attribution theory, may enhance our effectiveness in changing appraisals under severe conditions.

Modifying coping behavior is still another challenge. Coping behavior within the model is predicted by appraisal. However, evidence from people with chronic illnesses does not consistently document a link between the perceived stressor and coping behavior (Lewis and Hammond, 1992; Lewis, Hammond, and Woods, 1993). There is evidence instead that people with life-threatening chronic illness may adopt certain types of coping behavior and freeze on those behaviors, rather than modify their coping in response to different properties of the stressors (Lewis, 1999).

Social Influence and Interpersonal Communication

The chapter on Social Influence and Interpersonal Communication is new in this edition of *Health Behavior and Health Education*. Megan Lewis, Brenda DeVellis, and Betsy Sleath recommend the use of Interdependence Theory as a theoretical framework into which many theories of social influence and interpersonal communication can be efficiently organized. This larger framework moves us toward a broader view of interpersonal influence and communication processes than in prior editions. Although research on patient-provider communication and models of health professional power relationships are important components of this new chapter, they are only a small part of a much larger literature that needs to be considered when studying social influence processes.

The chapter contains two underlying hypotheses: first, relationship interdependence causes greater levels of influence between the focal person and others, and second, this heightened influence can produce changed health behavior in the focal persons. Both hypotheses deserve further testing and elaboration, especially beyond the evidence available on dyads. What can be done to increase relationship interdependence between providers and patients or between health educators and family members? How can relationship interdependence positively enhance health behavior?

The chapter authors suggest explicit ways to use three key concepts in Interdependence Theory—relationship interdependence, interdependence, and correspondence of outcomes—to affect health outcomes. For example, the concept of interdependence suggests that both interacting partners should be included in interventions that usually involve individuals. Coyne, Ellard, and Smith (1990) reported an excellent intervention with spouses, but much more research is needed with family members using Interdependence Theory. We know very little about how to use a family member's social influence to modify the health behavior of its members. At best we know that family members can influence the behavior of the focal person, but we know very little about how to structure that source and form of influence. For example, what can spouses or other family members do to help a relative modify his or her lifestyle or to better manage illness-related symptoms? Another needed area of research relates to families with either risk factors for illness or with documented genetic abnormalities. What can be done to enhance family member participation in screening programs when a relative has known risk factors?

Conclusion

The theory and theoretical frameworks in Part Three have direct applicability to asymptomatic populations, healthy populations, and those with serious acute or chronic life-threatening illnesses. Each theory and framework has sufficient development to guide both the form and structure of future descriptive as well as intervention studies.

Research is needed to evaluate the delivery of interventions with the theories in Part Three using new technologies, including interactive computer-mediated telephone or Web-based interventions. Previously held biases that symptomatic, distressed, or otherwise vulnerable or clinical populations are best served only through case-intensive direct services need to be empirically tested. For example, there is evidence that even persons with a recent cardiac arrest and a surgically implanted cardiac defibrillator can be assisted by a telephone-delivered intervention based on Social Cognitive Theory (Dougherty, Johnson-Crowley, Lewis, and Thompson, 2001). All the models in Part Three have sufficient conceptual structure to guide future descriptive and intervention research.

References

Andersen, R. E., Bartlett, S. J., Moser, C. D., Evangelisti, M. I., and Verde, T. J. "Lifestyle or Aerobic Exercise to Treat Obesity in Dieting Women." *Medical Science Sports Exercise* 1997, *29*(Supplement 5), S46.

Bandura, A. *Social Foundations of Thought and Action, A Social Cognitive Theory.* New Jersey: Prentice Hall, 1986.

Bandura, A. *Self-Efficacy: The Exercise of Control.* New York: W.H. Freeman, 1997.

Bandura, A. "Social Cognitive Theory: An Agentic Perspective." *Annual Review of Psychology,* 2001, *52,* 1–26.

Bennett, E., Cummings, P., Quan, L., and Lewis, F. M. "Evaluation of a Drowning Prevention Campaign in King County, Washington." *Injury Prevention,* 1999, *5,* 109–113.

Coyne, J. C., Ellard, J. H., and Smith, D. A. "Social Support, Interdependence, and the Dilemmas of Helping." In B. R. Sarason, I. G. Sarason, and G. R. Pierce (eds.), *Social Support: An Interactional View.* New York: Wiley, 1990.

Dougherty, C. M., Johnson-Crowley, N. R., Lewis, F. M., and Thompson, E. A. "Theoretical Development of Nursing Interventions for Sudden Cardiac Arrest Survivors Using Social Cognitive Theory." *Advances in Nursing Science,* 2001, *24,* 78–86.

Dunn, A. L., Anderson, R. E., and Jakicic, J. M. "Lifestyle Physical Activity Interventions: History, Short- and Long-Term Effects, and Recommendations." *American Journal of Preventive Medicine,* 1998, *15,* 398–412.

Dunn, A. L., and others. "Project Active: A Randomized Clinical Trial of Lifestyle and Structured Physical Activity Programs." *Medical Science Sports Exercise,* 1997a, *29,* S75.

Dunn, A. L., and others. "Reduction in Cardiovascular Disease Risk Factors: Six-Month Results from Project Active." *Preventive Medicine,* 1997b, *26,* 883–892.

Eggert, L. L., Thompson, E. A., Herting, J. R., and Nicholas, L. J. "Reducing Suicide Potential Among High-Risk Youth: Tests of a School-Based Prevention Program." *Suicide and Life-Threatening Behavior,* 1995, *25,* 276, 296.

Fang, C. J., Manne, S. L., and Pape, S. J. "Functional Impairment, Marital Quality, and Patient Psychological Distress as Predictors of Psychological Distress among Cancer Patients' Spouses." *Health Psychology,* 2001, *20,* 452–457.

Fawzy, F. I., and others. "A Structured Psychiatric Intervention for Cancer Patients: Changes over Time in Immunological Measures." *Archives of General Psychiatry,* 1990, *47,* 729–735.

Fawzy, F. I., and others. "Malignant Melanoma: Effects of an Early Structured Psychiatric Intervention, Coping and Affective State on Recurrence and Survival 6 Years Later." *Archive of General Psychiatry,* 1993, *50,* 681–689.

Goodwin, P. J., and others. "The Effect of Group Psychosocial Support on Survival in Metastatic Breast Cancer." *New England Journal of Medicine,* 2001, *345,* 1719–1726.

Herting, J. R., Eggert, L. L., and Thompson, E. A. "A Multidimensional Model of Drug Involvement." *Journal of Research on Adolescence,* 1996, *6,* 325–361.

Kiecolt-Glaser, J. K., and Glaser, R. "Psychoneuroimmunology and Health C Consequences: Data and Shared Mechanisms." *Psychosomatic Medicine,* 1995, *57,* 269–274.

Lewis, F. M. "The Relational Model of Functioning with Cancer: A Family Focused Framework for Nursing Practice." In *Cancer Across Health Care Sites.* St. Louis: Mosby Year Book, 1999.

Lewis, F. M., and Hammond, M. A. "Psychosocial Rehabilitation of the Family to Breast Cancer: A Longitudinal Analysis." *Journal of the American Medical Women's Association,* 1992, *47,* 194–200.

Lewis, F. M., and Hammond, M. A. "The Father's, Mother's and Adolescent's Functioning with Breast Cancer." *Family Relations,* 1996, *45,* 456–465.

Lewis, F. M., Hammond, M. A., and Woods, N. F. "The Family's Functioning with Newly Diagnosed Breast Cancer in the Mother: The Development of an Explanatory Model." *Journal of Behavioral Medicine,* 1993, *16,* 351–370.

Lewis, F. M., Zahlis, E. H., Shands, M. E., Sinsheimer, J. A., and Hammond, M. A. "The Functioning of Single Women with Breast Cancer and Their School-Aged Children." *Cancer Practice,* 1996, *4,* 15–24.

Lorig, K., Gonzalez, V. M., Laurent, D. D., Morgan, L., and Laris, B. A. "Arthritis Self-Management Program Variations: Three Studies." *Arthritis Care & Research*, 1998, *11*, 448–454.

Marcus, B. H., Owen, N., Forsyth, L. H., Cavill, N. A., and Fridinger, F. "Physical Activity Interventions Using Mass Media, Print Media, and Information Technology." *American Journal of Preventive Medicine*, 1998, *15*, 362–378.

Moore, J. E., Von Korff, M., Cherkin, D., Saunders, K., and Lorig, K. "A Randomized Trial of a Cognitive-Behavioral Program for Enhancing Back Pain Self-Care in a Primary Care Setting." *Pain*, 2000, *88*, 145–153.

Parcel, G. S., and others. "Self-Management of Cystic Fibrosis: A Structural Model for Educational and Behavioral Variables." *Social Science & Medicine*, 1994, *38*, 307–315.

PART FOUR

COMMUNITY AND GROUP MODELS OF HEALTH BEHAVIOR CHANGE

An understanding of the functioning of groups, organizations, large social institutions, and communities is vital to health enhancement. Designing health behavior and environmental change initiatives to serve communities and targeted populations, not just single individuals, is at the heart of a public health orientation. The collective well-being of communities can be fostered by creating structures and policies that support healthy lifestyles, and by reducing or eliminating health hazards and constraints in the social and physical environments. Both approaches require an understanding of how social systems operate, how change occurs within and among systems, and how community and organizational changes influence people's behavior and health.

Health behavior today occurs in the context of rapid technological change and important policy debates. Health concerns such as substance abuse, AIDS prevention and education, smoking prevention and control, bioterrorism, and new health care technologies raise issues that cannot be addressed adequately through individual or small group interventions alone (Smedley and Syme, 2000). Rather, health professionals need to view and understand health behavior and organizational changes in the context of social institutions and communities. The theories and frameworks in this part of *Health Behavior and Health Education* can help professionals understand the health behavior of large groups, communities, organizations, and coalitions, and can guide organizationwide and communitywide health promotion and education interventions. These social systems are both viable and essential units of practice when widespread, and long-term maintenance of behavior change and social change are important goals.

Community-level models are frameworks for understanding how social systems function and change and how communities and organizations can be activated. They complement individually oriented behavior change goals with broad aims that include advocacy and policy development. Community-level models suggest strategies and initiatives that are planned and led by organizations and institutions with missions to protect and improve health: schools, worksites, health care settings, community groups, and government agencies. Other institutions for which health enhancement is not a central mission, such as the mass media, also play a critical role.

The chapters in this section represent state-of-the-art descriptions of four models for behavior change and community development in social systems or large populations. Some of the chapters address theoretical perspectives on changing the health behavior of populations, whereas other chapters are concerned primarily with conceptual frameworks for intervention methods that are *based on* theoretical foundations from the social sciences.

In Chapter Thirteen, Meredith Minkler and Nina Wallerstein provide a comprehensive overview of principles and methods of community organization and community building for health improvement. They discuss the main theoretical and conceptual bases of community organization, processes and models for community organization, and emerging concepts and methods of community building for health. They also discuss progress and tools for measuring and evaluating community organizing and community building. Minkler and Wallerstein then describe two case studies of community organization. The Tenderloin Senior Organizing Project (TSOP) for low-income elderly in San Francisco illustrates a community organization program that grew and developed over more than fifteen years. The Adolescent Social Action Program (ASAP) in New Mexico is a youth-centered experiential prevention program that involved a collaboration between university, schools, and numerous community and health organizations that included empowerment education, leadership development, and community building.

In Chapter Fourteen, Brian Oldenburg and Guy Parcel present Diffusion Theory, which addresses how new ideas, products, programs, and social practices spread within a society or from one society (or social system) to another. They then focus on how Diffusion Theory was applied to increase diffusion of a school-based heart disease prevention program and a workplace health promotion program in Australia.

In Chapter Fifteen, Allen Steckler, Robert Goodman, and Michelle Kegler analyze three theories of organizational change: Stage Theory, Organizational Development Theory, and Interorganizational Relations Theory. Each of these theories suggests specific intervention strategies that are directed at levels of a single organization or at coalitions of multiple organizations, thus improving adoption and implementation of health promotion programs and community strategies. Further, strategies based on each of the three theories can be used simultaneously to produce optimal effects. Steckler and colleagues then illustrate how these theories can be used as a basis for health promotion interventions in school settings and in public health action in the community.

John Finnegan and K. Viswanath introduce the Media Studies Framework for health behavior change in Chapter Sixteen. Their chapter describes communication theories that are especially relevant to public health and health behavior change. Four perspectives on the effects of media are introduced: the Knowledge Gap hypothesis, Agenda Setting, Cultivation Studies, and Risk Communication. The authors then present applications of media studies to health in two areas: the day-to-day impact of media on health, and planned use of media communication for health improvement.

Part Four concludes with a summary, comparison, and critique of organizational and community interventions in health promotion and education. Chapter Seventeen discusses parallel elements in concept and strategies, and converging applications of community and group intervention models of health behavior change.

An understanding of theory, research, and practice in communities, systems, and organizations will be critical to wide improvement of health in the future. This part of *Health Behavior and Health Education* provides a diverse set of frameworks and applications for consideration of both researchers and practitioners.

Reference

Smedley, B. D., and Syme, S. L. (eds.). *Promoting Health: Intervention Strategies from Social and Behavioral Research*. Washington, D.C.: National Academy Press, 2000.

CHAPTER THIRTEEN

IMPROVING HEALTH THROUGH COMMUNITY ORGANIZATION AND COMMUNITY BUILDING

Meredith Minkler
Nina B. Wallerstein

Although a number of new approaches and change strategies have been developed and adapted by health education professionals in recent years, the principles and methods loosely referred to as community organization remain a central method of practice. For the purposes of this chapter, community organization will be defined as the process by which community groups are helped to identify common problems or goals, mobilize resources, and in other ways develop and implement strategies for reaching the goals they collectively have set. The newer and related concept of community building* will be seen, as Walter (forthcoming) suggests, not as a method so much as an orientation to the ways in which people who identify as members of a shared community engage together in the process of community change.

Implicit in both of these definitions is the concept of empowerment, viewed as an enabling process through which individuals or communities take control over their lives and their environment (Rappaport, 1984). Indeed, Murray Ross, widely regarded as the father of community-organizing practice, argued early on that com-

___

* The term *community building* is increasingly being used in fields such as urban planning but in a broader sense. Although placing a similarly strong emphasis on identifying and promoting community strengths and capacity, for example, this more macro conceptualization also emphasizes regional economic development and federal and state policy level reinvestment in local communities (Blackwell and Colmenar, 2000).

munity organization could not be said to have taken place unless community competence or problem-solving ability had been increased in the process (Ross, 1955).

Strict definitions of community organization also suggest that the needs or problems around which community groups are organized must of necessity be identified by the community itself and not by an outside organization or change agent. Thus, while a health education professional may borrow some principles and methods from community organization to help mount an AIDS organizing effort in the community, he or she can't be said to be doing community organization in the pure sense unless the community itself has identified AIDS as the problem area it wishes to address.

Community organization is important in health education in part because it reflects one of the field's most fundamental principles, that of "starting where the people are" (Nyswander, 1956). The health education professional who begins with the community's felt needs, rather than with a personal or agency-dictated agenda, will be far more likely to experience success in the change process and to foster real community ownership of programs and actions than if he or she were to impose an agenda from outside. Community organizing also is important in light of the evidence that social involvement and participation can themselves be significant psychosocial factors in improving perceived control, individual coping capacity, health behaviors, and health status (Eng, Briscoe, and Cunningham, 1990; Wandersman and Florin, 2000). Finally, the "rediscovery" of community, and the heavy emphasis being placed on community partnerships and community-based health initiatives by government agencies, foundations, and the like, suggest the need for further refining theory, methods, and measurement techniques in this area. In this chapter, key concepts and principles of community organization and community building will be examined for their relevance to health education and related disciplines. Following a brief historical look at the field and process of community organization and the emergence of community-building practice, the concept of community will be examined, and several models of community organization and community building will be presented. Key theoretical and conceptual bases of community organization and community building then will be explored, and two case studies will be presented and analyzed to demonstrate the relevance of these models in practice settings.

Community Organization and Community Building in Historical Perspective

The term *community organization* was coined by U.S. social workers in the late 1800s in reference to their efforts to coordinate services for newly arrived immigrants and the poor (Garvin and Cox, 2001). As Garvin and Cox have pointed out, however, although community organization typically is portrayed as having been born of the settlement house movement, several important milestones, which took place outside of social work, by rights should be included in any history of community organization practice. Prominent among these are (1) the post–Reconstruction Period organizing by African Americans to try to salvage newly won rights that were rapidly slipping away, (2) the Populist movement, which began as an agrarian revolution and became a multisectoral coalition and a major political force, and (3) the Labor Movement of the 1930s and 1940s, which taught the value of forming coalitions around issues, the importance of full-time professional organizers, and the use of conflict as a means of bringing about change (Garvin and Cox, 2001).

Within the field of social work, early approaches to community organization stressed collaboration and the use of consensus and cooperation as communities were helped to self-identify and to increase their problem-solving ability (Garvin and Cox, 2001; Ross, 1955). By the 1950s, however, a new brand of community organization, which stressed confrontation and conflict strategies for social change, was gaining popularity. Most closely identified with Saul Alinsky (1969, 1972), social action organizing emphasized redressing power imbalances by creating dissatisfaction with the status quo among the disenfranchised, building community-wide identification, and helping members devise winnable goals and nonviolent conflict strategies as means to bring about change.

From the late 1950s onward, strategies and tactics of community organization increasingly were being applied to the achievement of broader social change objectives, through the civil rights movement, the women's movement, the gay rights movement, anti–Vietnam War organizing, and the disability rights movement. The 1980s and early- to mid-1990s also witnessed the adaptation and development of new community organization tactics and strategies, in areas as diverse as the AIDS crisis and the New Right's organizing to ban abortions. The effective use of personal computer technology also has greatly increased, with groups across the political spectrum going online to build community and to identify and organize supporters on a mass scale.

In the health field, a major emphasis on community participation, beginning in the 1970s, culminated in the World Health Organization's adoption in 1986 of a new approach to health promotion that stressed increasing people's control over the determinants of their health, high-level public participation, and intersectoral cooperation (World Health Organization, 1986). Reflecting this new approach, the WHO-initiated Healthy Cities movement emerged and grew to involve thousands of healthy cities and communities worldwide. It aims to create sustainable environments and processes through which governmental and nongovernmental sectors work in partnership to create healthy public policies, achieve high-level participation in community-driven projects, and, ultimately, to reduce inequities and disparities between groups (Norris and Pittman, 2000).

Finally, alongside these developments has been a growing appreciation of the importance of facilitating *community building,* conceptualized as a process that people in a community engage in themselves, rather than solely community organizing, viewed typically from the vantage point of the outside organizer (Walter, forthcoming). The community-building orientation is reflected in efforts such as the National Black Women's Health Project, a twenty-year-old network of close to two dozen chapters with more than 10,000 members, which stresses empowerment through self-help and consciousness raising for social change (Avery, 1990; see also www.nationalblackwomenshealthproject.org). Community-building projects like this one are strength-based and grounded in feminist notions of "power to" and "power with," rather than the more masculine concept of "power over" frequently encountered in traditional organizing (French, 1986). They further borrow from feminist organizing an emphasis on the process of practice (Hyde, 1990) and on "integrating personal and political experiences through dialogue" (Gutierrez and Lewis, 1997, p. 218). Although theoretical work and practical applications and research in the area of community building remain in their infancy, community-building practice may become an increasingly important complement to more traditional notions of community organization in the years ahead. Following a look at the concept of community and at several models of community organization and community-building practice, the key principles and concepts underlying these approaches will be examined in more detail.

The Concept of Community

Integral to a discussion of community organization and community-building practice is an examination of the underlying concept of community. While typically thought of in geographical terms, communities may also be nonlocality identified and based instead on shared interests or characteristics such as ethnicity, sexual orientation, or occupation (Fellin, 2001). Communities indeed have been defined as (1) *functional spatial units* meeting basic needs for sustenance, (2) *units of patterned social interaction,* and (3) *symbolic units of collective identity* (Hunter, 1975). Eng and Parker (1994) add a fourth political definition of community as a social unit that is people coming together to act politically to make changes.

Two sets of theories are relevant for understanding the concept of community. The first of these, the *ecological system perspective,* is particularly useful in the study of autonomous geographical communities, focusing as it does on population characteristics such as size, density, and heterogeneity; the physical environment; the social organization or structure of the community; and the technological forces affecting it. In contrast, the *social systems perspective* focuses primarily on the formal organizations that operate within a given community, exploring the interactions of community subsystems (economic, political, and so on) both horizontally, within the community, and vertically, as they relate to other, extra-community systems (Fellin, 2001). Warren's (1963) classic approach to community clearly fits within the latter perspective, envisioning communities as entities that change their structure and function to accommodate various social, political, and economic developments. Similarly, Alinsky's view of communities as reflecting the social problems and processes of an urban society (Reitzes and Reitzes, 1980) provides a good example of a social systems perspective.

Clearly, the perspective on community that one adopts will influence his or her view of the appropriate domains and functions of the community organization process. Community development specialists (for example, agricultural extension workers and Peace Corps volunteers) thus have tended to focus on helping people identify with and bring about changes within their own geographical community, implicitly defining the latter as a unit unto itself (Khinduka, 1975; Rothman, 2001). By contrast, proponents of a broader approach, typified by Alinsky (1972) and other social action organizers, have encouraged organizing around issues such as public housing and unemployment, in recognition of the tremendous impact of those larger socioeconomic issues on local communities. Similarly, though communities are rich in diversity with multiple interacting subcommunities, whether one *views* the community as more or less heterogeneous will determine the strategies employed and often the types of organizing goals.

Finally, as Rivera and Erlich (1995) and Gutierrez and Lewis (1997) have suggested, an appreciation of the unique characteristics of communities of color should be a major consideration in thinking about organizing within such communities. In African American communities, for example, Cornel West (1993) argues that market exploitation has led to a shattering of the religious and civic organizations that have historically buffered these communities from hopelessness and nihilism. He calls for community change through re-creating a sense of agency and political resistance based on "subversive memory—the best of one's past without romantic nostalgia" (West, 1993, p. 19). A view of community that incorporates such a perspective would support building on preexisting social networks and structures and would emphasize self-determination and empowerment (Gutierrez and Lewis, 1997).

The different models of community organization and community building described in the following section illustrate how alternative assumptions about the nature and meaning of community heavily shape and determine how community organization and community building are conceptualized and practiced.

Models of Community Organization

While community organization frequently is treated as though it were a singular model of practice, several typologies of community organization have been developed on the premise that this phenomenon is in fact composed of various alternative change models. The best known of these typologies is Rothman's (2001) categorization of community organization as consisting of three distinct models of practice: locality development, social planning, and social action. Briefly, *locality development* is seen as heavily process oriented, stressing consensus and cooperation and aimed at building group identity and a sense of community. By contrast, *social planning* is viewed as heavily task oriented, and stressing rational-empirical problem solving—usually by an outside expert—as a means of problem solving. Finally, the *social action* model may be seen as both task and process oriented. It is concerned with increasing the problem-solving ability of the community and with achieving concrete changes to redress imbalances of power and privilege between an oppressed or disadvantaged group and the larger society (Rothman, 2001).

Originally arguing that most community-organizing efforts tended to fall into one or the other of these categories, Rothman more recently has suggested that many professionals use an intermixing of two or more of the models (Rothman, 2001) rather than relying solely or principally on any one. Feminist organizing, for example, may be seen as combining the goals and assumptions of social action organizing with methods that often are consistent with locality development (Rothman, 2001). Similarly, the heart health community trials and PATCH (Planned Action Toward Community Health) interventions have mixed social planning with elements of locality development (Farquhar and others, 1984; "PATCH," 1992; Bracht and Kingsbury, 1990), while many organizers in the Alinsky tradition have mixed social action and locality development in their community efforts (Marquez, 1990; Wechsler, 1990; Guillory, Willie, and Duran, 1988).

For close to three decades, Rothman's typology has remained the dominant framework within which community organization has been examined and understood, and as such, it has had a significant impact on practice (Walter, forthcoming). Despite its continued widespread application, however, the typology and its underlying assumptions have a number of important limitations. Use of the term *locality development*, for example, may be unnecessarily restrictive, discouraging a consideration of organizing along nongeographical lines. Second, inclusion of a model (social planning) that often relies heavily on outside technical experts and need not increase the problem-solving ability of the community appears to contradict one of the most basic criteria of effective organizing. Finally, the fact that this typology is problem-based and organizer-centered, rather than strength-based and community-centered, constitutes a philosophical and practical limitation that may be particularly problematic as organizing occurs increasingly in multicultural contexts.

In part in reaction to the perceived limitations of the Rothman typology, Walter (forthcoming) and others (Kaye and Wolff, 1995; Gardner, 1991; Himmelman, 1992; Labonte, 1994; Wallerstein and Sanchez-Merki, 1994) have suggested newer models of collaborative empowerment and community-building practice that provide important alternative approaches. These models can be seen partially as descendants of the community development model in their emphases on self-help and collaboration. Yet, they extend beyond the tradition within community development, which is externally driven and may implicitly accept the status quo. They take their parentage from community-driven development in which community concerns direct the organizing in a process that creates healthy and more equal power relations (Labonte, 1993; Purdey, Adhikari, Robinson, and Cox, 1994).

The newer community-building model emphasizes community strengths, not as nostalgia for the "good old days" but as a diversity of groups and systems that can identify shared values and nurture the development of shared goals (Gardner, 1991). Himmelman's (1992) "collaborative empowerment model," for example, includes many of the steps or activities stressed in more traditional organizing (for example, clarifying a community's purpose and vision, examining what others have done, building a community's power base) but puts its heaviest emphasis on enabling communities to play the lead role so that real empowerment, rather than merely "community betterment," is achieved. McKnight's (1987) notion of "community regeneration" has at its heart the enabling of people to recognize and contribute their "gifts," the totality of which represent the building blocks or assets of a community that enable it to care for its members.

Along similar lines, Walter's (forthcoming) community-building-practice approach is described not as a method but as "a way of orienting one's self in community" that places community "at the center of practice" (p. 74). Walter's concept of community building attempts to balance and blend such elements of community as historicity, identity, and autonomy with the dimensions of community development, community planning, community action, community consciousness, and "the commons" (which encompasses the relationship between community and its broader environment). As such, the community-building approach contrasts significantly with more traditional notions of community organization practice that are "community based," but not necessarily of and by the community (Kaye and Wolff, 1995; Walter, forthcoming).

Lying midway between older models of community organizing and newer conceptualizations of community building are models that incorporate some elements of each while putting the greatest accent on culturally relevant practice.

Among the best-known of these approaches in the health field is Braithwaite and colleagues' (Braithwaite, Bianchi, and Taylor, 1994; Braithwaite and others, 1989) Community Organization and Development (COD) model for health promotion in communities of color. Although aimed toward the outside organizer and admonishing him or her to engage in such initial steps as getting to know the community and its ecology through participatory ethnography and gaining entry and credibility, the central thrust of the COD model involves facilitating the development and effective functioning of a coalition board dominated and controlled by the community. The board in turn undertakes its own community assessment, sets policy, facilitates leadership development, and, on the basis of "bottom-up planning" and community problem solving, designs culturally relevant interventions. The COD model, in short, appears to move from initial reliance on more traditional community organizing to an incorporation of many of the principles of community-building practice, all the while stressing the cultural context within which both organizing and community building take place.

Finally, there is coalition building, alternately defined as a model of community organization practice and as a strategy or method used across models. Coalitions are increasingly popular in the health field in areas as diverse as chronic disease, drugs and alcohol, violence, and the fight against budget cuts (Goodman, Burdine, Meehan, and McLeroy, 1993; Kaye and Wolff, 1995) and have attracted heavy public- and private-sector funding, though they have only recently begun to be studied in a systematic fashion (see Chapter Fifteen).

In sum, several models of community organizing and community building have surfaced within the last decade to complement a long history of earlier organizing approaches. In Figure 13.1 we attempt to integrate new perspectives with the older models, presenting a typology that incorporates both needs- and strengths-based approaches. In the needs-based field, "community development," as primarily a consensus model, is contrasted with Alinsky's "social action" conflict-based model. The newer strength-based models contrast a community-building-capacity approach with an empowerment-oriented social action approach. Several concepts span these two strength-based approaches, such as community competence, leadership development, and the multiple perspectives on gaining power. Looking at primary strategies, consensus approaches, whether needs-based or strengths-based, primarily use collaboration strategies, whereas conflict approaches use advocacy strategies and ally-building to support advocacy efforts.

Community organizing and community building are fluid endeavors. Although some organizing efforts primarily have focused in one quadrant, the majority incorporate multiple tendencies, possibly starting as the result of a specific need or crisis and moving to a strength-based community capacity approach. Different organizing models, such as coalitions, lay health worker programs, political action

FIGURE 13.1. COMMUNITY ORGANIZATION AND COMMUNITY BUILDING TYPOLOGY.

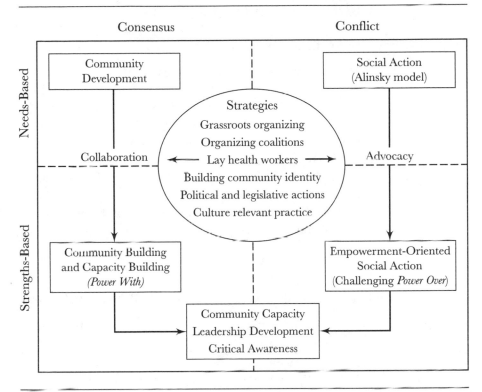

groups, or grassroots organizing may incorporate needs- or strengths-based approaches at different times as well, depending on the starting place and the ever-changing social dynamic. It is important, however, that organizing efforts clarify their assumptions and make decisions on primary strategies based on skills of group members, history of the group, willingness to take risks, or comfort level with different approaches.

Concepts in Community Organization and Community-Building Practice

While no single unified model of community organization or community building exists, some key concepts are central to affecting and measuring change on the community level. Several of these concepts and principles—empowerment and critical consciousness, community capacity, issue selection, and the evaluation and measurement issues—are presented in the following section and summarized in Table 13.1.

Empowerment and Critical Consciousness

Although the term *empowerment* has been justifiably criticized as a "catch-all phrase" in social science (Rappaport, 1984), it nevertheless represents a central tenet of community organization and community-building practice. Within public health, empowerment or community empowerment has been variously defined, with definitions running from communities achieving equity (Katz, 1984) to communities having the capacity to identify problems and solutions (Braithwaite and others, 1989; Cottrell, 1983) to participatory self-competence in the political life of the community (Wandersman and Florin, 2000; Kieffer, 1984).

Though many limit their definition to a narrow individual focus, similar to self-esteem or self-confidence, empowerment is, as noted below, a multilevel con-

TABLE 13.1. KEY CONCEPTS IN COMMUNITY ORGANIZATION AND COMMUNITY BUILDING.

Concept	Definition	Application
Empowerment	Social action process for people to gain mastery over their lives and the lives of their communities	Community members assume greater power or expand their power from within to create desired changes.
Critical consciousness	A consciousness based on reflection and action in making change	People engage in dialogue that links root causes and community actions.
Community capacity	Community characteristics affecting its ability to identify, mobilize, and address problems	Community members participate actively in the life of their community through leadership, social networks, and access to power.
Issue selection	Identifying winnable and specific targets of change that unify and build community strength	Issues are identified through community participation; targets are decided on as part of a larger strategy.
Participation and relevance	Community organizing that "starts where the people are" and engages community members as equals	Community members create their own agenda based on felt needs, shared power, and awareness of resources.

struct involving "participation, control, and critical awareness," whether one focuses on the individual, organizational, or broader community level (Zimmerman, 2000). Bearing this in mind, a broader definition is most useful—one that views empowerment as a social action process by which individuals, communities, and organizations gain mastery over their lives in the context of changing their social and political environment to improve equity and quality of life (Rappaport, 1984; Wallerstein, 1992).

Such a definition highlights issues of power, or the ability to create change on a personal, interpersonal, and political level (Gutierrez and Lewis, 1997). Labonte addresses power as a social relationship with contradictory elements (Bernstein and others, 1994; Labonte, 1990). "Power from within" and "power with" (the collective aspect of power from within) are moral, spiritual sources of power that can be constantly expanding as people empower themselves. "Power over" has a material base of domination through force or ideological hegemony. People without power cannot gain against exploitation without others losing their historic authority. Foucault argues that oppressive power, however, is not monolithic but composed of localized unstable relationships, which can be challenged by historically disenfranchised groups (Foucault, 1977). Empowerment therefore embraces both power taking (or resisting power structures through community organizing and advocacy) and community-building efforts that expand power through strengthening community relationships.

For health educators, these contradictory elements raise issues of their own practice. Many professionals have higher status positions than community members. Can people in positions of dominance or privilege—whether from culture, gender, race, or class—empower others, or must people empower themselves? If empowerment includes the dimension of transferring power to others, professionals may need to let go of their power to make it more available to others. In Labonte's words, "Empowerment . . . is a fascinating dynamic of power given and taken all at once, a dialectical dance between consensus and conflict, professional expertise and lay wisdom, hierarchic institutions and community circles" (Bernstein and others, 1994, p. 285).

As a theory and methodology, community empowerment is multilayered, representing both processes and outcomes of change for individuals, the organizations of which they are a part, and the community social structure itself (Zimmerman, 2000). At the level of the individual, "psychological empowerment" best illustrates a concept that extends intra-psychic self-esteem to include people's perceived control in their lives, their critical awareness of their social context, and their political efficacy and participation in change (Zimmerman, 1990, 2000). For individuals, empowerment challenges the perceived or real "powerlessness" that comes from the health injuries of poverty, chronic stressors, lack of control, and few resources, or what Len Syme has termed lack of "control over destiny" (Syme, 1988).

Organizational empowerment incorporates both the *processes* of organizations (for example, whether they are acting to influence societal change) and the *outcomes,* such as their effectiveness in gaining new resources. At the community level, as individuals engage in community-organizing efforts, community empowerment outcomes can include increased sense of community; greater participatory processes and community competence; and outcomes of actual changes in policies, transformed conditions, or increased resources that may reduce inequities. As communities become empowered and better able to engage in collective problem solving, key health and social indicators may reflect this with rates of alcoholism, divorce, suicide, and other social problems beginning to decline. Moreover, the empowered community that works effectively for change can bring about changes in some of the very problems that contributed to its ill health in the first place (Israel, 1985; Minkler, 1997).

The link between psychological, organizational, and community-level empowerment is strengthened through the development of critical consciousness, or "conscientization," a concept that comes from Brazilian educator Paulo Freire (1970, 1973). Freire developed a methodology for teaching illiterate peasants to read, by teaching them to "read" their political and social reality. His work has been a catalyst worldwide in the past three decades for programs in adult education, health, and community development (Hope and Timmel, 1984; Minkler and Cox, 1980; Wallerstein and Bernstein, 1994; Wallerstein and Weinger, 1992; Arnold and others, 1995).

Freire's central premise is that the purpose of education should be liberating, to transform the status quo in the classroom and in people's lives. He questions whether education reinforces powerlessness, by treating people as objects who receive knowledge, or whether education enables people to engage in active dialogue and to challenge the conditions that keep them powerless. Freire proposes a dialogical problem-posing process, with equality and mutual respect between learner-teachers and teacher-learners. Problem posing contains a cycle of listening-dialogue-action that enables all participants to engage in continuous reflection and action. Through structured dialogue, group participants listen for the issues contained in their own experiences, discuss common problems, look for root causes and the interconnections between the "problems behind the problem-as-symptom," and devise strategies to help transform their reality (Freire, 1970, 1973).

Conscientization is the consciousness that comes through the social analysis of conditions and peoples' roles in changing those conditions. This awareness enables community groups to analyze moments and open spaces to enact change or to understand those "limit situations" that may deter change (Barndt, 1989). Conscientization is a key ingredient to maintaining a broader vision and sustaining community-organizing efforts over time, and as such is one of the most important links between psychological and community empowerment.

Community Capacity

Closely related to the concept of empowerment is the notion of "community capacity," defined as "the characteristics of communities that affect their ability to identify, mobilize, and address social and public health problems" (Goodman and others, 1999, p. 259). In a recent conference sponsored by the CDC (Centers for Disease Control and Prevention) to strengthen our understanding of the concept, community capacity was articulated as having multiple dimensions: active participation, leadership, rich support networks, skills and resources, critical reflection, sense of community, understanding of history, articulation of values, and access to power (Goodman and others, 1999).

Definitions of community capacity have drawn from other related concepts, such as "community competence" and "social capital." Community competence is defined by Cottrell (1983) as "the various component parts of the community being able to collaborate effectively on identifying the problems and needs of the community; to achieve a working consensus on goals and priorities; to agree on ways and means to implement the agreed-upon goals; to collaborate effectively in the required actions." Important recent refinements in thinking about community competence have come with lay health worker programs that have incorporated community development and an emphasis on assessing the transformations such work may produce in lay health workers themselves, instead of only their impact on clients (Eng and Parker, 1994; Lorig, Lubeck, Kraines, Seleznick, and Holman, 1985; Ovrebo, Ryan, Jackson, and Hutchinson, 1994).

Social capital has more recently captured the imagination of public health. From its origins in political science, social capital is defined as the features of social organization that facilitate coordination and cooperation for mutual benefit (Putnam, 1996). In sociology, it is viewed as a resource stemming from the structure of social relationship that facilitates achievement of specific goals (Coleman, 1988). Within epidemiology, to date, social capital has been operationalized predominantly as a horizontal relationship between neighbors or community members, with variables such as trust, reciprocity, and civic engagement such as in voluntary organizations, soccer leagues, parent teacher organizations, and the like (Kawachi, Kennedy, Lochner, and Prothrow-Stith, 1997; Kreuter, Lezin, and Koplan, 1997). Lack of social capital has been correlated with poor health status through such things as increased homicide rates, all-cause mortality, and other morbidities, and may mediate the relationship between income inequality and health (Kawachi, Kennedy, Lochner, and Prothrow-Stith, 1997; Sampson, Raudenbush, and Earls, 1997).

Despite correlational associations with health outcomes, the ascendance of the construct, social capital, remains problematic. First, there is no evidence as yet that lack of social capital causes poor health outcomes independent from the material conditions that inform day-to-day experience (Lynch, Smith, Kaplan, and House, 2000). Second, when the focus is on horizontal relationships, the issues of power and vertical relationships between communities and the outside world may be ignored (Hawe and Shiell, 2000). Although Sampson's novel reconfiguration of social capital as collective efficacy, or the belief of community members that they have the capacity to create change, offers an important exception in the latter regard (Sampson and Morenoff, 2000), the tendency of many social capital advocates to deemphasize issues of power and relationships beyond the local community level is disconcerting (Hawe and Shiell, 2000). A third and related concern lies in the fact that the focus on social capital may reinforce a victim-blaming mentality: communities would be healthier if they just "got it together" themselves. Fourth, we have no information on how long social capital takes to develop or to change through planned intervention. Finally, social capital is not a new concept and is in fact often incorporated into the literature on community capacity through the operationalization of many of its key constructs, for example, social networks, social support, and neighborhood integration.

Social networks, or the web of relationships in which people are embedded, and social support, or the tangible and intangible resources they give and receive through these networks (Cohen and Syme, 1985) are important to consider within the context of community capacity building (see Chapter Nine for a fuller discussion of this topic). Social network techniques, for example, by which one can "map" individuals' social ties, can be employed to help identify natural helpers or leaders within a community, to help these natural leaders in turn identify their own networks, to identify high-risk groups within the community, and to involve network members in undertaking their own community assessment and actions necessary to strengthen networks within the community. A number of network assessment tools are available for mapping personal or community networks (McCallister and Fischer, 1978; Heitzmann and Kaplan, 1988) and other community assets (McKnight and Kretzmann, 1992; Sharpe, Greaney, Lee, and Royce, 2000) and offer important strategies to health education professionals concerned with understanding and helping to foster community capacity.

Finally, leadership development represents a key aspect of fostering community capacity. In particular, the development of leaders able to fulfill the roles of animator (stimulating people to think critically and to identify problems and new solutions) and facilitator (providing a process through which the group can discuss its own content in the most productive possible way) is key to building group capacity and effectiveness (Hope and Timmel, 1984) in both geographical and interest-based communities. As Gutierrez and Lewis (1997) suggest, an emphasis on leadership development may be especially important in communities of color where "a unidirectional outreach approach" often is taken, in which such communities are "targets of change rather than active participants and collaborators" (p. 226). By involving people of color in leadership roles from the outset, and nurturing the development of new leaders within these communities, health education professionals can make important contributions to capacity building that reflect feminist notions of strength through diversity (Gutierrez and Lewis, 1997).

Issue Selection

One of the most important steps in community organization practice involves the effective differentiation between *problems,* or things that are troubling, and *issues,* or problems the community feels strongly about (Miller, 1985). As Miller suggests, a good issue must meet several other important criteria as well. It must be *winnable,* to insure that working on the campaign doesn't simply reinforce fatalistic attitudes and beliefs. It must be simple and *specific,* so that any member of the group can explain it clearly in a sentence or two. It must *unite members* of the group and must *involve them in a meaningful way* in achieving problem resolution. It should *affect many people,* should *build up the community or organization* (giving leadership experience, increased visibility, and so on) and, finally, it should be *part of a larger plan or strategy.* A variety of methods familiar to health education professionals can be used to help a community group acquire the data needed for issue selection. Among those most popular currently is the focus group, through which a moderator, using a predetermined discussion guide or series of questions, elicits input from a small group of community members to determine their qualitative perceptions of key issues or concerns facing the community (Krueger and Casey, 2000). Like other face-to-face data collection processes, focus groups, depending on how they are developed and run, can be empowering for members and a valuable information source, or of little relevance to the community and its issue-selection efforts.

Nominal Group Process (NGP), a structured technique that allows a large number of people to have input in issue selection and related activities (Delbecq, Van de Ven, and Gustafson, 1975), door-to-door surveys, and other data-collection methods also can be useful in assessing felt needs and in increasing a sense of participation. Too often, however, community members are merely invited to express their relative agreement with the outside professionals' preconceived notion of what the problems of significance in the community really are. Surveys and other methods are useful for issue selection only to the extent that they enable the discovery of the real issues of concern to the community.

Even if organizers attempt to genuinely "start where the people are," they may lack access to the "hidden discourse" in a community and may misinterpret an apparent community apathy because of their own lack of cultural competence, lack of access to key stakeholders or cultural translators, or lack of self-reflection on the problematic nature of power dynamics between themselves and community members (Scott, 1990). They may have access to community discourse yet find community resistance and organizing strategies that challenge their own level of comfort. They may have a working relationship with community leaders yet find the group has chosen issues that are too broad to be winnable. In the case of issue selection, the organizer has the responsibility to pose questions to refocus the group on specific targets.

Further, as Labonte (1994) has suggested, the community's selection of an issue may reflect racism, sexism, homophobia, or other discriminatory attitudes (as when communities in California, Oregon, and Colorado organized to put anti–gay rights ballot initiatives on their state or local ballots). In cases like these, the health education practitioner's commitment to "starting where the people are" and to "community self-determination" must be tempered by concern with the paramount principle of social justice in the larger community, the interests of which would not be served by the parochial and prejudicial concerns and actions of one subgroup (Minkler, 1994).

An approach to issue selection that has proven especially helpful in overcoming some of these difficulties involves the use of Freire's (1970, 1973) dialogical problem-posing method. As noted previously, part of a Freirian approach involves engaging participants in identifying their core generative themes, those themes that elicit social and emotional involvement and therefore high-level motivation to participate. Community development approaches worldwide have adopted Freire's educational strategies to identify the core issues for starting organizing efforts (Arnold and others, 1995; Hope and Timmel, 1984).

Community organizers in the United States also have adopted strategies from organizational development in creating strategic action plans to prioritize issues by available resources, appropriate timelines, and barriers to reaching goals (French and Bell, 1990). In choosing an issue that may be feasible to win, politically minded organizers have included an analysis of the power brokers, allies, and resisters (Staples, 1984; Feldblum, Wallerstein, Varela, and Collins, 1994).

As suggested above, on the one hand issue selection processes, undertaken thoughtfully, can contribute to community empowerment and can serve as a positive force for social change. On the other hand, calls increasingly have been made for "a new process of community organizing—one relying less on issue-based mobilization and more on community education, leadership development and support, and building local sustainable organizations" (Traynor, 1993). Community-building practice increasingly is being looked to as this "new process of community organizing," and one which, as we have seen, is less concerned with community issue selection as with the identification, nurturing, and celebration of community strengths and the creation of a context, by people in community, for the sharing of those strengths (McKnight, 1987; Walter, forthcoming).

Among the useful new approaches to combining issue selection with this more positive emphasis on community strengths and assets is Wang's "photovoice" method (Wang and Burris, 1997). Using this technique, health education professionals provide cameras and skills training to community residents who then use the cameras to convey their own images of their community, including problems in need of redress and community strengths and assets. Participants then work together to select the pictures that best capture their collective wisdom, and use these to both tell their stories and stimulate change through local organizing and through institutional and policy-level action. Whether with homeless people in Detroit or rural women in China, this approach has been used with considerable success and offers new and "imaginative models for integrating community capacity, health concerns and the visual image" (Wang and Burris, 1997; Wang, Cash, and Powers, 2000).

Measurement and Evaluation Issues

A major limitation of most community-organizing and community-building efforts to date has been the failure to adequately address evaluation processes and outcomes. This typically stems from several sources, among them severe funding constraints and lack of knowledge about how to build a meaningful evaluation component into the organizing effort. The continually evolving nature of community-organizing initiatives, complex and dynamic contexts, and the fact that these projects often seek change on multiple levels make many traditional evaluative approaches inappropriate or ill-suited to such organizing endeavors (Goodman, 2000; Connell and others, 1995). Similarly, the focus of many standard evaluation approaches on long-term change in health and social indicators may miss the shorter-term system-level impacts with which community organizing is heavily concerned, such as improvements in organizational collaboration, community involvement and capacity, and healthier public policies or environmental conditions.

The lack of formal evaluations of most community-organizing efforts, coupled with the failure of many engaged in these projects to write up and publish their results, have made it difficult to amass a literature of "successful" and "unsuccessful" organizing efforts, and the hallmarks of each. Although some characteristics of successful community collaborations have been identified—such as shared vision, strong leadership, and an accent on process and not merely task achievement (Connell and others, 1995)—much remains to be examined and assessed. The careful evaluation and documentation of both successful and unsuccessful community-organizing projects must be a vital part of this new database.

Fortunately, the late 1980s and the 1990s brought important steps forward in evaluation of community organizing and related areas. Key among these was the convening of a "roundtable" on community initiatives for children and families, and its development of *New Approaches to Evaluating Community Initiatives* (Connell and others, 1995). This edited volume explored dilemmas commonly faced in the design, measurement, and interpretation of community initiatives, as well as a variety of options and strategies for evaluators working with such projects. A special volume of *Health Education Research* on community coalitions included several articles that addressed measurement and evaluation issues (Goodman, Burdine, Meehan, and McLeroy, 1993), and has been followed by research on those internal dynamics that may influence a coalition's effectiveness (Goodman, Wandersman, Chinman, Imm, and Morrissey, 1996; Butterfoss, 1998; Kegler, Steckler, McLeroy, and Malek, 1998; Helitzer, 2000).

Evaluation and measurement of community empowerment was brought to the fore by a two-part issue of *Health Education Quarterly* (Wallerstein and Bernstein, 1994) titled "Community Empowerment, Participatory Education and Health," which included both tools and case studies. Measurement of community empowerment, capacity, and social capital has proceeded slowly, but some measures exist for sense of community; community competence (Eng and Parker, 1994); multilevel perceived control (Israel, Checkoway, Schulz, and Zimmerman, 1994); social cohesion and social influence; trust, reciprocity, and civic engagement (Kreuter, Lezin, and Koplan, 1997; Kawachi, Kennedy, Lochner, and Prothrow-Stith, 1997); collective efficacy and social norm control (Sampson, Raudenbush, and Earls, 1997; Bandura, 1995); psychological empowerment beliefs of perceived control, critical understanding of one's social environment, and participation in social action (Zimmerman, 1990, 2000); and perceived neighborhood control and neighborhood participation (Parker and others, 2001).

Equally important is whether new capacities lead to health and health behavior outcomes—a process that may be both direct and indirect. Direct health outcomes may result from coalition or neighborhood activity to prevent siting of a toxic-waste facility or to pass a clean air ordinance that leads to reduced tobacco use. Indirectly, as a result of participation, social isolation may be diminished, leading to improved health, or people may develop the self-esteem and confidence needed to change their health behaviors.

Despite the advances in measurement for capturing these kinds of changes, however, there are limits to any tool or set of scales. Self-report measures of individuals cannot capture the full organizational and community-level processes over a period of time. Qualitative approaches therefore are needed to enhance understanding of the context, dynamics of change, and outcomes such as transformed conditions, new policies, participation, and political voice.

Equally important to the development of validated scales, however, may be the process by which communities develop their own sets of capacity and empowerment indicators. Some community groups have already developed indicators of capacity and sustainability (Norris, 1997; The Aspen Institute, 1996; Bauer, 1997). A useful resource for communities that wish to develop their own indicators can be found in the self-reflection workbook developed in New Mexico to evaluate community organizing and community building in the context of creating healthier communities (Maltrud, Polacsek, and Wallerstein, 1997). The workbook focuses on changes in community processes, such as grassroots participation, and changes in short-term system level outcomes, such as the development of new programs, as a result of the organizing experience. As noted before, it is these middle-level outcomes, rather than long-term changes in self-rated health and other health or social indicators, that are often most important in documenting changes in community capacity and empowerment.

A major contribution to the literature in this area lay in the publication of Fetterman, Kaftarian, and Wandersman's (1996) comprehensive volume *Empowerment Evaluation*. Empowerment evaluation is defined as "an interactive and iterative process by which the community, in collaboration with the support team, identifies its own health issues, decides how to address them, monitors progress toward its goals and uses the information to adapt and sustain the initiative" (Fawcett and others, 1996). Although some of the evaluation approaches described in this book (for example, evaluation of HIV-prevention evaluation initiatives) fit better into a social-planning rather than a true organizing approach to practice, most have immediate relevance for health education professionals concerned with the evaluation of community-organizing efforts.

Finally, recent work by Fawcett and his colleagues (1997, 2001) in the Work Group on Health Promotion and Community Development at the University of Kansas has helped tailor empowerment evaluation methods more directly to the evaluation of community coalitions for health and related organizing efforts. Stressing both processes (for example, community mobilization to address substance abuse) and outcomes (for example, changes in youth self-reports of decreased substance abuse and community-level impacts that can be attributed to coalition efforts), this approach uses multiple qualitative and quantitative measurement instruments and involves community members actively in the evaluation process. A Web site developed in part to help other groups use a "community tool-box" to better document their own community-organizing and community-building efforts in health promotion (ctb.lsi.ukans.edu) was created by the Work Group and is being widely used to foster more rigorous and empowering approaches to such evaluation (Fawcett and others, 2000).

The availability of new theoretical contributions and practical tools that lend themselves to evaluation of community organizing fails, of course, to solve the problem of insufficient funding or commitment to carrying out high-quality evaluative research. Yet the increased attention of both foundation and government funders to evaluation and measurement issues in community-organizing and community-based initiatives is encouraging. If translated into increased funding, this increased attention, together with the availability of new measurement tools and processes, should help spur major advances in the evaluation and documentation of community organizing and community building.

Applications of Community Organization and Community Building

The next section of this chapter describes two applications of the concepts and methods of community organizing and community building. The first case study is the Tenderloin Senior Organizing Project (TSOP), a sixteen-year community-organizing and community-building effort involving elderly residents of San Francisco's Tenderloin District. The second case study discusses the Adolescent Social Action Program (ASAP), a youth-centered experiential prevention program in communities throughout New Mexico.

The Tenderloin Senior Organizing Project

For the low-income elderly in America's single-room-occupancy (SRO) hotels, poor health, social isolation, and powerlessness often are intimately connected. This case study describes a community-organizing effort to address these interrelated problems by fostering social support and social action organizing among elderly residents of San Francisco's Tenderloin District.

Of the many health and social problems facing elders in the Tenderloin, poor nutrition and clinical depression have been among the most prevalent and important. A survey conducted in the early 1980s thus suggested that at least 40 percent of Tenderloin elders were malnourished or seriously undernourished (Wechsler and Minkler, 1986), while high rates of suicide, a problem drinking rate of 20 percent (Arean, 1994), and related health and social indicators suggested that clinical depression also is a frequent fact of life for elders in this neighborhood (Minkler, 1997).

Poverty, social isolation, physical illness and disability, and social stressors such as fear of facing crime when venturing outdoors are among the factors contributing to the high rates of both malnutrition and clinical depression observed (Minkler, 1997). Finally, the social marginalization of people in neighborhoods such as the Tenderloin, and their classification as "undeserving poor," place them at high risk for dependency on stigmatizing and miserly health and social programs (such as food stamps, Medicaid, and Supplemental Security Income, or SSI) that are frequent targets of budget cuts in times of fiscal retrenchment.

Originally known as the Tenderloin Senior Outreach Project, TSOP was established in 1979 by graduate students and faculty at UC Berkeley's School of Public Health with the dual goals of (1) improving physical and mental health by reducing social isolation and providing relevant health education and (2) facilitating, through dialogue and participation, a process through which residents were encouraged to work together to identify common problems and to seek solutions to these shared problems and concerns.

Student volunteers began in a single Tenderloin hotel, encouraging resident interaction and eventually forming an informal group that met weekly and included a core of twelve residents and two outside facilitators. As levels of trust and rapport increased, group members began to share personal concerns regarding such issues as fear of crime, loneliness, rent increases, and their own sense of powerlessness. Student facilitators used a combination of organizing and educational approaches to help residents select an initial issue on which they wanted to focus (crime and safety) and to foster group solidarity and social action organizing. A modified Freirian problem-posing process thus was used to help residents engage in dialogue about shared problems and their causes and to generate potential action plans. In addition, Alinsky's (1972) admonitions to create dissatisfaction with the status quo and help people identify specific, winnable issues were among the community-organization precepts followed, as were McKnight (1987, 1993) and Miller's (1993) emphases on identifying and building on community strengths. Finally, and drawing on social support theory stressing the importance of social interaction opportunities, the student facilitators attempted to create a group atmosphere conducive to meeting the purely social needs of residents as well as the more political and task-oriented concerns of some group members (Minkler, 1997).

As the first hotel group evolved into an established entity, seven additional groups were organized in other Tenderloin hotels. In all but one of these, empowerment was facilitated through decreased reliance on outside facilitators, with broader resident participation in discussion and decision making. A second trend observed in the groups, and one critical to TSOP's evolution, was the realization among residents of the need for looking beyond hotel boundaries and working with residents of other hotels and community groups on shared problems. TSOP residents in several hotels thus identified crime and safety as their key area of concern and formed an interhotel coalition to begin work on this problem. The coalition in turn started the Safehouse Project, recruiting during its first year forty-eight neighborhood businesses and agencies that agreed to display colorful posters indicating that they had become places of refuge where residents could go in time of emergency. Through this and other actions (for example, convincing the mayor to increase the number of beat patrol officers in the neighborhood), the coalition was credited with helping to bring about an 18 percent drop in crime during its first year of operation and a 26 percent drop by the end of year two ("Safehouses Now Easing the Fears of Elderly Residents," 1982). Concurrent changes in individual health and social behavior also were seen, with increased feelings of self-efficacy and social support leading some residents to quit smoking or cut down on problem drinking and others to demonstrate dramatic improvements in their mental health and self-esteem (Minkler, 1997).

Encouraged by the success of the Safehouse Project, TSOP members turned their attention to the problem of undernutrition and poor food access, establishing minimarkets in three hotels and a cooperative breakfast program in a fourth, and creating and widely disseminating a "no cook cookbook" for residents not allowed to cook in their rooms (Minkler, 1997). Alongside these and other tangible projects, TSOP engaged in significant leadership training, through one-on-one and small-group activities and a leadership training conference, and later by arranging for about twenty indigenous leaders to participate in four-day intensive organizer training workshops with other organizers around the country.

As Tenderloin residents became increasingly willing and able to take control of this project, TSOP staff and volunteers played a less visible role, serving primarily as resource persons and "sounding boards" for residents' ideas and strategy discussions. TSOP changed the "O" in its name from "Outreach" to "Organizing" in 1988 to reflect this change in orientation and increasingly defined its role as one of facilitating community empowerment by drawing out the competence, self-confidence, and leadership skills of elderly residents (Miller, 1993).

TSOP's key mechanism of action also changed over time from health-educator-facilitated support groups to resident-run tenant associations. Prior to its closing in 1995, TSOP had helped organize sixteen autonomous tenant associations and trained more than two hundred indigenous leaders. Their victories included getting hot water turned on in a building that had gone without for ten years; winning back rent for residents of a building whose elevator had been "out of service" for five months; pressuring to make one hotel wheelchair accessible; pressuring to get a vending machine selling nutritious foods in another; and getting security guards, trash pick-up, and other discontinued services reinstated in still other residences. Although small in and of themselves, each of these victories contributed to both the health and safety of residents, and to their feelings of empowerment, self-esteem, and community competence (Minkler, 1997).

TSOP was not without problems, including resident "burnout" on some issues they had earlier decided to tackle, occasional power conflicts within groups, and leadership turnover as a consequence of illness, transiency, and other problems. Evaluation of the project also proved difficult, because many residents harbored an understandable distrust of outside researchers and because project staff were committed to avoiding data-gathering activities that might confuse residents as to the true mission of the organization. A comprehensive external evaluation recently was completed, however, that attempted to explore residents' perceptions of individual and community control and involved informal interviews with a variety of key informants as well as structured interviews with 150 residents of both TSOP and comparison non-TSOP buildings. The evaluation was unable to document specific improvements in physical health status that could be directly linked to the project. However, significant increases in sense of control (making decisions that affect one's life), social interaction, morale, perceived safety, and perceived ability to improve one's housing conditions were among the outcomes demonstrated (Shaw, 1995).

Although TSOP was forced to close its doors in the mid-1990s as a consequence of funding constraints, a number of tenant organizations that TSOP helped get under way continue to organize in the Tenderloin. A detailed replication manual was produced and disseminated. Replication projects have included use of the early TSOP model by a disabled veteran in New York City to help organize chronically schizophrenic veterans in a residential treatment center and a Ministry of Health–funded project involving nine SRO hotels in Vancouver, British Columbia (Minkler, 1997). Through such replications, the TSOP model continues to make a difference in the lives of people for whom organizing and creating a sense of community can be an important route to improved health and quality of life.

The Adolescent Social Action Program (ASAP)

Youth today are confronted with multiple risks in their lives: fears about the future, lack of employment opportunities, media targeting by the alcohol and tobacco industries, family and community violence, and social norms of peer pressure to engage in risky behaviors. This case study illustrates how a university-community partnership is working with youth to address the interconnectedness of personal choices and social conditions through a mix of empowerment education and community-organizing strategies.

The Adolescent Social Action Program (ASAP) is a youth-centered experiential prevention program that has involved a collaboration between the University of New Mexico, the University hospital, the county detention center, and over thirty multiethnic schools and communities throughout New Mexico since 1982. ASAP's goals are to reduce excess morbidity and mortality among youth who live in high-risk environments, to encourage them to make healthier choices in their own lives, and to empower them to take an active political and social role in improving their neighborhoods and communities.

The ASAP program consists of a seven-week experience for small groups of youth who are brought into the hospital and detention center settings to interview and interact with patients and jail residents who have problems related to drug and alcohol abuse, interpersonal violence, and other risky behaviors (Wallerstein and Bernstein, 1988). Follow-up school and community-based organizing activities extend the length of the intervention for one semester, with a structured booster session at the end.

At the heart of the program is Freire's educational empowerment approach (Wallerstein and Sanchez-Merki, 1994). Through Freirian problem-posing-structured dialogue led by university health professional students trained as facilitators, the youths discuss the patients' and jail residents' life stories and their own experiences and lives, and examine the consequences of their actions and how to make healthier choices for themselves and their communities. Unlike "scared-straight" programs, which have been proven to be ineffective (Rogers and Mewborn, 1976; Job, 1988), ASAP also incorporates Protection-Motivation Theory directed at increasing students' threat appraisal and coping self-efficacy for behavior change (Rogers, 1984; Floyd, Prentice-Dunn, and Rogers, 2000; Stainback and Rogers, 1983). The integration of behavior and social change is especially important for youths of color who face poverty, discrimination, and unemployment, and who therefore are overrepresented in injury and mortality statistics.

Through Freirian empowerment education, ASAP incorporates a listening-dialogue-action model that links educational processes to community organizing. During the structured curriculum in the hospital or detention center, the dominant model is the development of critical consciousness toward the goals of leadership development and community building, as the youths develop empathy with each other and with their neighborhoods and school communities. Through listening to patient stories, the youths begin to dialogue critically about their own lives and their relationships to their communities. Active participation is a key tenet of ASAP in the issues youths bring to the dialogue and in their choice of follow-up activities.

As the seven-week curriculum ends, the ASAP program typically has offered the youths two possibilities: to enter a peer-education component or to work in social action. The peer-education program allows the youths to continue the educational model with younger elementary students. The social action model, however, is the one that extends into community organizing. For social action, the youths are encouraged to devise their own prevention projects for their school site with the aid of project staff. This approach has encouraged the youth to explore existing social and legal policies, the current prevention strategies for risky behaviors, and how to change alcohol norms in their own communities.

Early examples of ASAP social action projects included youth-panel discussions at the ASAP Summer Institutes, local booths at school fiestas, and red ribbon rallies. Issue selection has been added more recently, with youths connecting to citywide organizing and developing their own long-term initiatives, such as production of videotapes and photonovellas. The ASAP videos, including a recent music video, and the series of photonovellas have been conceptualized, written, and produced by groups of youths, who learned the technical skills and developed the issues they wanted to examine about their neighborhoods and society. These products have been distributed widely in the local schools and community centers as aids to other educational and organizing endeavors that promote youth problem solving and community competence.

Certain issues, such as gang activity, have demanded larger neighborhood and citywide attention. The Albuquerque South East Community Gang Task Force provides youths with the opportunity to act as Advisory Committee board members and Task Force members. Street Reach is a gang prevention project in which ASAP youth have shared the health information and coping strategies they have learned through ASAP. At the New Mexico State Fair in 1994, ASAP youths helped plan and participated in the program "A Day Without Alcohol Is Fair." In Albuquerque's Civic Plaza, youths participated in the program "A Day Without Colors" by directing activities and running the ASAP booth. ASAP youth have been involved in a local youth-produced TV station program on teenagers. They have helped cook and serve Thanksgiving dinner at a local community center.

In addition to the direct effects of youth-organizing and youth-produced curriculum, program effectiveness has been tracked over the years with a randomized design of intervention versus control students, measured through questionnaires administered at pretest, posttest, and six- or eight-month follow-up assessments. Cognitive variables, related to self- and other-protective behaviors, and self-reported drinking and other substance-abuse behaviors have been collected. Cognitive scales have included self-efficacy, response efficacy, intentions, empathy, and communication with others to influence risky behaviors.

The earliest study of ASAP participants at the high school level demonstrated increased awareness of riskiness of drinking and driving for participants, countering the normal developmental trend for teenagers (Bernstein and Woodall, 1987). In later research of middle school youths, a drug-free-schools randomized study of three conditions—social action, peer education, and control—found increased self-efficacy for protecting others over time for both participant groups versus a decrease in the control group, and greater decline of drinking for both girls and boys involved in social action over a peer-education curriculum. And a tobacco and alcohol drug-free-schools grant found participants to have a higher perception of severity of problems due to substance abuse, increased self-efficacy for communicating, and higher self-efficacy to influence friends' behaviors (Dow-Velarde, Starling, and Wallerstein, 2000). Data are currently being analyzed from a five-year NIAAA-funded (National Institute of Alcoholism and Alcohol Abuse) study of participants versus controls up to fifteen months postintervention.

Some core issues exist about the limits of community organizing within a program such as ASAP. The first issue is the ability of youths to assume full responsibility for organizing. Youths still depend on adults as mentors and to facilitate the logistics of organizing; middle school youths, in particular, need parental permission and basic transportation to organizing events. The hope is, however, that youths will develop a belief in group action, a belief in social responsibility, and a belief in themselves as leaders who can make a difference.

The second issue is that the school is the starting place for the program, which raises questions of community and one's base of organizing. Unfortunately, many youths today identify with their school, their neighborhood, or their gang, and will not work across these boundaries. Broader organizing would have to take these polarized subcommunities into account to help bridge the differences and build a "community of youths" who could have citywide policy impact.

The third organizing issue is that the majority of funding for ASAP is categorical—for alcohol and other drug prevention. Despite the potential narrowing of the issue, in practice, alcohol and drugs have been prominent concerns for teenagers, and the youths have been able to choose projects within the broad range of adolescent risky behaviors. One photonovella, for example, delves into the difficulties within adolescent relationships.

In sum, ASAP uses a comprehensive model that combines elements of empowerment education, critical consciousness, leadership development, community building, and high-level participation with some of the elements of traditional community organizing. Though the starting place is not directly community organizing, the ASAP model illustrates how it is possible to combine many of the principles with an overarching social change agenda.

Conclusion

The continued pivotal role of community organization in health education practice reflects not only its time-tested efficacy but also its high degree of philosophical fit with the most fundamental principles of effective community health education. Community organization stresses the principle of relevance, or starting where the people are; the principle of participation; and the importance of creating environments in which individuals and communities can become empowered as they increase their community competence or problem-solving ability.

Similarly, newer conceptualizations of community building stress many of the same principles, within an overall approach that focuses on community growth and change from the inside, through increased group identification; discovery, nurturing, and mapping of community assets; and creation of "critical consciousness," all toward the end of building stronger and more caring communities.

The San Francisco–based TSOP project is an example of an effort in which a relatively "pure" application of community-organizing principles and methods by health educators was undertaken with considerable success. Far more frequently, however, health and social service professionals are employed by an agency with specific agendas and often with categorical funding. The practitioner in this setting may find that he or she cannot undertake community organizing in the strictest sense of the word because an outside group rather than the community itself has identified the specific health problem(s) to be addressed. Yet professionals in such situations can apply with effectiveness many of the core principles and approaches of community organization and community-building practice. They thus can elicit high-level community participation or involvement, and can strive to build leadership skills and increase community competence as an integral part of the overall health education project. Further, as demonstrated by the ASAP case study, while the overall problem area (such as alcohol and substance abuse) may initially have been identified by an outside group or agency, the health education professional, using community-organizing and community-building skills and approaches, can help communities identify, within this broader framework, those specific issues they feel are of greatest relevance.

Most important, professionals can challenge themselves to examine their own dynamic of power, with their professional colleagues and members of the community, to understand the complexities of working in partnership toward the goals of community ownership of the projects undertaken and increased empowerment and community competence (Wallerstein, 1999). In sum, both community organization and newer conceptualizations of community-building practice have essential messages for health education professionals in a wide variety of settings, and may hold particular relevance in the changing sociopolitical climate of the twenty-first century.

References

Alinsky, S. D. *Reveille for Radicals.* Chicago, Ill.: University of Chicago Press, 1969.

Alinsky, S. D. *Rules for Radicals.* New York: Random House, 1972.

Arean, P. "Implications and Service Use of Mental Disorders in Older Medical Patients." Paper presented at the eighth annual meeting of the NIMH Conference on Psychiatric Disorders in the General Health Care Sector. Washington, D.C., November 1994.

Arnold, R., and others. *Educating for a Change.* Toronto: Between the Lines and Doris Marshall Institute for Education and Action, 1995.

The Aspen Institute. *Measuring Community Capacity Building: A Workbook-in-Progress for Rural Communities.* The Aspen Institute Rural Economic Policy Program, 1996.

Avery, B. "Breathing Life into Ourselves: The Evolution of the Black Women's Health Project." In E. White (ed.), *The Black Women's Health Book.* Seattle: Seal Press, 1990.

Bandura, A. "Exercise of Personal and Collective Efficacy." In A. Bandura, (ed.), *Self-Efficacy in Changing Societies.* New York: Cambridge University Press, 1995.

Barndt, D. *Naming the Moment: Political Analysis for Action.* Toronto: Jesuit Center for Social Faith and Justice, 1989.

Bauer, G. *Community Health Indicators on the Neighborhood Level: A Prototype for the Fruitvale/San Antonio Area in Oakland.* Oakland Community-Based Public Health Initiative (OCBPHI), 1997.

Bernstein, E., and Woodall, W. G. "Changing Perceptions of Riskiness in Drinking, Drugs, and Driving: An Emergency Department-Based Alcohol and Substance Abuse Prevention Program." *Annals of Emergency Medicine,* December 1987, *16*(12), 1350–1354.

Bernstein, E., and others. "Empowerment Forum: A Dialogue Between Guest Editorial Board Members." *Health Education Quarterly,* 1994, *21*(3), 281–294.

Blackwell, A. G., and Colmenar, R. "Community Building: From Local Wisdom to Public Policy." *Public Health Reports.* 2000, *113*(2 and 3), 167–173.

Bracht, N., and Kingsbury, L. "Community Organization Principles in Health Promotion: A Five-Stage Model." In N. Bracht (ed.), *Health Promotion at the Community Level.* Thousand Oaks, Calif.: Sage, 1990.

Braithwaite, R. L., Bianchi, C., and Taylor, S. E. "Ethnographic Approach to Community Organization and Health Empowerment." *Health Education Quarterly,* 1994, *21*(3), 407–419.

Braithwaite, R. L., and others. "Community Organization and Development for Health Promotion within an Urban Black Community: A Conceptual Model." *Health Education,* 1989, *2*(5), 56–60.

Butterfoss, F. D. *Coalition Effectiveness Inventory Self-Assessment Tool.* Charleston, S.C.: Center for Pediatric Research, Center for Health Promotion, 1998.

Butterfoss, F. D., Goodman, R. M., and Wandersman, A. "Community Coalitions for Prevention and Health Promotion: Factors Predicting Satisfaction, Participation, and Planning." *Health Education Quarterly,* 1996, *23*(1), 65–79.

Cohen, S., and Syme, S. L. (eds.). *Social Support and Health.* Orlando, Fla.: Academic Press, 1985.

Coleman, J. S. "Social Capital in the Creation of Human Capital." *American Journal of Sociology,* 1988, *94,* S95-S121.

Connell, J. P., and others. (eds.). *New Approaches to Evaluating Community Initiatives: Concepts, Methods and Contexts.* Washington, D.C.: The Aspen Institute, 1995.

Cottrell, L. S., Jr. "The Competent Community." In R. Warren and L. Lyon (eds.), *New Perspectives on the American Community.* Homewood, Ill.: The Dorsey Press, 1983.

Delbecq, A., Van de Ven, A. H., and Gustafson, D. H. *Group Techniques for Program Planning: A Guide to Nominal Group and Delphi Processes.* Glenview, Ill.: Scott, Foresman, 1975.

Dow-Velarde, L. D., Starling, R., and Wallerstein, N. "Identity in Early Adolescence via Social Change Activities: Experience of the Adolescent Social Action Program." In T. Brinthaupt (ed.), *Understanding the Self of the Adolescent.* Albany, N.Y.: New York State University Press, 2000.

Eng, E., Briscoe, J., and Cunningham, A. "The Effect of Participation in State Projects on Immunization." *Social Science and Medicine,* 1990, *30*(12), 1349–1358.

Eng, E., and Parker, E. "Measuring Community Competence in the Mississippi Delta: The Interface Between Program Evaluation and Empowerment." *Health Education Quarterly,* 1994, *21*(2), 199–220.

Farquhar, J., and others. "The Stanford Five City Project: An Overview." In J. D. Matarazzo, N. E. Miller, S. M. Weiss, and J. A. Herd (eds.), *Behavioral Health: A Handbook of Health Enhancement and Disease Prevention.* Silver Spring, Md.: Wiley, 1984.

Fawcett, S. B., and others. "Empowering Community Health Initiatives Through Evaluation." In D. Fetterman, S. Kaftarian, and A. Wandersman (eds.), *Empowerment Evaluation.* Thousand Oaks, Calif.: Sage, 1996.

Fawcett, S. B., and others. "Evaluating Community Coalitions for Prevention of Substance Abuse: The Case of Project Freedom." *Health Education and Behavior,* December 1997, *24*(6), 812–828.

Fawcett, S. B., and others. "The Community Tool Box. A Web-Based Resource for Building Healthier Communities." *Public Health,* 2000, *113*(2 and 3), 274–278.

Fawcett, S. B., and others. "Evaluating Community Initiatives for Health and Development." In I. Rootman, D. McQueen, L. Potvin, J. Springett, and E. Ziglio (eds.), *Evaluation in Health Promotion Approaches.* Copenhagen: WHO European Series No. 92, 2001.

Feldblum, M., Wallerstein, N., Varela, F., and Collins, G. (eds.). *Community Organizing: An Experience for Building Healthier Communities.* (3rd ed.) Albuquerque, New Mexico Department of Health, Public Health Division, 1994.

Fellin, P. "Understanding American Communities." In J. Rothman, J. Erlich, and J. Tropman (eds.). *Strategies of Community Intervention.* (5th ed.) Itasca, Ill.: F. E. Peacock Publishers, 2001.

Fetterman, D., Kaftarian, S., and Wandersman, A. (eds.). *Empowerment Evaluation.* Thousand Oaks, Calif.: Sage, 1996.

Floyd, D., Prentice-Dunn, S., and Rogers, R. "A Meta-Analysis of Research on Protection Motivation Theory. *Journal of Applied Social Psychology,* 2000, *30,* 407–429.

Foucault, M. *Power/Knowledge: Selected Interviews and other Writings.* C. Gordon (ed.), New York: Pantheon, 1977.

Freire, P. *Pedagogy of the Oppressed.* New York: Seabury Press, 1970.

Freire, P. *Education for Critical Consciousness.* New York: Seabury Press, 1973.

French, M. *Beyond Power: On Women, Men And Morals.* London: Abacus, 1986.

French, W., and Bell, C. *Organization Development: Behavioral Science Interventions for Organization Improvement.* (2nd ed.) Englewood Cliffs, N.J.: Prentice Hall, 1990.

Gardner, J. *Building Community.* Washington, D.C.: Independent Sector Leadership Studies Program, 1991.

Garvin, C. D., and Cox, F. M. "A History of Community Organizing Since the Civil War with Special Reference to Oppressed Communities." *Strategies of Community Intervention.* (5th ed.) Itasca, Ill.: Peacock Publishers, 2001.

Goodman, R. M. "Evaluation of Community-Based Health Programs: An Alternate Perspective." In N. Schneiderman, M. A. Speers, J. M. Silva, H. Tomes, and J. H. Gentry (eds.), *Integrating Behavioral and Social Sciences with Public Health.* Washington, D.C.: American Psychological Association Press, 2000.

Goodman, R. M., Burdine, J., Meehan, E., and McLeroy, K. "Coalitions." *Health Education Research,* 1993, *8*(3), 313–314.

Goodman, R. M., Wandersman, A., Chinman, M., Imm, P., and Morrissey, E. "An Ecological Assessment of Community-Based Interventions for Prevention and Health Promotion: Approaches to Measuring Community Coalitions." *American Journal of Community Psychology,* 1996, *24*(1), 33–61.

Goodman, R. M., and others. "Identifying and Defining the Dimensions of Community Capacity to Provide a Basis for Measurement." *Health Education and Behavior,* 1999, *25*(3), 258–278.

Guillory, B., Willie, E., Jr., and Duran, E. "Analysis of a Community Organizing Case Study: Alkali Lake." *Journal of Rural Community Psychology,* 1988, *9*(1), 27–35.

Gutierrez, L., and Lewis, E. "Education, Participation and Capacity Building in Community Organizing with Women of Color." In M. Minkler, (ed.), *Community Organizing and Community Building For Health.* New Brunswick, N.J.: Rutgers University Press, 1997.

Hawe, P., and Shiell, A. "Social Capital and Health Promotion: A Review." *Social Science and Medicine,* 2000, *51,* 871–885.

Heitzmann, C. A., and Kaplan, R. M. "Assessment of Methods for Measuring Social Support." *Health Psychology,* 1988, *7*(1), 75–109.

Helitzer, D. *Coalition Member Survey.* Albuquerque, New Mexico: Office of Evaluation, University of New Mexico, 2000.

Himmelman, A. "Communities Working Collaboratively for a Change." Unpublished paper, July 1992.

Hope, A., and Timmel, S. *Training for Transformation: A Handbook for Community Workers.* Gweru, Zimbabwe: Mambo Press, 1984.

Hunter, A. "The Loss of Community: An Empirical Test Through Replication." *American Sociology Review,* 1975, *40*(5), 537–552.

Hyde, C. "A Feminist Model for Macro Practice." *Administration in Social Work,* 1990, *13,* 145–181.

Israel, B. "Social Networks and Social Support: Implications for Natural Helper and Community Level Interventions." *Health Education Quarterly,* 1985, *12*(1), 66–80.

Israel, B., Checkoway, B., Schulz, A., and Zimmerman, M. "Health Education and Community Empowerment: Conceptualizing and Measuring Perceptions of Individual, Organizational, and Community Control." *Health Education Quarterly,* 1994, *21*(2), 149–170.

Job, R. "Effective and Ineffective Use of Fear in Health Promotion Campaigns." *American Journal of Public Health,* 1988, *78,* 163–167.

Katz, R. "Empowerment and Synergy: Expanding the Community's Healing Resources." *Prevention in Human Services,* 1984, *3,* 201–226.

Kawachi, I., Kennedy, B. P., Lochner, K., and Prothrow-Stith, D. "Social Capital, Income Equality, and Mortality." *American Journal of Public Health,* 1997, *87,* 1491–1497.

Kaye, G., and Wolff, T. *From the Ground Up: A Workbook on Coalition Building and Community Development.* Amherst, Mass.: AHEC/Community Partners, 1995.

Kegler, M., Steckler, A., McLeroy, K., and Malek, S. "Factors That Contribute to Effective Community Health Promotion Coalitions: A Study of 10 Project ASSIST Coalitions in North Carolina." *Health Education and Behavior,* 1998, *25*(3), 338–353.

Khinduka, S. K. "Community Development: Potentials and Limitations." In R. M. Kramer and H. Specht (eds.), *Readings in Community Organization Practice.* (2nd ed.) Englewood Cliffs, N.J.: Prentice Hall, 1975.

Kieffer, C. "Citizen Empowerment: A Developmental Perspective." In *Studies in Empowerment: Steps Toward Understanding and Action, Prevention in Human Services.* 1984, *3*(2 and 3), 9–36.

Kreuter, M. W., Lezin, N. A., and Koplan, A. N. *Social Capital: Evaluation Implications for Community Health Promotion.* Atlanta: World Health Organization, 1997.

Krueger, R. A., and Casey, M. A. *Focus Groups: A Practical Guide for Applied Research.* Thousand Oaks, Calif.: Sage, 2000.

Labonte, R. "Empowerment: Notes on Professional and Community Dimensions." *Canadian Review of Social Policy, 26,* 1990, 1–12.

Labonte, R. "Community Development and Partnerships." *Canadian Journal of Public Health,* 1993, *84*(4), 237–240.

Labonte, R. "Health Promotion and Empowerment: Reflections on Professional Practice." *Health Education Quarterly,* 1994, *21*(2), 253–268.

Lorig, K., Lubeck, D., Kraines, R. G., Seleznick, M., and Holman, H. R. "Outcomes of Self-Help Education for Patients with Arthritis." *Arthritis Rheum,* 1985, *28*(6) 680–685.

Lynch, J., Smith, G. D., Kaplan, G. A., and House, J. S. "Income Inequality and Mortality: Importance to Health of Individual Income, Psychosocial Environment, or Material Conditions." *British Medical Journal,* 2000, 320.

Maltrud, K., Polacsek, M., and Wallerstein, N. *Participatory Evaluation Workbook for Community Initiatives.* Albuquerque: University of New Mexico, Master's in Public Health Program, 1997.

Marquez, B. "Organizing the Mexican American Community in Texas: The Legacy of Saul Alinsky." *Policy Studies Review,* Winter 1990, 355–373.

McCallister, L., and Fischer, C. S. "A Procedure for Surveying Personal Networks." *Sociological Methods and Research,* 1978, *7,* 131–148.

McKnight, J. "Regenerating Community." *Social Policy,* Winter 1987, 54–58.

McKnight, J. "Local Social Community Development and Economic Development Issues." Presentation at the annual meeting of the American Public Health Association, San Francisco, October 27, 1993.

McKnight, J. L., and Kretzmann, J. P. *Mapping Community Capacity.* Evanston, Ill.: Center for Urban Affairs and Policy Research, Northwestern University, 1992.

Miller, M. "Turning Problems into Actionable Issues." Unpublished article. San Francisco: Organize Training Center, 1985.

Miller, M. "The Tenderloin Senior Organizing Project." In *A Journey to Justice.* Presbyterian Committee on the Self Development of People. Report of the Special Task Force. Louisville, Ky.: Presbyterian Church of the USA, 1993.

Minkler, M. "Ten Commitments for Community Health Education." *Health Education Research,* 1994, *9*(4), 527–534.

Minkler, M. "Community Organizing Among the Elderly Poor in San Francisco's Tenderloin District." In M. Minkler (ed.), *Community Organizing and Community Building for Health.* New Brunswick, N.J.: Rutgers University Press, 1997.

Minkler, M., and Cox, K. "Creating Critical Consciousness in Health: Applications of Freire's Philosophy and Methods to the Health Care Setting." *International Journal of Health Services*, 1980, *10*(2), 311–322.

Norris, T. *The Community Indicators Handbook: Redefining Progress.* Boulder, Colo.: Tyler Norris Associates, 1997.

Norris, T., and Pittman, M. "The Healthy Communities Movement and the Coalition for Healthier Cities and Communities." *Public Health Reports*, 2000, *113*(2 and 3), 118–124.

Nyswander, D. B. Education for Health: Some Principles and their Application. *Health Education Monographs*, 1956, *14*, 65–70.

Ovrebo, B., Ryan, M., Jackson, K., and Hutchinson, K. "The Homeless Prenatal Program: A Model for Empowering Homeless Pregnant Women." *Health Education Quarterly*, 1994, *21*(2), 187–198.

Parker, E. A., and others. "Disentangling Measures Of Individual Perceptions Of Community Social Dynamics: Results Of A Community Survey." *Health Education and Behavior*, 2001, *28*(4), 462–486.

"PATCH" (entire issue). *Journal of Health Education*, 1992, *23*(3).

Purdey, A., Adhikari, G., Robinson, S., and Cox, P. "Participatory Health Development in Rural Nepal: Clarifying the Process of Community Empowerment." *Health Education Quarterly*, 1994, *21*(3), 329–344.

Putnam, R. D. "The Strange Disappearance of Civic America." *The American Prospect*, 1996, *24*, 34–48.

Rappaport, J. "Studies in Empowerment: Introduction to the Issue." *Prevention in Human Services*, 1984, *3*(2 and 3), 1–7.

Reitzes, D. C., and Reitzes, D. C. "Saul Alinsky's Contribution to Community Development." *Journal of the Community Development Society*, 1980, *11*(2), 39–52.

Rivera, F., and Erlich, J. "An Option Assessment Framework for Organizing in Emerging Minority Communities." In J. Tropman and others (eds.), *Tactics and Techniques of Community Intervention.* (3rd ed.) Itasca, Ill.: Peacock Publishers, 1995, 198–213.

Rogers, R. "Changing Health-Related Attitudes and Behavior: the Role of Preventive Health Psychology." In R. McGlyn, J. Maddox, C. Stoltenbery, and R. Harvey (eds.), *Interfaces in Psychology.* Lubbock, Tex.: Texas Tech University Press, 1984.

Rogers, R., and Mewborn, C. "Fear Appeals and Attitude Change: Effects of a Threat's Noxiousness, Probability of Occurrence, and the Efficacy of Coping Responses." *Journal of Personality and Social Psychology*, 1976, *34*, 54–61.

Ross, M. *Community Organization: Theory and Principles.* New York: Harper, 1955.

Rothman, J. "Approaches to Community Intervention." In J. Rothman, J. L. Erlich, and J. E. Tropman (eds.), *Strategies of Community Intervention.* Itasca, Ill.: Peacock Publishers, 2001.

"Safehouses Now Easing the Fears of Elderly Residents." *Los Angeles Times*, Nov. 21, 1982.

Sampson, R. J., and Morenoff, J. D. "Public Health and Safety in Context: Lessons from Community-Level Theory on Social Capital." In B. D. Smedley and S. L. Syme (eds.), *Promoting Health Intervention Strategies from Social and Behavioral Research.* Washington, D.C.: National Academy Press, 2000.

Sampson, R. J., Raudenbush, S. W., and Earls, F. "Neighborhoods and Violent Crime: A Multilevel Study of Collective Efficacy." *Science*, 1997, *277*, 918–924.

Scott, J. *Domination and the Arts of Resistance: Hidden Transcripts.* New Haven: Yale University Press, 1990.

Sharpe, P. A., Greaney, M. L., Lee, P. R., and Royce, S. W. "Assets-Oriented Community Assessment." *Public Health Reports*, 2000, *113*(2 and 3), 205–211.

Shaw, F. "Tenderloin Senior Organizing Project Evaluation." Unpublished report for the California Wellness Foundation, November 1995.

Stainback, R., and Rogers, R. "Identifying Effective Components of Alcohol Abuse Prevention Programs: Effect of Fear Appeals, Message Style, and Source Expertise." *The International Journal of the Addictions*, 1983, *18*(3), 393–405.

Staples, L. *Roots to Power: A Manual for Grassroots Organizing.* New York: Praeger, 1984.

Syme, S. "Social Epidemiology and the Work Environment." *International Journal of Health Services*, 1988, *18*(4), 635–645.

Traynor, B. "Community Development and Community Organizing." *Shelterforce*, March-April 1993.

Wallerstein, N. "Powerlessness, Empowerment, and Health: Implications for Health Promotion Programs." *American Journal of Health Promotion*, 1992, *6*, 197–205.

Wallerstein, N. "Power Between Evaluator and Community: Research Relationships Within New Mexico's Healthier Communities." *Social Science and Medicine*, 1999, *49*, 39–53.

Wallerstein, N., and Bernstein, E. "Empowerment Education: Freire's Ideas Adapted to Health Education." *Health Education Quarterly*, 1988, *15*, 379–394.

Wallerstein, N., and Bernstein, E. (eds.). "Community Empowerment, Participatory Education and Health." *Health Education Quarterly*, Summer and Fall 1994, *21*(2 and 3).

Wallerstein, N., and Sanchez-Merki, V. "Freirian Praxis in Health Education: Research Results from an Adolescent Prevention Program." *Health Education Research*, 1994, *9*(1), 105–118.

Wallerstein, N., and Weinger, M. (eds.). *American Journal of Industrial Medicine*, 1992, *22*(5).

Walter, C. "Community Building Practice" In M. Minkler (ed.), *Community Organizing and Community Building to Improve Health*. New Brunswick, N.J.: Rutgers University Press, forthcoming.

Wandersman, A., and Florin, P. "Citizen Participation and Community Organizing." In J. Rappaport and E. Seidman (eds.), *Handbook of Community Psychology*. New York: Kluwer Academic/Plenum Publishers, 2000.

Wang, C., and Burris, M. A. "Photovoice: Concept, Methodology and Use for Participatory Assessment." *Health Education and Behavior*, June 1997, *24*(3), 369–387.

Wang, C., Cash, J., and Powers, L. "Who Knows the Streets as Well as the Homeless? Promoting Personal and Community Action Through Photovoice." *Health Promotion Practice*, January 2000, *1*(1), 81–89.

Warren, R. *The Community in America*. Chicago, Ill.: Rand McNally, 1963.

Wechsler, R. "Harnessing People Power: A Community-Based Approach to Preventing Alcohol and Drug Abuse." *Western City*, June 1990, 1–4.

Wechsler, R., and Minkler, M. "A Community-Oriented Approach to Health Promotion: The Tenderloin Senior Outreach Project." In K. Dychtwald (ed.), *Wellness and Health Promotion for the Elderly*. Rockville, Md.: Aspen Systems, 1986.

West, C. *Race Matters*. Boston: Beacon Press, 1993.

World Health Organization. Ottawa Charter for Health Promotion, 1986.

Wolff, T. "Coalition Building. Is This Really Empowerment?" Presentation to the annual meeting of the American Public Health Association. November 17, 1993.

Zimmerman, M. "Taking Aim on Empowerment Research: On the Distinction Between Individual and Psychological Conceptions." *American Journal of Community Psychology*, 1990, *18*, 169–177.

Zimmerman, M. "Empowerment Theory: Psychological, Organizational and Community Levels of Analysis." In E. S. Julian Rappaport (ed.), *Handbook of Community Psychology*. New York: Kluwer Academic/Plenum Publishers, 2000.

CHAPTER FOURTEEN

DIFFUSION OF INNOVATIONS

Brian Oldenburg
Guy S. Parcel

Although considerable effort and resources are devoted to developing and testing health behavior interventions, less attention is usually given to developing effective methods for their diffusion. Diffusion can maximize the exposure and reach of successful interventions, thus increasing their impact on public health. This chapter provides a conceptual framework for understanding the process of diffusion and its various stages, an overview of key methodological and research issues, and some applications of Diffusion Theory to the development and implementation of health behavior change innovations.

In the latest edition of his book, *Diffusion of Innovations,* Rogers notes that the literature on the topic of diffusion is broad and vast, representing almost four thousand publications on subjects ranging from agricultural research to research on contraceptives, consumer products, and modern math in schools and health promotion (Rogers, 1995). Nevertheless, many health behavior change innovations ultimately fail because of "the gap that is frequently left unfilled between the point where innovation-development ends and diffusion planning begins" (Orlandi, Landers, Weston, and Haley, 1990, p. 294). The assumption is often made that after an innovation is developed, and its efficacy and effectiveness demonstrated,

The authors wish to thank Nicola Burton for her contribution to the final manuscript.

widespread adoption and uptake will occur automatically. However, there is now ample evidence that even users' initial attempts at implementation do not typically lead to sustained use of an effective health education program, and that uptake by other users beyond this is typically even poorer.

Therefore, there is a need to focus on the broader public health impact of health behavior change interventions beyond the traditional emphasis on efficacy and effectiveness, and to plan for active dissemination of such innovations. Insufficient attention to program reach, adoption, implementation, and maintenance can lead to a waste of resources, discontinuity between phases of research, and failure to improve public health to the limits of our capacity (see Chapter Twenty-Four; Glasgow, Vogt, and Boles, 1999). For example, Lock and Kaner (2000) reported that of 614 eligible physicians offered the use of an effective screening and brief alcohol-intervention program, 52 percent took the program, and of those available to use it for three months, 41 percent actively considered doing so, but only 23 percent went on to use it, even for a short period of time.

Rates of initial program uptake, or adoption, implementation, and maintenance, can vary markedly as a result of the strategies used to disseminate the program actively and to train program adopters in its use. When an innovative Australian cardiovascular disease risk-reduction program called Fresh Start was actively disseminated to primary care physicians using workshops or education detailing, 80 percent of the physicians reported ongoing use of the program at twelve months, compared with only 42 percent of those physicians who had received the program in the mail (Salkeld, Phongsaven, and Oldenburg, 1996). The costs associated with different dissemination methods can also be quite different. Individual networking and detailing are very resource intensive, and these costs need to be evaluated against the differential results.

Even public health efforts that have been successfully implemented and diffused in the short term are not necessarily sustained over time. For example, the notable success of the United States with HIV risk-reduction programs during the first ten years of the AIDS epidemic was not maintained with all at-risk populations, and there has been limited diffusion to other population groups that practice HIV-risk behaviors (Kelly, Murphy, Silkema, and Kalichman, 1993). This has occurred despite implementation of the U.S. Centers for Disease Control and Prevention's HIV Prevention Community Planning program (Centers for Disease Control and Prevention, 1999) and support from relevant health department staff, representatives of affected communities, and staff and administrators from community-based organizations (DeGroff, 1996).

There are also examples of programs or "innovations" in which, despite limited evidence of both efficacy and effectiveness, the rates of spontaneous diffusion are very high. Rogers (1995) has noted that some drug abuse prevention programs may diffuse very widely for reasons that are largely unrelated to their proven effectiveness, and often before their effectiveness in reducing drug use has even been determined. In a retrospective analysis of the reasons for the rapid spread of the DARE Program and Project STAR during the 1980s—despite little evidence of effectiveness—Rogers (1995) identified a range of factors as being important influences. One key factor is that such programs often provide perceived solutions to a social problem that is a high political priority at a national or local level.

Description of Key Terms

Rogers (1983) defines an *innovation* as "an idea, practice or object that is perceived as new by an individual or other unit of adoption." *Diffusion* is defined as "the process by which an innovation is communicated through certain channels over time among the members of a social system," with the aim being to maximize the exposure and reach of innovations, strategies, or programs (Rogers, 1983). This process of diffusion typically involves five stages: innovation development, dissemination, adoption, implementation, and maintenance.

Innovation development includes "all the decisions and activities (and their impacts) that occur from the early stage of an idea through to its development and production" (Rogers, 1983). People from the user system should play a major role in identifying the relevant audiences, contributing to further development of the innovation and providing information and feedback on its content, design, and presentation. Promotional strategies and product design are also critical features of this stage. A social marketing framework can aid in further designing, targeting, refining, and implementing the innovation (see Chapter Nineteen). Other well-developed frameworks for designing theory- and evidence-based health behavior change programs include the PRECEDE/PROCEED Model (see Chapter Eighteen) and Intervention Mapping (Bartholomew, Parcel, Kok, and Gottlieb, 2001).

Dissemination is defined as "an active approach for knowledge transfer from the resource system to the user system" (Orlandi, Landers, Weston, and Haley, 1990). It involves the identification of communication channels and systems that are best used for the diffusion of an innovation to a given audience. For example, dissemination of a program for community-based cholesterol screening such as the Mount Vernon Cares Project described by Orlandi and associates may require use of both formal channels, such as public service announcements and press releases, and informal channels, such as community announcements at social and recreational events.

Adoption refers to the uptake of the program by the target audience, which requires moving through the stages of knowledge of the innovation, persuasion or attitude development, decision, implementation, and confirmation (Rogers, 1995). During adoption, several concerns require attention: the needs of the target adopters, their current attitudes and values, how they will respond to the innovation, what factors would increase the likelihood of adoption, how the potential adopters can be influenced to change their behavior and adopt a new one, what barriers exist to adoption of the innovation, and how these barriers can be overcome. The decision to adopt is influenced by three types of knowledge: *awareness knowledge* that the innovation exists, *procedural knowledge* about how to use the innovation, and *principles knowledge*, or understanding how the innovation works (Rogers, 1995).

Implementation refers to the initial use of the program in practice. A major focus here is on improving the self-efficacy and skills of adopters and encouraging a trial of the innovation. A *linkage agent* can play a key role in facilitating the smooth implementation of programs by providing training, troubleshooting problems that arise, and answering any questions (Orlandi, Landers, Weston, and Haley, 1990).

Maintenance refers to the ongoing implementation or continued use of the innovation in practice. Programs may be discontinued for many reasons. Health professionals therefore need to address reasons for termination—such as the lack of financial incentives for preventive medicine activities—and also encourage sustained use of the innovation. Bartholomew, Parcel, Kok, and Gottlieb (2001) describe this phase of diffusion as *sustainability* and make the distinction between *maintenance* and *institutionalization* as two different aspects of sustainability. Maintenance involves continued use, and institutionalization goes beyond this to involve incorporating the program into the routines of the organization.

Paulussen and others have examined these stages in the context of the diffusion of AIDS education curricula in schools in the Netherlands (Paulussen, Kok, and Schaalma, 1994). In their analysis, *dissemination* refers to the transfer of information about the innovation to potential users (the school teachers), *adoption* refers to the teachers' intentions to use the innovation (the curriculum), *implementation* refers to the actual use of the innovation, and the *continuation* or *maintenance* stage describes long-term use of the program.

Diffusion Theory and Practice

In the area of tobacco control, there are good examples of planned and organized program diffusion at a variety of levels—individual, organizational, and communitywide—and across multiple community settings. These efforts have contributed in turn to the significant decline in reported national rates of smoking in many developed countries over the past thirty years (Warner, 2000). Successful strategies have included smoking cessation programs for individuals in the community, programs to train health professionals to assist individuals to quit smoking, and programs involving smokefree policies in workplaces, restaurants, transport, and community recreational facilities. These efforts at diffusion have been further advanced by the increasing availability of nicotine replacement therapy and other pharmacological adjuncts.

Another example of diffusion at multiple levels and in a variety of settings is the uptake and adoption of safe sexual practices, including the use of condoms, in the general population (De Vroome, Paalman, Dingelstad, Kolker, and Sandfort, 1994), and the reduction of unsafe sex among gay men (Hospers and Kok, 1995). Examples of diffusion research in primary health care settings include identifying the predictors of adoption of a smoking cessation program (Cooke, Mattick, and Campbell, 1999) and an educational protocol to control pediatric asthma (Mesters and Meertens, 1999).

Rogers (1995) proposes that diffusion of innovations in organizations can be conceptualized as involving a particular application of the stages of diffusion, which include agenda setting, matching, redefining or restructuring, clarifying, and routinizing (see Table 14.1). Organizational-level application of diffusion is discussed in more detail in the context of organizational change strategies in Chapter Fifteen by Steckler, Goodman, and Kegler.

TABLE 14.1. STAGES OF DIFFUSION OF INNOVATIONS IN ORGANIZATIONS.

Stage	Description
Agenda setting	The agenda is triggered by (1) acknowledging organizational problems and prioritizing them for solution or (2) awareness of the existence of a certain innovation.
Matching	An innovation is selected to match an issue or problem and is tried out by the organization.
Redefining or restructuring	The organization molds the innovation to fit its objectives and structure.
Clarifying	The fit is formalized between organization and innovation.
Routinizing	The innovation is incorporated into organizational routine.

Planning for Diffusion: Innovation and Adopter Characteristics

Historically, the study of diffusion of innovations evolved from rural sociology, and some of the earliest applications included research directed at understanding how new agricultural techniques spread among farmers (Rogers, 1983). Since that time, Diffusion Theory, as it has been applied to health, has been used to study the uptake of a wide range of behaviors and programs including family planning, the use of new tests and technologies by health professionals, and the use of new pharmaceutical agents (Rogers, 1983, 1995).

Diffusion Theory derives from a body of research that has attempted to identify predictable patterns of program adoption and diffusion by a variety of population groups and across a broad range of innovations (Green, Gottlieb, and Parcel, 1987). Rogers (1983, 1995) has identified the attributes or characteristics of an innovation that are most likely to affect the speed and extent of the adoption and diffusion process (see Table 14.2). Given the importance of these characteristics, practitioners and researchers need to ensure that these features are considered and addressed at the *innovation development* stage and later communicated to potential adopters and users during dissemination.

Patterns of adoption can be described mathematically, and a number of key theoretical constructs have been identified as important through analyzing these patterns (Rogers, 1983; Green, Gottlieb, and Parcel, 1987). Rogers (1995) describes the process of adoption as a normal, bell-shaped distribution, with five adopter categories: innovators, early adopters, early majority adopters, late majority adopters, and laggards. Early and late majority adopters are within one standard deviation on either side of the mean or midpoint of the curve, adopters and laggards are two standard deviations away, and innovators are three standard deviations away. The identification of such adopter categories provides a basis for designing and implementing intervention strategies aimed at particular groups of individuals. The strategies can be based on the source of influence to which a particular group is most likely to respond. For example, Green, Gottlieb, and Parcel (1987) suggest that a cognitively oriented intervention may be most appropriate for early adopters, a motivational emphasis may be most effective for the majority adopters, and later adopters may require special efforts to overcome barriers.

Planning for Diffusion: Communication, Linkage, and Context

As Orlandi, Landers, Weston, and Haley (1990) have noted, "the adoption decision is only one step in a multi-step process that ranges from the first phases of innovation development to a point beyond adoption at which the innovation either

TABLE 14.2. ATTRIBUTES THAT ARE KEY DETERMINANTS OF DIFFUSION'S SPEED AND EXTENT.

Attribute	Key Question
Relative advantage	Is the innovation better than what it will replace?
Compatibility	Does the innovation fit with the intended audience?
Complexibility	Is the innovation easy to use?
Trialability	Can the innovation be tried before making a decision to adopt?
Observability	Are the results of the innovation observable and easily measurable?
Impact on social relations	Does the innovation have a disruptive effect on the social environment?
Reversibility	Can the innovation be reversed or discontinued easily?
Communicability	Can the innovation be understood clearly and easily?
Time	Can the innovation be adopted with a minimal investment in time?
Risk and uncertainty level	Can the innovation be adopted with minimal risk and uncertainty?
Commitment	Can the innovation be used effectively with only modest commitment?
Modifiability	Can the innovation be updated and modified over time?

succeeds or fails in achieving a lasting and meaningful impact" (p. 291). Recent examples of diffusing innovations through schools and other systems or settings illustrate this shift in focus from innovation attributes to adopter characteristics (Fullan, 1991; Rogers, 1995) to achieve the ideal fit between innovation and user. Maximizing this fit requires detailed consideration of the means used to communicate the innovation (*communication channels*), collaboration between the developers and users of a system (*linkage agents*), and the characteristics of the systems or environment in which this process takes place (*diffusion context*).

Effective diffusion involves the implementation of strategies through various settings and systems, using a variety of formal or informal media and communication channels, which can enhance the durability of an innovation and ensure its longer-term sustainability and institutionalization. Diffusion theorists view communication as a two-way process rather than as one of merely persuading an audience to take action. Communication is also seen as a product of both mass media and personal interactions. The *two-step flow of communication,* in which opinion leaders mediate the impact of mass media communications, emphasizes the value of social networks, or interpersonal channels, over and above mass media, for adoption decisions (Rogers, 1983).

Whereas program diffusion sometimes occurs in a passive and informal way, a more active, organized, and deliberate approach to program dissemination is recommended to improve uptake and ongoing use. A number of studies provide evidence to support the importance of inter-organizational collaboration and linkage agents to enhance the diffusion process (Monahan and Scheirer, 1988; Goodman, Steckler, and Kegler, 1996). This is a deliberate collaborative partnership between the group or individual promoting the program—the *resource system*—and the potential users of the program (the *user system*) (Orlandi, Landers, Weston, and Haley, 1990).

Recent research on understanding and improving rates of program adoption, implementation, and sustainability has looked at these same issues with respect to *program users*—such as school teachers—who are responsible for delivering health education and promotion programs to school students (Bartholomew, Parcel, Kok, and Gottlieb, 2001). Gatekeepers for delivery systems, such as school principals, can also be considered as important *program adopters,* because their support for the program may be critical to its adoption and implementation by teachers. In the school situation, the linkage might be a liaison group including representatives of the user system, representatives of the resource system, and a linkage agent facilitating the collaboration. Diffusion of the innovation may be carried out collectively by the members of the liaison group. The critical point is that the innovation-development and diffusion-planning processes should each improve the fit between the innovation and users to adapt innovations to practical possibilities and constraints and facilitate widespread implementation. It is very important to understand the environment or context in which the diffusion process occurs. This is because, in most organizations and systems where programs are being disseminated, the environment and social system are inevitably dynamic, unpredictable, and turbulent, rather than static and one-dimensional.

Diffusion as a Multilevel Change Process

Achieving satisfactory diffusion of an innovation to prevent disease and promote health involves a complex, multilevel change process (Parcel, Perry, and Taylor, 1990). The complexity arises from the need to consider change occurring at multiple levels, across many different settings, and resulting from the use of many different change strategies. At the level of the individual, family, or small group, uptake and implementation of a health behavior change innovation typically involves changes in lifestyle practices. At the organizational level, such as the workplace, school, or the health care setting, successful uptake of an innovation may require the introduction of particular programs or services, changes in policies or regulations, and changes in the roles and functions of particular personnel. At a broader communitywide or even societal level, such as in the area of tobacco control, the diffusion process can involve the use of the media, support from government policies and legislation, and coordination of a variety of other initiatives for individuals and groups. Most of the theories or models that have been used extensively to understand and describe change at an individual or small-group level, such as Social Cognitive Theory (see Chapter Eight) or the Theory of Planned Behavior (see Chapter Four), are also applicable to explaining the change and diffusion process at an organizational level (Parcel, Perry, and Taylor, 1990; Paulussen, Kok, and Schaalma, 1994). Other theories and models, including more ecological models and community organization theory, can also be useful.

Application of Diffusion of Innovations to Health Education

This section describes two applications of diffusion theory to health behavior change, illustrating the application of key constructs and of Diffusion Theory in both intervention research and explanatory research.

The CATCH Program

The Child and Adolescent Trial for Cardiovascular Health (CATCH) trial was a multisite, randomized, controlled field trial to assess the outcomes of health behavior interventions focusing on the elementary school environment, classroom curricula, and home programs for the primary prevention of cardiovascular disease. The CATCH intervention was able to modify the fat content of school lunches, increase moderate-to-vigorous physical activity in physical education classes, and improve eating and physical activity behaviors in children during third through fifth grades (Luepker and others, 1996). A follow-up study of the maintenance of improved diet and physical activity over a three-year period indicated that the behavioral changes initiated during the elementary school years persisted to early adolescence for self-reported diet and physical activity behaviors (Nader and others, 1999). Initial diffusion of the CATCH Program was conducted in the state of Texas. For more detailed information on the diffusion of CATCH, see Hoelscher and others (2002).

Planning for Diffusion: Innovation Characteristics.

Planning for Diffusion: Innovation Characteristics. Key innovation attributes were emphasized in the development of CATCH and the design and development of dissemination strategies. *Relative advantage* was demonstrated by emphasizing that CATCH had been designed using state-of-the-art intervention methods and strategies and that the program had demonstrated positive effects. The demonstrated effectiveness of CATCH was presented in dissemination material as an advantage over current practices or competing programs. *Compatibility* of the program with current practice was evidenced by the fact that in 1999, the Texas State Board of Education unanimously approved the CATCH materials for use as part of the school health curriculum under the Texas Education Code. CATCH physical education materials fit the state guidelines for physical activity, and the Eat Smart program was compatible with the USDA guidelines for school meal menus and recipes that were mandated through the School Meals Initiative.

The *complexity* of the program was minimized by developing CATCH curriculum and physical education materials that were designed to be "teacher friendly" and fun. The program was easy to adapt to different situations (outdoor versus indoor use), class sizes, or lesson length. CATCH curriculum lessons were formatted for easy use by teachers, with complete lesson instructions and script, copies of transparencies, and worksheet pages for the students.

Good *trialability* was indicated by the fact that CATCH materials were available during the dissemination phase as loaner copies of the CATCH package and through lessons and recipes available on the CATCH Web site. It was possible to show *observability* by illustrating the other attributes—relative advantage, compatibility, and complexity—through demonstration. Teachers and food service staff were able to observe CATCH activities through professional presentations around the state; through the recruitment, physical education, and foodservice training videotapes; and through the hands-on training sessions held throughout the state.

Planning for Diffusion: Adopter Characteristics.

Planning for Diffusion: Adopter Characteristics. Early adopters were identified and targeted through attendance at various professional conferences and through networking with national, state, and local decision makers. Generally, these innovators tended to be involved in local and state organizations, were better educated, and had leadership roles and the accompanying influence. Once these individuals were identified, relationships were formed and interpersonal and media channels employed. When possible, partnerships were formed with various organizations, including state health agencies, the state education agency, state and national organizations, and private health foundations. Because curriculum adoption decisions can be made at many levels within school districts, each level was targeted through CATCH promotional efforts. Regional and district administrators were reached through individual or professional meetings. Teachers were contacted through professional meetings and networks, as well as through training sessions.

Dissemination and Linkage Systems. The program was marketed as "A Coordinated Approach to Child Health" (CATCH), using the same acronym as the original trial but a name that did not signal a research focus or limit the intervention to cardiovascular disease. There was a national marketing effort conducted by the commercial publisher of the program, and the University of Texas School of Public Health conducted an intensive diffusion intervention study in Texas. The diffusion effort continued with increased involvement of the Texas Departments of Education and Health. A coalition of governmental agencies and health advocacy groups formed to support legislation to fund and support further expansion of efforts to encourage CATCH program adoption and implementation.

CATCH investigators partnered with the Texas Department of Health Diabetes Council to disseminate the program to Texas schools. As part of this partnership, CATCH staff conducted training sessions for schools that purchased the program materials. Statewide awareness and institutionalization of the program was further increased in 1999 when the Texas State Board of Education approved the CATCH materials as a diabetes education program that schools could use as part of their health curriculum under the Texas Education Code. A CATCH Web site was created that included samples of classroom lessons and school foodservice recipes. Investigators made presentations at state and national professional meetings to increase awareness of the program. A short video based on modeling methods and persuasive communication was made to recruit schools to adopt the program. Partnerships were also formed with a foundation in southwest Texas and the Child Nutrition Services of the Department of Education.

After two years of implementing the dissemination intervention, the program was adopted in Texas by 24 percent of elementary schools (728 out of 3,000), and reached about 435,000 school children. Over 900 school personnel at 578 schools have been trained to conduct CATCH. The majority of the people trained have been physical education teachers, with the physical education component most often the first implemented component of the program.

Communication Channels. Communication channels included both interpersonal networking between CATCH personnel and decision makers and media channels such as videos and print materials. Networking was the most time-intensive and costly component of the dissemination process, as it required one-on-one time with decision makers at all levels. Initially, networking occurred with directors of state health and education agencies; following that, individuals who dealt with schools, health education, physical education programs, chronic diseases, or nutrition were sought as appropriate partners. A systematic, sequential approach to reach one region at a time was more efficient than targeting the state as a whole. District administrators in large metropolitan school districts were contacted first, as these districts usually have more funding for health promotion and professional staff. Individuals were educated about the CATCH program and its results through a personal visit, a conference presentation or a group meeting, or a more informal meeting.

Other communication channels included recruitment and training videos, brochures detailing the benefits and outcomes of CATCH, personalized cover letters, and the CATCH Web site (sph.uth.tmc.edu/catch). The CATCH dissemination video proved to be an effective method to quickly convey the attributes of the program. The video used modeling to show successful implementation of the program, positive responses from the children, testimonials expressing the advantages of CATCH, and persuasive communication to make a case for expected outcomes and ease of implementation of the program.

Comments. Based on Diffusion Theory, this innovation was designed to address the factors that influence adoption, including the attributes of the innovation, characteristics of the adopter, and channels of communication. This application demonstrates the importance of networking and developing partnerships to develop and implement good *linkage systems*. The use of multiple channels for communications (including brochures, presentations, video, Web site) was very important to the intervention. Because the complexity of the CATCH program was a potential barrier to adoption, dissemination focused on individual program components such as physical education and food service. The classroom curriculum was more difficult to disseminate because it is more complex and time consuming, and competes with other priorities for limited instructional time. The experience with CATCH has shown that it is possible to disseminate a multicomponent, multiyear coordinated school health program in a large, diverse state. More work is needed to determine which factors significantly affect the diffusion process, how implementation and institutionalization can be enhanced, and whether the impact of the program that was found in the efficacy trial is achieved through the diffusion process.

The Australian National Workplace Health Project

The Australian National Workplace Health Project (NWHP) aimed to identify effective ways of promoting health at work and of preventing chronic diseases such as cancer and cardiovascular disease, through environmental and sociobehavioral intervention strategies (Simpson and others, 2000). The health behaviors on which the NWHP focused were physical activity, fruit and vegetable and fat consumption, alcohol consumption, and smoking. The intervention strategies built on strategies that had been previously evaluated in efficacy and effectiveness studies conducted with other work organizations, especially with emergency service workers (Gomel, Oldenburg, Simpson, and Owen, 1993; Gomel, Oldenburg, Simpson, Chilvers, and Owen, 1997). In the NWHP, twenty worksites were randomized into four groups using a two-by-two factorial design, with the two factors being socio-behavioral interventions and environmental interventions (Simpson and others, 2000). The environmental intervention component aimed to facilitate health behavior change by promoting high rates of program implementation, uptake, and sustainability in each intervention worksite. At those worksites that received the environmental and sociobehavioral intervention strategies, the environmental strategies were designed to facilitate dissemination and uptake of the socio-behavioral intervention strategies.

Diffusion Context. The NWHP was implemented in twenty predominantly blue-collar worksites, with a total of about 3,500 employees. These included four coal mines, eight mail and postal sorting centers, and eight workplaces responsible for the organization and supply of electrical power. Each of these three types of work organizations was quite different. The mail and postal sorting centers were large public sector worksites with a relatively high proportion of employees from non-English-speaking backgrounds. The four coal mines were privately owned and employed personnel who typically lived in less urban and more remote communities.

Multilevel Change Process. Three key levels of the workplace were targeted for change—the physical environment, the information environment, and the policy environment. Examples of change at the level of the physical environment to encourage healthy eating included the placing of posters at strategic points around the workplace and adding low-fat, high-fiber food choices to vending machines. Change at the level of the information environment to promote healthy eating included point-of-purchase messages about healthy food choices and take-home messages for health lunch tips in employees' pay slips. Change at the policy level to promote healthy eating involved reviewing existing policies relating to employee health and then incorporating specific statements about providing access to healthy food choices.

Planning for Durability and Diffusion. As a precursor to facilitating good, long-term diffusion within each work organization, five steps were used for innovation development and to gain access, support, and commitment within each work organization (Harris, Oldenburg, and Owen, 1999; see Table 14.3). Key employees from each work organization also played an important role in systematically addressing each of the steps outlined in Table 14.3.

TABLE 14.3. INNOVATION DEVELOPMENT STRATEGIES OF THE NWHP.

Initial Access	Support	Commitment
Making initial contact • Telephone contact with managers • Letter of invitation	Making presentations at management and supervisor meetings • Tailoring and benefits emphasized	Presenting consistent messages • Written and rehearsed scripts for project team
Holding the first meeting • Program director and liaisons in attendance • Draft proposal and potential benefits presented	Establishing worksite task groups • Assist with planning; role models • Representatives from management, unions, OHS, and work groups	Using multiple entry points • Every worker entitled to participate at any time
Gaining approval • Draft proposal to gain "in principle" approval • Formal presentation to executive and OHS management groups	Identifying key contacts at worksites • Make liaisons, arrange events, encourage participation, provide feedback • Identify position of influence such as manager	Timing program delivery • Aimed to maximize participation, fit with work schedules, and encourage staff acceptance
Creating the draft agreement • Made between university and organization • Outlined services to be received, costs, support, permission for participation		Locating activities • Held onsite for least work disruption and maximum exposure and publicity • Created challenges such as privacy
Establishing maintenance • CEO to be kept informed • Senior-level steering committee to participate in program design, planning, and problem solving		Consulting • Written workforce survey to assess health concerns, program preferences • Ongoing communication via quarterly newsletters

Source: Adapted from Harris, Oldenburg, and Owen, 1999.

To influence the program adopters and program delivery system in each organization, strategies were developed to gain and maintain ongoing access to the workplace. The program coordinator needed to gain access so that he could interact freely with employees. The degree to which access was achieved and maintained within an organization was likely to determine the quantity and quality of contact between the program coordinator and the workforce, which would have an impact, in due course, on program diffusion. The point of initial access was primarily senior-level management, although the initial entry point for contact with this group often occurred through occupational health or human resource channels.

To gain support for the program within each organization, the NWHP employed the strategy of identifying workplace *gatekeepers*. Gatekeepers were identified by the program coordinator and included line managers, supervisors, union and occupational health and safety (OHS) representatives, and significant spokespersons for key work groups. Direct support from line managers was important because, although senior management could provide access at an organizational level, the line managers generally determined the amount and quality of access to the workforce on a unit-specific basis. The health program was sometimes viewed as a threat to productivity that could, in turn, reflect poorly on the line managers' and supervisors' effectiveness. For this reason, the NWHP coordinator needed to develop a good working knowledge of the nature of the work and the responsibilities of the line managers and supervisors before interacting with them and their staff.

Several strategies were implemented to develop and win the commitment of employees. The coordinator's main role was to help the project team win the trust and endorsement of the workforce for the program, and, eventually, to have the workforce assume ownership of the program. It is usually very challenging and time-consuming to achieve and sustain such commitment in the long term. For example, many workplace health promotion programs commenced with a "kick-off" event and reported good-to-excellent participation rates. However, it is rare for high participation to be sustained in later stages of the program. The environmental interventions were implemented by task groups that met once a month at each worksite. Their meetings were facilitated by an NWHP employee.

Program Dissemination. Measures of program adoption, implementation, maintenance, and diffusion of various program components were tracked throughout the program. Logbook records indicated satisfactory adoption and implementation of all components of the environmental intervention in each worksite, with, on average, 80 percent of the environmental intervention components being implemented across all worksites by the task groups themselves (range equals 71 to 88 percent). However, for the worksites that received both the sociobehavioral *and* environmental interventions, rates were higher than for the environmental intervention-only worksites. Good rates of employee recall were recorded for most of the environmental intervention strategies, with the most recalled components being posters and policy information for each of the four health-related behaviors. After twenty-four months, recall of each of the intervention components among all employees in the intervention worksites was significantly greater than for control worksites (73 versus 50 percent of employees). Moreover, changes in recall rates from twelve to twenty-four months reflected the chronological order in which the various components were put in place. Also, there were significant changes in the physical, policy, and information environments between the intervention and control worksites, as measured by environmental audits.

Comments. Most published evaluations of workplace health promotion provide little information regarding the formative stages of program development, how organizational linkages were formed and developed, and how the established relationships affected subsequent program implementation and diffusion. The stage of *innovation development* is a key determinant of implementation and dissemination of the innovation, as are the linkages that are formed during this phase between the *resource system* and *user system*. Linkages are particularly important given the potential of workplaces as organized systems for diffusion. This includes the steps involved in negotiating and recruiting worksites to participate and in establishing support and *communication channels* within the worksites prior to the implementation of the program intervention. Planning for long-term maintenance, sustainability, and institutionalization of worksite health programs, or what Bracht, Thompson, and Winner (1996) have called *durability*, should be a key ingredient in all stages of the planning process (Sorensen and others, 1998; Patterson and others, 1998). The experience with NWHP has shown that it is possible to disseminate a multicomponent, coordinated workplace health program in a variety of blue collar worksites. Environmental change strategies can be used to support and complement more traditional sociobehavioral methods. More work is needed to determine which factors significantly affect this process, and how implementation and institutionalization can be enhanced.

Future Directions and Challenges for Research and Practice

Diffusion as Both a Passive and an Active Process

While many innovations, particularly those in health behavior change interventions, have a substantial product component, most complex innovations for promoting health also consist of procedures, regulations, and practice. This is why many of the concepts from marketing, particularly social marketing, have been applied usefully to disseminating innovations. A major challenge for both practitioners and researchers is to identify ways to activate the change process at a personal, organizational, or communitywide level, rather than rely solely on passive diffusion.

Recent applications of Diffusion Theory demonstrate the importance of using relevant theories in large-scale efforts to reduce communitywide death and disability. For example, Howze and Redman (1992) reported that in one statewide coalition, the Health Promotion and Education Council of Virginia, diffusion of innovations and other social science theories were applied through legislative action, work with opinion leaders, the creation of information-exchange relationships, and the use of advocacy to increase the impact of effective health promotion practice. Well-organized large-scale communitywide programs for diffusion of programs across multiple levels will become more common as the emphasis on linking health promotion strategies and interventions to improve population health outcomes increases in many developed countries. As Sorensen, Emmons, Hunt, and Johnston (1998) note, widespread and multilevel diffusion is the means by which small changes at the individual level may result in large benefits at the population level.

Determinants of Diffusion Across Settings

With an increasing focus on the importance of socioenvironmental and ecological factors as determinants of rates of diffusion and of adoption, implementation, and maintenance, it will be important to better understand whether the determinants of diffusion are specific to particular settings. Determinants of health curriculum adoption, implementation, and maintenance in schools may be unique to formal educational environments. The extent to which other determinants identified from school settings are relevant in other settings has not yet been well researched (Smith, Steckler, McCormick, and McLeroy, 1995). For example, the unpredictability of the diffusion context, sometimes called environmental turbulence, has been identified as a very important influence for dissemination within the school environment (Smith, Steckler, McCormick, and McLeroy, 1995) and may also be important in other settings, such as workplace organizations.

Studies have clearly identified factors necessary for increasing the uptake and maintenance of preventive medicine practice by physicians. Elford, Jennett, Bell, Szafran, and Meadows (1994) have called the key set of factors a "sustaining office system in prevention," with the key components being (1) a practice coordinator for prevention, (2) clear, clinical prevention-related job descriptions, (3) an information-management system that reinforces prevention, and (4) a practice feedback and problem-solving strategy. More generally, health care systems throughout the world are recognizing the challenge of how best to improve the linkages between the science and practice of medicine (Dunn, Norton, Stewart, Tudiver, and

Bass, 1994). Moulding, Silagy, and Weller (1999) have used a range of key concepts from social and behavioral sciences to develop a conceptual framework for effective management of change in clinical practice, including the improved dissemination and implementation of clinical practice guidelines.

The Evidence Base for Diffusion and Dissemination

Diffusion research has not kept up with the demand by practitioners and policymakers. For example, an audit of thirteen leading public health and health promotion journals published during the year 1994 found that few published empirical papers at that time were pertinent to the stages of research beyond descriptive, methods development or intervention studies (Oldenburg, Sallis, French, and Owen, 1999; Oldenburg, French, and Sallis, 2000). A follow-up review of these same journals indicated that between 1994 and 1999–2000 there has been a negligible increase in diffusion studies. Similarly, a thematic analysis of editorials and content analysis of all the articles in three leading health education journals from 1989 to 1994 (*Health Education Research: Theory and Practice, Health Education Quarterly,* and *Health Promotion International*) concluded that dissemination studies were underrepresented in spite of being regularly identified in the editorials as a very important priority for professionals (Rychetnik, Nutbeam, and Hawe, 1997). This deficit of evidence is problematic for effective practice. However, as Sorensen and others (1998) have noted, dissemination research is typically asking different questions than efficacy or effectiveness research, and consequently requires different research designs and measurement systems.

Economic evaluation of different dissemination strategies and methods are also needed. This type of evaluation can yield valuable information to help further develop strategies to enhance the likelihood of diffusion. For example, when the various strategies used to disseminate the Fresh Start cardiovascular disease risk-reduction program were subjected to an economic evaluation, the workshop method was shown to be the most expensive, as it involved more of the physician's time for travel and participation than did educational detailing, which took place in the physician's office (Salkeld, Phongsavan, and Oldenburg, 1996; Salkeld and others, 1997).

A System-Wide Approach to Dissemination and Diffusion

Jonathan Lomas (1993) has been writing for many years about the ways in which information flows from a source, how such information is received by individuals and organizations and becomes knowledge, and how that in turn influences individuals and organizations to change their behavior. These issues have been studied

extensively in relation to the behavior of physicians and other health professionals, to identify the conditions under which research findings are most likely to be
implemented into practice (Dunn, Norton, Stewart, Tudiver, and Bass, 1994). As
applied to the behavior of physicians, the concepts of diffusion, dissemination,
and implementation are distinguishable as progressively more-active steps in the
process of translating valid and reliable research findings into routine clinical practice (Dunn, Norton, Stewart, Tudiver, and Bass, 1994).

For example, in an adapted stage model of behavioral change by Lomas
(1993), diffusion is seen as a precursor for subsequent dissemination activities,
which in turn predispose physicians to consider change in their practices. However, diffusion methods, including journal publications, really only affect the most
highly motivated health professionals, though such low-intensity messages might
still generate changes in awareness, attitudes, and knowledge as precursors to subsequent behavior change. More-active dissemination activities include the development of practice guidelines, consensus statements, and other forms of tailored
information. Local implementation activities capitalize on these earlier stages by
enabling and subsequently reinforcing the desired behavior change in health care
practice. These activities generally include a combination of academic detailing,
audit and feedback, strategic use of opinion leaders, patient-mediated intervention, decision-support systems, and many others. Different skills and tools are
clearly required for each of these stages. From the work of Lomas and others who
have been at the forefront of developments related to the burgeoning field of
evidence-based medicine—defined by Sackett, Straus, Richardson, Rosenberg,
and Haynes (2000) as the "integration of best research evidence with clinical expertise and patient values"—medical journals are identified as diffusion agents;
collaboration between researchers, academics, and medical organizations is best
suited to the dissemination stage; and local organizations, with appropriate resources, are best equipped for implementation activities. The development and
elaboration of such systems to improve the uptake of research findings into routine clinical practice have drawn heavily from the "social influences" literature,
studies of the diffusion of innovations, adult learning theory, marketing theory,
and, more recently, models of technology diffusion (Geroski, 2000).

At the core of this relatively new field of evidence-based medicine is an improved understanding of how new knowledge and research findings can be translated better into improved clinical practice, as it is now well-documented that the
availability of research findings does not in itself guarantee good, effective practice in the field. Given that the gap between knowledge generation and knowledge
use in the fields of public health and health education is just as problematic, if not
more so, there is much to be gained by applying what has been learned from the
field of evidence-based medicine to the diffusion and dissemination of those health

behavior interventions that can lead to very significant improvements in health at a population level.

For this to occur, a coordinated and strategic systemwide effort is required. This type of effort would identify the current and preferred dissemination practices and linkage systems between those groups of individuals who are involved in the research system and those who are responsible for implementation as practitioners, managers, or policymakers.

As with biomedical or clinical innovations, the effective dissemination of health behavior and public health interventions is also influenced by the level of interest generated by new programs, the attributes of the innovation, and the capacity for their widespread implementation. However, the nature of the public health, health education, and health behavior evidence base and the complex nature of its practice also need to be considered, because there are many barriers and obstacles (Rimer, Glanz, and Rasband, 2001). A key component of such a multistrategy approach to dissemination is a specific focus on the linkages between research and practice systems to identify potential dissemination failure points, as well as strategies for preventing or overcoming these barriers.

Conclusion

An improved understanding of how new programs, strategies, practices, or innovations are spread is critical to maximize the population impact of health behavior change programs. Given that documented successful diffusion is more the exception than the rule, there is a great need for more diffusion research in health behavior and health education. This research requires innovative approaches to study design and measurement, despite the challenges posed by using rigorous research designs on a large scale. Also, measurement can be intrusive and reactive, and control over contextual factors is often poor. Moreover, such intervention studies are by their very nature large and often costly, and take a number of years to complete.

Most important though, at the practice level, the planning of health behavior change programs should also incorporate a systematic approach to planning for program adoption, implementation, and sustainability. This planning should be an integral part of the original innovation development rather than a process that is only thought about when one is ready to disseminate the program or innovation.

Finally, diffusion is not just an important concept to those in the health field. Rather, it is of interest to the whole of society, because at any point in time there are many different products, messages, or ideas that individuals and groups want to see advanced and widely disseminated. An understanding of how some products, ideas, and ways of behaving suddenly cross a threshold or "tipping point" and take off is an important idea that can be applied to the health field as well as to other domains (Gladwell, 2000).

References

Bartholomew, L. K., Parcel, G. S., Kok, G., and Gottlieb, N. H. *Intervention Mapping: Designing Theory and Evidence-Based Health Promotion Programs.* Mountain View, Calif.: Mayfield, 2001.

Bracht, N., Thompson, B., and Winner, C. *Planning for Durability: Keeping the Vision Alive.* Rockville, Md.: Prospect Associates, 1996.

Centers for Disease Control and Prevention. *HIV Prevention Community Planning: Shared Decision Making in Action.* Atlanta: Centers for Disease Control and Prevention, 1999.

Cooke, M., Mattick, R. P., and Campbell, E. "The Dissemination of a Smoking Cessation Program to 23 Antenatal Clinics: The Predictors of Initial Program Adoption by Managers." *Australian and New Zealand Journal of Public Health,* 1999, *23,* 99–103.

DeGroff, A. "Is Prevention Research Reaching Front-Line Prevention Programs? A Descriptive Study from San Francisco." Presented at the Eleventh International Conference on AIDS, Vancouver, B.C., 1996.

De Vroome, E. M., Paalman, M. E., Dingelstad, A. A., Kolker, L., and Sandfort, T. G. "Increase in Safe Sex Among the Young and Non-Monogamous: Knowledge, Attitudes and Behavior Regarding Safe Sex and Condom Use in The Netherlands from 1987 to 1993." *Patient Education and Counseling,* 1994, *24,* 179–288.

Dunn, E. V., Norton, P. G., Stewart, M., Tudiver, F., and Bass, M. (eds.). *Disseminating Research/Changing Practice.* London: Sage, 1994.

Elford, R. W., Jennett, P., Bell, N., Szafran, O., and Meadows, L. "Putting Prevention into Practice." *Health Reports,* 1994, *6,* 142–153.

Fullan, M. G. *The New Meaning of Educational Change.* New York: Teachers College Press, 1991.

Geroski, P. A. "Models of Technology Diffusion." *Research Policy,* 2000, *29,* 603–625.

Gladwell, M. *The Tipping Point: How Little Things Can Make a Big Difference.* London: Little, Brown, 2000.

Glasgow, R. E., Vogt, T. M., and Boles, S. M. "Evaluating the Public Health Impact of Health Promotion Interventions: The RE-AIM Framework." *American Journal of Public Health,* 1999, *89,* 1322–1327.

Gomel, M. K., Oldenburg, B., Simpson, J. M., Chilvers, M., and Owen, N. "Composite Cardiovascular Risk Outcomes of a Work-Site Intervention Trial." *American Journal of Public Health,* 1997, *87,* 673–676.

Gomel, M., Oldenburg, B., Simpson, J., and Owen, N. "Worksite Cardiovascular Risk Reduction: Randomized Trial of Health Risk Assessment, Risk Factor Education, Behavioral Counseling and Incentive Strategies." *American Journal of Public Health,* 1993, *83,* 1231–1238.

Goodman, R. M., Steckler, A., and Kegler, M. C. "Mobilizing Organizations for Health Enhancement: Theories of Organizational Change." In K. Glanz, F. M. Lewis, and B. K. Rimer (eds.), *Health Behavior and Health Education: Theory, Research, and Practice.* (2nd ed.) San Francisco: Jossey-Bass, 1996.

Green, L. W., Gottlieb, N., and Parcel, G. "Diffusion Theory Extended and Applied." In W. B. Ward (ed.), *Advances in Health Education and Promotion.* Greenwich, Conn.: JAI, 1987.

Harris, D., Oldenburg, B., and Owen, N. "Australian National Workplace Health Project: Strategies for Gaining Access, Support, and Commitment." *Health Promotion Journal of Australia,* 1999, *9,* 49–54.

Hoelscher, D. M., Kelder, S. H., Murray, N., Cribb, P. W., Conroy, J., and Parcel, G. "Dissemination and Adoption of the Child and Adolescent Trial for Cardiovascular Health (CATCH): A Case Study in Texas." *Journal of Public Health Management and Practice,* 2002.

Hospers, H. J., and Kok, G. "Determinants of Safe and Risk-Taking Sexual Behavior Among Gay Men: A Review." *AIDS Education and Prevention,* 1995, *7,* 74–96.

Howze, E. H., and Redman, L. J. "The Uses of Theory in Health Advocacy: Policies and Programs." *Health Education Quarterly,* 1992, *19,* 369–383.

Kelly, J. A., Murphy, D. A., Silkema, K. J., and Kalichman, S. C. "Psychological Interventions to Prevent HIV Infection Are Urgently Needed." *American Psychologist,* 1993, *48,* 1023–1034.

Lock, C. A., and Kaner, E.F.S. "Use of Marketing to Disseminate Brief Alcohol Intervention to General Practitioners: Promoting Health Care Interventions to Health Promoters." *Journal of Evaluation in Clinical Practice,* 2000, *6,* 345–357.

Lomas, J. "Diffusion, Dissemination, and Implementation: Who Should Do What?" *Annals of New York Academy of Sciences,* 1993, *703,* 226–235.

Luepker, R. V., and others for the CATCH Collaborative Group. "Outcomes of a Field Trial to Improve Children's Dietary Patterns and Physical Activity: The Child and Adolescent Trial for Cardiovascular Health (CATCH)." *Journal of the American Medical Association,* 1996, *275,* 768–776.

Mesters, I., and Meertens, R. M. "Monitoring the Dissemination of an Educational Protocol on Pediatric Asthma in Family Practice: A Test of Associations Between Dissemination Variables." *Health Education and Behavior,* 1999, *26,* 103–120.

Monahan, J. I., and Scheirer, M. A. "The Role of Linking Agents in the Diffusion of Health Promotion Programs." *Health Education Quarterly,* 1988, *15,* 417–433.

Moulding, N. T., Silagy, C. A., and Weller, D. P. "A Framework for Effective Management of Change in Clinical Practice: Dissemination and Implementation of Clinical Practice Guidelines." *Quality in Health Care,* 1999, *8,* 177–183.

Nader, P. R., and others. "Three-Year Maintenance of Improved Diet and Physical Activity: The CATCH Cohort." *Archives of Pediatrics and Adolescent Medicine,* 1999, *153,* 695–704.

Oldenburg, B., French, M. L., and Sallis, J. F. "Health Behavior Research: The Quality of the Evidence Base." *American Journal of Health Promotion,* 2000, *14,* 253–257.

Oldenburg, B., Sallis, J., French, M., and Owen, N. "Health Promotion Research and the Diffusion and Institutionalization of Interventions." *Health Education Research,* 1999, *14,* 121–130.

Orlandi, M. A., Landers, C., Weston, R., and Haley, N. "Diffusion of Health Promotion Innovations." In K. Glanz, F. M. Lewis, and B. K. Rimer (eds.), *Health Behavior and Health Education: Theory, Research, and Practice.* San Francisco: Jossey-Bass, 1990.

Parcel, G. S., Perry, C. L., and Taylor, W. C. "Beyond Demonstration: Diffusion of Health Promotion Innovations." In Bracht, N. (ed.), *Health Promotion at the Community Level.* Thousand Oaks, Calif.: Sage, 1990.

Patterson, R. E., and others. "Durability and Diffusion of the Nutrition Intervention in the Working Well Trial." *Preventive Medicine,* 1998, *27,* 668–673.

Paulussen, T. G., Kok, G., and Schaalma, H. P. "Antecedents to Adoption of Classroom-Based AIDS Education in Secondary Schools." *Health Education Research,* 1994, *9,* 485–496.

Rimer, B. K., Glanz, K., and Rasband, G. "Searching for Evidence About Health Education and Health Behavior Interventions." *Health Education and Behavior,* 2001, *28,* 231–248.

Rogers, E. M. *Diffusion of Innovations.* New York: Free Press, 1983.

Rogers, E. M. *Diffusion of Innovations.* (4th ed.) New York: Free Press, 1995.

Rychetnik, L., Nutbeam, D., and Hawe, P. "Lessons from a Review of Publications in Three Health Promotion Journals from 1989 to 1994." *Health Education Research,* 1997, *12,* 491–504.

Sackett, D. L., Straus, S. E., Richardson, W. S., Rosenberg, W., and Haynes, R. B. *Evidence-Based Medicine: How to Practice and Teach EBM.* New York: Churchill Livingston, 2000.

Salkeld, G., Phongsavan, P. H., and Oldenburg, B. "Getting Your Message Across to GPs, Efficiently." *Health Promotion Journal of Australia,* 1996, *6,* 8–13.

Salkeld, G., and others. "The Cost-Effectiveness of a Cardiovascular Risk Reduction Program in General Practice." *Health Policy,* 1997, *41,* 105–119.

Simpson, J., and others. "The Australian National Workplace Health Project: Design and Baseline Findings." *Preventive Medicine,* 2000, *31,* 249–260.

Smith, D., Steckler, A., McCormick, L., and McLeroy, K. "Lessons Learned About Disseminating Health Curricula to Schools." *Journal of Health Education,* 1995, *26,* 37–43.

Sorensen, G., Emmons, K., Hunt, M. K., and Johnston, D. "Implications of the Results of Community Intervention Trials." *Annual Review of Public Health,* 1998, *19,* 379–416.

Sorensen, G., and others. "Durability, Dissemination, and Institutionalisation of Worksite Tobacco Control Programs: Results from the Working Well Trial." *International Journal of Epidemiology,* 1998, *5,* 335–351.

Warner, K. "The Need for, and Value of, a Multi-Level Approach to Disease Prevention: The Case of Tobacco Control." In B. D. Smedley and S. L. Syme (eds.), *Promoting Health: Intervention Strategies from Social and Behavioral Research.* Washington, D.C.: National Academy Press, 2000.

CHAPTER FIFTEEN

MOBILIZING ORGANIZATIONS FOR HEALTH ENHANCEMENT

Theories of Organizational Change

Allan Steckler
Robert M. Goodman
Michelle Crozier Kegler

Organizational change is important to health promotion researchers and practitioners for several reasons: (1) often, new health promotion programs are created and implemented within organizations—for example, a worksite physical fitness program for employees; (2) frequently, organizations adopt and implement new health promotion policies—for example, a school policy banning smoking on its campus; (3) usually, health promotion practitioners work within organizations that must change and adapt for the practitioner to be able to create and implement new programs, services, and policies; and, (4) increasingly, health promoting organizations collaborate with other organizations in their communities to reach goals no single organization can accomplish alone. In all of these instances, the practitioner who understands the theories and principles of organizational change, and who has tools and skills for analyzing and facilitating such change, is likely to be more successful than his or her counterpart who does not possess such knowledge and proficiencies.

Organizational theory is like a Chinese box puzzle. When the key is found and the box unlocked, another box is revealed within that requires a different key. In the smaller box is another box, and another still, each requiring a separate key. Organizational theory, like the box puzzle, can be penetrated on many levels.

Organizations are layered. Their strata range from the surrounding environment at the broadest level to the overall organizational structure to the management within to work groups to each individual member. Change may be influenced at each of these strata (Kaluzny and Hernandez, 1988), and health promotion strategies that are directed at several levels simultaneously may be most durable in producing the desired results (McLeroy, Bibeau, Steckler, and Glanz, 1988). The practitioner who understands the ecology of organizations and who can apply appropriate strategies has powerful tools for stimulating change.

In a similar vein, public health organizations exist in a larger social environment, or social ecology. In the past decade, the social ecology perspective gained currency as a framework for community-based public health. The social ecology framework holds that individual, interpersonal, community (including cultural, social, and economic factors), organizational, and governmental factors influence health directly and through individual behavior (Israel, Checkoway, Schulz, and Zimmerman, 1994; McLeroy, Bibeau, Steckler, and Glanz, 1988). That is, individual lifestyle choices and behaviors are more likely to be health promoting when social ecology factors are taken into account, because such factors have a direct influence on lifestyle and behavior choices. As Stokols, Allen, and Bellingham (1996) write, the "interdependencies between socioeconomic, cultural, political, environmental, organizational, psychological, and biological determinants of health and illness" (p. 247) are addressed by ecologically informed programs. They envision the shift to comprehensive ecological formulations as a needed transformation for program implementation, because pockets of ill health persist in communities when interventions are limited in scope.

Increasingly, public health organizations use ecological frameworks to guide the development of their activities. Interventions that are informed by this perspective are directed mainly at social factors such as community norms and the structure of community services, including their comprehensiveness, coordination, and linkages, in addition to individual motivations and attitudes (Israel, Checkoway, Schulz, and Zimmerman, 1994; McLeroy, Bibeau, Steckler, and Glanz, 1988).

In this chapter, we analyze three theories of organizational change: Stage Theory, Organizational Development Theory, and Interorganizational Relations Theory. These theories were selected for several reasons. First, they illustrate how theory can be directed at different organizational levels. Second, they suggest specific intervention strategies. Thus, the practitioner can translate these theories into prescriptions for action. Third, the strategies that extend from these theories are directed at levels of the organization at which health promotion may be most influential. Fourth, the strategies can be used simultaneously, thus creating synergistic results.

Two cases are presented in this chapter to illustrate how the theories may be used together and at the different organizational strata. Before the cases are presented, the origins and elements of each theory are described.

Stage Theory of Organizational Change

Stage Theory of Organizational Change explains how organizations innovate new goals, programs, technologies, and ideas (Kaluzny and Hernandez, 1988; it is not related to Prochaska and DiClemente's Stages of Change [1983]; see also Chapter Five). Stage Theory is a type of "contingency" theory, so categorized because organizational approaches are contingent on socioenvironmental factors, some of which are outside the organization's control. Furthermore, as organizations innovate, they pass through a series of organizational steps or stages. Each stage requires a unique set of strategies if the innovation is to grow and to mature. Strategies that are effective at one stage may be misapplied at the next, thereby disabling the innovation. Thus, the most effective strategies are contingent upon the organization's stage of change in adopting, implementing, and sustaining new approaches. Therefore, the skillful application of Stage Theory requires an accurate assessment of the nature of the social environment, an assessment of an innovation's current stage of development, and the selection of strategies that are appropriate for each stage.

History

Stage Theory emerges from two research traditions. The first extends from the work of Lewin, who developed one of the earliest stage models (Lewin, 1951). Lewin's model, which emphasizes factors resisting change efforts, has three stages. (1) unfreezing of past behavior and attitudes; (2) moving by exposure to new information, attitudes, and theories; and (3) refreezing through processes of reinforcement, confirmation, and support for the change.

The second influence on the development of Stage Theory is Diffusion Theory (See Chapter Fourteen). In the 1950s, Diffusion Theory focused on how individuals such as farmers, teachers, and physicians adopted innovations (Rogers, 1983). In the 1960s, innovation theorists realized that individuals often adopt innovations as members of organizations, and that such individuals seldom adopt an innovation until it is first accepted by the organization.

Modern Stage Theory

Beyer and Trice (1978) have developed a comprehensive, well-defined, and contemporary model of Stage Theory that consists of seven stages:

1. *Sensing of unsatisfied demands on the system.* Some part of the system receives information indicating a problem or potential problem.

2. *Search for possible responses.* Elements in the system try to find alternative solutions.

3. *Evaluation of alternatives.* The various alternatives are compared.

4. *Decision to adopt a course of action.* An alternative is chosen from among those evaluated. Operative goals and means are specified; that is, a strategy is adopted.

5. *Initiation of action within the system.* A policy or other directive for implementing the change is formulated. Resources necessary for implementation are acquired.

6. *Implementation of the change.* Resources are allocated for implementation. The innovation is carried out.

7. *Institutionalization of the change.* The innovation becomes part of routine organizational operations.

How Stage Theory Operates

How innovations "move" from one stage to the next is still an open question. Most studies measure the dynamics within stages, but only a few suggest what mechanisms might lead from one stage to the next (Steckler and others, 1992).

In their study of innovations in schools, Huberman and Miles (1984) demonstrated that different actors play leading roles at different innovation stages: senior-level administrators are important at the problem definition and early adoption stages; mid-level administrators, such as curriculum coordinators and principals, are important actors at the adoption and early implementation stages; teachers are instrumental at the implementation stage; and senior-level administrators once again play a key role at the institutionalization stage. This example illustrates that strategies which organizations apply are contingent on the innovation's stage of change and on the social environment surrounding the innovation. For instance, schools may take different approaches within any stage depending on such factors as the level of involvement in the schools of parent organizations, churches, or other local organizations concerned with education (Smith, Steckler, McCormick, and McLeroy, 1995).

Future Challenges

Stage Theory holds promise for guiding the practitioner's efforts to nurture health promotion programs, but more precise specification of the number of stages within the model is desirable. Currently, the number of stages varies depending on which model is employed. Better definition of the stages will lead to greater precision of strategies for each stage.

Second, the completeness of stage models has been questioned. To date no models extend beyond institutionalization. Yet evidence indicates that beyond institutionalization is renewal, a stage during which well-established programs evolve to meet changing demands (Goodman and Steckler, 1989).

Third, those factors known to enable a program's development at each stage should be expanded to include contingencies in the social ecology. As additional ecological factors are identified as important at each developmental stage, both researchers and practitioners will find a greater array of strategies for enhancing program development.

Fourth, not all programs go through all stages, and others may advance from one stage to the next, only to reverse course. A better understanding of when and why stages may be bypassed or reversed will increase precision in applying the most opportune strategies at each stage.

Organizational Development Theory

Organizational development (OD) is defined as the application of behavioral sciences to improve organizational effectiveness, and it has the dual goals of improving organizational performance and improving the "quality of work life." These goals generally are accomplished through interventions directed at organizational processes and structures and at worker behavior (Brown and Covey, 1987). The interventions often are stimulated by an OD consultant who is engaged by management, and who implements a set of strategies to help the organization diagnose, evaluate, and address its perceived concerns.

History

Organizational Development Theory is rooted in the human relations perspective that emerged in the 1930s. Before the 1930s, organizational effectiveness was equated with structural efficiencies, such as establishing precise lines of authority (Weber, 1964). In the 1920s and 1930s, research that became known as the Hawthorne studies (Roethlisberger and Dickson, 1939) demonstrated that increasing the attention paid to workers also increased productivity. These studies resulted in an expanded view of organizational effectiveness as influenced largely by worker motivation.

Developments in social science in the late 1940s and 1950s provided the theoretical and philosophical basis for management that is worker-concerned (Margulis and Adams, 1982). Paramount here is Lewin's scientific and humanizing influence on the field of organizational behavior. In emphasizing practical applications, Lewin's action research converted organizations into vibrant laboratories for scientific and self-discovery (Cooperrider and Srivastva, 1987). His stage model of unfreezing, moving, and refreezing is the basis for action research and the precursor of most contemporary organizational change theories.

Like Lewin, Argyris (1957) rejected classical bureaucracy, arguing that individual needs must be fulfilled in the contexts of work and organization. MacGregor (1960) also rejected bureaucratic organization, which he termed Theory X, a set of axioms that held that managers must exert control if workers were to comply with organizational goals. MacGregor proposed an alternative, Theory Y, which held that work is natural to human activity, and that workers will readily fulfill the management's requirements given a supportive environment.

Modern Organizational Development Theory

By the 1960s, the term *organizational development* emerged in the literature and was characterized by interventions directed at either the organization's design and technologies or its human processes. Today, the emphasis has evolved to include environmental influences and how the norms and values of entire organizations are transformed (Brown and Covey, 1987). Three concepts—organizational climate, organizational culture, and organizational capacity—are useful in informing the development of organizational design, technologies, norms, values, and environment.

Organizational Climate. The concept of organizational climate has been present in the literature for nearly forty years, yet no standard definition exists. In general terms, it can be conceptualized as the mood or personality of an organization (O'Keefe, 1999). According to several researchers (Forehand and Gilmer, 1964), organizational climate can be thought of as the personality of an organization; just as each individual has his or her own unique personality, so do organizations (O'Keefe, 1999). Tagiuri (1968, p. 23) notes, "A particular configuration of enduring characteristics of the ecology, milieu, social system and culture would constitute a climate, as much as a particular configuration of personal characteristics constitute a personality." Gilmer (1966, p. 57) defines organizational climate as "those characteristics that distinguish an organization from other organizations and that influence the behavior of people in the organization." Other key elements to understanding organizational climate are individual and collective perceptions of an organization. Members' shared perceptions, attitudes, and beliefs about their organization create the overall organizational climate (Hoy and Miskel, 1987). Litwin and Stringer (1968, p. 1) echo the belief that perception is a key element of organizational climate, so they define it as "a set of measurable properties of the work environment, based on the collective perceptions of the people who live and work in the environment and demonstrated to influence their behavior."

Clearly, the climate of an organization influences whether new programs are successfully implemented. In an organization in which staff feels unsupported and apathetic, it is unlikely that they will put in the extra effort required to adapt, implement, and maintain new programs (O'Keefe, 1999). For instance, in regard to school change, Cullen and others (1999, p. 376) noted that teachers who report high job satisfaction and principal support may work in environments more supportive of behavioral change programs than do teachers who report low job satisfaction and low support.

Organizational Culture. This concept is closely related to organizational climate, but with important differences. Organizational culture is often also conceptualized as "the deeper level of basic assumptions and beliefs that are shared by members of an organization, that operate unconsciously, and that define in a basic 'taken-for-granted' fashion an organization's view of itself and its environment" (Schein, 1985, p. 6). The lines between culture and climate are blurred when compared with contemporary definitions of organizational climate, such as "a system of shared orientations that hold the unit [organization] together and give it a distinctive identity" (Hoy, Tarter, and Kottkamp, 1991, p. 5). Clearly, the concepts are linked, but important yet subtle distinctions may be drawn. Ashforth (1985) describes organizational climate as "shared perceptions" and organizational culture as "shared assumptions." Climate is dynamic and directly affected by any number of changing factors. Culture, in contrast, forms slowly over time and is more stable and resistant to change. To the members of an organization, it is often unnoticeable. In many instances, these two concepts affect one another (O'Keefe, 1999). In teaching about organizational climate and culture, we often use the analogy that climate is the psychology of an organization, and culture is its anthropology.

Organizational Capacity. Both organizational climate and organizational culture influence an organization's capacity to function efficiently and effectively. Katz and Kahn (1978) provide a helpful framework for organizational capacity as an optimum level of functioning within an organization's subsystems: *production* of services or products, *maintenance* of organizational operations, *support* from the social and political environments in which an organization operates, *adaptation* of organizational operations based on everchanging environmental conditions, and *management* of these subsystems as a coherent whole. McLeroy and others (1995) extend organizational capacities beyond these subsystems to include (1) coordination and linkages among local organizations to provide a comprehensive range of services and (2) linkages between social organizations and local citizenry.

Some research on organizational capacity has focused on public health agencies. For instance, Schwartz, Smith, Speers, and Schmidt (1993) include the following elements as central to the core capacity of state health departments: appropriate personnel; effective oversight of programs; ability to plan and evaluate; ability to acquire resources for local programs; and expertise in community organization, needs assessment, data applications, and priority setting. In addition, Schwartz, Smith, Speers, and Schmidt describe the role of state health departments as linking agents between the federal government and local organizations.

How Climate, Culture, and Capacity May Operate as Components of Organizational Development Theory.

Changes in organizational climate or organizational culture can affect the organization's capacity to function effectively. As climate and especially culture are difficult to change, approaches that incorporate Lewin's unfreezing, moving, refreezing strategy seem most useful. Action research is one such popular approach that consists of four steps: diagnosis, action planning, intervention, and evaluation (Argyris, Putnam, and Smith, 1985).

Diagnosis. Diagnosis can be equated with Lewin's unfreezing. Diagnosis aids an organization in identifying problems or gaps that may impede its functioning. The diagnosis is often conducted by an outside consultant who helps the organization identify its most salient problems. The most traditional diagnostic technique is a formal survey of members of the organization (Sommer, 1987). A more recent technique examines cultural gaps between management and work groups, to reduce such gaps (Kilmann, 1986). Variables commonly studied include environmental factors; the organization's mission, goals, policies, procedures, structures, technologies, and physical setting; social and interpersonal factors; desired outcomes (Porras and Robertson, 1987); and readiness to take action (Weisbord, 1988).

Action Planning. Diagnosis is often followed by action planning or the development of strategies or interventions for addressing the diagnosed problems. Porras and Robertson (1987) describe a two-step process for selecting interventions. In the first step, several possible interventions are identified based on the gaps or problem areas that are diagnosed. In the second step, the number of interventions is narrowed based on three criteria: the organization's readiness to adopt a proposed strategy (for example, climate factors include administrative support, time commitment, and sufficiency of resources); the availability of leverage points, that is, where and how to intervene within the organization; and the skill of the OD practitioner in applying the chosen interventions. The two-step process contains the essential ingredient of action planning: the practitioner and members of the organization assess the feasibility of different strategies for change. By so doing, the practitioner helps to raise the organization's commitment to the chosen course of action. Action planning that is informed by social ecology principles holds that community members and other stakeholders outside of the implementing organization should be involved in planning community-based programs (Hawe and Shiell, 2000).

Intervention. The literature is richest in describing OD interventions. Lewin is credited with the development of T-groups, originally used to encourage managers to improve climate by becoming more aware of their interpersonal style and impact. Other interventions include management building, structural redesign, process consultation (Schein, 1969), and group development (Bradford, 1978). In process consultation, the consultant helps members of the organization identify problems, questions, and barriers to a desired change, and then works with the organization to address these potential impediments (Lippitt, Langseth, and Mossop, 1985). The consultant usually does not offer specific solutions, but rather facilitates problem solving among members. Face-to-face contact and group interaction is integral to this approach. Process consultation is employed in one of the case applications described below.

Evaluation. The final step in action research is evaluation, which assesses the planned change effort. Several evaluation techniques measure planned change in organizations. An essential feature of evaluation is that the organization takes stock of its progress in moving to a new state and determines whether additional alterations are needed (Goodman and Wandersman, 1994). Evaluation often allows the changes in an organization to settle, or refreeze.

Future Challenges

Organizational development can benefit from refinements in both theory and practice. To illustrate, Weisbord (1988) questions Lewin's premise that organizations that are stuck can become unfrozen. This challenges one of the basic assumptions upon which organizational development theory rests, that is, that supportive conditions make it possible for changes in organizational climate and culture to be applied to best advantage in increasing the organization's capacity to function effectively.

Health promotion programs may fail to develop sufficient capacity due to nonsupportive organizational climates and cultures. However, such failures are often attributed to other factors because the importance of climate and culture is not understood or assessed. The field of health behavior and health education often overemphasizes individual-level factors and ignores or minimizes factors at other levels. This is particularly true for the organizational level and in relation to the role of organizational change in the success or failure of health promotion programs. Key challenges for the future are to increase understanding of organizations' roles and to include measures of organizational factors and social context in health promotion research and practice.

Finally, most OD interventions are not specific to the stage of development of the organizations at which they are directed. Although the two cases presented in this chapter are quite distinctive, the first being experimental and the second being a multiple-case study, they both demonstrate how OD strategies can be tailored to fit an organization's stage of development.

Interorganizational Relations Theory

Interorganizational Relations(IOR) Theory is a branch of organizational theory that focuses on how organizations work together. Thus, IOR Theory is directed at the social ecology of multiple organizations that operate within communities. Collaboration among organizations often leads to a more comprehensive and coordinated approach to public health than can be achieved by one organization. As with Stage Theory of Organizational Change, IOR Theory also is a contingency theory. That is, the increasing complexity of health and social issues, economic and political factors, and other demands such as increased competition require that organizations link efforts and form networks to create more comprehensive and effective responses. Examples of interorganizational linkages range from grassroots coalitions of leaders from rural black churches (Sutherland, Cowart, and Harris, 1997) to multihospital systems that reduce competition and provide flexibility in the face of accelerated changes in technology (Zuckerman, Kaluzny, and Ricketts, 1995).

History

Focus on IOR grew out of organizational theory in the 1960s, as more attention was devoted to the impact of the environment on organizational behavior. Researchers became interested in how organizations decreased uncertainty in the environment by working together. Early research focused on factors that influence an organization's decision to enter into a collaborative relationship and was based largely on an assessment of the benefits versus the costs of the relationship (Gray, 1989). Major benefits of collaboration include access to new information, ideas, materials, and other resources; potential to minimize duplication of services and to use existing resources more efficiently; potential to maximize power and influence by combining forces; ability to address issues beyond a single organization's domain; and shared responsibility across organizations for complex or controversial issues (Alter and Hage, 1993; Butterfoss, Goodman, and Wandersman, 1993). Potential costs associated with an organization's participation in collaborative relationships include diversion of an organization's resources to IOR; dilution of an organization's position or focus on issues that are central to its mission; incompatibility with a policy or position taken by the IOR Theory; and delays in taking action due to the often slow and cumbersome consensus development process by which IOR Theory frequently operates (Alter and Hage, 1993).

Other factors important in the formation of IOR Theory include recognition of interdependence and the need for coordination; acknowledgment that an organizational goal is more likely to be achieved through collaboration; resources such as time, staff, and expertise for maintaining a coordinated process; mandates from a powerful outside force such as a funding agency or regulating body; clear and mutually shared goals; awareness of potential partners and geographic proximity; similar organizational interests and values; a positive attitude toward cooperation and norms for collaboration; and successful previous experience in working together (Gray, 1989; D'Aunno and Zuckerman, 1987; Alter and Hage, 1993). Several of these factors, such as mutually shared goals and successful previous experience in working together, help explain why interorganizational networks such as coalitions in public health often have core groups of the "usual players" from the health, education, and voluntary sectors (Florin, Mitchell, and Stevenson, 1993; Kegler, Steckler, McLeroy, and Malek, 1998).

Development of Interorganizational Relations as Informed by Stage Theory.
Recently, researchers have broadened their focus from factors contributing to the formation of IOR to IOR maintenance and continued development (Bazzoli and others, 1997). Stage Theory has been used to explain the ongoing development of these collaborative relationships (Alter and Hage, 1993; Florin, Mitchell, and Stevenson, 1993; Gray, 1989). For example, Alter and Hage (1993) propose a three-stage model of network development as a continuum from informal to formal linkages. The three stages are *exchange or obligational networks*, composed of loosely linked organizations devoted to resource exchange with few joint activities and that are maintained by individuals who coordinate and integrate tasks across organizations; *action or promotional networks* of organizations that share and pool resources to accomplish concerted action, but whose interorganizational activities tend to be peripheral to member organizations' goals; and *systemic networks* of organizations that have long-term formal links to abet the joint production of goods or services.

Evolution of IOR as Informed by Contingency Theory of Organizations.
As previously mentioned, organizational development largely focuses on enhancing structure and processes. The formation of IOR structure and processes is based on Contingency Theory of Organizations, which postulates that organizational design reflects the degree of complexity of the environment in which the organization operates (Shortell and Kaluzny, 1988). Alter and Hage (1993) apply the principles of Contingency Theory to designs. They have developed a model for understanding the structure and operational processes of IOR as contingent on

selected characteristics of the environment and the nature of the work to be undertaken. The structure and operational processes, in turn, influence the level of conflict between the participating organizations and the perceived effectiveness of the network in producing desired outcomes. For instance, Alter and Hage (1993) assert that the degree of external control influences the structure of the IOR. To illustrate, if an interorganizational network is dependent on a single funding source, such as a federal or state public health agency, Alter and Hage postulate that the resulting structure will tend to be highly centralized, or dominated by a single or small group of organizations. This is because centralized structures enhance the funding agency's ability to regulate work objectives and to control costs.

Future Challenges

Interorganizational Relations Theory has the potential to provide valuable insights into the effective use of interorganizational arrangements such as multiagency networks and community coalitions. The field, however, is still relatively new and several challenges remain. First, future research should acknowledge the complexity of interorganizational relations by distinguishing the type of partnership and stage of development. Many types of IOR exist and, throughout their evolution, they are likely to be influenced by different factors. Second, greater understanding of the stages through which interorganizational relations develop is needed. Existing models are inconsistent in the number of stages, and research on health coalitions has focused largely on the earlier stages (Chinman, Anderson, Imm, and Wandersman, 1996). Third, more research is needed on the contextual factors that influence IOR functioning at each stage. Although research in this area is expanding, contextual factors have not been adequately examined among interorganizational partnerships in public health (Gray, 1996; Provan, Milward, and Brinton, 1995; Blau and Rabrenovic, 1991).

A final remaining challenge for IOR Theory is the selection and definition of IOR outcomes. Alter and Hage (1993) discuss four categories in which to measure IOR effectiveness: the extent to which goals are met, the extent to which needed resources are acquired, the extent to which smooth internal functioning is exhibited, and the extent to which all constituents are minimally satisfied. The literature on health promotion coalitions and interorganizational partnerships has focused mainly on internal functioning and member satisfaction (Butterfoss, Goodman, and Wandersman, 1996; Kegler, Steckler, McLeroy, and Malek, 1998) and less so on long-term outcomes such as systems change and health outcomes (Roussos and Fawcett, 2000; Kreuter, Lezin, and Young, 2000).

Table 15.1 summarizes the organizational change concepts discussed in this section.

TABLE 15.1. SUMMARY OF ORGANIZATIONAL CHANGE CONCEPTS.

Concept	Definition	Application
Stages of change	Organizations pass through specific steps as they change	Help organizations move through all the stages; do not stop at just adoption
Problem definition* (Awareness stage)	Problems recognized and analyzed; solutions sought and evaluated	Involve management and other personnel in awareness-raising activities
Initiation of action* (Adoption stage)	Policy or directive formulated; resources for beginning change allocated	Provide process consultation to inform decision makers and implementers of what adoption involves
Implementation of change*	Innovation is implemented, reactions occur, and roles change	Provide training, technical assistance, and problem-solving aid
Institutionalization of change*	Policy or program becomes entrenched in the organization; new goals and values are internalized	Identify high-level champion, work to overcome obstacles to institutionalization, and create structures for integration
Organizational development	An approach that tries to improve the quality of work life	Identify aspects of work life— through organizational diagnosis—that positively and negatively affect workers
Organizational climate	The personality of an organization	Use existing measures as part of change efforts
Organizational culture	Assumptions and beliefs that are shared by members of an organization and that operate unconsciously	Require an outsider to gauge culture; use deeper understanding to plan interventions
Organizational capacity	Optimum functioning of an organization's subsystems	Identify an organization's strengths and weaknesses as part of program planning
Action research	Four steps for improving organizations: diagnosis, action planning, intervention, and evaluation	Based on organizational diagnosis, develop and implement a plan for change
Organizational development interventions	Specific techniques such as t-groups that are used to help improve organizations	Use techniques such as surveys, cultural inventories, t-groups, and process consultation

TABLE 15.1. SUMMARY OF ORGANIZATIONAL CHANGE CONCEPTS, Continued.

Concept	Definition	Application
Interorganizational relations	How organizations collaborate to solve problems of mutual interest	Determine which organizations in a community are concerned about a given health problem
Stages of interorganizational collaboration	The steps that organizations go through as they attempt to collaborate	Develop strategies to help collaborating organizations overcome barriers at each stage; for example, process evaluation of coalition effectiveness

Note: * From Glanz and Rimer, 1995.

Applications of Organizational Change Theories

The following sections illustrate how organizational change theories have been applied by researchers and practitioners to understand and influence health promotion efforts in school and community settings. The first example describes a program of research to integrate tobacco use prevention into public schools. The second is an analysis of programs to enhance state health departments' capacity for cancer prevention and control programs.

Application: Integrating Tobacco Prevention into School Systems

Each year cigarette smoking is responsible for over 390,000 deaths and is reported to be the leading preventable cause of death and disability in the United States (U.S. Department of Health and Human Services, 1989). Health curricula with effective smoking-prevention components can help to substantially reduce adolescent smoking (Perry, Murray, and Klepp, 1987). Yet, the rate of tobacco use among adolescents generally has remained constant over the past decade (Johnston, O'Malley, and Bachman, 1991). Due primarily to a failure of dissemination and effective implementation, effective school health curricula reach only a small portion of adolescents in the United States (Parcel, Perry, and Taylor, 1990).

In 1987 the National Cancer Institute funded a large-scale project to test the effectiveness of health curricula dissemination strategies (NCI Grant No. R01CA45997). The five-year study, called the North Carolina School Health and Tobacco Education Project, was designed to assess and influence schools' curriculum awareness, adoption, implementation, and institutionalization. Of the 140 school districts in North Carolina, 28 were randomly selected and subsequently contacted about participating in the study. After 22 districts agreed to participate, they were randomly assigned to either an experimental or control condition (Goodman, Smith, Dawson, and Steckler, 1991). The treatment group received intensive intervention strategies, while the control districts received just enough attention to retain them in the study. To give schools a choice, three curricula were used.

Four-Stage Model. Stage Theory informed the interventions for disseminating the health curricula to schools. Different intervention strategies were employed at each of the four stages: awareness, adoption, implementation, and institutionalization. Furthermore, Organizational Development Theory was the basis for the strategies used during the adoption, implementation, and institutionalization stages.

Awareness Stage. Because senior-level administrators are most influential in decisions to adopt new programs (Huberman and Miles, 1984), the project directed its initial strategies at increasing administrator awareness and concern for tobacco prevention. Two intervention strategies were used to accomplish this. The first was incorporated into an annual, week-long conference to which school districts sent teams of administrators and teachers. At this conference, the awareness and adoption of the eight components of comprehensive school health were emphasized (Girven and Cottrell, 1987). The second awareness strategy was a site visit by members of the research team with senior administrators of the school districts that were asked to participate in the project.

Both awareness interventions were evaluated. The evaluation of the statewide conference included pre- and posttest measures of administrator and teacher awareness and concern for tobacco-use prevention among adolescents (Smith and others, 1991; Steckler and others, 1992). The statewide conference was successful in increasing teachers' and administrators' awareness and concern about comprehensive school health. The individual site visits were evaluated using a case study and indicated that administrators' awareness and concern regarding tobacco prevention increased when the research team identified a local intermediary who could help establish legitimacy for the research project and when the investigators were able to arrange for more than one meeting with the district administrators to continue discussions about the project (Goodman, Smith, Dawson, and Steckler, 1991).

Adoption Stage. Once a school district's administrators agreed to participate, the research team offered each school district a choice of one of three curricula; both experimental and control districts were given this choice. The experimental districts in addition were exposed to the organizational development technique known as *process consultation,* in which an outside agent works with organization personnel to identify problems, questions, and barriers and then helps resolve the identified concerns by facilitating desired changes (Schein, 1969). For experimental districts, the process consultation consisted of a three-hour workshop with district personnel, at least one follow-up meeting, and telephone contacts. In contrast, the researchers mailed written material about the three curricula to the control districts, instructing them to write to the project indicating which curriculum they wanted to adopt.

The adoption stage was evaluated in several ways. Whether a school district actually adopted one of the study curricula was signified by a letter of agreement between the district and project indicating which of the three curricula had been selected, when it would be taught, and which teachers would teach it. The time of adoption was signified by the number of weeks that elapsed between the process consultation (or receipt of written materials) and the signing of the letter of agreement. Case studies of the adoption process were conducted in a sample of experimental and control districts. The average length of time of adoption was fifteen weeks, with no significant difference between experimental and control districts in time or in the number of districts that adopted. The decision to adopt was influenced by the degree to which a teacher or health supervisor championed the curriculum and by the active support of the champion by a central office administrator (Goodman, Tenney, Smith, and Steckler, 1992).

Implementation Stage. The main implementation intervention was intensive training for teachers in using the adopted curriculum. A three-part training was employed that included a pretraining consultation meeting with experimental districts to plan for the upcoming teacher training; a training workshop conducted by nationally recognized specialists in each of the three study curricula and lasting from two to four days, depending on the curriculum adopted; and a posttraining consultation with teachers and administrators about one month after the workshop that was intended to boost skills and help each district plan for curriculum implementation (Smith, McCormick, Steckler, and McLeroy, 1993). The control districts received the adopted curriculum in the mail, but no training was conducted.

Evaluation results indicated that more experimental than control district teachers taught the adopted curricula and that they taught more lessons than control district teachers. The study also found that school districts with an active health coordinator and a supportive administrator had greater implementation of the curricula (Smith, McCormick, Steckler, and McLeroy, 1993). In addition, larger school districts were more likely to implement one of the three study curricula than were smaller districts. The researchers surmised that larger districts had more resources available to support implementation activities (McCormick, Steckler, and McLeroy, 1995).

Institutionalization Stage. After a school district had taught one of the study curricula for one school year, the researchers employed a process consultation for institutionalization that consisted of the dissemination of a guidebook to program champions (for instance, school health coordinators) on how to institutionalize curricula; consultative meetings with these champions; and a two-hour meeting with superintendents, assistant superintendents, middle school coordinators, health coordinators, principals, teachers who had taught the curriculum, and teachers who might teach it in the future. The main purpose of this meeting was to assess experiences with the adopted curriculum and to determine necessary steps to maintain and increase its use in the future.

The study produced no difference in institutionalization between experimental and control districts. In both conditions institutionalization was moderate to low due to a number of factors: the fact that process consultation for institutionalization was a weak intervention; "turbulence" in the school environment (for example, teacher and administrator turnover, change in school format from junior high to middle schools, and inadequate overall funding); lack of strong leadership for health among school administrators; the combining of health instruction with physical education or science; inadequate K–12 planning for health instruction or comprehensive school health; and lack of training for teachers beyond that provided by the research project (Smith, Steckler, McCormick, and McLeroy, 1995).

Organizational Change Theories. *Project Strengths.* By using an experimental design, the health curriculum dissemination project randomized intervention and control school districts. Thus, the effectiveness of the strategies was compared across two similar groups in which only one received an intervention, and bias that often influences retrospective explanations for a program's outcomes was reduced.

Perhaps the project's most important contribution is that Stage and OD Theories were intertwined, and the related strategies were directed at multiple organizational levels. The application of process consultation illustrates how OD techniques can be applied to specific stages of organizational change. At the adoption stage, the project had to overcome three major impediments: the project was sponsored by outsiders who were trying to influence schools to adopt one of three new health curricula, school personnel had limited knowledge about the curricula being offered and the requirements for instruction, and tobacco prevention was not a priority in schools.

At the implementation stage, process consultation was combined with training to help prepare teachers for using the curriculum that their district had adopted. The combination of process consultation and traditional training proved effective in leading to greater implementation among experimental school districts.

At the institutionalization stage, process consultation focused on the political skills of those individuals, such as school health coordinators, who championed the program. Skill development centered on building coalitions of program advocates so that the program could become entrenched within the school system.

In addition to contouring OD techniques to fit specific stages, the curriculum dissemination study intervened at different organizational levels. For instance, the onsite visits were directed exclusively at district level administrators; the visits were focused on increasing the administrators' awareness of tobacco-use prevention among youths and on their concern for addressing the problem in their school district. The process consultation for adoption included administrators and teachers; the administrators were from both the district and building levels. The training and consultation for implementation was primarily at the teacher level. At institutionalization, the focus was once again on administrators.

Project Weaknesses. Despite the curriculum dissemination project's strengths in conceptualization and design, it also illustrates areas in which the application of theory can be improved. For instance, in both the onsite awareness visits and the process consultation for adoption the research team had a preplanned agenda; for example, getting schools to recognize the need for tobacco-use prevention curricula, getting them to participate in the project, and getting them to adopt one of the three study curricula. The traditional approach to OD is less directed in that the consultant is more generally interested in identifying gaps between actual and desired practice. At the awareness stage in particular, process consultation strategies could have been used more effectively to help the organization assess its own needs.

At the institutionalization stage, focusing on the political and organizational skills of the program champion and holding a one-meeting process consultation for adoption proved to be a weak intervention. Institutionalization itself is a process that occurs over a number of organizational cycles (school years in this case). To be effective, institutionalization interventions need to be multifaceted and should occur over several school years.

Application: Enhancing State Health Departments' Capacity for Cancer Prevention and Control

To help state health departments adopt a new role in cancer prevention and control, The National Cancer Institute (NCI) initiated the Data-Based Intervention Research program (DBIR). The goal of DBIR was to stimulate data-driven activities and to build organizational capacity within state health departments to ensure the translation of cancer prevention and control science into practice. NCI's objective reflected the readiness of cancer control research for public health application, the paucity of cancer control activity within public health settings, and the recognition that state health departments could play a critical role in the effective transfer of research results into public health practice. The DBIR project began in 1987, with twenty-two state health departments eventually participating. The states were funded in three annual rounds; the first round received five years of funding and the second and third rounds received seven years (Goodman, Steckler, and Alciati, 1997).

Enhancing Organizational Capacity

The goal of the NCI in developing the DBIR project was to increase the organizational capacity of state health departments to be able to engage in data-driven cancer prevention and control programming. The use of an external catalyst is consistent with many OD approaches to organizational change. NCI used two important catalysts in stimulating and assessing changes in state-level capacities to deliver cancer prevention and control programs. The first was to use the funding of the DBIR model (described in following sections) as an external policy lever to influence change in the structure and functions of state health departments. The second was the funding of an external evaluation to assess DBIR's influence of state-level capacities to deliver cancer-related initiatives.

The DBIR Model. The DBIR model consisted of four phases: (1) identifying and analyzing relevant data, (2) using these data to develop a state cancer control plan for high priority intervention areas, (3) implementing interventions, and (4) evaluating interventions. Specific requirements were established for each phase. These phases parallel those elaborated earlier for action research (that is, diagnosis, action planning, intervention, and evaluation). During Phase 1 of DBIR, states were to use only existing data sources and to collaborate with experts, both within the health department and throughout the state, to analyze and review data. In Phase 2, states were to use the data results from Phase 1 to establish appropriate goals and objectives for the state. To accomplish this, states were required to involve a consortium representing the state public health community in the planning process. This was a form of interorganizational relations, as discussed earlier. The final products of the planning phase, the cancer control and intervention plans, were to serve as the basis for local interventions to be carried out during Phase 3. Finally, evaluations of the interventions were to be conducted in Phase 4. The NCI required that the interventions include an initiative with state legislators, informing them of the nature and extent of the cancer problem in the state, the potential for intervening, and the resources available.

The DBIR model was directed at the development of both organizational structure and process capacities. Structural elements in the model included increasing state health departments' capacities to identify cancer-related data sources for more effective program prioritization and planning, to implement community-oriented cancer prevention and control programs, and to evaluate program efforts and effects. Process elements in the model included increasing the health departments' capacities to generate interorganizational relations and to collaborate among linked organizations, to communicate effectively with state legislators in support of cancer prevention initiatives, and to disseminate project results for possible replication (Goodman, Steckler, and Alciati, 1997).

Evaluation of DBIR. An evaluation was conducted to determine how DBIR had been implemented and what effect it had on the capacities for cancer prevention and control of the twenty-two participating state health departments. Data were collected in three ways: review of archival records; in-person, in-depth interviews; and a survey. Over one hundred archival records such as state health department's funding applications, annual reports, and cancer plans were reviewed by the evaluators. Presentation materials and correspondence as well as NCI program summary documents were also reviewed (Goodman, Steckler, and Alciati, 1997; Steckler, Goodman, and Alciati, 1997).

Based on the review of archival records, an open-ended interview guide was developed and four representative states were visited by the evaluators. States were visited for two days, during which in-depth interviews were conducted. (Goodman, Steckler, and Alciati, 1997). Based on the results of the site visits, a detailed survey was developed. The survey was sent to all twenty-two state health departments that had received funding for DBIR. Responses were received from all twenty-two states, for a 100 percent response rate (Steckler, Goodman, and Alciati, 1997).

Results

While the evaluation study had a number of findings, what is of interest here is the extent to which the DBIR program enhanced state health department's capacities for cancer prevention and control activities and how these capacities may be understood as occurring across the organizational subsystems of production, maintenance, support, adaptation, and management, as well as interorganizational networks. In this regard, DBIR was more successful in some areas than in others. For instance, DBIR was successful in enhancing the health departments' linkage capacity with other relevant organizations and agencies in their states. DBIR was also successful in increasing states' capacities in program planning, especially in the area of identifying and using existing cancer data, and their capacity to develop cancer prevention and control plans, which many previously did not have. For many states, DBIR was the first time they had done data-based planning for chronic disease prevention and control. The states indicated that they found both the planning process and the product (that is, the plan) to be beneficial in a number of important ways. Most indicated they would continue to use data for cancer control planning and that they would maintain the new relationships established in the DBIR planning process. These findings strongly suggest that DBIR would have a lasting effect on enhancing important aspects of state health departments' capacity for cancer prevention and control planning (Goodman, Steckler, and Alciati, 1997; Steckler, Goodman, and Alciati, 1997).

DBIR was less successful in enhancing state health departments' capacities for program planning and implementation, and in the management function of evaluating interventions at the local level. Despite the emphasis given to this aspect of cancer prevention by NCI and the DBIR model, states found implementing and evaluating local programs to be problematic. The evaluation results suggest several reasons for this lack of success. While cancer data were useful in narrowing the targets for intervention, suggesting a focus on a particular type of cancer and identifying high-risk groups, they were generally less helpful in guiding states to specific interventions. The NCI goal that the DBIR program generate publishable research results about the application of cancer control science was a departure from the traditional role of state health departments and was perceived to reflect a lack of understanding of the mission and function of state agencies (Goodman, Steckler, and Alciati, 1997; Steckler, Goodman, and Alciati, 1997). In essence, the incompatibility between NCI and state health department expectations for DBIR may be understood as a gap between two distinct organizational cultures.

In conclusion, the evaluation of the DBIR program suggests that federal agencies can have a positive effect on enhancing state health departments' organizational capacities in important public health areas. Enhancements in capacity are reflected in adjustments throughout an organization's subsystems and interorganizational linkages. However, these adjustments are most likely to occur when the funding agency has a good understanding of the culture and climate of the grantee agencies' missions, roles, procedures, rules, rewards, and sanctions. The DBIR experience also suggests that structural and process capacities and interorganizational relations of organizations, such as state health departments, can be enhanced through planned, externally originated change efforts such as action research. Organizational capacity, therefore, is mutable and malleable, but the process often is more long- than short-term (Goodman, Steckler, and Alciati, 1997; Steckler, Goodman, and Alciati, 1997).

Conclusion

Organizational change theories, such as those presented in this chapter, have not often been applied, or reported, as foundations for health promotion or public health programs. We can only speculate on why this might be so. Perhaps it is because individual change theories and strategies are more developed and easier to test than organizational theories. Health education and health promotion are dominated by and heavily reliant on well-developed social-psychological theories of individual change. Perhaps, unlike social psychologists, few organizational psychologists or organizational development specialists apply their expertise to health behavior. This, in turn, may explain why few faculty in health education and health promotion have expertise in organizational change, leading to a dearth of courses or even sections of courses devoted to careful examination of the role of organizations in health behavior and promotion in graduate education programs. Perhaps it is because considering organizational factors introduces a new level of complexity in the needs assessment, program planning, implementation, and evaluation process that researchers and practitioners are unable to consider due to the time and cost constraints. Or perhaps it is because organizational change, particularly Stage Theory, is similar to other more familiar theories, such as Diffusion Theory (Chapter Fourteen).

This chapter has illustrated the importance of organizational change to health promotion researchers and practitioners and offered some of the conditions for successfully guiding organizational change. Three theories of organizational change were analyzed: stage, organizational development, and interorganizational relations. The impact of climate, culture, and the social ecology on organizations was described for each theory. The theories were applied to two distinct cases. The first case, a randomized experimental study, illustrated how OD techniques may be used to intervene at different stages of an innovation's development. The second, a case study, illustrated how an external agent, such as a federal agency, can use organization development to affect change in climate, culture, capacity, and interorganizational relations of organizations such as state health departments.

Whether directing change strategies from within or from outside an organization, health practitioners are presented with unique challenges. Organizational change theories suggest strategies to mediate such challenges and those discussed in this chapter, when applied effectively, can influence change.

References

Alter, C., and Hage, J. *Organizations Working Together.* Thousand Oaks, Calif.: Sage, 1993.

Argyris, C. *Personality and Organization.* New York: McGraw-Hill, 1957.

Argyris, C., Putnam, R., and Smith, D. M. *Action Science: Concepts, Methods, and Skills for Research and Intervention.* San Francisco: Jossey-Bass, 1985.

Ashforth, S. J. "Climate Formations: Issue and Extensions." *Academy of Management Review,* 1985, *25*(4), 837–947.

Bazzoli, G., and others. "Public-Private Collaboration in Health and Human Service Delivery: Evidence from Community Partnerships." *The Milbank Quarterly,* 1997, *75*(4), 533–561.

Beyer, J. M., and Trice, H. M. *Implementing Change: Alcoholism Policies in Work Organizations.* New York: Free Press, 1978.

Blau, J., and Rabrenovic, G. "Interorganizational Relations of Nonprofit Organizations: An Exploratory Study." *Sociological Forum,* 1991, *6*(2), 327–347.

Bradford, L. P. (ed.). *Group Development.* (2nd ed.) La Jolla, Calif.: University Associates, 1978.

Brown, L. D., and Covey, J. G. "Development Organizations and Organization Development: Toward an Expanded Paradigm for Organization Development." In R. W. Woodman and W. A. Pasmore (eds.), *Research in Organizational Change and Development.* (Vol. 1.) Greenwich, Conn.: JAI Press, 1987.

Butterfoss, F., Goodman, R., and Wandersman, A. "Community Coalitions for Prevention and Health Promotion." *Health Education Research: Theory and Practice,* 1993, *8*(3), 315–330.

Butterfoss, F., Goodman, R., and Wandersman, A. "Community Coalitions for Prevention and Health Promotion: Factors Predicting Satisfaction, Participation and Planning." *Health Education Quarterly,* 1996, *23*(1), 65–79.

Chinman, M., Anderson, C., Imm, P., and Wandersman, A. "The Perceptions of Costs and Benefits of High Active Versus Low Active Groups in Community Coalitions at Different Stages in Coalition Development." *Journal of Community Psychology,* 1996, *24*(3), 263–274.

Cooperrider, D. L., and Srivastva, S. "Appreciative Inquiry in Organizational Life." In R. W. Woodman and W. A. Pasmore (eds.), *Research in Organizational Change and Development.* (Vol. 1.) Greenwich, Conn.: JAI Press, 1987.

Cullen, K. W., and others. "Influence of School Organizational Characteristics on the Outcomes of a School Health Promotion Program." *Journal of School Health,* 1999, *69*(9), 376–380.

D'Aunno, T., and Zuckerman, H. "A Life-Cycle Model of Organizational Federations: The Case of Hospitals." *Academy of Management Review,* 1987, *12*(3), 534–545.

Florin, P., Mitchell, R., and Stevenson, J. "Identifying Technical Assistance Needs in Community Coalitions: A Developmental Approach." *Health Education Research,* 1993, *8,* 417–432.

Forehand, G. A., and Gilmer, B. "Environmental Variation in Studies of Organizational Behavior." *Psychological Bulletin,* 1964, *62,* 361–381.

Gilmer, B. "The Company Personality." *Management Review,* 1966, *48,* 69–76.

Girven, J. T., and Cottrell, R. "The Impact of the Seaside Health Education Conference on Middle School Health Programs in Oregon." *Health Education,* 1987, *18*(5), 78–82.

Glanz, K., and Rimer, B. K. *Theory at a Glance.* Washington, D.C.: National Cancer Institute, 1995.

Goodman, R. M., Smith, D. W., Dawson, L., and Steckler, A. "Recruiting School Districts into a Dissemination Study." *Health Education Research: Theory and Practice,* 1991, *6,* 373–385.

Goodman, R. M., and Steckler, A. "A Framework for Assessing Program Institutionalization." *Knowledge in Society: The International Journal of Knowledge Transfer,* 1989, *2*(1), 52–66.

Goodman, R. M., Steckler, A., and Alciati, M. H. "A Process Evaluation of the National Cancer Institute's Data-Based Intervention Research Program: A Study of Organizational Capacity Building." *Health Education Research,* 1997, *12*(2), 181–197.

Goodman, R. M., Tenney, M., Smith, D. W., and Steckler, A. "The Adoption Process for Health Curriculum Innovations in Schools: A Case Study." *Journal of Health Education*, 1992, *23*(4), 215–220.

Goodman, R. M., and Wandersman, A. "FORECAST: A Formative Approach to Evaluating the CSAP Community Partnerships." *Journal of Community Psychology*, 1994, CSAP special issue, 6–25.

Gray, B. *Collaborating: Finding Common Ground For Multiparty Problems.* San Francisco: Jossey-Bass, 1989.

Gray, B. "Cross-Sectoral Partners: "Collaborative Alliances Among Businesses, Government and Communities." In C. Husham (ed.), *Creating Collaborative Advantage.* London: Sage, 1996.

Hawe, P., and Shiell, A. "Social Capital and Health Promotion: A Review. *Social Science and Medicine*, 2000, *51*, 871–885.

Hoy, W. K., and Miskel, C. G. *Educational Administration: Theory, Research and Practice.* (3rd ed.) New York: Random House, 1987.

Hoy, W. K., Tarter, C. J., and Kottkamp, R. B. *Open Schools/Healthy Schools: Measuring Organizational Climate.* Thousand Oaks, Calif.: Sage, 1991.

Huberman, A. M., and Miles, M. B. *Innovation Up Close: How School Improvement Works.* New York: Plenum Press, 1984.

Israel, B. A., Checkoway, B., Schulz, A., and Zimmerman, M. "Health Education and Community Empowerment: Conceptualizing and Measuring Perceptions of Individual, Organizational and Community Control." *Health Education Quarterly*, 1994, *21*(2), 149–170.

Johnston, L., O'Malley, P. M., and Bachman, J. G. *Drug Use Among American High School Senior, College Students and Young Adults: 1975–1990.* Washington, D.C.: United States Department of Health and Human Services, National Institute for Drug Abuse, 1991.

Kaluzny, A. D., and Hernandez, S. R. "Organization Change and Innovation." In S. M. Shortell and A. D. Kaluzny (eds.), *Health Care Management: A Text in Organization Theory and Behavior.* (2nd ed.) New York: Wiley, 1988.

Katz, D., and Kahn, R. *The Social Psychology of Organizations.* (2nd ed.) New York: Wiley, 1978.

Kegler, M., Steckler, A., McLeroy, K., and Malek, S. "Factors That Contribute to Effective Community Health Promotion Coalitions: A Study of 10 Project ASSIST Coalitions in North Carolina." *Health Education and Behavior*, 1998, *25*(3), 338–353.

Kilmann, R. H. "Five Steps for Closing Culture-Gaps." In R. H. Kilmann, and others (eds.), *Gaining Control of the Corporate Culture.* San Francisco: Jossey-Bass, 1986.

Kreuter, M., Lezin, N., and Young, L. "Evaluating Community-Based Collaborative Mechanisms: Implications for Practitioners." *Health Promotion Practice*, 2000, *1*(1), 49–63.

Lewin, K. *Field Theory in Social Science.* New York: HarperCollins, 1951.

Lippitt, G. L., Langseth, P., and Mossop, J. *Implementing Organizational Change.* San Francisco: Jossey-Bass, 1985.

Litwin, G. H., and Stringer, R. A. *Motivation and Organizational Climate.* Boston: Graduate School of Business Administration, Harvard University, 1968.

MacGregor, D. *The Human Side of Enterprise.* New York: McGraw-Hill, 1960.

Margulis, N., and Adams, J. "Introduction to Organizational Development." In N. Margulis and J. Adams (eds.), *Organizational Development in Health Care Organizations.* Reading, Pa.: Addison-Wesley, 1982.

McCormick, L. K., Steckler, A., and McLeroy, K. R. "Diffusion of Innovations in Schools: A Study of Adoption and Implementation of School-Based Tobacco Prevention Curricula." *American Journal of Health Promotion*, 1995, *9*(3), 210–219.

McLeroy, K. R., Bibeau, D., Steckler, A., and Glanz, K. "An Ecological Perspective on Health Promotion Programs." *Health Education Quarterly*, 1988, *15*(4), 351–378.

McLeroy, K. R., and others. "Creating Capacity: Establishing a Health Education Research Agenda for Special Populations." *Health Education Quarterly*, 1995, *22*(3), 390–405.

O'Keefe, K. "An Analysis of a Process Evaluation and School Climate Assessment for a School-Based Health Promotion Intervention Targeting Native-American Children." Unpublished paper, School of Public Health, University of North Carolina at Chapel Hill, 1999.

Parcel, G., Perry, C., and Taylor, W. "Beyond Demonstration: Diffusion of Health Innovation." In N. Bracht (ed.), *Health Promotion at the Community Level*. Thousand Oaks, Calif.: Sage, 1990.

Perry, C. L., Murray, D. M., and Klepp, K. I. "Predictors of Adolescent Smoking and Implications for Prevention." *Morbidity and Mortality Weekly Report*, 1987, *36*(45), 41–45.

Porras, J. I., and Robertson, P. J. "Organization Development Theory: A Typology and Evaluation." In R. W. Woodman and W. A. Pasmore (eds.), *Research in Organization Change and Development*. (Vol. 1.) Greenwich, Conn.: JAI Press, 1987.

Prochaska, J. O., and DiClemente, C. C. "Stages and Processes of Self-Change of Smoking: Toward an Integrative Model of Change." *Journal of Consulting and Clinical Psychology*, 1983, *51*, 390–395.

Provan, K., Milward, H., and Brinton, H. "A Preliminary Theory of Interorganizational Network Effectiveness: A Comparative Study of Four Community Mental Health Systems." *Administrative Science Quarterly*, 1995, *40*(1), 1–33.

Roethlisberger, F. J., and Dickson, W. J. *Management and the Worker*. Cambridge, Mass.: Harvard University Press, 1939.

Rogers, E. M. *Diffusion of Innovations*. (3rd ed.) New York: Free Press, 1983.

Roussos, S., and Fawcett, S. "A Review of Collaborative Partnerships as a Strategy for Improving Community Health." *Annual Review of Public Health*, 2000, *21*, 369–402.

Schein, E. H. *Process Consultation: Its Role in Organization Development*. Reading, Pa.: Addison-Wesley, 1969.

Schein, E. H. *Organizational Culture and Leadership*. San Francisco: Jossey-Bass, 1985.

Schwartz, R., Smith, C., Speers, M. A., and Schmidt, T. "Capacity Building and Resource Needs of State Health Agencies to Implement Community-Based Cardiovascular Disease Programs." *Journal of Public Health Policy*, 1993, *14*, 480–494.

Shortell, S. M., and Kaluzny, A. D. "Organization Theory and Health Care Management." In S. M. Shortell and A. D. Kaluzny (eds.), *Health Care Management: A Text in Organization Theory and Behavior*. (2nd ed.) New York: Wiley, 1988.

Smith, D. W., McCormick, L. K., Steckler, A., and McLeroy, K. R. "Teachers' Use of Health Curricula: Implementation of Growing Healthy, Project SMART, and the Teenage Health Teaching Modules." *Journal of School Health*, 1993, *63*(8), 349–354.

Smith, D. W., Steckler, A., McCormick, L. K., and McLeroy, K. R. "Lessons Learned About Disseminating Health Curricula to Schools." *Journal of Health Education*, 1995, *26*, 37–43.

Smith, D. W., and others. "Promoting Comprehensive School Health Programs Through Summer Health Promotion Conferences." *Journal of School Health*, 1991, *61*(2), 69–74.

Sommer, R. "An Experimental Investigation of the Action Research Approach." *Journal of Applied Behavioral Science*, 1987, *23*(2), 185–199.

Steckler, A., Goodman, R. M., and Alciati, M. H. "The Impact of the National Cancer Institute's Data-Based Intervention Research Program on State Health Agencies." *Health Education Research*, 1997, *12*(2), 199–211.

Steckler, A., and others. "Measuring the Diffusion of Innovative Health Promotion Programs." *American Journal of Health Promotion,* 1992, *6*(3), 214–224.

Stokols, D., Allen, A. J., and Bellingham, R. L. "The Social Ecology of Health Promotion: Implications for Research and Practice." *American Journal of Health Promotion,* 1996, *10,* 247–251.

Sutherland, M., Cowart, M., and Harris, G. "Jackson County Partnership: Developing an Effective Coalition." *International Quarterly of Community Health Education,* 1997, *17*(4), 405–415.

Tagiuri, R. "The Concept of Organizational Climate." In R. Tagiuri and G. W. Litwin (eds.), *Educator's Handbook: A Research Perspective.* New York: Longman, 1968.

U.S. Department of Health and Human Services. *Reducing the Health Consequences of Smoking— 25 Years of Progress: A Report of the Surgeon General.* Washington, D.C.: Centers for Disease Control, Center for Health Promotion and Education, Office on Smoking and Health, U.S. DHHS, Public Health Service, 1989.

Weber, M. *The Theory of Social and Economic Organization.* New York: Free Press, 1964.

Weisbord, M. R. "Towards a New Practice Theory of OD: Notes on Snap Shooting and Moviemaking. In R. W. Woodman and W. A. Pasmore (eds.), *Research in Organizational Change and Development.* (Vol. 2.) Greenwich, Conn.: JAI Press, 1988.

Zuckerman, H., Kaluzny, A., and Ricketts, T. "Strategic Alliances: A Worldwide Phenomenon Comes to Health Care." In A. Kaluzny, H. Zuckerman, and T. Ricketts (eds.), *Partners for the Dance: Forming Strategic Alliances in Health Care.* Ann Arbor: Health Administration Press, 1995.

CHAPTER SIXTEEN

COMMUNICATION THEORY AND HEALTH BEHAVIOR CHANGE

The Media Studies Framework

John R. Finnegan Jr.
K. Viswanath

According to the Oxford English Dictionary, the word *communication* comes from the Latin "to make common to many" or "to give to another as a partaker." It incorporates three concepts: (1) the conveyance or exchange of intangible elements such as information, ideas, and meaning; (2) a union or relationship implying mutual revelation, discovery, and effects; and (3) a recognition that these processes occur at all levels of human experience. The word entered common English usage at about the same time that printing technology emerged in fifteenth-century Europe and made possible the growth and diffusion of knowledge on a previously unprecedented scale.

Today we define communication as the production and exchange of information and meaning by use of signs and symbols (Gerbner, 1985). It involves processes of encoding, transmission, reception (decoding), and synthesis of information and meaning. As political psychologist Harold D. Lasswell (1948) put it, to study an act of communication is to pose the question, "Who Says What In Which Channel To Whom With What Effect?" Thus, Lasswell identified some key components of communication study: the sender (who encodes and transmits), the content or message (communication substance), the channel (the medium through which content is transmitted), the receiver or audience (who decodes communication to derive meaning), and the effect (a measurable outcome of the process).

Because of the centrality of communication in human affairs, many fields claim its study as an empirical, critical, and applied phenomenon, public health included. Applied communication perspectives particularly influence public health. That is, how do communication processes add to or detract from health behavior change? Second, how can communication strategies be used in a planned way to influence health behavior change?

The purpose of this chapter is to describe communication theories especially relevant to public health and health behavior, to review and critique their application in the study of health behavior effects, and to provide examples of how communication theory informs health behavior change interventions. For reasons that will be made clear, we emphasize communication theory in a media studies context applied to public health.

Organization of Communication Studies

Communication scholar George Gerbner (1985) described a widely accepted framework for communication studies that includes three main branches. The first is the study of how signs and symbols combine into "codes" to create messages that convey meaning in different social contexts. This branch is called "semiotics," the science of symbols, signs, and codes. This branch of communication studies is often concerned with the construction of meaning. How do signs, symbols, and codes combine to "construct reality"—that is, influence us to think about things in some ways and constrain us from thinking about them in other ways? Language, for example, is a "code" that may be analyzed by its constituent signs and symbols to understand how it builds meaning. There are also aural and visual codes that communicate meaning (consider, for example, how slow motion in a film sequence communicates the ideas of beauty and grace).

Gerbner described the second branch as the study of behavior and interaction through exposure to messages. Here the emphasis is on measuring, explaining, and predicting communication effects on cognitions, beliefs, attitudes, and public opinion. The fields of psychology and social psychology influence this approach.

The third branch is the study of how communication is organized through large-scale social institutions and systems, their history, regulation, and policy-making impact.

Levels of Study

Within each branch, communication study may be further broken down to examine effects at various levels of human experience on a "micro to macro" continuum. For example, at the level of the individual we may study how a person processes information about health and converts it into action. At the interpersonal (dyadic) level, we may examine how two people interact and influence one another relevant to some health behavior outcome. At the group or organizational level, we may examine how formal or informal communication among many people influences health behavior change including, perhaps, the effective delivery of a health-related service. Finally, at the level of the community, society, or culture, we may examine how communication contributes to health behavior change within the constraints of social structure.

It is important to recognize that just as there is no single, unifying theory that explains and predicts all human behavior, there is also no such theory that explains and predicts all communication effects. Theories tend to diverge along the levels of analysis just described but also according to effects relevant to each discipline that studies communication. Some view this as symptomatic of fragmentation in our understanding of communication. Others view this as a healthy theoretical diversity necessary to understand human activity in many complex dimensions (Finnegan and Viswanath, 1989). In either case, current trends in communication research increasingly seek to connect and to integrate effects across levels of analysis from the "micro" to the "macro" (Hawkins, Weimann, and Pingree, 1988).

All three branches and levels of study are important to understanding health behavior change. The applied emphasis of public health means that our approach to human communication is necessarily eclectic. Most chapters in this book illustrate this diversity in their treatments of health behavior change theories. Whether studied in individual, group, or community contexts, most health behavior change theories implicate critical roles and effects of communication. It is not the aim of this chapter to repeat these insights but to carry the discussion of communication and health behavior change into an area of growing interest in public health: mass communication and its research framework, media studies.

The reasons for this emphasis are several. First, as Clarke and Evans (1983) have described, a media studies framework cuts across Gerbner's three branches of communication theory as well as "micro to macro" levels of analysis. It "consists in the study of media by which information and entertainment are delivered in society, the conditions and processes by which this content is shaped, and the effects that content and form exert on individuals . . . groups," communities, societies, and cultures. Above all, communication in this context is "distinguished . . . by its social complexity and self-conscious organization and use of technological instruments to extend and preserve symbolic exchange in time and space." These processes have important effects on public health in light of the mass media's ubiquity and their role as primary sources of information about health and most other human activities.

Second, communication effects on health behavior may be studied in this framework from the perspective of day-to-day interactions but also as planned use of mass communication to influence health behavior. Third, the community-based intervention campaign approach to influence health behavior change has gained currency in public health during the past twenty years. This approach recognizes the need to seek change in health behavior across multiple levels of human experience—from the individual to the community (Rogers and Storey, 1987).

Interventions are planned, multistrategy efforts that seek different kinds of change leading to population shifts in health outcomes (see especially the chapters in this book on planning and process models for fuller treatment of this approach). Mass communication has become a key part of this approach, whether the object of change is to build the community's agenda for prevention, to change public policy, or to educate individuals about specific health behavior changes. Media institutions play a crucial role in health behavior change because they are key gatekeepers for disseminating information in social systems and because, as socializing agents, they have a powerful effect on legitimizing social norms of behavior.

Evolution of Communication Media

Anthropologists tell us that communication is as old as the human species. Almost as soon as humans began to communicate with each other, they began developing tools to extend their contact beyond interpersonal speech. It is likely that early drums were the first instruments intended to carry messages to other humans at a distance. In a sense, mass media are an extension of those ancient drums, yet they are relatively recent phenomena in human history. They emerged less than two centuries ago (as did virtually all of modern society) in that spectacular release of creative and physical energy historians call the Industrial Revolution. Although the printing press was invented in fifteenth-century Europe, it was not until the early nineteenth century that steam power was harnessed to the printing press for mass production and distribution of information. Mass circulation daily newspapers, cheap enough for all to afford at a penny per copy, first appeared in 1833 in New York City and soon all over the world. In 1844, the speed of information for the first time in human experience exceeded the speed of the fastest form of transportation. In that year, information was first transmitted electronically over wires in Britain and the United States, broken down into a series of dots and dashes. If you understood this "Morse Code," you could use this new "telegraph" to both send and receive information as far as the wires could reach. By 1869, they reached across the Atlantic Ocean, first linking the European and North American continents. The nineteenth century also gave birth to other communication technology: the photograph, the telephone, recorded sound, moving pictures, and the first wireless transmission of sound. The twentieth century built on these advances by creating radio, television, the computer, global satellite networks, and the World Wide Web, not to mention vast improvements in older technologies (Emery, Emery, and Roberts, 1996).

Although technology itself makes communication physically possible on a mass scale, it is human organization of activity into a *media system* that is key. That is, the media are interconnected large-scale organizations that systematically gather, process, and disseminate news, information, entertainment, and advertising worldwide. Many are small operations like your neighborhood newspaper, while others are large corporations operating chains of media outlets and employing tens of thousands of workers. Still others are global media empires operating in many countries and cultures simultaneously. In some parts of the world, the media are owned and operated by government rather than private enterprise. No matter the size or form of ownership, the media today are all around us. They influence almost all aspects of human life: economic, political, social, and behavioral. From a public health perspective, the miracles of communication technology and the evolving influence of the media in our lives pose both great promise and worrisome perils.

Major Study Areas

There is a widespread popular and academic perception that media are powerful, that they play influential roles in promoting, discouraging, or even inhibiting healthy behaviors. To understand the nature of these roles requires us to evaluate how, where, and with whom media interact and with what consequences.

Two areas of research are germane. One deals with message production. It asks the question, What are the social and organizational factors involved in media work that may affect the creation of media messages influencing behavior change? Here, we are interested in message production through processes of creating news, information, advertising, and entertainment. In Lasswell's (1948) terms, these are the *sender* and *channel* characteristics of mass media that form media work and content.

The second area of research asks, What are the consequences of media exposure on individuals, groups, institutions, and social systems? This question has been traditionally studied as *media effects*. Here, we are interested in some of the major media effects hypotheses and their relevance to health behavior change.

Media Message Production

Mass media organizations are bureaucracies in which tasks are specialized and routinized to achieve efficiency in creating news, advertising, and entertainment. For example, journalists seek established or official sources routinely to gather information that is used to create "news" (Sigal, 1987). The criteria for using sources are usually straightforward: they should be credible, available, and able to supply reliable information when needed. Sources essentially subsidize the process of gathering information (Gandy, 1982). Sources may be established spokespersons for government agencies, businesses, or other powerful groups and elites in the social system (Hilgartner and Bosk, 1988; Donohue, Tichenor, and Olien, 1995). Journalists routinize their news-gathering process to ensure predictability in an idiosyncratic world. However, reliance on a regular supply of information from established sources means that groups without social power are often less likely to gain access to news making and therefore have less influence.

What becomes news is the product of the interaction of sources and media professionals. Sources perform the key role of identifying social problems and bringing them to the attention of the media. Whether representing campaigns, government agencies, advocacy groups, or other interests, sources compete for media and therefore also for public attention in seeking to define and to increase the public profile of an issue or problem. For example, the U.S. Surgeon General's office, a major official source of public health information, regularly releases reports on the status of smoking and its effects on U.S. health. From year to year, the reports emphasize different aspects of the smoking problem that the Public Health Service wishes to bring to the attention of news media and the general public (for example, increased smoking among young women). Despite their dependence on official sources, media professionals also enjoy some autonomy in defining the problem particularly in the ways they construct news stories. The definition of a social problem is crucial to how the public understands it, the actions individuals or communities are likely to take to ameliorate the problem, the attention given the problem by different groups, and the knowledge they acquire (Viswanath, Finnegan, Hannan, and Luepker, 1991).

Media Effects

The outcomes of media dissemination of images, ideas, themes, and stories are commonly discussed under the rubric of *media effects* (Bryant and Zillman, 1994). At first blush, the term seems to imply the unidirectional study of the media on some outcome (knowledge, opinion, attitude, behavior) among individuals, groups, institutions, or communities that are regarded as more or less passive recipients of the effect (McLeod, Kosicki, and Pan, 1991). However, media effects research also looks at effects flowing in the opposite direction—from audiences to the media. Moreover, strong traditions in media research regard audiences not as passive recipients but as active seekers and users of information (Blumler and Katz, 1974).

Media studies, like other social and behavioral sciences, also vary in the level of analysis applied in research—from the individual to groups, communities, and social systems. Table 16.1 provides an overview of this variety in media studies research. Major theories and concepts are organized by level of analysis. At each level, we provide a few key studies and also the disciplinary origin and relationship to other fields.

At the individual level of analysis, media studies emphasize effects on motivations, cognitions, involvement, attitudes, and behaviors resulting from exposure to media messages. A long-standing interest is the relationship between individuals' knowledge, attitudes, and behaviors. Important theories drawn from psychology and social psychology include hierarchies of effects, persuasion, and social cognitive theories. These types of media studies have dominated the field since the 1930s.

Specifically, researchers have looked at *learning hierarchies,* in which knowledge change affects attitudes that in turn affect behavior (K-A-B). Others have noted different hierarchies: *dissonance attribution,* in which behavior change affects attitude change which in turn affects knowledge (B-A-K), and the *low-involvement* hierarchy, in which knowledge change affects behavior, which in turn influences attitudes (K-B-A). More recently, researchers have suggested that there are not three distinct hierarchies of effects but a single continuum (Chaffee and Roser, 1986). The order of effects will depend on where individuals or groups are positioned at the start with respect to some outcome.

Early persuasion studies by Hovland, Janis, and Kelley at Yale (1953) were controlled experiments testing various conditions under which opinion or attitude change would occur in the context of such variables as source credibility, fear, organization of arguments, the role of group membership in resisting or accepting communication, and personality differences. This line of research continues today with an emphasis on cognitive processing of information leading to persuasion (Perloff, 1993).

Since the 1960s, media effects research has changed its dominant focus from attitude change to studying cognitive impact (Beniger and Gusek, 1995) and has also emphasized community and social systems levels of analysis. The latter happened partly because of Latin American scholars' interest in developing new approaches to the use of mass communication in guided social change projects in developing countries (Lee, 1980). Units of observation in this macro-level perspective have included populations in diverse community settings, groups, organizations, social institutions, and large-scale social systems including communities and nations. It has an obvious connection to public health, in which guided social change and community-based health interventions have become ideal settings for testing macro-social applications of communication strategies.

TABLE 16.1. SELECTED COMMUNICATION THEORIES AND LEVELS OF ANALYSIS.

Level of Analysis	Theory or Concept	Major Studies and Reviews	Disciplinary Origin
Individual	Hierarchies of effects	Ray and others (1973) McGuire (1984) Chaffee and Roser (1986)	Psychology Social psychology
	Persuasion theories	Hovland, Janis, and Kelley (1953) Roloff and Miller (1980) Petty and Cacioppo (1981) McGuire (1985) Perloff (1993)	Psychology Social psychology
	Social cognitive theory	Bandura (1994)	Social psychology
Organization	News gatekeeping	Donohue, Tichenor, and Olien (1995) Shoemaker (1991)	Sociology of organizations
	Reporter-source relations	Sigal (1973; 1987)	Sociology
	Media work routines	Roshco (1975) Tuchman (1978)	Sociology
	Media message systems	Gerbner, Gross, Morgan, and Signorielli (1980) Turow (1992)	Sociology of organizations
Communities and social systems	Diffusion of innovations	Rogers (1995)	Sociology Social psychology
	The knowledge gap	Tichenor, Donohue, and Olien (1980) Gaziano (1983) Viswanath and Finnegan (1996)	Sociology Structural functionalism Social conflict
Mass society and culture	Cultivation studies	Gerbner, Gross, Morgan, and Signorielli (1994)	Sociology of mass society
Cross-level analysis	Agenda setting	McCombs and Shaw (1972) Kosicki (1993)	Sociology Psychology Political science
	Definition, framing of social problems	Iyengar and Kinder (1987) Entman (1993) Gamson and Modigliani (1987) Hilgartner and Bosk (1988)	Sociology Psychology
	Risk communication	Weinstein (1984) Sandman (1987) Slovic, Fischoff, and Lichtenstein (1981) Glanz and Yang (1996)	Sociology Psychology

Because of their relevance to public health efforts to guide social and behavioral change, we review and critique in greater detail four of the media-effects perspectives listed in Table 16.1: the Knowledge Gap, Agenda Setting, Cultivation Studies, and Risk Communication.

The Knowledge Gap. Conventional wisdom long held that persistent social problems could be resolved through public education. To paraphrase the film *Field of Dreams,* the assumption was "if you tell them, they will know." However, studies examining public knowledge on a variety of topics and issues have shown that "they" did not always know. Moreover, knowledge and information turned out not to be equally distributed across populations. Studies showed that people with more formal education learned and knew more about many issues than did people with less formal education (Hyman and Sheatsley, 1947; Mosteller and Moynihan, 1972).

These findings were formally presented as the knowledge gap hypothesis by Minnesota researchers Tichenor, Donohue, and Olien (1970, 1980). They proposed that an increasing flow of information into a social system (from a media campaign, for example) is more likely to benefit groups of higher socioeconomic status (SES) than those of lower SES. Increasing the information available in the system would likely exacerbate already existing differences between these groups. They supported this proposition using studies of several topics including health. The disturbing implications were, of course, that public information campaigns would only perpetuate inequities. Because this called into question the entire basis of guided social change efforts, it attracted the attention of scholars and policy makers.

As a media studies perspective, knowledge gap research arose from a long-standing sociological tradition emphasizing how the structure and organization of communities and societies function as means of social control and management of conflict. This tradition has long considered the mass media as important institutions of social control and conflict management. The hypothesis advanced media effects insights in at least two important ways. It contradicted conventional wisdom that social interventions are a simple panacea for resolving social problems, and it suggested that media have differential impact on audiences—impact that is importantly mediated by the social-structural conditions in which audiences live. It was thus one of the first media studies hypotheses to focus attention on the role of environment in media effects on individuals (Viswanath and Finnegan, 1996).

Fortunately, subsequent studies found that knowledge gaps were not intractable. Researchers discovered a variety of contingent and contributory conditions that could affect knowledge gaps and also present opportunities for applications in public health campaigns (Table 16.2): content domains, channel influence, social conflict and community mobilization, the structure of communities, and individual motivational factors (Donohue, Tichenor, and Olien, 1975; Ettema and Kline, 1977; Gaziano, 1983; Viswanath and Finnegan, 1996).

TABLE 16.2. KNOWLEDGE GAP CONCEPTS, DEFINITIONS, AND APPLICATIONS.

Concept	Definition	Application
Knowledge gap	Difference in knowledge between groups of differing socioeconomic status (SES)	Potential unintended consequence of campaigns to increase "gaps" over time
Knowledge	Information leading to understanding or for taking informed action	Communication of information about causes and prevention of disease and health skills
Information flow	Degree of information availability on an issue in a social system such as a community or organization	Increasing opportunities (through multiple channels) to encounter health information
Socioeconomic status (SES)	Populations characterized by differing education, income, wealth, or occupation	Emphasis on information and channels relevant to different SES groups
Social structure/ pluralism	Differentiation and interdependence among community sub-systems including institutions, organizations, interest groups	Large communities increase competition for public attention to health information and require more communication resources than smaller communities
Social conflict	Conflict over an issue or problem; often a struggle for power and influence among social groups	Controversy attracts media attention, especially in highly differentiated communities; increases public interest
Mobilization	Organized activity to focus community power and influence to address a problem or issue	Publicity about health issues often driven by social groups and leaders
Motivation	Factors influencing individuals to attend to and act upon information and knowledge	Emphasize strategies to increase motivation to acquire and use information

Content and Channel Factors. Although studies have found SES-based knowledge gaps in the content domain of health, others have suggested that as a general topic, "health" may appeal more broadly to all SES groups (Ettema, Brown, and Luepker, 1983; Snyder, 1990; Yows, Salmon, Hawkins, and Love, 1991; Zandpour and Fellow, 1992). That is, audiences may be more involved in the topic because, a priori, it affects everyone in some way. This aspect, however, does not account for other factors influencing knowledge gaps. For example, studies of channel influence show that people who obtain their news from print media are usually more knowledgeable than are those who receive it from other media (Viswanath and Finnegan, 1996). There is, of course, a slight tendency for newspaper readers to have more formal education than do nonreaders. Television has the potential to be a knowledge equalizer among SES groups as the cost of access through cable, digital satellite, and the Internet becomes more affordable. An additional modifiable aspect of channel influence has to do with the link between media and interpersonal communication. Tichenor, Donohue, and Olien (1980) have suggested, for example, that interpersonal discussion is helpful in narrowing knowledge gaps by reinforcing information received from the media.

Social Conflict and Mobilization. Media studies have also shown that significant knowledge gaps are less likely to be found where social conflict or community mobilization occur (Donohue, Tichenor, and Olien, 1975). Social conflict, an engine of social change, appears to increase public attention to issues encouraging greater interpersonal communication. Mobilization of community groups, institutions, and advocates to address a public problem has a similar effect even if overt conflict is not present (Gaziano, 1983).

Community Structure and Pluralism. An important though largely nonmodifiable factor affecting knowledge gaps is the structure of communities themselves. Large communities are characterized by greater specialization in interest groups, services, and institutions including government, business, the media, and other organized centers of power. The potential for conflict is higher in these pluralistic communities because of such diversity and specialization. Small towns are less specialized and differentiated across all these sectors. Thus, knowledge gaps are more likely in larger, more complex communities and less likely in smaller, less pluralistic communities (Donohue, Tichenor, and Olien, 1975; Shinghi and Mody, 1976; Ettema, Brown, and Luepker, 1983; Gaziano, 1988). However, some recent studies in health communication have reported findings counter to this: gaps were more likely to be found in smaller communities (Viswanath, Finnegan, Hertog, Pirie, and Murray, 1994). It has been suggested that in certain content domains such as health, the greater availability of diverse sources may work to the advantage of residents of larger communities (Viswanath and Finnegan, 1996).

Motivational Factors. An important set of modifiable factors affecting knowledge gaps was proposed by Ettema and Kline (1977). They argued that gaps between higher and lower SES groups were not necessarily due to the effects of less formal education or economic deprivation, but to differential levels of motivation, interest, and salience in specific topics. They shifted the focus in knowledge gap studies to the role of variables of individual difference. Support for this alternative explanation appeared in several studies reporting that the association between knowledge and individual variables such as interest, salience, motivation, and involvement was greater than the association between knowledge and education (Ettema, Brown, and Luepker, 1983; Zandpour and Fellow, 1992; Fredin, Monnett, and

Kosicki, 1994). Contrary evidence has been reported by other studies (Griffin, 1990; Snyder, 1990; Viswanath, 1990; Yows, Salmon, Hawkins, and Love, 1991; McLeod and Perse, 1994). Viswanath, Kahn, Finnegan, Hertog, and Potter (1993), in a study of a dietary health campaign, reported that even among those motivated, the more educated knew more about diet and nutrition than did the less educated.

Despite conflicting evidence on the role of motivational factors, it is clear that both individual-level and social-structural variables are important in explaining knowledge gaps. However, future studies need to do a better job in linking these different levels of analysis (Viswanath and Finnegan, 1996).

The importance of these recent studies is that they have given back to guided social change efforts some modifiable factors that, if appropriately understood and addressed, restore some of our optimism about the use of interventions to address public problems. However, unlike the unbounded optimism of the early days of public campaigns, these studies urge us to be "sober and wiser" in considering structural factors that pose barriers to public campaigns. Public health regards it as an ethical precept to address problems of the whole population, whether they are information rich or information poor.

Agenda-Setting. Mass communication research has long been concerned with the influence of mass media on public opinion, especially as they affect politics and policymaking. Early writers such as Walter Lippmann (1922) saw media's behavior as a "restless searchlight" panning from one issue to the next while seldom lingering long on any single issue. Later, researchers such as Berelson (1948) noted that although the media influence public opinion, the reverse is also true: public opinion influences what the media report. Paul Lazarsfeld and colleagues (1948) also noted that media attention itself confers status on issues and raises their importance. These insights coalesced in the 1970s as a focus on the mass media's role and influence in setting the public agenda of important issues and problems.

Agenda setting has received much scholarly attention in part because of the reemergence of media models that predict powerful media effects (McCombs and Shaw, 1972). An axiom underlying this area of study is that mass media are not very successful in telling us *what* to think, but they are surprisingly successful in telling us what to think *about*. The key idea here is that mass media are powerful in setting the public agenda of important issues and problems.

Studies have shown high correlations between media coverage of issues and the public's opinion of the importance of those issues. This implies a strong if not direct link between the media's agenda of important issues (reflected in news coverage) and the public's agenda of important issues (the causal direction flowing from the media to the public). Agenda setting also presents a number of opportunities for applications of media in public health interventions (Table 16.3).

TABLE 16.3. AGENDA SETTING CONCEPTS, DEFINITIONS, AND APPLICATIONS.

Concept	Definition	Application
Media agenda setting	Institutional roles, factors, and processes that influence the definition, selection, and emphasis of issues in the media	Work with media professionals to understand their needs and routines in gathering and reporting news
Public agenda setting	The link between issues portrayed in the media and the public's priorities	Work with media via advocacy or partnerships to build the public agenda for important health issues
Policy agenda setting	The link between issues developed in policymaking institutions and issues portrayed by the media	Work with community leaders and policymakers to increase importance of health issues on the media's and public's agenda
Problem identification, definition	Factors and process leading to the identification of an issue as a "problem" by social institutions	Community leaders, advocacy groups, organizations define an issue and solutions
Framing	Organized public discourse about an issue leading to the selection and emphasis of features and the exclusion of others	Advocacy groups "package" an important health issue for the media and the public

Kosicki (1993) has identified three types of agenda setting research: (1) public agenda setting that examines the link between media portrayal of issues and their impact on issue priorities assigned by the public, (2) policy agenda setting that examines the connection between media coverage and the legislative agenda of policymaking bodies, and (3) media agenda setting that focuses on factors influencing the media to cover certain issues.

Recent research has proposed refining agenda-setting theory (Kosicki, 1993). Initial simple studies have given way to more empirically sophisticated designs with clearer causal links (Iyengar and Kinder, 1987; Demers, Craff, Choi, and Pessin, 1989). This approach also is being further refined through several changes in the agenda-setting perspective. According to this changing view, the media not only tell us what is important in a general way, they also provide ways of thinking about specific issues by the signs, symbols, terms, and sources they use to define the issue in the first place. In this view, public problems are social constructions. That is, groups, institutions, and advocates compete to identify problems, to move them onto the public agenda, *and* to define the issues symbolically (Gamson and Modigliani, 1987; Hilgartner and Bosk, 1988; Entman, 1993). This refinement is important because it suggests that the media's agenda-setting function is not completely independent but is built by various community groups, institutions, and advocates. It also has a basis in the sociology of knowledge that emphasizes processes involved in the social construction of reality (Berger and Luckmann, 1966). This has implications and applications for those in public health who seek to use the mass media to raise the salience and awareness of specific health problems.

Cultivation Studies. Cultivation studies emphasize the impact that mass media have on our perceptions of reality. The pervasiveness of television and visual media and their power to alter perception is the starting point of this approach. Simply stated, researchers proposed that heavy exposure to television often leads individuals to accept the world portrayed by television as real (Gerbner, Gross, Morgan, and Signorielli, 1980; Stossel, 1997). The more the exposure to television, the greater the congruence between viewers' perception of reality and the mythical reality portrayed by television (Gerbner, Gross, Morgan, and Signorielli, 1994; Weimann, 2000). In essence, television cultivates a stilted view of the world.

Cultivation studies have evolved two types of research. The first, *message system analysis,* seeks to examine the world that television constructs. For example, Gerbner, Gross, Morgan, and Signorielli (1980, 1994), in a long series of studies, have been tracking television's violent content. They defined violence as "overt expression of physical force" by characters to compel victims to act against their will, and measured the frequency of these acts. In an early report (Gerbner, Gross, Morgan, and Signorielli, 1980), they demonstrated an average of five violent acts per hour of prime-time programming and twenty acts of violence on weekend daytime television. They also tracked and recorded the gender, age, ethnicity, and occupation of characters who frequent television dramas. They reported that in the world portrayed on television, men outnumber women, young people and senior citizens are underrepresented, and professional and law enforcement personnel are overrepresented.

The second type of research is *cultivation analysis.* Gerbner and his colleagues (1994) proposed that heavy exposure to television has a profound effect on viewers' perception of social reality. Heavy viewers were more likely to give "television answers" to opinion and knowledge questions as compared with light viewers. They were also more likely to perceive the world as violent and frightening out of proportion to reality, to be less trusting of others, to overestimate the number of people employed in law enforcement, and to fear that they are more likely than statistically true to become victims of crime. They also are likely to be more accepting of violence as a means of dealing with social problems.

This cultivation of the television worldview is believed to occur through two distinct mechanisms: *mainstreaming* and *resonance.* Mainstreaming is the sharing of commonality of outlooks. Interestingly, irrespective of sociodemographic background, heavy viewers of television tend to share this worldview. As Gerbner and his colleagues (1980) asserted, heavy viewing "may serve to cultivate beliefs of otherwise disparate and divergent groups toward a more homogeneous 'mainstream' view."

Resonance is regarded as the more powerful mechanism. That is, the "reality" of television programs for certain groups may in fact be congruent with the reality of their lives. In such cases, they receive a double dose of the cultivation effect: television has stronger effects for these groups. At least one study has suggested that in some cases the source of resonance effects actually may be audience affinity. For example, some audience segments may identify so highly with crime victims in the news who resemble themselves that they then develop unreasonable fears about their own risk as victims (Chiricos, Eschholz, and Gertz, 1997).

Although other research has raised questions about the nature of evidence supporting the cultivation hypothesis, most researchers agree that television affects our perception of reality depending on the level of exposure (Potter, 1999). Subsequent studies have added several contingent conditions that could affect cultivation. For example, some research suggests that the cultivation effects of television become weaker or disappear when controlled for factors such as age, gender, education, income, hours worked per week, social ties, and the size of one's community. The fear of crime supposedly cultivated by heavy viewing of television may be explained by the number of heavy viewers living in high-crime areas and staying home watching more television. Some have also argued that cultivation effect could be nonlinear. That is, television viewing may lead to a cultivation of a "television worldview" but only up to a point (Potter, 1999). Still others argue that entertainment programming is not the only culprit in the distortion of worldviews. The news media, politicians, government, and social and political advocacy groups often seek to further their ends by raising public fear and concerns out of proportion to reality (Dorfman, Woodruff, Chavez, and Wallack, 1997; Glassner, 1999).

Risk Communication. Communication about risk is a field of special concern in public health that bridges individual and community levels of analysis. At the individual level, scholars have focused on understanding cognitive processes, and the development of expert and mental models of communication (Fischoff, 1999; Maibach, 1999; Weinstein, 2000); issues of individual innumeracy (Lipkus, Rimer, Halabi, and Strigo, 2001; Weinstein, 1984); confusion and misinformation (Weinstein, 2000); the efficacy of individualized counseling and tailoring

(Rimer, Glanz, and Rasband, 2001); and the advantages of intensive, calibrated, and directed communication (Rimer and Glassman, 1999).

Moreover, at the individual level, researchers also emphasize the cognitive mechanisms by which individuals are exposed to and attend to information about risk, how they interpret risk information in relation to themselves, and whether and how they act upon risk information to alter their behavior (Slovic, Fischoff, and Lichtenstein, 1981; Weinstein, 1984; Glanz and Yang, 1996). This approach to the study of risk communication owes much of its theoretical base to sociopsychological models of behavior (discussed elsewhere in this volume), including value expectancy theories such as the Health Belief Model, the Theory of Reasoned Action, and the Precaution Adoption Process Model (for example, perception of personal risk susceptibility and severity) and also to self-regulatory models, including Social Cognitive Theory (for example, self-efficacy beliefs that one can take effective action to reduce personal risk). This approach is also a staple of communication research at the individual level that examines media effects on knowledge, beliefs, and behavior.

Significant developments in the study of risk communication have also occurred at the community level of analysis. Recent work on social problems and the accompanying discourse in the public arena has attracted considerable attention. At the community level, studies of communication about risk focus on the interaction of populations and social institutions (such as government agencies, advocacy groups, and the mass media) in the formation and management of public opinion and policymaking about risk. Here, risk communication studies owe much of their theoretical basis to the agenda-setting and agenda-building perspectives but also to research into the definition and framing of public issues. Risk communication research in this vein has noted that risk is a social construction; that is, a product of communication activity of social institutions, advocates, and the public (Hilgartner and Bosk, 1988; Sandman, 1987; Griswold and Packer, 1991; Glanz and Yang, 1996).

Public definitions of risk will usually include some form of scientifically assessed risk information (objective) mediated by the political and social context of the risk (the "outrage" factor). Social conflict is a critical variable in drawing attention to social problems and leading to arousal and salience of the issue possibly leading to social action (Tichenor, Donohue, and Olien, 1980; Viswanath and Demers, 1999). This can have both negative and positive consequences depending on whether the actual risk is low or high contrasted with whether public "outrage" is low or high. "Outrage" is a form of community conflict that can have the effect of quickly propelling important information through the population at all socioeconomic levels (this phenomenon relates to the knowledge gap discussed earlier). In such cases, there will be little difference in information holding among all socioeconomic groups (Viswanath and Finnegan, 1996). Where outrage is low (or there is little publicity), one might expect to find socioeconomic group differences in knowledge about risk. Either situation may have an impact on policy-making about risk, whether the public is well- or ill-informed. Further, community level of definition could be crucial to social action by powerful actors in the interest of ameliorating an unacceptable condition, as in the case of AIDS in Africa.

Following the events of September 11, 2001, and the advent of modern bioterrorism, there is little doubt that this research has gained new importance. Of special concern are the media's effects on public perceptions of risk in an environment of rapidly occurring sensational and unfamiliar events, the context of a vulnerable open society, and information uncertainty.

Media Studies Applications in Health

In this section, we review examples of how some of these perspectives are useful in understanding and evaluating health promotion and disease prevention efforts. Application of communication theories to health behavior in the media studies framework occurs mainly along the two dimensions described earlier: (1) effects of day-to-day interaction with media on health outcomes and (2) effects of the purposive use of media to achieve some health outcome, usually in the context of a planned campaign intervention.

Day-to-Day Impact of Media on Health

The first category linked media studies and public health for much of the twentieth century and shows little sign of abating, to judge by the amount of research generated. Its major concern is the effect of media use itself on health-related behavior (DeFleur and Dennis, 1985). In the 1930s, the Payne Fund sponsored some of the first empirical studies examining the effects on youth of exposure to movies. The concern was whether movies engendered violent or other antisocial behavior. These studies approached the question more from a psychological or socio-psychological perspective, but more recently investigators have used the cultivation studies approach. The emphasis on vulnerable groups in such studies also stems from the fact that children and the elderly are the most frequent users of television.

Violence and the Media. Concern about media impact grew dramatically after commercial television first went on the air in 1946. By the early 1970s, the U.S. Department of Health, Education, and Welfare (1972) was expressing great concern about the effects of television violence on children and youth. The

Surgeon General's report found disturbingly consistent associations between exposure to violent television content and aggressive behavior, a link amplified by thousands of subsequent studies (Kelly, 1996; Wilson and others, 1997; Singer and Singer, 2001). This long-standing concern has not abated in the age of digital media. Despite content-rating systems implemented by the industry in the late 1990s, researchers continue to find high rates of violent television programming and accuse the industry of specifically marketing violence to young people (Gerbner, 1998; Federal Trade Commission, 2000). In addition, studies show how young people's media-use habits are changing with the introduction of new media including music CDs, videogames, computers, and the Internet integrated with older media such as television and radio (Livingstone and Bovill, 2001). A recent study of youth media habits by the Kaiser Family Foundation (1999) found that the average American child now spends about five-and-a-half hours per day outside of school with media of all kinds. At the same time, few parents have media-use rules for their children and spend little time supervising their media use, the study found.

A key continuing challenge for this research, however, is the issue of causality: does youth exposure to media violence cause violence in the real world? Because media are ubiquitous, it may not be possible to design a study that will ever solve this puzzle decisively. While many researchers point to the consistency of exposure-aggression associations in myriad studies and the media's continuing obsession with violence (Willis and Strasburger, 1998; American Academy of Pediatrics, 1999), real-world youth violent crime has declined strikingly in the United States since the mid-1990s to the lowest levels in almost thirty years (Snyder, Sickmund, and Bilchik, 1999). So, it is evident that the relationship of media exposure to behavior is complex and variable (Hogben, 1998; Felson, 1996). If direct causal links are elusive, many researchers have noted cumulative exposure effects leading to other equally disturbing outcomes such as desensitization toward real-world violence or negative changes in perceptions about one's vulnerability to violence (mean-world syndrome). In a provocative departure from mainline research in this area, one investigator has suggested that media violence may actually have a beneficial cathartic effect as an outlet for aggressive impulses before they are acted upon in the real world (Fowles, 1999). In addition, he views the struggle over media violence as part of the nation's recurring "culture wars" over values in popular culture.

Advertising and Entertainment. Advertising has raised additional public health issues, also with an emphasis on vulnerable groups such as children and adolescents. Both the sociopsychological and cultivation studies approaches to communication effects have informed research in this area. Recent studies have suggested, for example, that cigarette advertising is extremely appealing to youths and plays a role in influencing their decisions to start smoking (Ammerman, Ott, and Tarter, 1999). Studies of alcohol advertising and depiction of drinking in entertainment programming suggest that their effect on youths is to alter perceptions in favor of the product's use by implying a false norm that "everybody drinks" and by suggesting falsely that one can't have a good time unless one drinks alcohol, and may also be linked to drinking-related aggression (Grube and Wallack, 1994; Caswell and Zhang, 1998; Robinson, Chen, and Killen, 1998).

Other studies have illustrated concerns that excessive television use influences children's adoption of sedentary lifestyles and may be partly responsible for increased rates of childhood obesity, poor eating patterns, high cholesterol, eating disorders, and other mental health problems (Myers and Biocca, 1992; Singer and Singer, 2001). Many of these studies also have public policy ramifications. For example, some public health advocates have proposed major restrictions on advertising and entertainment content or counteradvertising as solutions to the negative impact of media exposure on the health of children (Sidney and others, 1994; Stevens, 1990).

Applications in the Planned Use of Media

Studies have also examined the positive effects of media use on health (Barker, Pistrang, Shapiro, Davies, and Shaw, 1993; Suman and Rossman, 2000). These studies note that whereas mass media, especially television, may have negative impact, they can and should be used to create positive impact in public health. This view especially imbues the second dimension of media studies and health: effects of the purposive use of media in the context of planned interventions.

The planned use of media communication to accomplish some health outcome predates the founding of the United States itself (Paisley, 1989). This American penchant for public media campaigns continues unabated today but with a deeper understanding of, and more systematic approach to, the role of planning.

Many of the media communication theories discussed earlier are relevant to public health community-based campaigns. In intervention planning models (discussed in Part Five), many media studies theories are useful in formative-analysis and strategy-development stages, and in evaluating outcomes. In this section we provide examples of such applications.

Heart Disease Prevention and Media Communication. Beginning in the 1950s, epidemiological studies discovered that rates of heart disease varied greatly around the world. It became apparent that these differences were due largely to socially acculturated behavior patterns (Kromhout, Menotti, and Blackburn, 1994). To reduce mass levels of disease, investigators reasoned, would require multiple prevention strategies aimed at change in whole populations. The rationale underlying this approach was a chain of causal links hypothesizing that increasing exposure to such a campaign would increase participation and involvement leading to behavior change (Mittelmark and others, 1986). This in turn would result in increasing change in heart disease risk factors and eventually disease reduction.

In the United States, federally funded communitywide prevention campaigns were started by investigators in California, Minnesota, and Rhode Island. Multiple strategies were used, in which media communication played an important role. The idea of using multiple strategies was also informed by the idea of synergy. That is, strategies used together are more powerful in accomplishing behavior change than if each were used alone (the effect of the whole being greater than the sum of the parts). This is based on the idea that each individual strategy has strengths and weaknesses in the achievement of health behavior change. For example, group educational settings (such as classes) are strong in presenting an intensive, interactive experience but weak in their capacity to reach a high proportion of the population. Mass media, on the other hand, are strong in their capacity to reach large numbers of people but weaker in their capacity to provide an intense, interactive experience. Campaign-planning frameworks seek to offset this individual weakness through the strengths of diverse strategies.

Media were used initially in each of the campaigns to increase public awareness of the problem of heart disease, its major risk factors and associated lifestyle change strategies, and the programs themselves. In this sense, media were used first to build the community agenda for heart disease prevention as a major concern worthy of public attention. A strength of mass media is their capacity to expose many persons simultaneously to the same information, and thus it is not surprising that public awareness of prevention messages and programs increased dramatically and rapidly (Viswanath, Finnegan, Hertog, Pirie, and Murray, 1994). A key issue for these and all public health campaigns is the extent to which they attain exposure of all socioeconomic status segments of the community because exposure is regarded as a contingent condition for some kind of effect to occur (McGuire, 1989). Yet health campaign planners are confronted with a number of important factors that influence exposure leading to behavior change. As the knowledge gap makes clear, the tendency is for higher-SES groups to acquire more information faster than lower-SES groups. Also, people living in communities of varying size and complexity may be differentially exposed to campaigns because of differences in communication systems. This requires health campaign planners to ensure in the development and evaluation of campaigns that social-structural factors are considered, so that they do not pose serious barriers to the diffusion of exposure, other intermediate effects, and behavioral outcomes.

Exposure and Cardiovascular Disease Prevention Information. In the heart disease prevention campaigns, a number of studies examined the question of exposure, intermediate effects such as the distribution of prevention information, and behavioral change itself. To measure intermediate exposure to the campaign, the Minnesota program tracked changes in community awareness and the ability of the public to recall the program name. Of course, neither of these intermediate outcomes was necessary to achieve behavioral change, but they functioned importantly as a process measure of campaign delivery. That is, due to the campaign, were people aware of the cardiovascular disease (CVD) prevention activity, and could they recall (unaided) the name of the specific institutional source of this activity? More important, did these effects vary by SES group?

During the five-year campaign, random population surveys were conducted in each of three communities about every six months to monitor such changes (Viswanath, Finnegan, Hertog, Pirie, and Murray, 1994). Awareness in the smallest community (population 28,651) increased rapidly from 42 percent at six months to a peak of 91 percent at three years and 88 percent at five years. In the regional community (population 137,574), awareness increased from 30 percent at six months to a peak of about 86 percent at two years and 76 percent at five years. In the suburb (population 81,831), awareness increased from about 30 percent at six months to a peak of 84 percent at three years and 71 percent at five years. Recall of the program name grew at about the same rate but was lower in each community overall due certainly to the more difficult task of recalling a name without prompting. The data were suggestive of the more difficult task posed in conducting campaigns in more complex communities. In the regional community and the suburb (part of a metropolitan area of two million), much more media communication was required to maintain levels of awareness and name recall, which in any case were somewhat lower than the smallest community in the study. The level of media communication required was more intense due to the complexity of the larger communities: there are more available channels and more "noise" and distractions than in the smallest community. But what about effects by SES segment?

The study showed that, as predicted by the knowledge gap, CVD awareness and program name recall were highest among high-SES groups (measured by formal education) over the course of the five years. However, importantly, the less educated groups showed net gains that were actually larger than the highest group. So although the gaps still existed, the campaign succeeded in narrowing them to a great extent as the result of targeted communication efforts (Finnegan, Viswanath, Kahn, and Hannan, 1993). Moreover, it is important to recognize that changes among lower-SES groups can and do occur but frequently lag behind higher-SES groups. In our view, the reason for this is primarily one of equal access to channels of communication and education, which even further raises the importance of channel-influence analysis in campaign planning stages—that is, What channels are used most and are most effective with which groups (Finnegan, Viswanath, Kahn, and Hannan, 1993)?

Future Directions

There are several important issues in the application of media studies theory in health that will continue to influence research in the new century. The first is continuing study of the media's influence on vulnerable audiences such as children and adolescents. Today, people are exposed to television unrelentingly almost from birth and now face heavy exposure to the Internet and other new information technologies. While we recognize that the media have powerful socializing effects for good, we also recognize that the media's purpose is not primarily to support the goals of public health improvement. The media's goals frequently collide with the goals of public health. Can the mass media as message producers be encouraged to do a better job—for example, to improve content beneficial to public health goals?

The answer is an equivocal "maybe." There have been successes, notably efforts by public health advocates to encourage television producers to include positive messages in their programs. Further successes in encouraging the media to modify content at odds with public health will depend in large measure on the effectiveness of public health advocates in building relationships with the media for such changes.

A second issue that will continue in the new century is the planned use of mass media to achieve health behavior change. Specifically, community health settings will continue to provide an ideal environment to examine communication effects across levels of analysis. Of particular interest is how communication at each level of analysis may influence or link to communication at other levels. There undoubtedly are both structural- and individual-level factors responsible. The power of any single channel of communication (mass media or interpersonal) may depend on the complexity of the behavior change being sought (Bandura, 1994). On one hand, the less complex the change, the more the influence of a single channel leading to performance of the behavior (Bandura, 1994). On the other hand, the more complex the behavior, the greater the need for multiple exposure to multiple sources. In this setting, the influence of any single channel is relatively less.

Third is the issue of health disparities and how communication may be both a contributory cause and a contributory solution. *Healthy People 2010* (U.S. Department of Health and Human Services, 2000), which guides the nation's health objectives for the decade, declared elimination of racial- and socioeconomic-based health disparities as one of its major goals. Studies show that minorities and families with lower income and education suffer from a greater disease burden compared with whites and those with higher income and education. They are also less often exposed to prevention information, despite the fact that the current media environment is rich in channels and information. While new communication technologies such as the World Wide Web provide new sources of health information (Rainie and others, 2001), it is clear that not all Americans are benefiting equally. Studies have drawn attention to the "digital divide," which shows less access to new technologies among the poor (U.S. Department of Commerce, 2000; Viswanath, McDonald, and Lavrakas, 2000). The issue of quality of access is a related concern.

Finally, in light of the current preference in public health for community-based interventions, is there a place for national media campaigns in public health? Some suggest that national campaigns are a waste of time and that resources could be better spent mobilizing local communities for health behavior change. Our judgment is that national media campaigns are important because they help build a national prevention agenda on specific issues. They can amplify local prevention efforts that are typically more targeted and intense. The most suitable issues for national media campaigns are those that are of concern to every community, big or small. But national media campaigns should not be regarded as a substitute for community prevention, nor should they be expected in themselves to accomplish widespread behavior change without local partnerships.

References

American Academy of Pediatrics, Committee on Public Education. "Media Education." *Pediatrics*, August 1999, *104*(2), 341–343.

Ammerman, R. T., Ott, P. J., and Tarter, R. E. (eds.). *Prevention and Societal Impact of Drug and Alcohol Abuse*. Mahwah, N.J.: Erlbaum, 1999.

Bandura, A. "Social Cognitive Theory of Mass Communication." In J. Bryant and D. Zillmann (eds.), *Media Effects: Advances in Theory and Research*. Mahwah, N.J. Erlbaum, 1994.

Barker, C., Pistrang, N., Shapiro, D. A., Davies, S., and Shaw, I. "You in Mind: A Preventive Mental-Health Television Series." *British Journal of Clinical Psychology*, September, 1993, *32*(3), 281–293.

Beniger, J. R., and Gusek, J. A. "The Cognitive Revolution in Public Opinion and Communication Research." In T. L. Glasser and C. T. Salmon (eds.), *Public Opinion and the Communication of Consent*. New York: Guilford Press, 1995.

Berelson, B. "Communications and Public Opinion." In W. Schramm (ed.), *Communications in Modern Society*. Urbana, Ill.: University of Illinois Press, 1948.

Berger, P. L., and Luckmann, T. *The Social Construction of Reality: A Treatise in the Sociology of Knowledge*. New York: Doubleday, 1966.

Blumler, J. G., and Katz, E. (eds.). *The Uses of Mass Communication: Current Perspectives on Gratifications Research.* Thousand Oaks, Calif.: Sage, 1974.

Bryant, J., and Zillman, D. (eds.). *Media Effects: Advances in Theory and Research.* Mahwah, N.J.: Erlbaum, 1994.

Caswell, S., and Zhang, J. F. "Impact of the Liking for Advertising and Brand Allegiance on Drinking and Alcohol-Related Aggression: A Longitudinal Study." *Addiction,* August 1998, *93*(8), 1209–1217.

Chaffee, S., and Roser, C. "Involvement and Consistency of Knowledge, Attitudes and Behaviors." *Communication Research,* 1986, *13*(3), 373–400.

Chiricos, T., Eschholz, S., and Gertz, M. "Crime, News and Fear of Crime: Toward an Identification of Audience Effects." *Social Problems,* August 1997, *44*(3), 342–357.

Clarke, P., and Evans, S. "Field Definitions: Mass Communication." In *1984–85 U.S. Directory of Graduate Programs.* Princeton, N.J.: Educational Testing Services, 1983.

DeFleur, M., and Dennis, E. *Understanding Mass Communication.* (2nd ed.) Boston: Houghton-Mifflin, 1985.

Demers, D., Craff, D., Choi, Y. H., and Pessin, B. M. "Issue's Obtrusiveness and the Agenda-Setting Effect of National Network News." *Communication Research,* 1989, *16,* 793–812.

Donohue, G. A., Tichenor, P. J., and Olien, C. N. "Mass Media and the Knowledge Gap: A Hypothesis Reconsidered." *Communication Research,* 1975, *2,* 3–23.

Donohue, G. A., Tichenor, P. J., and Olien, C. N. "A Guard Dog Perspective on the Role of Media." *Journal of Communication,* 1995, *45*(2), 115–132.

Dorfman, L., Woodruff, K., Chavez, V., and Wallack, L. "Youth Violence on Local Television News in California." *American Journal of Public Health,* 1979, *87,* 1311–1316.

Emery, M., Emery, E., and Roberts, N. L. *The Press and America: An Interpretive History of the Mass Media.* Boston: Allyn & Bacon, 1996.

Entman, R. M. "Framing: Toward Clarification of a Fractured Paradigm." *Journal of Communication,* 1993, *43*(4), 51–58.

Ettema, J. S., Brown, J., and Luepker, R. V. "Knowledge Gap Effects in a Health Information Campaign." *Public Opinion Quarterly,* 1983, *47,* 516–527.

Ettema, J. S., and Kline, F. G. "Deficits, Differences and Ceilings: Contingent Conditions for Understanding the Knowledge Gap." *Communication Research,* 1977, *4,* 179–202.

Federal Trade Commission. *Marketing Violent Entertainment to Children: A Review of Self-Regulation and Industry Practices in the Motion Picture, Music Recording, and Electronic Games Industries.* Washington, D.C.: Federal Trade Commission, September 2000. Available at http://www.ftc.gov/opa/2000/09/youthviol.htm.

Felson, R. "Mass Media Effects on Violent Behavior." *Annual Review of Sociology,* 1996, *22,* 103–128.

Finnegan, J. R., and Viswanath, K. "Health and Communication: Medical and Public Health Influences on the Research Agenda." In E. Berlin-Ray and L. Donohew (eds.), *Communication and Health: Systems and Applications.* Mahwah, N.J.: Erlbaum, 1989.

Finnegan, J. R., Viswanath, K., Kahn, E., and Hannan, P. "Exposure to Sources of Heart Disease Prevention Information: Community Type and Social Group Differences." *Journalism Quarterly,* 1993, *70,* 569–584.

Fischoff, B. "Why Cancer Risk Communication Can Be Hard." *The Journal of National Cancer Institute Monographs,* 1999, *25,* 7–13.

Fowles, J. *The Case for Television Violence.* Thousand Oaks, Calif.: Sage, 1999.

Fredin, E., Monnett, T. H., and Kosicki, G. M. "Knowledge Gaps, Social Locators, and Media Schemata: Gaps, Reverse Gaps, and Gaps of Disaffection." *Journalism Quarterly,* 1994, *71,* 176–190.

Gamson, W., and Modigliani, A. "The Changing Culture of Affirmative Action." In R. G. Braungart and M. M. Braungart (eds.), *Research in Political Sociology.* (Vol. 3) Greenwich, Conn.: JAI Press, 1987.

Gandy, O. H., Jr. *Beyond Agenda-Setting.* Norwood, N.J.: Ablex, 1982.

Gaziano, C. "Knowledge Gap: An Analytical Review of Media Effects." *Communication Research,* 1983, *10,* 447–486.

Gaziano, C. "Community Knowledge Gaps." *Critical Studies in Mass Communication,* 1988, *5,* 351–357.

Gerbner, G. "Field Definitions: Communication Theory." In *1984–85 U.S. Directory of Graduate Programs.* Princeton, N.J.: Educational Testing Services, 1985.

Gerbner, G. "New Television Rating System Is Extremely Flawed." *The Progressive.* http://www.progressive.org/mpgerbnermrch98.htm. Viewed March 10, 1998.

Gerbner, G., Gross, L., Morgan, M., and Signorielli, N. "The 'Mainstreaming' of America: Violence Profile no. 11." *Journal of Communication,* 1980, *30,* 10–29.

Gerbner, G., Gross, L., Morgan, M., and Signorelli, N. "Growing Up with Television: The Cultivation Perspective." In J. Bryant and D. Zillmann (eds.), *Media Effects: Advances in Theory and Research.* Mahwah, N.J.: Erlbaum, 1994.

Glanz, K., and Yang, H. "Communicating About Risk of Infectious Diseases." *Journal of the American Medical Association,* 1996, *275*(3), 253–256.

Glassner, B. *The Culture of Fear: Why Americans Are Afraid of the Wrong Things.* New York: Basic Books, 1999.

Griffin, R. "Energy in the Eighties: Education, Communication and the Knowledge Gap." *Journalism Quarterly,* 1990, *67,* 554–566.

Griswold, W., and Packer, C. "The Interplay of Journalistic and Scientific Conventions in Mass Communication About AIDS." *Mass Communication Review,* 1991, *18*(3), 9–20, 47.

Grube, J. W., and Wallack, L. "Television Beer Advertising and Drinking Knowledge, Beliefs, and Intentions Among Schoolchildren." *American Journal of Public Health,* February 1994, *84*(2), 254–259.

Hawkins, R. P., Weimann, J. M., and Pingree, S. (eds.). *Advancing Communication Science: Merging Mass and Interpersonal Processes.* Thousand Oaks, Calif.: Sage, 1988.

Hilgartner, S., and Bosk, C. L. "The Rise and Fall of Social Problems: Public Arenas Model." *American Journal of Sociology,* 1988, *94,* 53–77.

Hogben, M. "Factors Moderating the Effects of Televised Aggression on Viewer Behavior." *Communication Research,* April 1998, *25*(2), 220–247.

Hovland, C. I., Janis, I. L., and Kelley, H. H. *Communication and Persuasion: Psychological Studies of Opinion Change.* Westport, Conn.: Greenwood Press, 1953.

Hyman, H. H., and Sheatsley, P. B. "Some Reasons Why Information Campaigns Fail." *Public Opinion Quarterly,* 1947, *11,* 412–423.

Iyengar, S., and Kinder, D. R. *News That Matters.* Chicago: University of Chicago Press, 1987.

Kaiser Family Foundation. *Kids and the Media @ the New Millennium.* Publication no. 1536. Menlo Park, Calif.: Kaiser Family Foundation, 1999. http://www.kff.org

Kelly, P. T. *Television Violence: A Guide to the Literature.* Commack, N.Y.: Nova Science Publishers, 1996.

Kosicki, G. M. "Problems and Opportunities in Agenda-Setting Research." *Journal of Communication,* 1993, *43,* 100–127.

Kromhout, D., Menotti, A., and Blackburn, H. B. *The Seven Countries Study: A Scientific Adventure in Cardiovascular Disease Epidemiology.* Utrecht, The Netherlands: Brouwer Offset, 1994.

Lasswell, H. D. "The Structure and Function of Communication in Society." In L. Bryson (ed.), *The Communication of Ideas.* New York: Institute for Religious and Social Studies, 1948.

Lazarsfeld, P., Berelson, B., and Gaudet, H. *The People's Choice*. New York: Columbia University Press, 1948.

Lee, C. C. *Media Imperialism Reconsidered*. Thousand Oaks, Calif.: Sage, 1980.

Lipkus, I. M., Rimer, B. K., Halabi, S., and Strigo, T. S. "Can Tailored Interventions Increase Mammography Use Among HMO Women?" *American Journal of Preventive Medicine*, 2001, *18*(1), 1–10.

Lippmann, W. *Public Opinion*. New York: MacMillan, 1922.

Livingstone, S., and Bovill, M. (eds.). *Children and Their Changing Media: A European Comparative Study*. Mahwah, N.J.: Erlbaum, 2001.

Maibach, E. "Cancer Risk Communication: What We Need to Learn." *Journal of the National Cancer Institute, Monographs*, 1999, *25*, 179–181.

McCombs, M. E., and Shaw, D. "The Agenda-Setting Function of the Mass Media." *Public Opinion Quarterly*, 1972, *36*, 176–187.

McGuire, W. J. "Public Communication as a Strategy for Inducing Health Behavior Change." *Preventive Medicine*, 1984, *13*, 299–319.

McGuire, W. J. "Attitudes and Attitude Change." In G. Lindzey and E. Aronson (eds.), *Handbook of Social Psychology*. (3rd ed., Vol. 2) New York: Random House, 1985.

McGuire, W. J. "Theoretical Foundations of Campaigns." In R. E. Rice and C. K. Atkin (eds.), *Public Communication Campaigns*. (2nd ed.) Thousand Oaks, Calif.: Sage, 1989.

McLeod, J. M., Kosicki, G. M., and Pan, Z. "On Understanding and Misunderstanding Media Effects." In J. Curran and M. Gurevitch (eds.), *Mass Media and Society*. London: Edward Arnold, 1991.

McLeod, J. M., and Perse, E. M. "Direct and Indirect Effects of Socioeconomic Status on Public Affairs Knowledge." *Journalism Quarterly*, 1994, *71*, 433–442.

Mittelmark, M. B., and others. "Community-Wide Prevention of Cardiovascular Disease: Education Strategies of the Minnesota Heart Health Program." *Preventive Medicine*, 1986, *15*(1), 1–17.

Mosteller, F., and Moynihan, D. P. *On Equality of Educational Opportunity*. New York: Random House, 1972.

Myers, P. N., and Biocca, F. A. "The Elastic Body Image: The Effect of Television Advertising and Programming on Body Image Distortions in Young Women." *Journal of Communication*, June 1992, *42*(3), 108–133.

Paisley, W. "Public Communication Campaigns: The American Experience." In R. E. Rice and C. K. Atkin (eds.), *Public Communication Campaigns*. (2nd ed.) Thousand Oaks, Calif.: Sage, 1989.

Perloff, R. M. *The Dynamics of Persuasion*. Mahwah, N.J.: Erlbaum, 1993.

Petty, R. E., and Cacioppo, J. T. *Attitudes and Persuasion: Classic and Contemporary Approaches*. Dubuque, Iowa: William C. Brown, 1981.

Potter, J. *On Media Violence*. Thousand Oaks, Calif.: Sage, 1999.

Rainie, L., and others. "More Online, Doing More: 16 Million Newcomers Gain Internet Access in the Last Half of 2000 as Women, Minorities, and Families with Modest Incomes Continue to Surge Online." Washington, D.C.: The Pew Internet & American Life Project, February 2001. Available online at http://www.pewinternet.org/

Ray, M., Sawyer, A., Rothschild, M., Heeler, R., Strong, E., and Reed, J. "Marketing Communication and the Hierarchy of Effects." In P. Clarke (ed.), *New Models for Mass Communication Research*. Thousand Oaks, Calif.: Sage, 1973.

Rimer, B. K., Glanz, K., and Rasband, G. "Searching for Evidence About Health Education and Health Behavior Interventions." *Health Education & Behavior,* 2001, *28*(2), 231–248.

Rimer, B. K., and Glassman, B. "Is There a Use for Tailored Print Communications in Cancer Risk Communication?" *The Journal of National Cancer Institute Monographs,* 1999, *25,* 140–148.

Robinson, T. N., Chen, H. L., and Killen, J. "Television and Music Video Exposure and Risk of Adolescent Alcohol Use." *Pediatrics,* November 1998, *102*(5), E541–E546.

Rogers, E. M. *Diffusion of Innovations.* (4th ed.) New York: Free Press, 1995.

Rogers, E. M., and Storey, J. D. "Communication Campaigns." In C. R. Berger and S. H. Chaffee (eds.), *Handbook of Communication Science.* Thousand Oaks, Calif.: Sage, 1987.

Roloff, M. E., and Miller, G. R. (eds.). *Persuasion: New Directions in Theory and Research.* Thousand Oaks, Calif.: Sage, 1980.

Roshco, B. *Newsmaking.* Chicago: University of Chicago Press, 1975.

Sandman, P. M. "Apathy Versus Hysteria: Public Perception of Risk." In L. R. Batra and W. Klassen (eds.), *Public Perception of Biotechnology.* Bethesda, Md.: Agricultural Research Institute, 1987.

Shinghi, P., and Mody, B. "The Communication Effects Gap: A Field Experiment on Television and Agricultural Ignorance in India." *Communication Research,* 1976, *3,* 171–190.

Shoemaker, P. J. *Gatekeeping.* Thousand Oaks, Calif.: Sage, 1991.

Sidney, S., and others. "Television Viewing and Cardiovascular Risk Factors in Young Adults: The CARDIA Study." *Annals of Epidemiology,* March 1996, *6*(2), 154–159.

Sigal, L. V. *Reporters and Officials: The Organization and Politics of Newsmaking.* Lexington, Mass.: Heath, 1973.

Sigal, L. V. "Sources Make the News." In K. Manoff and M. Schudson (eds.), *Reading the News.* New York: Pantheon, 1987.

Singer, D. G., and Singer, J. L. (eds.). *Handbook of Children and the Media.* Thousand Oaks, Calif.: Sage, 2001.

Slovic, P., Fischoff, B., and Lichtenstein, S. "Perceived Risk: Psychological Factors and Social Implications." In F. Warner and D. H. Slater (eds.), *The Assessment and Perception of Risk.* London: The Royal Society, 1981.

Snyder, H. N., Sickmund, M., and Bilchik, S. *Juvenile Offenders and Victims: 1999 National Report.* Washington, D.C.: U.S. Department of Justice, 1999. Available at http://www.ncjrs.org/html/ojjdp/nationalreport99/toc.html

Snyder, L. B. "Channel Effectiveness Over Time and Knowledge and Behavior Gaps." *Journalism Quarterly,* 1990, *67,* 875–886.

Stevens, C. "Designing an Effective Counteradvertising Campaign—California." *Cancer,* 1998, *83*(12 Supplement), 2736–2741.

Stossel, S. "The Man Who Counts the Killings." *Atlantic Monthly* (Atlantic Online), May 1997. Available online at http://www.theatlantic.com/issues/97may/gerbner.htm

Suman, M., and Rossman, G. (eds.). *Advocacy Groups and the Entertainment Industry.* Westport, Conn.: Praeger, 2000.

Tichenor, P. J., Donohue, G. A., and Olien, C. N. "Mass Media Flow and Differential Growth in Knowledge." *Public Opinion Quarterly,* 1970, *34,* 159–170.

Tichenor, P. J., Donohue, G. A., and Olien, C. N. *Community Conflict and the Press.* Thousand Oaks, Calif.: Sage, 1980.

Tuchman, G. *Making News: A Study in the Construction of Reality.* New York: Free Press, 1978.

Turow, J. *Media Systems in Society: Understanding Industries, Strategies, and Power.* New York: Longman, 1992.

U.S. Department of Commerce. *Falling Through the Net: Towards Digital Inclusion: A Report on Americans' Access to Technology Tools.* Washington, D.C.: Department of Commerce, 2000.

U.S. Department of Health, Education, and Welfare. *Television and Growing Up: The Impact of Televised Violence. Report to the Surgeon General, United States Public Health Service.* Rockville, Md.: National Institute of Mental Health, U.S. Department of Health, Education, and Welfare, 1972.

U.S. Department of Health and Human Services. *Healthy People 2010: Understanding and Improving Health.* Washington, D.C.: Department of Health and Human Services, 2000. Available online at http://www.health.gov/healthypeople/

Viswanath, K. *Knowledge Gap Effects in a Cardiovascular Disease Prevention Campaign: A Longitudinal Study of Two Community Pairs.* Ph.D. Dissertation. Minneapolis, Minn.: University of Minnesota, 1990.

Viswanath, K., and Demers, D. "Mass Media from a Macrosocial Perspective." In D. Demers and K. Viswanath (eds.), *Mass Media, Social Control, and Social Change: A Macrosocial Perspective.* Ames, Iowa: Iowa State University Press, 1999.

Viswanath, K., and Finnegan, J. R. "The Knowledge Gap Hypothesis: Twenty-Five Years Later." In B. Burleson (ed.), *Communication Yearbook.* (Vol. 19) Thousand Oaks, Calif.: Sage, 1996.

Viswanath, K., Finnegan, J. R., Hannan, P. J., and Luepker, R. V. "Health and Knowledge Gaps: Some Lessons from the Minnesota Heart Health Program." *American Behavioral Scientist,* 1991, *34,* 712–726.

Viswanath, K., Finnegan, J. R., Hertog, J., Pirie, P., and Murray, D. "Community Type and the Diffusion of Campaign Information." *Gazette,* 1994, *54,* 39–59.

Viswanath, K., Kahn, E., Finnegan, J. R., Hertog, J., and Potter, J. "Motivation and the "Knowledge Gap": Effects of a Campaign to Reduce Diet-Related Cancer Risk." *Communication Research,* 1993, *20,* 546–563.

Viswanath, K., McDonald, D. G., and Lavrakas, P. J. "Class Versus Place: Contrasting Models of Diffusion and Adoption of New Communication Technologies." Paper presented at the 55th annual AAPOR Conference, Portland, Oregon, May 18–21, 2000.

Weimann, G. *Communicating Unreality: Modern Media and the Reconstruction of Reality.* Thousand Oaks, Calif.: Sage, 2000.

Weinstein, N. D. "Why It Won't Happen to Me: Perceptions of Risk Factors and Susceptibility." *Health Psychology,* 1984, *3,* 431–457.

Weinstein, N. D. "Perceived Probability, Perceived Severity, and Health-Protective Behavior." *Health Psychology,* 2000, *19*(1), 65–74.

Willis, E., and Strasburger, V. C. "Media Violence." *Pediatric Clinics of North America,* 1998, *45*(2), 319ff.

Wilson, B. J., and others. (eds.). *The National Television Violence Study.* (Vols. 1 and 2) Thousand Oaks, Calif.: Sage, 1997.

Yows, S., Salmon, C. T., Hawkins, R., and Love, R. "Motivational and Structural Factors in Predicting Different Kinds of Cancer Knowledge." *American Behavioral Scientist,* 1991, *34,* 727–741.

Zandpour, F., and Fellow, A. R. "Knowledge Gap Effects: Audience and Media Factors in Alcohol-Related Health Communication." *Mass Communication Review,* 1992, *19*(3), 34–41.

CHAPTER SEVENTEEN

PERSPECTIVES ON GROUP, ORGANIZATION, AND COMMUNITY INTERVENTIONS

Karen Glanz

The chapters in Part Four have presented four models for health behavior change in groups, organizations, and communities. The aim of these chapters is to demonstrate the utility and promise of each theory or framework in health behavior and health education. This chapter highlights new concepts and strategies included in this third edition of *Health Behavior and Health Education,* discusses similarities among the models, draws common themes, and critiques their usefulness for research and practice in health promotion.

The central theme of Part Four is that we need to understand, predict, and know how to work with people through the social structures that are the context for their health behavior. We also need to be able to foster change and to assist populations in their efforts to create healthier institutions and communities. The concepts of social networks, change within and among systems, organizational processes, and communication channels are apparent across each of the chapters.

New Concepts and Strategies for Macro-Level Change

The chapters in this section bring together longstanding ideas with new concepts and strategies for understanding behavior and facilitating change. In Chapter Thirteen, Minkler and Wallerstein update the idea of distinct models of community organization and explain that there is an increasing emphasis on combining more than one model, for example social action plus locality development. They also note that the concept of community building is increasingly recognized as part of mainstream public policy development by government agencies and philanthropic foundations. The renewed emphasis on social capital is discussed as similar to the idea of community capacity. Chapter Thirteen also discusses new developments in measurement and evaluation of community organization and related processes. Emerging methodologies and crosscutting research issues will be discussed later in this chapter.

Chapter Fourteen, by Oldenburg and Parcel, analyzes Diffusion Theory, its main concepts, and its applications in school and worksite settings. This chapter is particularly noteworthy because one of its authors is from Australia and the other from the United States; they demonstrate that some organizational issues cross geographical boundaries and that many health education challenges are shared internationally. The authors also examine diffusion as a multilevel change process and underscore the organizational processes of adoption and implementation.

Steckler, Goodman, and Kegler present and analyze three theories of organizational change in Chapter Fifteen: Stage Theory, Organizational Development Theory, and Interorganizational Relations Theory. Stage Theory has much in common with Diffusion Theory. Interorganizational Relations Theory overlaps with community organizing and community building and thus reveals how these models are complementary. This chapter raises intriguing questions about the uncontrollability of many aspects of community health practice, as well as about what types of outcomes health promotion experts need to examine.

In Chapter Sixteen, Finnegan and Viswanath synthesize the extensive literature on communication theories and focus on theories and hypotheses with special relevance to public health and health behavior change. They emphasize the Media Studies Framework as distinct from interpersonal communication (which is covered in Part Three). Four media effects perspectives are introduced: the knowledge gap hypothesis, agenda setting, cultivation studies, and risk communication. These models cut across a range of considerations about mass media: its differential impact on high and low socioeconomic status populations; its application in social action and advocacy; its impact on people's worldviews; and its relationship to health risks, especially those risks with broad public health implications.

These four chapters offer expanded and updated coverage of long-standing theory, research, and practice in health education and also introduce new concepts and strategies. The constraints of the present chapter preclude in-depth coverage of all the issues at hand. However, this synthesis focuses on similarities among the models, draws common themes, and critiques their usefulness for research and practice in health behavior and health education.

Multiple Levels of Influence and Action

A central premise of this book is that improvements in health require both an understanding of the multilevel determinants of health behavior and a range of change strategies at the individual, interpersonal, and macro levels (Marmot, 2000). Critiques of the tendency for health education and health promotion programs to focus excessively on individuals abound in the literature (Orleans, Gruman, Ulmer, Emont, and Hollendonner, 1999; Smedley and Syme, 2000). Indeed there is substantial overlap between public health and health promotion approaches and disease prevention and control strategies in clinical settings (Rimer, Glanz, and Lerman, 1991). Nevertheless, the view that societal-level changes and supportive environments are necessary to address major health problems successfully *and* to maintain individual-level behavioral changes is now widely endorsed (Smedley and Syme, 2000; McKinlay and Marceau, 2000; Emmons, 2000). The chapters in this section clearly exemplify a multilevel perspective, which builds on intrapersonal and interpersonal theories to explain or affect community change.

Minkler and Wallerstein describe the Adolescent Social Action Program (ASAP) as drawing on Protection Motivation Theory, an individual-level model, along with empowerment education and community-building approaches. Oldenburg and Parcel describe a cardiovascular risk-reduction intervention in school settings that was based on Social Cognitive Theory (Parcel and others, 1995). Steckler, Goodman, and Kegler begin with the premise that organizations have multiple levels or layers, and carry through with the theme of the ecology of organizations. Finally, Finnegan and Viswanath organize their review of communication studies according to multiple levels, from intrapersonal processes (for example, information processing) and interpersonal interactions (for example, patient-provider communication) to the level of community and macro social structure. They advance the central thesis that various levels of analysis are appropriate to considering various types of effects and aims of interventions.

An important message at the heart of these chapters is that the broader, community- or organization-level models and concepts are not intended to stand alone at the expense of neglecting the individuals comprised in groups, organizations, and communities. Nor should the charge of excessive focus on individuals cause us to turn away from well-established theories and strategies. It is collectives of *individuals* who create organizational structures, provide leadership in communities, choose to participate—or not participate—in coalitions, and make decisions about local, state, and federal policies and priorities. Also, it would be a mistake to assume that the answers to all health promotion challenges lie in policy development, social action, and environmental change. For example, a recent evaluation of thirty-seven community AIDS prevention projects found that the health promotion strategies rated most effective were small-group discussions, outreach workers, trained peers or volunteers, and the provision of safer-sex kits. These small-group and individually oriented strategies were also more likely to be implemented, in contrast with education of policymakers and protest marches, which were either seldom done or were rated ineffective (Janz and others, 1996). Thus, the most suitable approaches, and not necessarily the most far-reaching methods, should be adopted for health behavior change initiatives.

Models for Change

The chapters in Part Four examine models for community activation, planned change, and collaboration.

Community Activation and Planned Change

Two general domains help define the scope of the models that are included in this section: social activation and processes for changing attitudes, behaviors, and policies. The former is usually characterized by internal or intragroup stimuli for change, whereas the latter are more likely to inform external change agents about how to facilitate changes that they identify a need for or deem desirable. None of the models is pure in this sense, but all break down roughly into these categories. These generalized approaches reflect implicit assumptions about power and social control versus empowerment and self-control.

Social activation is central to community organization, organizational development, interorganizational relations, and media advocacy. As Minkler and Wallerstein note in Chapter Thirteen, several of the key principles of community organizing relate directly to creating the conditions for change: empowerment, community competence, and the principles of participation and relevance. Two of the three models of community organization originally proposed by Rothman (2001)—locality (community) development and social action, as well as community building—stress consensus, cooperation, group identity, and mutual problem solving.

Organizational Development (OD) Theory aims to improve organizational performance and the quality of work life. Its roots are in human relations and humanistic psychology. It is concerned with members of organizations, and organizational problems are diagnosed by gathering information directly from the members or workers through formal surveys, interviews, and other methods. OD interventions include strategies such as team building, group development, and T-groups to promote interpersonal exchanges. As Steckler, Goodman, and Kegler point out in Chapter Fifteen, face-to-face contact and group interaction are integral to this approach.

Agenda-setting approaches to media communication involve telling people *what to think about*. Media advocacy strategies are an extension of these techniques, in which advocacy groups in the community define, identify, and frame a problem and stimulate media coverage of the problem as a public health issue (Wallack, 1990). Media advocacy activates forces in a social system (that is, media coverage) to help stimulate public concern and action.

Processes for facilitating large-scale *changes in attitudes and behaviors* are the province of Diffusion Theory, Stage Theory of Organizational Change, and the branch of communication studies that emphasizes changes in cognitions, beliefs, and behavior. Each of these frameworks offers guideposts for professionals wishing to promote specific changes in individuals in a larger society and within organizations. The term *diffusion of innovations* describes the spread of ideas, products, and behaviors within a society or from one society or social system to another. Stage Theory is closely allied to diffusion of innovations because it focuses on understanding and matching the organizational stages of change with efforts to introduce or encourage organizational change. The communication studies areas of message production and media effects are rooted in theory and research on communication and persuasion dating back to the work of Lasswell (1948) and Hovland, Janis, and Kelley (1953) almost fifty years ago.

These contrasting orientations to change—social activation and planned change—raise issues about power and control, who defines needs and problems, and the extent to which existing institutions (including the mass media) act as instruments of social control. As Kipnis (1994) noted, there has been a recent surge in behavioral techniques based on reducing restraints against change (for example, social support, empowerment, personal growth) rather than pushing people to change. But even when these methods are used to promote social justice, there remains an exercise of power that may be disquieting to some audiences (Kipnis, 1994). Of particular interest is the paradox that Minkler and Wallerstein suggest: that community needs and wants should be superceded by social justice concerns in cases in which communities are mobilizing to restrict civil rights (such as anti–gay rights legislation). This underscores the dilemma faced by professionals whose personal values are not consistent with those of a given community.

Collaboration

Collaboration, through partnerships of health promotion experts and other providers (such as educators, medical personnel, media producers), or through coalitions with interorganizational representation, emerges as a strategy for change across the chapters of Part Four. The relevance of social support and social networks concepts underpins these strategies. It is logical to expect that there is strength in numbers and that partnerships and coalitions can mobilize material and human resources and be more effective at achieving desired goals than individuals working alone. Collaborations also have enormous potential for community and systems change; they can achieve valued public health outcomes while also transforming power relations and revitalizing a sense of shared power and shared responsibility (Himmelman, 1992). Yet collaborative efforts are complex, successful coalitions are not easy to develop, and the processes and outcomes of collaboration may be imperfectly correlated. There is a small but growing literature that may reveal the best practices in developing partnerships and helping them to succeed in achieving desirable changes. Minkler and Wallerstein describe an increased emphasis on coalition effectiveness, as distinct from merely forming coalitions.

Interorganizational Relations (IOR) Theory, discussed in Chapter Fifteen, articulates several stages for developing and sustaining community coalitions. The extent of external control and coalition structures affect the task orientation, extent of conflict, and effectiveness of coalitions. Butterfoss, Goodman, and Wandersman (1996) studied the determinants of participation and satisfaction in coalitions for alcohol, tobacco, and other drug abuse prevention, and their association with the quality of resultant plans. Community leadership, shared decision making, linkages with other organizations, and a positive organizational climate were correlated with participation and satisfaction among coalition members. However, neither these factors nor satisfaction were related to the quality of coalition plans (Butterfoss, Goodman, and Wandersman, 1996). Similarly, the example in Chapter Fifteen showed that the Data-Based Intervention Research (DBIR) model for cancer prevention and control was not very successful at improving the health departments' program planning and evaluation capacities. The National Cancer Institute, which funded the DBIR, had required states to use interventions of proven efficacy, and these interventions were not readily identified merely by analyzing cancer data (Alciati and Glanz, 1996). These results remind us that a satisfied, active coalition with better linkages to other community organizations does not guarantee effective products or results any more than worker happiness ensures high productivity.

Collaborations take many forms and proceed in many different ways. For a coalition in Virginia that was advocating for public health efforts to reduce premature and preventable death and disability, Diffusion Theory was a valuable practical tool. It helped coalition members shape a work plan, guide their work with opinion leaders, tailor the innovation to achieve its objectives, and create information exchange relationships (Howze and Redman, 1992). While the results of the Virginia coalition are described in terms of Diffusion Theory, they might also be viewed as Interorganizational Relations Theory. Mobilization of a coalition in an African American community for tobacco control was achieved through heavy reliance on community-organizing and community-building strategies (Ellis, Reed, and Scheider, 1995).

Approaches to Defining Needs, Problems, and Aims

The roots of change efforts for health enhancement begin in the early phases of needs assessment or problem definition. Several philosophical and methodological questions for developing and implementing health promotion strategies are either explicitly decided or implicitly addressed when defining needs, problems, and program aims or objectives. *Who* will decide what is a problem? What is the balance of professional (outsider or change agent) definition of needs and the lay community (insider or target audience) expression of needs? The concepts of felt ownership, participation, and relevance are shared in community organizing, organizational change, diffusion of innovations, and media communication studies, but their applications vary significantly.

Once needs or problems are defined (by whomever, by whatever methods), strategies are identified to achieve certain aims and objectives—usually to improve the situation or to prevent, reduce, or eliminate the problem(s). The questions that parallel these issues involve defining the appropriate or desirable outcome(s). Is a smoothly functioning participatory process sufficient in itself? Is adoption of a health curriculum enough? Is awareness of a health issue or program a meaningful endpoint? Must we aim for improvements in specific health behaviors, health risks, or health status outcomes, or are these impacts compromised because of their narrow definition of physical health? Is it enough to accomplish change in health-related policies or environments, even if those changes do not translate into improved health behaviors? Pressures for accountability for health improvement and even cost savings are growing at the same time that some health educators contend that these expectations are inappropriately narrow and limiting.

Indeed, a fundamental ideological conflict about the goal of health education and health promotion has arisen: should health promotion improve health status, serve as an instrument of social change, or both? Labonte (1994) comments that health promotion, while not a social movement per se, is a professional response to the challenges of social movements. He suggests that it is both empowering and disempowering, but he critiques the narrow view that focuses on physical and categorical health outcomes as disempowering *unless* they are combined with a view of clients in terms of their family, community, and economic lives as well (Labonte, 1994). While professional training in health education usually includes community-organizing techniques, it may not equip graduates to be any more than consultants in areas as diverse as health services, social welfare, human services, criminal justice, and urban planning. Robertson and Minkler (1994) suggest that what appears as an ideological conflict may be best understood as boundary issues, and that health promotion benefits by using multiple frameworks. They stress the importance of evaluating and demonstrating the benefits (or lack thereof) of whichever methods are chosen, a point I will return to later.

Similarities Between Models

Each theory and model in Part Four is distinctive in its perspective, emphasis, and research base. At the same time, there are many similarities between the models, as well as similarities to the intrapersonal and interpersonal models of health behavior presented earlier in this book. This section highlights some of those similarities and the related differences in the models. It compares and contrasts (1) community organization and organizational change, (2) diffusion of innovations and organizational change, (3) diffusion of innovations and Social Cognitive Theory, and (4) diffusion of innovations and communication-persuasion models of attitude change. The question of stages, steps, and phases across models is also addressed. This chapter does not offer in-depth analyses of these related models, because each comparison would require a chapter in itself (and these tasks have been accomplished in other books).

Community Organization and Organizational Change

Chapter Thirteen presents key principles and models of community organization and community building along with the theoretical foundations that form a base for these activities. There is no single theory of community organization that applies adequately to health promotion work (Bracht, 1990). Rather, we must borrow from other theories; some of these theories are integral to the organizational change frameworks discussed in Chapter Fifteen. Theories of social support, community development, and network analysis are most pertinent to OD Theory as a component of organizational change. Interorganizational Relations Theory is consonant with coalition building as it is used in community organizing. Another important consideration relates to the final stage of Stage Theory that Steckler, Goodman, and Kegler present. That phase, institutionalization, is the adoption of an innovation (a new idea or practice) as an ongoing part of an organization's structure and activities. The relationship to community organization lies in the virtual necessity of considering community organization principles (such as participation, relevance, and community competence) if institutionalization is to occur.

Diffusion of Innovations and Organizational Change

Chapters Fourteen and Fifteen put forth concepts from Diffusion Theory and organizational change that bear remarkable resemblances to one another. Oldenburg and Parcel emphasize diffusion of health promotion innovations through organizational structures, notably schools and workplaces. Both chapters include multistage models (adoption, implementation, maintenance, and so on). Also, both describe trials of interventions to promote adoption, implementation, and institutionalization of health promotion strategies of demonstrated efficacy, with diffusion or organizational change occurring with varying degrees of success. A recent analysis of the diffusion of a school-based drug abuse prevention program by Rohrbach, Graham, and Hansen (1993) reflects a combined application of diffusion and organizational change theories. They note the need for different strategies at different stages of the diffusion process, and describe system and innovation barriers to diffusion.

Diffusion of Innovations and Social Cognitive Theory

Albert Bandura's 1986 volume on Social Cognitive Theory (SCT) includes a chapter on social diffusion and innovation. In it, Bandura notes that "understanding how new ideas and social practices spread . . . has important bearing on personal and social change" (1986, p. 142). Even before this relatively recent attention to diffusion, the linkages between social learning (or cognition) and diffusion were set in place. The most apparent difference, which is reflected in the structure of this book, is that diffusion concepts and research emphasize the macro nature of social change, whereas social learning emphasizes intrapersonal and interpersonal factors, that is, the micro level. Similarities between diffusion and SCT include the focus on behavioral change, the importance of interpersonal networks for behavioral change, the essential role of information exchange, and the movement toward two-way influence processes. SCT and diffusion differ in their research traditions, as reflected in the dominant measurement methods and research designs. Historically, diffusion research has primarily involved naturalistic field surveys, whereas SCT research designs are primarily experimental and often conducted in the laboratory. However, these two traditions may be coming closer together, as suggested by some of Bandura's recent writing that emphasizes agentic transactions and collective efficacy (Bandura, 1997; Bandura, 2001). The convergence of thinking and the increasing attention to people as both producers and products of social systems heralds an increasing tendency to conduct multilevel analyses of health behavior, and to employ multilevel approaches for changing health-related behaviors and environments (Smedley and Syme, 2000).

Diffusion of Innovations and Communication-Persuasion

Diffusion frameworks are useful in understanding how the mass media contribute to the spread of innovations in populations. The phases of diffusion can also be examined as phases of psychological change in individuals. The correspondence suggests parallels between models of communication and persuasion and information processing at the individual level, and the community framework of adoption and diffusion. Communications can be designed to promote effects on individuals at each stage of the individual models and disseminated to promote optimal diffusion in social systems (Rogers, 1983).

Stages, Steps, and Phases

The chapters on diffusion of innovations and organizational change (Chapters Fourteen and Fifteen) include explicit discussions of staged models of organizational and social change. The diffusion process in the Australian National Workplace Health Project in Chapter Fourteen used a staged approach to health behavior change in worksites that involved initial access, support, and commitment. Chapter Sixteen, on communication theory, describes multistage processes as they apply to some of the communication models with relevance to public health. The influence of Lewin's work (Lewin, 1951), in particular his stage model of unfreezing, moving, and refreezing, is basic to concepts of group and organizational change. The exact number of stages varies across the models. Steckler, Goodman, and Kegler propose the need for greater consensus, or better specification, of the number of stages. While this might add precision and clarity to a given model, it may also be arbitrary. The editors of this book believe that a pragmatic approach serves well at this stage of the field: the number of stages (steps, or phases) should fit the situation and behavior while striving for parsimony as much as possible without losing meaning.

Research Issues

Each of the theories and action models presented in Part Four is complex and multimodal, and aims to influence not only large groups of individuals but organizational structures as well. An assessment of the impact of interventions based on these frameworks typically requires more complex and less controlled designs than the designs used at the intrapersonal or interpersonal level. Such evaluations may also require unusually large numbers of people to allow detection of statistically significant differences, especially if organizations or communities are used as the unit of randomization and analysis. Further, access to information at the organizational level may be difficult to obtain and even more difficult to validate, given the divergent perspectives of managers and workers or members and constituents or clients of an organization.

Action research has been proposed as an integral approach to intervention and evaluation in community organization and organizational change theories. Participatory research methods, which are often used in action research, include active roles for clients or consumers in defining their own health needs, setting priorities, and evaluating health-improvement efforts (Green and others, 1995). These methods are consistent with community participation, shared decision making, and facilitating ownership of change strategies, but they also pose great challenges in establishing valid and unbiased results from evaluations. Community intervention research and evaluation require a balance of scientific rigor and dynamic community environments with ethical concerns (Glanz, Rimer, and Lerman, 1996). Partnership research models are not all-or-nothing phenomena; they are a continuum with varying degrees of community and scientist participation and control (Wallerstein, 1999).

The use of both quantitative, hypothesis-testing research methods and qualitative methodologies is illustrated in each chapter in this section. These methods complement each other, and both lend strength to our understanding of the processes and impacts of health behavior change efforts. New developments in measurement are increasing our toolbox of community level indicators (Goodman and others, 1998; Cheadle, Wagner, Koepsell, Kristal, and Patrick, 1992), thus enabling better assessments of whether environments have changed and examination of the associations between individual- and community-level effects.

Additional research challenges involve the study of community change and societal change as two-way processes, the need to attend to personal influence as well as to the content of interventions, and the need to ensure that evaluation occurs prospectively, thus minimizing bias and ensuring that valuable information is not lost. We have an obligation to use our professional skills and resources for high-quality evaluation, even in the most process-driven change efforts. Models that work warrant wide dissemination, and models and strategies that are ineffective need to be improved or discarded (Rimer, Glanz, and Rasband, 2001). It is a disservice to the field of health education and health behavior to promulgate models based on ideology alone if they are not useful in achieving worthwhile aims.

Conclusion

Societal, community, and institutional factors are critical to promoting health because they can provide a fertile environment for health enhancement as well as directly shape individuals' health behavior. The power of policy is evident in health education settings such as workplaces and schools. Both broad social changes and specific organizational and governmental policies have been linked to individual behavior and perceptions. The impact of social historical events on individuals is complex: such events appear to interact with individual receptivity to change as reflected in life stages and other key developmental markers. The impacts can be seen, for example, in changes in women's work, family roles, and health-related behaviors as they differentially affect each generation of women (Stewart and Healy, 1989).

Macro-level approaches complement intrapersonal and interpersonal methods of health education and health behavior. Blended models suggest integrated strategies for reaching various units of practice in communitywide programs. Some health issues, for example infectious disease control and environmental protection through control of hazardous waste, cannot be influenced through individual-level efforts alone. However, they may be affected positively through methods based on individual-behavior-analysis frameworks combined with two-way communication with public health leaders and media efforts to promote wide awareness and prompt community action (Glanz and Yang, 1996; Weinstein and Sandman, 1993).

The integration of group, organization, and community intervention frameworks with individual and interpersonal models of health behavior has potential for real-world impact that exceeds the use of any one approach. Our most challenging public health problems require increased attention to organizational and environmental factors. Because behavior is highly influenced by settings, rules, organizational policy, community norms, and opportunities for action, changes in these factors are promising targets for change. Individual change will follow successful organizational and environmental changes, provided that these changes are both intensive enough and sustained over time.

Ideally, comprehensive health education efforts build on strategies that have been tried and found effective for reaching health and health behavior goals. However, while strategies have been shown to be effective in many behavioral arenas (for example, marketing or political arenas), there are currently few health issues for which a variety of demonstrably effective strategies is known. Smoking prevention and control is one of the few areas for which effective interventions have been developed and evaluated at each level of change (Warner, 2000). It is hoped that the armamentarium of effective strategies for other health behaviors will grow to the same level.

The theories and methods of community organization and community building, diffusion of innovations, organizational change, and media communication provide a strong foundation for understanding and positively influencing health behavior. Advances in research will clarify the operation mechanisms of these theories and models and refine our understanding of how best to use them. Health education and health behavior change strategies will achieve greater success through informed application of these frameworks for social activation and community attitude and behavioral change.

References

Alciati, M. H., and Glanz, K. "Using Data to Plan Public Health Programs: Experience from State Cancer Prevention and Control Programs." *Public Health Reports*, 1996, *111*, 165–172.

Bandura, A. *Social Foundations of Thought and Action: A Social Cognitive Theory*. Englewood Cliffs, N.J.: Prentice Hall, 1986.

Bandura, A. *Self-Efficacy: The Exercise of Control*. New York: Freeman, 1997.

Bandura, A. "Social Cognitive Theory: An Agentic Perspective." *Annual Review of Psychology*, 2001, *52*, 1–26.

Bracht, N. (ed.). *Health Promotion at the Community Level*. Thousand Oaks, Calif.: Sage, 1990.

Butterfoss, F. D., Goodman, R., and Wandersman, A. "Community Coalitions for Prevention and Health Promotion: Factors Predicting Satisfaction, Participation, and Planning." *Health Education Quarterly*, 1996, *23*(1), 56–79.

Cheadle, A., Wagner, E., Koepsell, T., Kristal, A., and Patrick, D. "Environmental Indicators: A Tool for Evaluating Community-Based Health-Promotion Programs." *American Journal of Preventive Medicine*, 1992, *8*(6), 345–350.

Ellis, G., Reed, D., and Scheider, H. "Mobilizing a Low-Income African American Community Around Tobacco Control: A Force-Field Analysis." *Health Education Quarterly*, 1995, *22*(4), 443–457.

Emmons, K. "Health Behaviors in Social Context." In L. F. Berkman and I. Kawachi (eds.), *Social Epidemiology*. New York: Oxford University Press, 2000.

Glanz, K., Rimer, B., and Lerman, C. "Ethical Issues in the Design and Conduct of Community-Based Intervention Studies." In S. Coughlin and T. Beauchamp (eds.), *Ethics in Epidemiology*. New York: Oxford University Press, 1996.

Glanz, K., and Yang, H. "Communicating About Risk of Infectious Diseases." *Journal of the American Medical Association*, 1996, *275*(3), 253–256.

Goodman, R. M., and others. "Identifying and Defining the Dimensions of Community Capacity to Provide a Basis for Measurement." *Health Education and Behavior*, 1998, *25*, 258–278.

Green, L. W., and others. *Study of Participatory Research in Health Promotion: Review and Recommendations for the Development of Participatory Research in Health Promotion in Canada*. Vancouver: University of British Columbia, 1995.

Himmelman, A. T. "On the Theory and Practice of Transformational Collaboration: Collaboration as a Bridge from Social Service to Social Justice." *Communities Working Collaboratively for Change.* Minneapolis: The HIMMELMAN Consulting Group, 1992.

Hovland, C., Janis, I., and Kelley, H. *Communication and Persuasion: Psychological Studies of Opinion Change.* Westport, Conn.: Greenwood Press, 1953.

Howze, E. H., and Redman, L. J. "The Uses of Theory in Health Advocacy: Policies and Programs." *Health Education Quarterly,* 1992, *19*(3), 369–383.

Janz, N., and others. "Evaluation of 37 AIDS Prevention Projects: Successful Approaches and Barriers to Program Effectiveness." *Health Education Quarterly,* 1996, *23*(1), 80–97.

Kipnis, D. "Accounting for the Use of Behavior Technologies in Social Psychology." *American Psychologist,* 1994, *49*(3), 165–172.

Labonte, R. "Health Promotion and Empowerment: Reflections on Professional Practice." *Health Education Quarterly,* 1994, *22*(2), 253–268.

Lasswell, H. D. "The Structure and Function of Communication in Society." In L. Bryson (ed.), *The Communication of Ideas.* New York: Institute for Religious and Social Studies, 1948.

Lewin, K. *Field Theory in Social Science.* New York: HarperCollins, 1951.

Marmot, M. "Multilevel Approaches to Understanding Social Determinants." In L. F. Berkman and I. Kawachi (eds.), *Social Epidemiology.* New York: Oxford University Press, 2000.

McKinlay, J. B., and Marceau, L. D. "To Boldly Go. . ." *American Journal of Public Health,* 2000, *90,* 25–33.

Orleans, C. T., Gruman, J., Ulmer, C., Emont, S. L., and Hollendonner, J. K. "Rating Our Progress in Population Health Promotion: Report Card on Six Behaviors." *American Journal of Health Promotion,* 1999, *14,* 75–82.

Parcel, G. S., and others. "Measurement of Self-Efficacy for Diet-Related Behaviors Among Elementary School Children." *Journal of School Health,* 1995, *65,* 23–27.

Rimer, B., Glanz, K., and Lerman, C. "Contributions of Public Health to Patient Compliance." *Journal of Community Health,* 1991, *16*(4), 225–240.

Rimer, B. K., Glanz, K., and Rasband, G. "Searching for Evidence About Health Education and Health Behavior Interventions." *Health Education and Behavior,* 2001, *28,* 231–248.

Robertson, A., and Minkler, M. "New Health Promotion Movement: A Critical Examination." *Health Education Quarterly,* 1994, *21*(3), 295–312.

Rogers, E. M. *Diffusion of Innovations.* (3rd ed.) New York: Free Press, 1983.

Rohrbach, L. A., Graham, J. W., and Hansen, W. B. "Diffusion of a School-Based Substance Abuse Prevention Program: Predictors of Program Implementation." *Preventive Medicine,* 1993, *22,* 237–260.

Rothman, J. "Approaches to Community Intervention." In J. Rothman, J. Erlich, and J. Tropman (eds.), *Strategies of Community Intervention.* Itasca, Ill.: Peacock, 2001.

Smedley, B. D., and Syme, S. L. (eds.). *Promoting Health: Intervention Strategies from Social and Behavioral Research.* Washington, D.C.: National Academy Press, 2000.

Stewart, A., and Healy, J. "Linking Individual Development and Social Changes." *American Psychologist,* 1989, *44,* 30–42.

Wallack, L. "Media Advocacy: Promoting Health Through Mass Communication." In Glanz, K., Lewis, F. M., and Rimer, B. K. (eds.), *Health Behavior and Health Education: Theory, Research, and Practice.* San Francisco: Jossey-Bass, 1990.

Wallerstein, N. "Power Between Evaluator and Community: Research Relationships Within New Mexico's Healthier Communities." *Social Science and Medicine,* 1999, *49,* 39–53.

Warner, K. "The Need for, and Value of, a Multi-Level Approach to Disease Prevention: The Case of Tobacco Control." In B. D. Smedley and S. L. Syme (eds.), *Promoting Health: Intervention Strategies from Social and Behavioral Research.* Washington, D.C.: National Academy Press, 2000.

Weinstein, N. D., and Sandman, P. M. "Some Criteria for Evaluating Risk Messages." *Risk Analysis,* 1993, *13,* 103–114.

PART FIVE

USING THEORY IN RESEARCH AND PRACTICE

One of the greatest challenges to public health professionals is to learn to analyze the "fit" of a theory or model for issues and populations with whom one is working. A working knowledge of a handful of theories and how they have been applied is the first step. Mastering the challenges of using theories appropriately and effectively is the logical next step. Effective practice depends on marshaling the most appropriate theory or theories and practice strategies for a given situation. Theory-based research and evaluation further require appropriate designs, measures, and procedures for the health problem, organization, and unique population at hand, as well as the development of appropriate interventions.

No one theory or model will be right in all cases. Depending on the unit of practice and type of health behavior or issue, different theoretical frameworks will be appropriate, practical, and useful. Often, more than one theory is needed to adequately address an issue. For comprehensive health promotion programs, this is almost always true. It is also evident in the use and description of applied theories in the professional literature. However, using too many theories may be counterproductive.

The preceding sections of this book make clear that theories often overlap, and that some fit easily within broader models. Generally, theories can be used most effectively if they are integrated within a comprehensive planning framework. Such a system assigns a central role to research as input to determine the situation and needs of the population to be served, the resources that are available, and the progress and effectiveness of the program at various stages. Planning is a continuous process in which new information is gathered to build or improve the program.

Part Five gives specific examples of combining theories for greater impact. PRECEDE-PROCEED, a well-developed planning model that can be used to integrate and apply diverse theoretical frameworks, is discussed in this section. In Chapter Eighteen, Andrea Gielen and Eileen McDonald describe the PRECEDE-PROCEED Model for health promotion planning and present a case study of theory-driven program planning for a comprehensive injury prevention program at a well-child clinic that used the PRECEDE-PROCEED planning model.

In Chapter Nineteen, Ed Maibach and colleagues describe the purpose, key components, and methods of social marketing. They illustrate the application of social marketing in the National High Blood Pressure Education Program and in a program to reduce binge drinking on a college campus. An important feature of these case examples is that they demonstrate both large- and small-scale social marketing programs.

Chapter Twenty, by James Sallis and Neville Owen, describes the current status of ecological models for health promotion and proposes principles that should be followed if these models are to contribute substantially to health promotion research and practice. Ecological models are comprehensive multilevel frameworks for health promotion. This chapter clarifies the various ecological models that have been advanced, their historical development, and implications for health behavior and health education. The authors focus on needs for greater clarity, precision, and understanding about how these models operate.

Chapter Twenty-One identifies issues to be considered when applying health behavior theory to culturally diverse and unique populations. Ken Resnicow and his coauthors challenge all health professionals to become aware of the importance of diverse characteristics of individuals and communities and elucidate how theories can and should assist practitioners and researchers in developing programs that are culturally sensitive for diverse populations. This chapter provides applied examples addressing the issues of individualism versus communalism, religiosity, and tobacco control among American Indian populations.

Chapter Twenty-Two describes recent developments in communication technology and their features that are most relevant to health behavior change. This is a new chapter in this edition of the book, and is included for two reasons: first, these emerging technologies have made possible a wide range of new strategies for health communication and education, and second, the editors believe that using theories and models of health behavior to guide technology-driven strategies will increase their success and improve the precision of evaluation research. Neville Owen, Michael Fotheringham, and Bess Marcus illustrate how theories and models can be used with communication technology, provide a few in-depth examples, and raise issues of concern to health education practice and research.

Chapter Twenty-Three describes the RE-AIM Model, an evaluation model that has proven useful for evaluating theory-based interventions and examining them in a broader public health perspective. In this new chapter for the third edition of *Health Behavior and Health Education*, Russell Glasgow offers tools and perspectives that are potentially valuable for planning, implementing, evaluating, and interpreting the results of studies of health behavior change interventions.

Using theory thoughtfully and appropriately is not simple but it can be most rewarding. Our aim in Part Five is to bring together many constructs and models and equip readers to work effectively with them in their own practice settings.

CHAPTER EIGHTEEN

USING THE PRECEDE-PROCEED PLANNING MODEL TO APPLY HEALTH BEHAVIOR THEORIES

Andrea Carlson Gielen
Eileen M. McDonald

Individual theories. Interpersonal theories. Community change theories. Pamphlets. Videotapes. Counseling. Support groups. Public service announcements. Grassroots organizing.

These represent but a few of the tools available to health professionals for designing, implementing, and evaluating health behavior change programs. The appropriate selection and application of these tools can mean the difference between program success and failure. Typically, a problem affecting a particular population has been identified and the health professional must *do something* to fix the problem. Examples include inappropriate use by enrollees of urgent-care facilities for nonurgent problems in a health maintenance organization, low birthweight rates in a geographically defined area, or high rates of smoking among pregnant women seen in a prenatal clinic. The health professional's ability to apply theories of health behavior is one of the most critical skills needed in designing programs to address such problems.

The SAFE Home Project was funded by the Maternal and Child Health Bureau (MCJ-240638), with additional support provided by the Johns Hopkins Center for Injury Research and Policy, which is funded by the Centers for Disease Control and Prevention, National Center for Injury Prevention and Control (R49/CCR302486). The needs assessment was supported by the Faculty Development Fund of the Johns Hopkins University. The authors would like to thank Drs. Lawrence Green and Marshall Kreuter for helpful comments on earlier versions of this chapter.

A planning model like PRECEDE-PROCEED can help guide this process (Green, Kreuter, Deeds, and Partridge, 1980; Green and Kreuter, 1991; Green and Kreuter, 1999). Unlike the theories described in previous chapters, PRECEDE-PROCEED does not attempt to predict or explain the relationship among factors thought to be associated with an outcome of interest. Rather, it provides a structure for applying theories so that the most appropriate intervention strategies can be identified and implemented. PRECEDE-PROCEED can be thought of as a road map and theories as the specific directions to a destination. The road map presents all the possible avenues, while the theory suggests certain avenues to follow. Although the emphasis in PRECEDE-PROCEED is typically on service programs delivered in practice settings, the framework may be equally useful to researchers conducting health behavior change intervention trials.

This chapter begins with an overview of PRECEDE-PROCEED, which includes a description of each step in the process as well as examples from the literature on how the process has been applied to health promotion programs. Descriptions of the steps presented here are summarized from the work of the model's creators, and readers are referred to their textbooks for more detailed information (Green, Kreuter, Deeds, and Partridge, 1980; Green and Kreuter, 1991; Green and Kreuter, 1999). In the second section of the chapter, we present a case study of theory-driven program planning that used the PRECEDE-PROCEED planning model to develop a comprehensive injury prevention program for a well-child clinic. The objectives of the chapter are to enable readers to use PRECEDE-PROCEED to choose and apply relevant health behavior change theories in their work and to incorporate constructs from theories described in previous chapters into their planning processes.

Overview of PRECEDE-PROCEED

The PRECEDE framework was developed in the 1970s by Green and colleagues (Green, Kreuter, Deeds, and Partridge, 1980; www.lgreen.net/precede/preapps.htm). The acronym stands for Predisposing, Reinforcing, and Enabling Constructs in Educational/Environmental Diagnosis and Evaluation. PRECEDE is based on the premise that just as medical diagnosis precedes a treatment plan, so should educational diagnosis precede an intervention plan. This approach addressed a concern among some professionals that health education focused too much on implementing interventions and too little on designing interventions that were strategically planned to meet demonstrated needs (Bartholomew, Parcel, Kok, and Gottlieb, 2001).

In 1991, PROCEED (Policy, Regulatory, and Organizational Constructs in Educational and Environmental Development) was added to the framework to recognize the importance of environmental factors as determinants of health and health behaviors (Figure 18.1). Over the past two decades, the significant contribution of lifestyle factors to the public's health and well-being has been increasingly recognized (McGinnis and Foege, 1993). Falling under the rubric of "lifestyle" are general patterns of diet, exercise, cigarette and alcohol use, sexual practices, and stress, all of which have been linked to longevity and quality of life. While these are considered individual behaviors, they are not wholly volitional behaviors. Rather, they are in many ways influenced by powerful forces outside of the individual, such as industry, media, politics, and social inequalities. Understanding this larger context that constrains or facilitates individual behavior is a hallmark of health promotion programming and is a central focus of ecological approaches to health promotion (McLeroy, Bibeau, Steckler, and Glanz, 1988; Simons-Morton and others, 1989).

FIGURE 18.1. THE PRECEDE-PROCEED PLANNING MODEL.

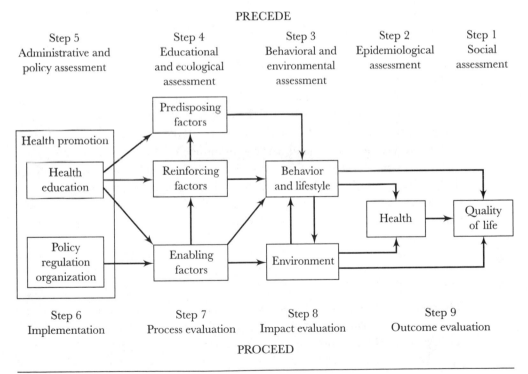

Source: Green and Kreuter, 1999, p. 34.

The PRECEDE-PROCEED process rests on a fundamental principle of practice, the principle of participation, which states that success in achieving change is enhanced by the active participation of the intended audience in defining their own high-priority problems and goals and in developing and implementing solutions (Green and Kreuter, 1999; Freudenberg and others, 1995). This principle derives from the community development roots of the profession (Steckler, Dawson, Israel, and Eng, 1993), as well as the empowerment-education models exemplified by Freire's early work and by the more recent work of Minkler, Wallerstein, Israel, and others (Wallerstein, 1992; Wallerstein and Bernstein, 1994; Israel, Checkoway, Schulz, and Zimmerman, 1994; see also Chapter Thirteen). Accordingly, at each step in a PRECEDE-PROCEED assessment, efforts should be made to include input from the program's intended audience.

The planning process begins with the proposition that health behaviors are complex, multidimensional, and influenced by a variety of factors (Green and Kreuter, 1999). As Freudenberg and others (1995) have noted, "the danger, however, in recognizing that a problem has many causes is that there is no method of assigning priorities to the importance of different causes and no rational way for allocating limited resources to address the most significant causes. A good theory should assist in this task" (p. 293). While PRECEDE-PROCEED is not considered a theory, per se, but rather a planning model or a conceptual framework for practice (Clark and McLeroy, 1995), its systematic approach offers specific guidelines for priority setting. In this way, intervention resources can be more efficiently and effectively used because different intervention strategies are appropriate for different types of influencing factors. For example, a high-fat diet is a health behavior problem with many determinants, two of which are a lack of public understanding of the problem and not knowing how to cook with low-fat alternatives. A well-designed public service announcement could inform the public about the health consequences of a high-fat diet, but would be insufficient to teach skills in low-fat cooking. PRECEDE-PROCEED is a nine-step planning process that begins at the end, focusing on the health-related outcomes of interest and working backward to diagnose which combination of intervention strategies will best achieve the objectives.

Step 1: Social Assessment

The social assessment determines people's perceptions of their own needs and quality of life (Green and Kreuter, 1999). At this stage, the planners expand their understanding of the community in which they are working by conducting multiple data-collection activities, such as interviews with key opinion leaders, focus groups with members of the community, observations, and surveys. The term *community* is typically used to mean a geographical area with defined boundaries; more generally, it may be used to describe a group with shared characteristics, interests, values, and norms (see Chapter Thirteen). In addition to articulating the community's needs and desires, a social assessment also considers the community's problem-solving capacity, its strengths and resources, and its readiness to change (Kretzmann and McKnight, 1993).

A social assessment is important for many reasons. First, the relationship between health and quality of life is reciprocal, with each affecting the other (Green and Kreuter, 1999). For example, living in poverty is associated with poor health and being unhealthy makes it more difficult to escape impoverished living conditions. People value their health not simply as an end in itself, but because being healthy enables them to achieve other goals (for example, enjoyment of work and recreation). By understanding the intended audience's concerns, the planner is more likely to develop a program that is relevant, which will increase its chances of being well received and effective. Including an assessment of problem-solving capacity will foster the development of intervention components that include strengthening capacity to address other issues in the future. Focusing on community strengths in addition to problems allows the planners and community members to form more effective and meaningful partnerships that will help to support both initial and sustained commitment to the program (Bartholomew, Parcel, Kok, and Gottlieb, 2001).

At this step in the program-planning process, community-organizing theories and principles are relevant (Table 18.1). Community organization "emphasizes the active participation and the development of communities that can better evaluate and solve health and social problems" (Glanz and Rimer, 1995, p. 25). Minkler's (1985) work in the Tenderloin Project with low-income older adults and Eng and Blanchard's (1991) work conducting a community action diagnosis in a rural county are good examples of the importance of social assessment and the use of community-organizing strategies. Kretzmann and McKnight (1993) provide useful tools for conducting an assets-based community assessment.

Programs are often predetermined with regard to audience, health problem, and health behavior problem. Even in this context, planners are well advised to learn as much as possible about the community, to work in partnership with the community members to build the program, and to link the community's concerns about quality-of-life issues to the program objectives. Developing a planning committee, holding community forums, and conducting focus groups or surveys are all examples of helpful activities to engage the audience in planning and are necessary regardless of where a planner begins in the PRECEDE-PROCEED process.

TABLE 18.1. PRECEDE-PROCEED MODEL AS AN ORGANIZING FRAMEWORK FOR APPLICATION OF THEORIES AND PRINCIPLES.

Change Theories and Principles by Level of Change	Precede-Proceed Planning Phases				
	Step 1 Social Assessment	Step 2 Epidemiological Assessment	Step 3 Behavioral and Environmental Assessment	Step 4 Educational and Ecological Assessment	Step 5 Administrative and Policy Assessment
Community level					
Participation and relevance	X	X	X	X	X
Community organization	X		X		
Organizational change				X	X
Diffusion of innovation				X	X
Interpersonal level					
Social Cognitive Theory			X	X	
Adult learning				X	
Interpersonal communication				X	
Individual level					
Health Belief Model				X	
Stages of Change			X	X	
Theory of Reasoned Action				X	
Theory of Planned Behavior			X	X	
Information processing				X	

Source: Adapted from Glanz and Rimer, 1995.

Step 2: Epidemiological Assessment

An epidemiological assessment helps determine which health problems are most important for which groups in a community (Green and Kreuter, 1999). This assessment, when linked with quality-of-life concerns of the audience, also makes clear that limited resources are being used to address health problems that contribute significantly to larger societal problems. The epidemiological assessment does not typically draw on specific theories (Table 18.1), although community-level theories may apply when the community is involved in the process of choosing the health problems to be addressed.

In an epidemiological assessment, planners can conduct secondary data analysis using existing data sources (such as vital statistics, state and national health surveys, medical and administrative records). These data provide indicators of morbidity and mortality in a population and can help to specify subgroups at particularly high risk. Subgroups may be characterized by age, gender, ethnicity, occupation, education, income, family structure, geographical location, and so on. Sometimes it is inappropriate to extrapolate from national data to a smaller region, in which case original data collection will be necessary. For example, household surveys of a nationally representative sample may have inadequate numbers of respondents from a single state to provide reliable state-level data. Data collection and analysis from an epidemiological assessment should yield reliable and valid indicators for setting measurable program objectives.

With data on the community's health problems, a planner is ready to set priorities and write program goals and objectives. Decisions should be guided by the desires of the community members themselves, with consideration given to health problems with the greatest impact, those that have been previously underserved, and those for which solutions are realistically available. A program goal is a statement of the program's ultimate benefit (for example, improve family health and quality of life by reducing infant mortality), whereas program objectives should answer the question, "Who will receive how much of what health benefit by when?" (for example, infant mortality will be reduced by 25 percent in County X by the Year 2010). Measurable program objectives are essential to guide the allocation of resources and to evaluate the program's success. The availability of national and regional policy documents should be investigated for guidance in setting reasonable targets for change. For example, the United States Public Health Service's Year 2010 health objectives—*Healthy People 2010*—provide data and objectives on the major health problems for the nation as a whole and for some age, gender, and race or ethnicity sub-groups (U.S. Department of Health and Human Services, 2000).

Step 3: Behavioral and Environmental Assessment

Step 3, the behavioral and environmental assessment, involves assessing factors that contribute to the health problem under consideration (Green and Kreuter, 1999). Behavioral factors are those behaviors or lifestyles of the individuals at risk that contribute to the occurrence and severity of the health problem. Environmental factors are those social and physical factors external to the individual, often beyond his or her personal control, that can be modified to support the behavior or influence the health outcome. Modifying environmental factors usually requires strategies other than education. For example, poor nutritional status among schoolchildren is a function of poor dietary habits (behavioral factor), which in turn is at least partly affected by the availability of unhealthy foods in schools (environmental factor). While an educational program could effectively teach students about healthy diets, policy and organizational changes at the institutional level would be required to increase the availability of healthy foods in schools.

While both biological and genetic factors contribute to health problems, these are not changeable through a health promotion program. They may be helpful, however, in identifying specific high-risk groups for intervention. For example, a breast cancer screening promotion program might include special efforts to reach women with a family history of the disease.

Using theory, literature, and the wisdom of the planning group, an inventory should be made of behavioral and environmental influencing factors. Interpersonal theories of health behavior change can be useful at this stage of the **PRECEDE-PROCEED** framework because of the emphasis on the interaction between individuals and their environment (Table 18.1). For example, Social Cognitive Theory posits that behavior, cognition, and other personal factors have reciprocal relationships with environments, so they continually influence one another (Bandura, 1986). In addition, an individual's behavior is influenced by observing others and by receiving reinforcement for behavioral change, both of which speak to the importance of the individual's social environment. Thus, at this stage of the assessment, planners should consider how these constructs help specify behavioral and environmental factors that contribute to the health problem of interest. For example, in the assessment for a program to reduce low birth weight, consideration should be given to whether there are women in the community who model appropriate use of prenatal care and whether community leaders and health professionals reinforce it.

Each of the enumerated factors is rated in terms of its importance to the health problem. The most important factors are those that are highly prevalent or strongly associated with the health problem. Allowing the community to rank factors is consistent with principles of community organization (for example, participation and relevance) and helps ensure that selected factors are indeed important to the intended audience.

Each factor is also rated in terms of its changeability. Theories of organizational change, community organization, and diffusion of innovations are helpful for estimating changeability (Erlich, Rothman, and Teresa, 1999; Rogers, 1995). Organizational change theories are particularly relevant when the policies and practices of formal organizations have been identified as environmental factors to be changed. For example, in a worksite, policies restricting smoking may need to be strengthened; planners need to understand how organizational policy can be changed if they are to make a reasonable estimate of the changeability of this environmental factor. Community organization may be used to effect change in environmental conditions that directly affects individuals' health or that influences health behaviors (Brown, 1991). Similarly, Diffusion Theory describes and predicts the process by which new ideas are adopted in a community (Rogers, 1995; see Chapter Fourteen). If, for example, the assessment at this point suggests that an important behavioral factor is bicycle-helmet use, then evaluating its changeability according to Diffusion Theory would consider such features of helmets as their observability by others, perceptions of their relative advantage, and how compatible their use is with existing norms. Intervention foci are chosen by combining importance and changeability ratings. Directing program resources toward those factors that are most important *and* most changeable helps to ensure program efficiency and effectiveness. Finally, measurable objectives are written to specify the desired behavioral impact (Who will do how much of what by when?) and environmental change (How much of what—conditions, circumstances, policies—will be changed by when?).

Step 4: Educational and Ecological Assessment

After selecting the appropriate behavioral and environmental factors for intervention, step 4 identifies the antecedent and reinforcing factors that must be in place to initiate and sustain the change process. These factors are classified as *predisposing, reinforcing,* and *enabling,* and they collectively influence the likelihood that behavioral and environmental change will occur. "*Predisposing factors* are antecedents to behavior that provide the rationale or motivation for the behavior" (Green and Kreuter, 1999, p. 153). They include individuals' knowledge, attitudes, beliefs, personal preferences, existing skills, and self-efficacy beliefs. "*Reinforcing factors* are those factors following a behavior that provide continuing reward or incentive for the persistence or repetition of the behavior" (Green and Kreuter, 1999, p. 153). Examples include social support, peer influence, significant others, and vicarious reinforcement. "*Enabling factors* are antecedents to behavior that allow a motivation to be realized" (Green and Kreuter, 1999, p. 153). Enabling factors can affect behavior directly or indirectly through an environmental factor. They include programs, services, and resources necessary for behavioral and environmental outcomes to be realized and, in some cases, new skills that are needed to enable health behavior change. As in the previous step, these factors are enumerated, rated in terms of importance and changeability, and priority targets for intervention are selected. Finally, measurable objectives are written: How many will know, believe, or be able to do what by when? How much of what resource will be available to whom by when? This process, as in all of the previous steps, should be driven by a thorough knowledge of the relevant empirical literature, with input from the intended audience through their participation in planning or through original data collection such as surveys and focus groups.

Green and Kreuter stress that "the decision to place a factor in one category or another is less important than ranking the factor as an influence or determinant of behavior worthy of attention and finding a way to address it in the program" (Green and Kreuter, 1999, p. 157). Classifying determinants of behavior into the general categories of predisposing, reinforcing, and enabling factors facilitates thinking about how best to address audience needs, because each category leads to different types of intervention strategies and methods. These constructs have demonstrated utility across a wide array of health behaviors, they provide a framework for incorporating more specific theories, and they help to organize the planning process.

All three levels of change theories—community, interpersonal, individual— can be useful at this stage of the planning process (Table 18.1). For example, in a community with high teen pregnancy and sexually transmitted disease (STD) rates, community norms and teen attitudes may support the use of contraception, but teens may not have access to confidential reproductive planning services. In this case, organizational change theories will provide more effective guidance than will individually oriented theories. Individually oriented theories would suggest ways to change attitudes when, in this example, these are already favorable. Alternatively, organizational change theories would suggest ways to enable the delivery of services to the intended audience. Enhancing the delivery of services, whether it is through onsite school-based clinics or through other structures in the community, would require a thorough understanding of the organization's policies, procedures, and processes of change.

In another example, planners of a program to promote bicycle-helmet use might learn that children find helmets uncomfortable, fear "looking nerdy," and believe that they won't get hurt on their bikes. This would suggest, from a Diffusion Theory perspective, that the relative advantage, compatibility, and observability attributes of helmet use need to be addressed in order to shape more favorable attitudes among children in the community. Drawing also on the inter-personal-level Social Cognitive Theory, these findings would suggest that social influence plays an important role in both predisposing and reinforcing helmet use. Finally, if children's personal beliefs are that bike riding is not dangerous, an in-dividual-level theory such as the Health Belief Model (Janz and Becker, 1984) will help. The Health Belief Model includes the construct of perceived susceptibility, which would be an important predisposing factor for helmet use in this hypo-thetical example.

The reason for making determinations about the relative importance of pre-disposing, reinforcing, and enabling factors and for incorporating different theo-retical orientations is to choose appropriate intervention strategies. In general, individual-level theories are most appropriate for addressing predisposing factors. They help planners identify messages for direct communication methods such as mass media and face-to-face education, as well as for newer technologies such as computer-tailoring of health messages (Kreuter, Farrell, Olevitch, and Brennan, 2000). Interpersonal-level theories are most appropriate for reinforcing factors, and they suggest indirect communication channels (for example, through significant others, social networks) and methods (for example, train-the-trainer models, social support enhancement). Community-level theories are most appropriate for en-abling factors, and they suggest environmental changes (such as organization and delivery of services; availability of products; policies, laws, and regulations that gov-ern products and behaviors) and methods such as grassroots organizing and ad-vocacy (Clark and McLeroy, 1995). Because of the complexity of lifestyle-related health problems typically addressed by health behavior change programs, multi-ple levels of factors and methods are generally needed. At this stage, intervention mapping steps may be particularly helpful for matching methods and strategies to the theoretically and empirically identified audience needs (Bartholomew, Parcel, Kok, and Gottlieb, 2001).

Step 5: Administrative and Policy Assessment

Delineating the intervention strategies and final planning for their implementa-tion occurs in step 5, the administrative and policy assessment. Its purpose is to identify policies, resources, and circumstances prevailing in the program's orga-nizational context that could facilitate or hinder program implementation. Green and Kreuter (1999) define the PRO in PROCEED as follows: *policy* is the set of objectives and rules guiding the activities of an organization or administration, *regulation* is the act of implementing policies and enforcing rules or laws, and *orga-nization* is the bringing together and the coordination of resources necessary to implement a program.

At this stage, intervention strategies are enumerated based on the previous steps, and planners must assess the availability of necessary resources (time, people, funding). Barriers to implementation, such as staff commitment or lack of space, should be assessed, and plans to address them put in place. Also, any organizational policies or regulations that could affect program implementation should be considered and planned for accordingly. Administrative and policy diagnosis is specific to the context of the program and the sponsoring organization(s) and requires as much political savvy as theoretical or empirical knowledge.

Administrative and policy assessment can be informed by community-level theories (Table 18.1). Community-organization theories encourage health planners to involve key community members. The definition and identification of those "key" members will differ for every community and health issue. Organizational change theory informs public health practitioners about the processes and strategies for creating and sustaining changes in health policies and procedures that influence the success of health promotion programs.

Steps 6 to 9: Implementation and Evaluation

At this point, the health promotion program is ready for implementation (step 6). Data collection plans should be in place for evaluating the process, impact, and outcome of the program, the final three steps in the PRECEDE-PROCEED planning model (steps 7–9). Typically, process evaluation determines the extent to which the program was implemented according to protocol. Impact evaluation assesses change in predisposing, reinforcing, and enabling factors, as well as in the behavioral and environmental factors. Finally, outcome evaluation determines the effect of the program on health and quality-of-life indicators. Generally, the measurable objectives that are written at each step of the PRECEDE-PROCEED planning model serve as milestones against which accomplishments are evaluated. Because the emphasis in this chapter is on the application of theory to program planning, the details of these steps will not be reviewed. Rather, their application will be described in a case study.

Summary of PRECEDE-PROCEED

The stepwise process outlined in the PRECEDE-PROCEED model enables program planners and their communities to find *"common ground"* (Green and Kreuter, 1999, p. 58). The social assessment leads to an understanding of the community's perceived needs; the epidemiological, behavioral, and educational assessments document actual needs. The starting points for intervention are where these needs intersect. The administrative and policy assessments define the parameters within which an intervention can operate. Following the sequential steps of PRECEDE-PROCEED helps ensure that program development can be replicated, and that steps in the process can be documented for later critique. However, at each step it is wise to consider the impact of current programmatic decisions on previous decisions. Program planning is usually an iterative process in which prior decisions are constantly being evaluated in light of new data, resources, and other decisions.

PRECEDE-PROCEED is a widely used planning model that has guided the design of programs for numerous health problems (Clarke, Frankish, and Green, 1997; Dignan and others, 1998; Howat, Jones, Hall, Cross, and Stevenson, 1997; Hendrickson and Becker, 1998; Morisky and others, 1983; Worden and others, 1990; Bertera, 1990; Bertera, 1993; Windsor, 1986; Windsor and others, 1993; Eriksen and Gielen, 1983; Rimer, 1995; Gielen, 1992). In a review of the most recent edition of Green and Kreuter's textbook, Glanz calls the model "logical, robust, and intuitively appealing" (Glanz, 2000, p. 104). Programs that have used this model as a basis for interventions have demonstrated significant improvements in health indicators for high blood pressure control (Morisky and others, 1983), breast cancer screening (Rimer, 1995), breast self-examination (Worden and others, 1990), smoking cessation (Windsor and others, 1993), worksite health promotion (Bertera, 1993), and correct use of car safety seats (Gielen, Bernstein-Cohen, and Radius, 1985). The model has also been incorporated into national policy documents for community health (Centers for Disease Control, 1992) and injury control (National Committee for Injury Prevention and Control, 1989). An interactive computerized version of the model, called EMPOWER, has been developed to assist in the development of community-level cancer prevention and control interventions. A bibliography of citations in published literature related to PRECEDE-PROCEED and more information on EMPOWER are available on the Web site www.ihpr.ubc.ca/precede.html.

Despite its considerable success, potential users of PRECEDE-PROCEED should be aware of some of the challenges in applying it. The model is heavily data driven, and its application may require greater financial and human resources than are available in some situations. For example, Bertera's (1990) experience using the model for a worksite health promotion program in the DuPont company led him to conclude that smaller companies might have difficulty implementing the model because of the need for record keeping, conducting surveys, and engaging skilled health education staff. An evaluation of four PATCH programs (which incorporate much of the PRECEDE-PROCEED model) found that the process of planning was slow and that planners needed substantial training or technical assistance to carry it out (Orenstein and others, 1992). Because of the heavy emphasis on up-front assessment, local coalitions may become frustrated with the PRECEDE-PROCEED framework and impatient for interventions. Program planners should be alert to this concern and should conduct their planning activities to ensure some early, visible successes to keep their partners engaged and enthusiastic.

The PRECEDE-PROCEED Model planning process also does not emphasize the specifics of intervention development. Planners may feel the need for additional guidance on methods and strategies for addressing the selected predisposing, reinforcing, and enabling factors. *Intervention mapping* is a new planning technique that holds promise for filling this gap (Bartholomew, Parcel, Kok, and Gottlieb, 2001). Intervention mapping describes an intervention method as "a theory-based technique to influence behavior or environmental conditions, whereas a strategy is a way of organizing and operationalizing the intervention methods. The translation of selected methods into action is completed through the development of strategies" (Bartholomew, Parcel, Kok, and Gottlieb, 2001, p. 11). For example, a PRECEDE-PROCEED assessment may determine that the absence of role models for a particular behavior is a reinforcing factor to be addressed in a program. Intervention mapping would identify role modeling as a theory-based (derived from Social Cognitive Theory) *method* to be used in the program; a *strategy* for using role models could be the development and distribution of stories about role models. Subsequent planning steps are described in the intervention mapping process to provide guidance on producing program materials.

Because PRECEDE-PROCEED is an integrative planning model that includes constructs from many theories, it has not been systematically evaluated in comparison with other theoretical models of health behavior. The one exception is a study conducted in 1981 by Mullen and colleagues. In a longitudinal study of 326 adults who were interviewed twice over an eight-month interval, the authors compared PRECEDE, the Health Belief Model, and the Theory of Reasoned Action in terms of the models' predictive power, parsimony, acceptability to respondents, and specificity for program planning. The outcomes were self-reported changes in smoking, exercise, and consumption of sweet and fried foods. The results demonstrated that PRECEDE explained more of the variance in all outcomes (except attempts to quit smoking) and that it was the most inclusive of the models, although it required a considerably larger number of variables than the Health Belief Model. This study found that PRECEDE could sensitize planners to certain categories of variables, but that it does not specify relationships among variables, especially in the broad class of predisposing variables (Mullen, Hersey, and Iverson, 1987, p. 978). While this may be a limitation when one seeks a parsimonious, predictive model of health behavior, the inclusion of multiple types and levels of factors is a strength of the model for planning comprehensive, ecologically oriented health promotion programs, as illustrated in the case study that follows.

Case Study: The SAFE Home Project

This case study illustrates how the PRECEDE-PROCEED framework and behavioral science theories were helpful in the development of the SAFE Home Project, an intervention trial aimed at reducing in-home childhood injury risk among low-income, inner-city families. This example highlights how the framework was used not only in program planning but also in applying and integrating theory within real-world constraints. Finally, the case study demonstrates the model's usefulness for guiding evaluation activities.

In practice, a new program must fit into an existing context. This program's context was the Johns Hopkins Bloomberg School of Public Health and the Johns Hopkins Children's Center. Specifically, several faculty members had a long-standing interest in the prevention of childhood injury and had collaborated to develop this program by sharing their multiple disciplinary expertise (in such areas as pediatrics, behavioral sciences, health education, injury prevention, biostatistics, communication sciences), and professional roles, responsibilities, and access to resources. The focal point for the program was a pediatric continuity clinic that provides medical care to children living in the East Baltimore community, one of the most impoverished areas of the city. Although the program was designed to serve this particular clinic's population, an overarching goal was that the intervention strategies developed would be feasible in a variety of other pediatric care settings.

Social and Epidemiological Assessment (Steps 1 and 2)

The health problem (pediatric injuries) and its associated impact on quality of life were defined at the outset (Figure 18.2). Injury prevention was a funding priority for the sponsoring agency and the pediatric faculty involved in the project were advocates of its importance to the families seen in their clinic. In-home injuries were a special focus because they are numerous, costly, and often preventable with relatively simple safety practices.

The first two steps of PRECEDE-PROCEED—the social and epidemiological assessment—relied heavily on a review of the literature and data on injuries among our intended audience. Following is a sample of the data we found:

Injury is the leading cause of death for U.S. children and children from birth to age four are particularly vulnerable to injuries (Baker, 1992).

In 1985, there were over four million medically attended injuries (Rice and MacKenzie, 1989) and numerous nonmedically attended injuries among the preschool population. In 1995, 3,067 children from birth to

FIGURE 18.2. APPLICATION OF PRECEDE-PROCEED TO INJURY PREVENTION.

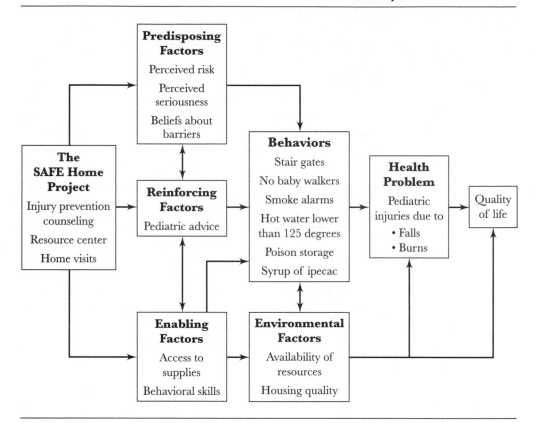

age four died as a result of unintentional injuries and one out of every four emergency department visits was due to an injury (Fingerhut and Warner, 1997).

Motor vehicle crashes are the leading cause of fatal injuries; falls, poisonings, and burns are the leading cause of nonfatal injuries for preschoolers. Most of the nonfatal injuries happen in and around the home (Baker, 1992; Rice and MacKenzie, 1989).

The American Academy of Pediatrics (AAP) recommends that pediatricians promote specific injury prevention practices to parents (American Academy of Pediatrics, 1994).

The extent to which pediatricians provide injury prevention counseling was not known, although recent studies indicated that, when provided, it could be effective (Bass and others, 1993; Miller and Galbraith, 1995).

We also assessed the prevalence of injuries in patients being seen at either the pediatric clinic or the pediatric emergency department for the year 1993. Both locations were selected because they are two of the clinical training sites for pediatric residents. More than six thousand injury diagnoses were made during this one-year period alone.

In preparing data collection instruments for the intervention trial, we confirmed that injury prevention was an important topic to families by conducting small, informal surveys in the clinic waiting room. Parents were asked to identify "things that concern you as a parent." Respondents generated from three to eight concerns, and child health and safety issues were frequently mentioned. When asked specifically to rank childhood injury in terms of its overall importance, about half the parents identified it as among their "most important" concerns.

These two steps in the process were conducted essentially without any specific guidance from a theory of health behavior change. However, we were cognizant of the important principles of health promotion practice, *participation* and *relevance*. To the extent that our resources allowed, we spoke with parents to confirm that injury prevention was a relevant topic to be addressed in this community. Parent input continued to be important and widely sought, as described in the subsequent steps.

Behavioral, Environmental, Educational, and Ecological Assessment (Steps 3 and 4).

Based on the literature and on advice from pediatricians, the most important and most changeable behavioral factors associated with in-home injuries in preschool children were found to be a cluster of behaviors, commonly referred to as "childproofing" (Wilson and others, 1991). For falls, burns, and poisonings, this includes using stair gates, not using baby walkers, having working smoke alarms, turning down the hot water temperature to less than 125 degrees, keeping poisonous substances locked away, and having syrup of ipecac in the home. There was little guidance in the literature about the relevant environmental factors associated with childproofing or with children's in-home injury experience. To clarify our understanding of the determinants of in-home injuries to preschool children, we supplemented our literature review with parent interviews (Gielen and others, 1995) and analysis of audiotapes of pediatric visits (Gielen, McDonald, Forrest, Harvilchuck, and Wissow, 1997). The results of this preliminary research are summarized in the following paragraphs.

Data from Parents. Parent interviews were guided by the Theory of Planned Behavior (Ajzen, 1991; see Chapter Four) because of its successful application to understanding a variety of other health-related behaviors. The theory directed us to examine the roles of personal beliefs about the consequences of childproofing, general attitudes toward childproofing, subjective norms, and barriers and facilitators of childproofing, including environmental factors.

The first step in applying this theory is to conduct elicitation interviews with a sample that represents the target population. The elicitation interview used semistructured items to elicit parents' perceptions of childproofing, what the term meant, its advantages and disadvantages and barriers and facilitators, and whose opinions about childproofing were important to parents. The results of these informal interviews were used to develop a structured interview that was administered to a convenience sample of 150 parents in the clinic (Gielen and others, 1995) to provide quantifiable data on parents' injury prevention practices (behavioral factor) and associated environmental factors, as well as predisposing, reinforcing, and enabling determinants.

We found that 88 percent of parents did not have syrup of ipecac, 63 percent did not know if their hot water temperature was at a safe setting, 59 percent did not use a stair gate, 27 percent did not have a smoke alarm, and 11 percent did not store poisonous substances safely. Only 5 percent of respondents reported doing all five childproofing practices. Despite these low rates of safety practices, virtually all respondents expressed favorable personal beliefs and attitudes about childproofing and the majority reported positive subjective norms favoring childproofing. In terms of environmental factors, housing quality, income, and barriers to childproofing such as not having help from others and moving often were significantly associated with the number of childproofing practices reported.

Constructs from the Theory of Planned Behavior were helpful in demonstrating the importance of barriers to parents but did not help to identify key beliefs that distinguished parents who practiced childproofing from those who did not. The Health Belief Model (Janz and Becker, 1984; see Chapter Three) and Weinstein's Precaution Adoption Process Model (Weinstein, 1988; see Chapter Six) suggest that parents' perceptions of the *risk of injury* and the *salience of this threat* might better explain their adoption of safety practices, as also was suggested by other published research (Glik, Kronenfeld, and Jackson, 1993).

From these data we concluded that disadvantaged living conditions, including a lack of resources and skills, interfere with parents' ability to implement safety practices, and uniformly favorable attitudes and norms suggest that a risk-oriented theory may be more useful for influencing parents' safety practices.

Data from Pediatricians. One of the reinforcing factors suggested by the parent interviews was routine injury prevention counseling by pediatricians. Although parents reported that their pediatricians thought childproofing was extremely important, discussions among the project team revealed that pediatricians received very little education about injury prevention during residency training. Pragmatically, because the intervention being planned was going to be delivered in the clinic, the role of the pediatrician was central. Theoretical and empirical support for their role was bolstered by evidence that the communication style of physicians has an impact on patient outcomes, and that adherence to principles of adult learning in counseling increases the chances of behavioral change (Roter, 1989; U.S. Preventive Services Task Force, 1996; Green and Kreuter, 1999). Thus, we needed a better understanding of pediatricians' current injury prevention counseling skills and efforts.

A prior study of mental health issues, conducted by a member of the project team, had included audiotaping all pediatric medical visits to the clinic over a one-year period (Wissow, Roter, and Wilson, 1994). From these, we selected all well-child visits for children under the age of five ($N = 214$) and developed a coding protocol to document the types of injury topics discussed and the communication skills used (Gielen, McDonald, Forrest, Harvilchuck, and Wissow, 1997). The majority (61 percent) of visits did not include any discussion of injury prevention. Among the remaining eighty-three visits in which families received any counseling, the average length of time spent on injury topics was 1.08 minutes per child. The most common communication pattern used by physicians was information giving, with little involvement of parents in any discussion.

From our analysis of these tapes, we concluded that injury prevention counseling was not a routine component of pediatric well-child care, potentially effective behavior change counseling skills were not widely evident, and prioritizing injury topics and enhancing communication skills should help pediatricians use limited time effectively and efficiently.

At this point in the PRECEDE-PROCEED planning process, data collection and planning had incorporated numerous theoretical constructs and principles of practice. Involvement of the population of interest included the primary audience, parents, and an equally important secondary target audience—pediatricians. Both individual-level theories (Theory of Planned Behavior, Health Belief Model, Precaution Adoption Process) and principles derived from interpersonal-level theories (adult learning, interpersonal communication) were incorporated into the data collection and analysis strategies. A considerable amount of data had been generated about injury prevalence; parents' childproofing knowledge, attitudes, and practices; and residents' clinical skills related to injury prevention counseling. The PRECEDE-PROCEED model prompted us to organize these data into predisposing, enabling, and reinforcing factors, which in turn allowed us to identify possible interventions likely to influence the health behaviors related to the health problem.

In the case of predisposing factors, parents had extremely favorable attitudes toward childproofing and we hypothesized that their perceptions about the

likelihood and seriousness of the risk of injury would be more important determinants of their childproofing behaviors. Parents' beliefs about barriers had also
emerged as important predisposing factors. With regard to reinforcing factors, our
needs assessment suggested that some reinforcements were in place. For instance,
mothers reported that their social support networks felt childproofing the home
was important. Professional associations endorsed injury prevention counseling
by pediatricians during well-child visits. One potentially important reinforcing factor was clearly missing: effective pediatric advice regarding childproofing. Finally,
in terms of enabling factors, access to safety supplies and the skills or assistance
to use them effectively were identified as important. The next step in the process
was translating these findings into effective intervention strategies.

Administrative and Policy Assessment and Implementation (Steps 5 and 6)

An administrative and policy assessment identified the resources needed, as well
as the barriers and supports available within the organization, to positively influence parents' childproofing practices. Three distinct yet related interventions were
identified: enhancing pediatricians' injury prevention counseling, developing a
clinic-based safety resource center, and conducting home visits. Planning for each
of these interventions again incorporated several theories and principles of practice, as described in the following paragraphs.

Enhanced Pediatric Counseling. The enhanced pediatric counseling was designed to address predisposing and reinforcing factors that influence parents' childproofing practices. Pediatric residents attended training sessions that covered
developmentally appropriate injury-prevention topics (falls, burns, poisonings) to
discuss with parents and specific communication skills to use for greater success
in improving parents' adoption of safety behaviors. As a result of the training, residents were expected to provide enhanced anticipatory guidance on injury prevention as a routine part of well-child care.

Implementing the training program within the organizational constraints of
the clinic schedule and the residency training program required support from the
pediatric faculty. Fortunately, they were integral members of the project team and
were committed to making it possible for the residents to attend. In fact, three pediatric faculty members served as trainers who provided effective role modeling,
reinforcement, and credibility.

A number of theories were useful in the development and implementation of
the enhanced pediatric counseling component. The primary objective was to enable pediatricians to heighten parents' perceptions about the risk and seriousness

of childhood injuries and to help them overcome specific barriers to injury prevention that are associated with living conditions in the inner city. In addition to drawing on these issues identified in the parent interview, we also drew on constructs from Stages of Change and information processing in the training. We educated pediatricians about the notion that health behavior change is a process and individuals are at different levels of readiness to change (Prochaska, DiClemente, and Norcross, 1992; see Chapter Five). Incorporating ideas from information-processing capacity, specifically that people are limited in the amount of information they can use and remember (Rudd and Glanz, 1990), we taught pediatricians how to select the most important injury-prevention advice to communicate.

Principles of adult learning and Social Cognitive Theory were used to successfully implement the enhanced pediatric counseling training. First, because residents brought to the training a considerable amount of experience in communicating with parents, we drew on their experiences in discussions during the training. We used a number of experiential teaching techniques, such as "skills stations," for hands-on practice with safety supplies (for example, smoke detectors, stair gates), shopping trips (for example, to purchase syrup of ipecac), and demonstrations (for example, falling down stairs in a walker). We also provided role-playing opportunities for residents to both observe and model effective communication and counseling skills. As residents practiced integrating new communication skills and safety messages into their counseling repertoire in the role plays, faculty trainers observed them and provided immediate feedback and critiques.

Onsite Safety Resource Center. The safety resource center focused primarily on reducing barriers of access to and costs of safety supplies, those enabling factors identified in earlier diagnostic steps. However, because education was provided by a trained health educator at the center, predisposing factors were also addressed. Advice from the health educator may also have served to reinforce the pediatrician's anticipatory guidance.

The objectives of the center are to increase the accessibility and affordability of home safety supplies for low-income families; to provide personalized, skills-oriented education that reinforces and supplements pediatric advice about child safety; and to elevate the priority given to injury prevention in medical care settings. Parents who come to the Children's Safety Center receive personalized home safety risk assessments and education, and can purchase safety products at reduced cost.

Many administrative and organizational constraints surfaced during the planning for this intervention component: space in the clinic for the center, renovation costs for the space, staffing, selecting and stocking supplies and educational materials, and access to the center by families who did not receive care in the clinic. A full year of planning was devoted to these issues before the center opened in March 1997 (McDonald and others, forthcoming).

The principles of participation and relevance were high priorities for developing the Children's Safety Center. Focus groups with parents were conducted to obtain their ideas about the role of the center, the supplies it should carry, and its operating policies and procedures. The notion of "empowerment" from community organization also influenced this component of the project. The clinic's Parent Advisory Board was consulted about plans for the center and also for the home-visiting component (described in the next section). Because pediatric residents made referrals to the center, they were also interviewed to allow them opportunities to shape the policies and procedures of the center.

Home Visits. The third intervention, home visits, addressed another recognized enabling factor—skills to adopt childproofing practices. Home visits were conducted by community health workers who described and demonstrated appropriate safety practices, such as changing a smoke alarm battery and testing the water temperature, and then allowed mothers to practice and master these skills. The community health worker did not actually install products because of liability concerns. Throughout the visit, efforts were made to emphasize predisposing factors, such as perceptions of injury risk and seriousness. Health workers also reinforced education that may have been provided by the pediatrician or health educator in the Children's Safety Center.

The administrative and organizational aspects of implementing this intervention were challenging. Training, supervising, and providing for the safety of community health workers making home visits required time and commitment from administrative staff. Safety protocols for the health workers and lists of community referrals were developed before the home visits began. It was especially important to develop a mechanism to make referrals for housing code violations, because poor housing quality had been identified by parents as a barrier to implementing safety practices.

Community empowerment and capacity building were evidenced by employing health workers from the community where the families resided. Moreover, the tasks of the community health workers were informed by the Social Cognitive Theory constructs of role modeling and self-efficacy.

Process, Impact, and Outcome Evaluation (Steps 7–9)

The final three steps in the PRECEDE-PROCEED planning model address evaluation of the intervention's process, impact, and outcome.

Evaluation Design. The SAFE Home Project was evaluated using a randomized controlled trial involving two cohorts of pediatricians and their patients' parents, who were enrolled during visits to the Harriet Lane Clinic when the infants were between birth and six months of age. Families enrolled in the evaluation were followed until their child was twelve to eighteen months old. Baseline and follow-up surveys of parents' knowledge, beliefs, and barriers (predisposing, reinforcing, enabling factors) were completed, and home observations were used to document safety practices and household hazards (behavioral and environmental factors). Because injuries are rare events and funding was limited, we could not follow families long enough to assess injury outcomes. Only a brief synopsis of the evaluation activities is provided here. Interested readers should refer to other sources for more details (Gielen and others, 2001, 2002; McDonald and others, forthcoming).

Cohort 1 pediatricians (and their patients' parents) were randomized to either a control or intervention group. All pediatricians received a one-hour seminar on pediatric injuries provided by the director of general pediatrics as part of their routine pediatric education. Pediatricians in the intervention group also participated in the special training in enhanced injury-prevention counseling, as described above. When the twelve-to-eighteen-month follow-up with this group was completed, the onsite Children's Safety Center was opened and Cohort 2 pediatricians (and their patients' parents) were recruited and randomly assigned to one of two intervention groups. Pediatricians in both intervention groups in Cohort 2 received the same special training in enhanced injury prevention counseling that was used in Cohort 1, and all of their patients' parents had access to the Children's Safety Center. One-half of these Cohort 2 pediatricians were randomly assigned to the home-visit intervention group, and their patients' parents were then offered the home visit when their babies were six to nine months old.

Process Evaluation. Process evaluation data are critical because they document how well program components are being implemented as planned and intended audiences are being reached. Process evaluation is particularly important in an intervention trial because it helps with both interpretation of the impact evaluation and replication of the intervention. In the SAFE Home Project, all pediatric visits with families enrolled in the project were audiotaped, and after each visit both the parent and physician completed checklists to record reactions to the visit and the counseling. These data were used to document whether enhanced injury-prevention counseling actually took place as well as parents' satisfaction. Based on analysis of audiotapes of medical visits in Cohort 1, we found that families in the intervention group received significantly more injury-prevention counseling than did families in the standard-care group and more counseling was provided for five out of six safety practices studied. Also, exit surveys completed after each visit showed that families cared for by pediatricians in the intervention group were significantly more satisfied with the amount of help they received about safety from their pediatrician, compared to families in the control group (Gielen and others, 2001).

Impact and Outcome Evaluation. Although families in the Cohort 1 intervention group were more satisfied than those in the control group with their pediatrician's counseling, there were no differences between the groups on their home-safety knowledge, beliefs, and self-reported practices, or on observed safety practices. We concluded that low-income families need additional support, such as improved access to safety products and additional reinforcement of educational messages, to affect behavioral change (Gielen and others, 2001). In Cohort 2, we found no evidence for an effect of the home-visit intervention on observed safety practices. However, when comparing families who visited the Children's Safety Center ($N = 75$) with those who did not ($N = 74$) we found statistically significant positive effects, even after adjusting for exposure to the other intervention components (such as counseling and home visits) and testing for potential selection differences between the two groups. Children's Safety Center visitors were using significantly more safety products and practices than non-visitors (Gielen and others, 2002). The results of these evaluation activities suggest that of the theoretical constructs used to guide program design, the enabling factors were paramount for the issue of home safety in this low-income, urban sample. The PRECEDE-PROCEED model guided the development of both the intervention components and the instruments used for evaluation. Thus, the follow-up interviews will provide important information about the relative importance of the predisposing, reinforcing, and enabling factors associated with the childproofing behaviors under study. We are continuing to analyze the parent interviews to further assess the relationship between these factors and parents' safety behaviors.

Conclusion

As with many professional endeavors, health education and health promotion include both *art* and *science*. There will always be a need for sound professional judgment in making decisions about program design, as part of the art of the discipline. The PRECEDE-PROCEED model is part of the science of the field. Using a systematic, theory-based planning model distinguishes the technician from the health behavior change professional. Technical experts start with a technique and apply it to whatever problem is presented, whereas health behavior change professionals draw selectively and advisedly from various techniques to solve problems. (Lawrence Green, personal communication, February 12, 2001). The PRECEDE-PROCEED planning framework was first developed partly because its originators felt that technical aspects were overemphasized relative to finding the right match between technique and audience needs.

For public health professionals, the usefulness of theory is in its application to solving real-world problems. The PRECEDE-PROCEED planning model helps in this process. It provides an approach to health promotion program planning that is both structured and flexible. Its careful diagnostic approach forces planners to think critically about where and how to intervene. The categories of behavioral determinants are sufficiently broad to incorporate the most relevant theoretical constructs for the problem under study, while at the same time helping to ensure a comprehensive approach to problem solving. By incorporating different levels of analysis of the problem and by linking determinants to intervention methods, the process broadens health promotion planning beyond constructs that are typically included in any single theory. PRECEDE-PROCEED should not be confused with a predictive theory but rather considered an integrative planning model that can be used to assist in the rigorous application of theory to practice.

References

Ajzen, I. "The Theory of Planned Behavior." *Organizational Behavior and Human Decision Processes,* 1991, *50,* 179–211.

American Academy of Pediatrics. *TIPP: The Injury Prevention Program: A Guide to Safety Counseling in Office Practice.* Chicago, Ill.: American Academy of Pediatrics, 1994.

Baker, S. P., O'Neill, B., Ginsburg, M. J., and Li, G. *The Injury Fact Book.* (2nd ed.) New York: Oxford University Press, 1992.

Bandura, A. *Social Foundations of Thought and Action: A Social Cognitive Theory.* Englewood Cliffs, N.J.: Prentice Hall, 1986.

Bartholomew, L. K., Parcel, G. S., Kok, G., and Gottlieb, N. H. *Intervention Mapping: Designing Theory and Evidence Based Health Promotion Programs.* Mountain View, Calif.: Mayfield, 2001.

Bass, J. L., and others. "Childhood Injury Prevention Counseling in Primary Care Settings: A Critical Review of the Literature." *Pediatrics,* 1993, *92*(4), 544–550.

Bertera, R. L. "Planning and Implementing Health Promotion in the Workplace: A Case Study of the DuPont Company Experience." *Health Education Quarterly,* 1990, *17*(3), 307–327.

Bertera, R. L. "Behavioral Risk Factor and Illness Day Changes with Workplace Health Promotion: Two-Year Results." *American Journal of Health Promotion,* 1993, *7*(5), 365–373.

Brown, E. R. "Community Action for Health Promotion: A Strategy to Empower Individuals and Communities." *International Journal of Health Education,* 1991, *21*(3), 441–456.

Centers for Disease Control, National Center for Chronic Disease Prevention and Health Promotion. "PATCH: Planned Approach to Community Health." *Journal of Health Education,* 1992, *23*(3), 129–192.

Clark, N. M., and McLeroy, K. R. "Creating Capacity through Health Education: What We Know and What We Don't." *Health Education Quarterly,* 1995, *22*(3), 273–289.

Clarke, V. A., Frankish, C. J., and Green, L. W. "Understanding Suicide Among Indigenous Adolescents: A Review Using the PRECEDE Model," *Injury Prevention,* 1997, *3*(2), 126–134.

Dignan, M. B., and others. "Health Education to Increase Screening for Cervical Cancer Among Lumbee Indian Women in North Carolina." *Health Education Research,* 1998, *13*(4), 545–556.

Eng, E., and Blanchard, L. "Action-Oriented Community Diagnosis: A Health Education Tool." *International Quarterly of Community Health Education,* 1991, *11*(2), 93–110.

Eriksen, M. P., and Gielen, A. C. "The Application of Health Education Principles to Automobile Child Restraint Programs." *Health Education Quarterly,* 1983, *10*(1), 30–55.

Erlich, J. L., Rothman, J., and Teresa, J. G. *Taking Action in Organizations and Communities.* (2nd ed.) Dubuque, Iowa: Eddie Bowers, 1999.

Fingerhut, L. A., and Warner, M. *Injury Chartbook. Health, United States, 1996–97.* Hyattsville, Md.: National Center for Health Statistics, 1997.

Freudenberg, N., and others. "Strengthening Individual and Community Capacity to Prevent Disease and Promote Health: In Search of Relevant Theories and Principles." *Health Education Quarterly,* 1995, *22*(3), 290–306.

Gielen, A. C. "Health Education and Injury Control: Integrating Approaches." *Health Education Quarterly,* 1992, *19*(2), 203–218.

Gielen, A. C., Bernstein-Cohen, L., and Radius, S. "Case Study of Program Evaluation Activities for Child Passenger Safety Programs in Local Health Department Settings." Paper presented at the 113th Annual Meeting of the American Public Health Association, Washington, D.C., November 1985.

Gielen, A. C., McDonald, E. M., Forrest, C. B., Harvilchuck, J. D., and Wissow, L. "Injury Prevention Counseling in an Urban Pediatric Clinic: Analysis of Audiotaped Visits." *Archives of General Pediatrics and Adolescent Medicine,* 1997, *151,* 146–151.

Gielen, A. C., and others. "In-Home Injury Prevention Practices for Infants and Toddlers: The Role of Parental Beliefs, Barriers, and Housing Quality." *Health Education Quarterly,* 1995, *22*(1), 85–95.

Gielen, A. C., and others. "Randomized Trial of Enhanced Anticipatory Guidance for Injury Prevention." *Archives of General Pediatrics and Adolescent Medicine,* 2001, *155,* 42–49.

Gielen A. C., and others. "Effects of Improved Access to Safety Counseling, Products and Home Visits on Parents' Safety Practices." *Archives of General Pediatrics and Adolescent Medicine,* 2002, *156*(1), 33–40.

Glanz, K. "Book Review. Health Promotion Planning: An Educational and Ecological Approach, (3rd ed.), by L. W. Green and M. W. Kreuter, 1999." *American Journal of Preventive Medicine,* 2000, *18,* 104–105.

Glanz, K., Lewis, F. M., and Rimer, B. K. "Theory, Research, and Practice in Health Education: Building Bridges and Forging Links." In K. Glanz, F. M. Lewis, and B. K. Rimer (eds.), *Health Behavior and Health Education: Theory, Research, and Practice.* (2nd ed.) San Francisco: Jossey-Bass, 1996.

Glanz, K., and Rimer, B. K. *Theory at a Glance: A Guide for Health Promotion Practice.* National Institutes of Health Publication Number 95–2896, 1995. Available at: http://oc.nci.nih.gov/services/Theory_at_glance/HOME.html

Glik, D., Kronenfeld, J., and Jackson, K. "Safety Behaviors Among Parents of Preschoolers." *Health Values,* 1993, *17*(1), 18–27.

Gottlieb, N. H., and McLeroy, K. R. "Social Health." In M. O'Donnell and J. Harris (eds.), *Health Promotion in the Workplace.* (2nd ed.) Albany, N.Y.: Delmar, 1994.

Green, L. W., and Kreuter, M. W. *Health Promotion Planning: An Educational and Ecological Approach.* (3rd ed.) Mountain View, Calif.: Mayfield, 1991.

Green, L. W., and Kreuter, M. W. *Health Promotion Planning: An Educational and Environmental Approach.* (2nd ed.) Mountain View, Calif.: Mayfield, 1999.

Green, L. W., Kreuter, M. W., Deeds, S. G., and Partridge, K. B. *Health Education Planning: A Diagnostic Approach.* Mountain View, Calif.: Mayfield, 1980.

Hendrickson, S. G., and Becker, H. "Impact of a Theory-Based Intervention to Increase Bicycle Helmet Use in Low-Income Children." *Injury Prevention,* 1998, *4*(2), 126–131.

Howat, P., Jones, S., Hall, M., Cross, D., and Stevenson, M. "The PRECEDE-PROCEED Model: Application to Planning a Child Pedestrian Injury Prevention Program." *Injury Prevention,* 1997, *3*(4), 282–287.

Israel, B. A., Checkoway, B., Schulz, A., and Zimmerman, M. "Health Education and Community Empowerment: Conceptualizing and Measuring Perceptions of Individual, Organizational and Community Control." *Health Education Quarterly,* 1994, *21*, 149–170.

Janz, N. K., and Becker, M. H. "The Health Belief Model: A Decade Later." *Health Education Quarterly,* 1984, *11*, 1–47.

Kretzmann, J. P., and McKnight, J. L. *Building Communities from the Inside Out: A Path Toward Finding and Mobilizing a Community's Assets.* Evanston, Ill.: The Asset-Based Community Development Institute, 1993.

Kreuter, M. K., Farrell, D., Olevitch, L., and Brennan, T. *Tailoring Health Messages: Customizing Communication with Computer Technology.* Mahwah, N.J.: Erlbaum, 2000.

McAlister, A. "Social Learning Theory and Preventive Behavior." In N. D. Weinstein (ed.), *Taking Care: Understanding and Encouraging Self-Protective Behavior.* Cambridge, Mass: Cambridge University Press, 1987.

McDonald, E. M., and others. "Evaluation Activities to Strengthen an Injury Prevention Resource Center for Urban Families." *Health Promotion Practice,* forthcoming.

McGinnis, J. M., and Foege, W. H. "Actual Causes of Death in the United States." *Journal of the American Medical Association,* 1993, *270*(18), 2207–2212.

McLeroy, K. R., Bibeau, D., Steckler, A., and Glanz, K. "An Ecological Perspective on Health Promotion Programs." *Health Education Quarterly,* 1988, *15*(4), 351–377.

Miller, T. R., and Galbraith, M. "Injury Prevention Counseling by Pediatricians: A Benefit-Cost Comparison." *Pediatrics,* 1995, *96*(1), 1–4.

Minkler, M. "Building Supportive Ties and Sense of Community Among the Inner-City Elderly: The Tenderloin Senior Outreach Project." *Health Education Quarterly,* 1985, *12*, 303–314.

Minkler, M. "Improving Health Through Community Organization." In K. Glanz, F. M. Lewis, and B. K. Rimer (eds.), *Health Behavior and Health Education: Theory, Research, and Practice.* (2nd ed.) San Francisco: Jossey-Bass, 1996.

Morisky, D. L., and others. "Five-Year Blood Pressure Control and Mortality Following Health Education for Hypertensive Patients." *American Journal of Public Health,* 1983, *73*(2), 153–162.

Mullen, P. D., Hersey, J. C., and Iverson, D. C. "Health Behavior Models Compared." *Social Science and Medicine,* 1987, *24*(11), 973–981.

National Committee for Injury Prevention and Control. *Injury Prevention: Meeting the Challenge.* New York: Oxford University Press, 1989.

Orenstein, D., and others. "Synthesis of the Four PATCH Evaluations." *Journal of Health Education,* 1992, *23*(3), 187–193.

Prochaska, J. O., DiClemente, C. C., and Norcross, J. C. "In Search of How People Change: Applications to Addictive Behaviors." *American Psychologist,* 1992, *47*(9), 1102–1114.

Rice, D. P., and MacKenzie, E. J. "Cost of Injury in the United States: A Report to Congress." San Francisco: Institute for Health and Aging, University of California and Injury Prevention Center, The Johns Hopkins University, 1989.

Rimer, B. "Audiences and Messages for Breast and Cervical Cancer Screenings." *Wellness Perspectives,* 1995, *11*(2), 13–39.

Rogers, E. M. *Diffusion of Innovations.* (4th ed.) New York: Free Press, 1995.

Roter, D. "Which Facets of Communication Have Strong Effects on Outcome—A Meta-Analysis." In M. Stewart and D. Roter (eds.), *Communicating with Medical Patients.* Thousand Oaks, Calif.: Sage, 1989.

Rudd, J., and Glanz, K. "How Individuals Use Information for Health Action: Consumer Information Processing." In K. Glanz, F. M. Lewis, and B. K. Rimer (eds.), *Health Behavior and Health Education: Theory, Research, and Practice.* San Francisco: Jossey-Bass, 1990.

Simons-Morton, B. G., and others. "An Ecological Approach to the Prevention of Injuries Due to Drinking and Driving." *Health Education Quarterly,* 1989, *16*(3), 397–411.

Steckler, A. B., Dawson, L., Israel, B. A., and Eng, E. "Community Health Development: An Overview of the Works of Guy W. Steuart." *Health Education Quarterly,* 1993, Supplement 1, S3-S20.

U.S. Department of Health and Human Services. *Healthy People 2010: National Health Promotion and Disease Prevention Objectives.* DHHS Publication No. (PHS) 91–50213. Washington, D.C.: Government Printing Office, 2000.

U.S. Preventive Services Task Force. *Guide to Clinical Preventive Services.* (2nd ed.) Baltimore, Md.: Williams and Wilkins, 1996.

Wallerstein, N. "Powerlessness, Empowerment, and Health: Implications for Health Promotion Programs." *American Journal of Health Promotion,* 1992, *6*(3), 197–205.

Wallerstein, N., and Bernstein, E. (eds.), "Community Empowerment, Participatory Education, and Health—Part I and Part II." *Health Education Quarterly,* 1994, *21*(2 and 3).

Weinstein, N. D. "The Precaution Adoption Process." *Health Psychology,* 1988, *7*(4), 355–386.

Wilson, M.E.H., and others. *Saving Children: A Guide to Injury Prevention.* New York: Oxford University Press, 1991.

Windsor, R. A. "An Application of the PRECEDE Model for Planning and Evaluating Education Methods for Pregnant Smokers." *International Journal of Health Education,* 1986, *5,* 38–43.

Windsor, R. A., and others. "Health Education for Pregnant Smokers: Its Behavioral Impact and Cost Benefit." *American Journal of Public Health,* 1993, *83*(2), 201–206.

Wissow, L. S., Roter, D. L., and Wilson, M.E.H. "Physician Interview Style and Mothers' Disclosure of Psychosocial Issues Important to Child Development." *Pediatrics,* 1994, *93,* 289–295.

Worden, J. K., and others. "A Community-Wide Program in Breast Self-Examination Training and Maintenance." *Preventive Medicine,* 1990, *19,* 254–269.

CHAPTER NINETEEN

SOCIAL MARKETING

Edward W. Maibach
Michael L. Rothschild
William D. Novelli

In the first edition of *Health Behavior and Health Education,* William D. Novelli's chapter on social marketing (1990) opened with a passage about the allure of marketing in public health. "For a long time, nonbusiness managers have looked at marketing and speculated about its application to social change. As was asked (fifty) years ago, 'Why can't you sell brotherhood like soap?'" (Wiebe, 1951–52). The allure of marketing is still alive and well in the field of public health.

R. Craig Lefebvre and Lisa Rochlin's (1996) chapter in the second edition of this book opened by documenting the ways in which social marketing had come of age since 1990, especially in the field of public health. The evidence cited included the establishment of a peer-reviewed journal and two annual conferences and the proliferation of review articles and books on the subject. Most important, they cited the fact that "[the use of] social marketing has expanded from a few federal, state, and private-sector agencies to virtually all federal agencies with a charge to conduct public health education efforts, . . . voluntary health organizations, and numerous private-sector agencies." Indeed, this expansion of social marketing programs has continued unabated to date.

Unfortunately, despite its allure and dramatic growth, social marketing remains poorly understood by many in the field of public health. Being misunderstood, especially in the context of growing demand, may pose a serious threat to the future of social marketing. William Smith (1993), one of the field's leading practitioners, described the threat in the following way: "I think the future of social marketing is in doubt. [Unless] we do something now, it will either pass away as just another fad of the 80s, or worse yet, be institutionalized as a new bureaucratic routine of the 90s. In both cases it may die, or become fossilized, without ever having been understood. The problem with social marketing is clear. There is often little or no marketing [in social marketing]."

This concern appears to be more relevant today than ever. There is still often little or no marketing in social marketing. Social marketing will continue to be misunderstood, and may as a result fail to live up to its promise, if nonmarketing-based health education and health behavior programs continue to proliferate under the banner of social marketing and if true marketing-based health education programs are few and far between.

Our goal for this chapter, therefore, is twofold: (1) to describe social marketing in a manner that will be clearly understood, and (2) to enable health education practitioners to harness elements of marketing practice in their behavioral change programs. To that end, we will present definitions of social marketing, discuss certain key concepts, and illustrate its use through two case studies. We will also differentiate social marketing from other approaches to behavioral influence (specifically education and legal approaches). The ability to distinguish between what social marketing is and what it isn't can help to eliminate misconceptions.

Defining Social Marketing

Many definitions of social marketing have been promulgated. For the purpose of reducing misunderstandings, we feel it important to harness elements of various definitions into a redefinition of social marketing. The three definitions we have drawn most directly from are

> "[Social marketing is] a program planning process that promotes the voluntary behavior of target audiences by offering benefits they want, reducing barriers they are concerned about, and using persuasion to motivate their participation in program activity" (Kotler and Roberto, 1989).

> "Social marketing is the application of commercial marketing technologies to the analysis, planning, execution, and evaluation of programs designed to influence the voluntary behavior of target audiences in order to improve their personal welfare and that of their society" (Andreasen, 1995).

> "[Social] [m]arketing consists of voluntary exchange between two or more parties, in which each is trying to further its own perceived self-interest while recognizing the need to accommodate the perceived self-interest of the other to achieve its own ends" (Rothschild, 1999).

These three definitions overlap completely with regard to one important point: the primary objective of social marketing is to influence the voluntary behavior of target market members. This influence that social marketers attempt to wield can include both efforts to change people's behavior (for example, to help people to quit smoking), and efforts to maintain people's current behavior (for example, to prevent people from initiating the smoking habit).

Kotler and Roberto's (1989) definition introduces a second critical attribute. Social marketing programs seek to influence behavior by offering target market members an attractive package of benefits and by reducing barriers that would otherwise discourage them from engaging in the behavior. Social marketers may attempt to alter the benefits and barriers associated with choices currently available to members of the target market or may create and deliver new alternative choices. Regardless, offering attractive benefits and reducing critical barriers are hallmarks of the social marketing approach.

Andreasen's (1995) definition introduces a third critical attribute. The primary beneficiaries of social marketing programs are members of the target market themselves, or society at large, rather than the person or the organization that initiated the marketing program. This distinction is important in that it differentiates social marketing from commercial marketing. By way of example, promoting handwashing among food preparation workers could qualify as social marketing, whereas promoting a specific brand of hand soap for food preparation workers (versus competitive brands of hand soap) probably would not.

Rothschild's (1999) definition introduces two final concepts we see as critical attributes of social marketing: fulfilling self-interests and voluntary exchange. It is human nature that people attempt to fulfill their own interests, and it is the nature of successful organizations that they too exist to fulfill their self-interests (as defined by the people who run the organization). Thus, both parties—the marketing organization and members of the target market—are attempting to fulfill their own interests. Effective marketers (and effective marketing organizations) learn to offer products, services, or ideas that members of the target market perceive to be in their own best interest. Target market members reciprocate by purchasing the product or service, or in some other way behaving (that is, using their resources) in a manner that fulfills the marketer's definition of self-interest. In other words, organizations succeed at marketing (that is, fulfilling their own self-interest) by assessing and meeting the perceived needs of their target market (by accommodating the self-interest of members of the target market).

This basic point in the Rothschild definition—that the heart of the marketing concept is the mutual fulfillment of self-interest through voluntary exchange—also suggests an alternative, and perhaps more distinct, way to differentiate social from commercial marketing. The marketing organization's definition of success is what differentiates social from commercial marketing. Commercial marketing occurs when the marketing organization defines success primarily in terms of financial gain, and social marketing occurs when the marketing organization defines success primarily in terms of benefits to members of the target market or to society as a whole. Both forms of marketing can yield benefits to members of the target market, and financial profit, but the point of distinction is the primary motivation of the marketing organization.

We use these critical attributes to derive the following definition: social marketing is a process that attempts to create voluntary exchange between a marketing organization and members of a target market based on mutual fulfillment of self-interest. The marketing organization uses its resources to understand the perceived interests of target market members; to enhance and deliver the package of benefits associated with a product, service, or idea; and to reduce barriers that interfere with the adoption or maintenance of that product, service, or idea. Target market members, in turn, expend their resources (such as money, time, or effort) in exchange for the offer when it provides clear advantages over alternative behaviors. Success of the social marketing program is defined primarily in terms of its contribution to the well-being of target market members, or to society as a whole.

Differentiating Social Marketing from Other Approaches to Behavioral Influence

Social marketing is a process that seeks to influence the behavior of target market members for their own benefit. There are also, however, nonmarketing approaches to influencing target market behavior. Understanding the differences between these approaches can clarify what social marketing is and what it isn't. For this purpose, Rothschild (1999) distinguished marketing from two other major options for influencing behavior: education and law. In the following section, we discuss the three options.

Education

Education refers to the delivery of information intended to inform or persuade members of a target market to voluntarily behave in a particular manner. As such, it can raise awareness of the benefits of a given behavior, but it cannot directly deliver those benefits. Defined in this manner, education is often a component of marketing, but is not synonymous with marketing.

Education alone can be sufficient to influence behavior under certain conditions. When the benefits of a recommended behavior are sufficiently attractive, when the barriers to performance are sufficiently minor, or when the alternative behaviors offer relatively less attractive benefits, education alone can have a powerful influence on behavior. Consider, for example, the dramatic reduction of Sudden Infant Death Syndrome (SIDS) since 1993 in the United States and in many other countries around the world. Merely educating parents to place their babies on their backs to sleep was sufficient to cause widespread behavior change and subsequent reductions in the incidence of SIDS (American Academy of Pediatrics, 2001). The same was true with regard to the reduction of Reyes Syndrome, a serious condition caused by administration of aspirin to children with high fevers (Soumerai, Ross-Degnan, and Kahn, 1992). In both instances, the recommended behavior offers highly valued benefits (that is, the continued life and good health of a child), the barriers to performance are minimal as the behaviors themselves are simple and easy to perform, and the alternative behaviors do not offer a compelling package of benefits.

Conversely, education alone often will not be sufficient to create behavioral change. This is typically the case when the recommended behavior's package of benefits is less compelling, the barriers to performance are more significant, or the alternative behaviors offer equal if not more compelling benefits. Consider, for example, smoking during pregnancy, binge drinking on college campuses, or the rapidly increasing rates of obesity due to a combination of increased caloric intake and reduced physical activity. These problems have shown remarkable resistance to behavior change through educational approaches alone.

Marketing

A marketing approach to behavioral change involves elements that go beyond education. Social marketers attempt to modify the relative attractiveness of specific behavioral options through the use of incentives and other benefits that positively reinforce the desired behaviors and through the reduction of barriers or costs associated with the behavior. In this way, social marketing seeks to "tip the scales" in the eyes of the target audience toward one choice and away from competing choices.

Every effort is made in social marketing to provide direct immediate benefits (in other words, positive reinforcement), either when an exchange is completed or when consumption occurs, so as to confirm that the exchange was indeed in the target market member's self-interest. Providing direct and immediate reinforcement is important specifically because immediate reinforcement has greater potential to shape behavior than does the expectation of (even more highly valued) benefits in the distant future.

Social marketing programs also make every effort to identify and reduce or remove barriers likely to interfere with a target market member's motivation or ability to perform the desired behavior. These barriers may be personal (for example, low sense of self-efficacy to perform the behavior), social (for example, loved ones or peers who are not supportive of the behavior change), economic (for example, money), or environmental (for example, lack of access to products or services needed to perform the behavior).

Social marketing programs attempt to ensure that all persons and organizations expected to play a role in the program will further their own interests as a result of participation. Not only must members of the target market further their self-interest as a result of the recommended behavior, but the other people and organizations involved in the target market's performance of the behavior must advance their interests as well. If means to do so are not inherent in the program (or in the exchange), the program is unlikely to support or facilitate the behavior being recommended to members of the target market.

Consider a reminder program intended to increase adherence with mammography guidelines among members of an HMO. Clinicians or office managers will be motivated to implement the program to the extent that it helps them fulfill their self-interests, and they will be resistant to the extent that it interferes with fulfillment of their interests. For example, the program is more likely to be implemented if it is perceived as offering a savings of time to HMO staff (a direct benefit to staff members) and improved mammography adherence (a direct benefit to patients and to the HMO because it helps them achieve HEDIS [Health Plan Employer Data and Information Set] requirements). Conversely, the program is less likely to be implemented if it improves mammography adherence but at the expense of additional time on the part of HMO staff.

Law

The use of laws is another approach to behavioral influence distinct from but of potential relevance to marketing solutions. Certain types of laws use coercion to achieve behavioral change in a nonvoluntary manner by threatening penalties for noncompliance. Examples include monetary fines for violations of seat-belt, child-restraint, and motorcycle-helmet laws. When such laws are deemed to be in society's best interest, they could be thought of as an exchange based on mutual fulfillment of self-interest. The distinction between use of these types of laws and marketing is the coercive versus voluntary nature of the exchange as well as the difference between rewarding compliant behavior and punishing undesirable behavior.

Laws and public policies also can be used in noncoercive ways. "Sin taxes" and price subsidies, for example, are uses of law to influence the relative attractiveness of one behavioral option versus another through monetary incentives or disincentives. Another noncoercive set of laws includes measures that increase nonmonetary barriers to a behavior (for example, access). An example of this approach is when alcohol sales are prohibited after a certain time of day.

The opportunities to use marketing, education, or law can be thought of as a continuum bounded at one end by "prone to behave as desired" and at the other end by "resistant to behave as desired." Different target markets for any public health or social issue may lie at many points along this continuum (Figure 19.1).

There will also be target markets that are neither prone nor resistant to influence but are closer to the middle of the continuum. They are open to good offers. Marketing can be used to increase benefits, to reduce barriers, to provide incentives, or to change the opportunities that exist as a way of encouraging a particular behavior.

FIGURE 19.1. CONTINUUM OF MARKETING, EDUCATION, AND LAW.

Prone to Behave as Desired		Resistant to Behave as Desired
Easy to see or convey self-interest	Need to manage and show benefits	Can't see and can't convey self-interest or benefits
Education	Marketing	Law
|←— Continue behavior —→| |←— Change behavior —→|	
no or weak competition	passive-active competition	unmanageable competition

1. Any issue can be placed on the continuum.
2. Any target within an issue can be placed on the continuum.

Combinations of Marketing, Education, and Law

For any health issue, there may be target markets requiring different combinations of marketing, education, and law. For example, most parents when told that their children should be immunized against childhood diseases immediately agree and only need to be told where to go for the immunization. Education is sufficient for this target market, as the infrastructure already exists to accommodate them. A second target consists of parents who see the benefit of having their children immunized but fail to do so as a result of economic or environmental barriers. Here, we may use marketing to provide free immunizations and increased access to immunization clinics. A third target consists of parents resistant to the concept of immunizations or who for some other reason do not respond to education and marketing efforts. Because society has deemed immunization to be in nearly every child's best interest, states pass laws that mandate immunization as a prerequisite for school or day-care entry (with exceptions made only for medical, religious, and in some cases philosophical reasons). The combination of education, marketing, and law is needed to protect children from serious infectious disease.

Key Elements of Social Marketing Practice

Certain key elements of social marketing practice differentiate it from other forms of health promotion intervention (see Table 19.1). Recognizing, assessing, and harnessing all elements of the marketing mix are fundamental aspects of social marketing practice. The elements of the marketing mix—also known as the 4 Ps of marketing—are product, price, place, and promotion.

Product (The Bundle of Benefits)

Social marketers assess the degree to which products, services, or ideas can be offered to target market members to increase the likelihood of eliciting a desired behavior from them. The more benefits of interest offered, the greater the likelihood that members of the target market will voluntarily surrender some of their resources in exchange for those benefits.

Thus, from a process perspective, the social marketer begins by identifying the benefits of greatest interest to target market members. Then, using resources available, the social marketer creates new products or services, or alters existing products or services, in a manner that will deliver as many of the desired benefits as possible to target market members.

Consider, for example, a county public health agency that seeks to reduce the prevalence of smoking among pregnant women. Consumer research with preg-

TABLE 19.1. SOCIAL MARKETING CONCEPTS.

Concept	Definition	Application
Mutual fulfillment of self-interest	Creating an exchange between the marketing organization and the target market that advances the interests of both groups	Create behavior change among members of a target market by developing opportunities for them to further their self-interest in a manner that is consistent with the mission of the marketing organization
Consumer orientation	The use of information to understand target market members and thereby develop marketing offers that respond to their perceptions of self-interest	Conduct audience research to understand consumer perceptions and competitive analysis to understand the environment in which a marketing offer will be introduced
Segmentation	The process of subdividing larger, more heterogeneous markets into smaller, more homogeneous market segments	Use attributes of market members (demographics, behaviors, and beliefs) to create segments based on between-group differences that will most influence program design and outcome
Marketing mix	The four basic elements of a marketing program: product, price, place, and promotion	Develop marketing programs that offer an attractive bundle of benefits, at an acceptable cost, at the time and place when or where target market members will be most open to the offer; inform and persuade target market members that the offer is in their self-interest

nant smokers shows that they understand the health risks of smoking, both to themselves and to their unborn children, but that smoking provides them with a number of important benefits (in addition to satisfying their addiction). One of these benefits is the opportunity to bond with friends over a cigarette. Another is the opportunity to gain some solitude for at least five minutes at a time by stepping outside for a smoke while someone else watches the children. Smoking cessation classes and other traditional forms of counseling may teach pregnant women cessation skills, but they are unlikely to replace highly valued benefits of smoking. As an alternative to a counseling-based intervention, a health department might offer a simple cessation brochure (to teach cessation skills) along with a "mommy respite" program to pregnant women who agree to quit smoking. The respite program could offer thirty minutes of daily baby-sitting services, at no cost, during the course of pregnancy so that women in the process of quitting can have a quiet moment each day for friendship, exercise, or solitude. This product-based approach offers pregnant smokers the opportunity to maintain the benefits of smoking that they value most, while also directly reinforcing them for giving up the harmful behavior.

Price (Reducing the Bundle of Barriers or Costs)

An equally important element in the social marketing process is the assessment of the barriers or costs involved in adopting the behavior (that is, purchasing the product or making the exchange) for members of the target market. As mentioned previously, these costs can be economic, psychological, social, and environmental. Identifying which costs create the most significant barriers for target market members allows the social marketer to make informed decisions about the best use of limited resources to maximize cost reduction. The more that costs of concern can be reduced or eliminated, the greater the likelihood that members of the target market will voluntarily incur the remaining costs in exchange for the benefits offered.

From a process perspective, the social marketer conducts consumer research with target market members to identify perceptions about product-related costs, including which of those costs are perceived to be the most significant barriers. Then, within the constraints of resources available, the social marketer designs the product in a manner that reduces or eliminates as many of those costs as possible.

Consider, for example, the use of price to promote more nutritious versus less nutritious snack selections from vending machines (French and others, 2001). By lowering the monetary price of more nutritious options (while holding stable the price of less nutritious items), marketers can increase sales of nutritious snacks considerably. In a test of this premise, the pricing strategy successfully influenced behavior as intended and effectively did so at zero cost to the marketing organization. Price reductions led to an increase in sales volume, and the increased volume of sales at a lower profit margin allowed the total level of profit to remain constant.

Place (Delivering the Benefits and Costs to the Right Place at the Right Time)

In consumer marketing, the distribution channel—getting the product in front of the customer—often may be the most important element of the marketing mix. Consider, for example, Coca-Cola's placement strategy: the consumer should never be more than an arm's length away from a Coke. Social marketers have no less of a need to make their products accessible and convenient.

From a process perspective, taking full advantage of the placement element requires a detailed understanding of where target market members spend their time, when and where they make their decisions, and who has access to them during those critical periods. Social marketers make decisions about how best to use their limited resources to place products in front of target market members as frequently as possible and in as close proximity as possible to the time in which the product will be used. This is often done in cooperation with other organizations (in other words, distribution partners) that have access to the target market.

Consider, for example, interventions to encourage condom use as a means to prevent HIV and other sexually transmitted infections among men who have sex with men. The probability of condom use increases to the extent that condoms are distributed in close proximity to when and where people have sex. Placement interventions that increase ready access to condoms when and where they are needed have been shown to increase rates of condom usage among individuals at high risk of HIV infection (Cohen and others, 1999; Centers for Disease Control AIDS Community Demonstration Projects Research Group, 1999).

Promotion (Informing and Persuading About the Costs and Benefits)

Target market members can only be expected to voluntarily exchange their resources for a product when aware that the product offers them attractive benefits at a reasonable price and that it is available at a convenient location. Creating this awareness is the role of the promotion element of social marketing.

The promotion element involves communication or education and is often mistaken to be synonymous with the whole of the social marketing concept. Promotional elements in social marketing can include advertising, public relations and publicity, entertainment media, direct mail and telemarketing, e-mail and Web-based approaches, word of mouth and other opinion-leader strategies, third-party endorsements, point-of-purchase materials, and the use of a "sales force" (that is, people who are provided an incentive to communicate with target market members about the product). Social marketing does not, however, use these tactics in a stand-alone effort but rather as part of an integrated effort involving all elements of the marketing mix.

Consider, for example, the promotional elements of the national 5 a Day for Better Health program, a joint marketing effort of the National Cancer Institute (NCI) and the produce manufacturing and retailing industries to increase consumption of fruit and vegetables (Lefebvre and others, 1995). To complement and effect its product, pricing, and placement efforts, the program mounted a concerted promotional campaign through outreach to news media, point-of-purchase materials, and comarketing to increase target market awareness. Between 1991 (the first year of the program) and 1997, awareness of the program's message increased nearly 150 percent, and the proportion of the adult population that ate five or more servings of fruit and vegetables per day increased by approximately 10 percent (Stables and others, under review).

Developing a salesforce, people who actively create opportunities to "sell" the product directly to members of the target market, is a potentially important yet often overlooked strategy for increasing the effectiveness of social marketing programs. An example of the impact of a sales force comes from a 5 a Day for Better Health research project conducted to test the efficacy of a telephone-counseling intervention (Marcus and others, 1998). People who called the NCI's Cancer Information Service (CIS) for reasons unrelated to 5 a Day for Better Health were proactively offered tailored promotional messages intended to persuade callers to increase their fruit and vegetable consumption. Direct "selling" in this manner resulted in significant increases in fruit and vegetable consumption.

Other Aspects of Social Marketing

Social Marketing as a Consumer-Oriented Process

Members of the target market are free to choose, or to reject, the behavior being promoted in a social marketing program. Because the power of choice ultimately resides with consumers, social marketers must focus their activities on understanding and responding to the consumer's perspectives. Thus, social marketing is a consumer-oriented process. This has several direct implications for the practice of social marketing.

The Use of Research. The consumer orientation in social marketing is largely driven by two distinct types of research. The first type of research—which is interchangeably termed consumer research, audience research, and formative research—generates a better understanding of members of the target market with regard to the behavior the marketer seeks to promote and focuses on understanding perceived needs, benefits sought, barriers of concern, and opportunities to make offers to members of the target market.

The second type of research—competitive analysis or environmental analysis—generates a better understanding of the environment in which consumers are making their decisions. It focuses on identifying competitive offers being made to members of the target market, as well as on identifying significant social, environmental, or economic forces that influence the context in which consumers make their choices. Both types of understanding, consumer insights and environmental insights, are critical in informing marketing decisions. Kotler and Andreasen (1996) and Weinreich (1999) feature excellent discussions of how to conduct this research.

Segmentation. Implicit in the research discussion above is the assumption that a social marketer can, through consumer research, develop insight into the motivations and behaviors of a target market. This assumption is obviously not valid in situations in which the target market is defined in an overly broad manner. People are different, and the environments in which they make choices are different. To avoid defining their target market(s) in an overly broad manner, social marketers segment (or subdivide) the larger and more heterogeneous market into smaller more homogeneous market segments (Andreasen, 1995; Slater, 1995).

Larger markets can be segmented using criteria including demographical variables (such as age, sex, income, ethnicity), geographical variables (such as urban, suburban, rural), psychological variables (such as self-efficacy, motivations, readiness to change), and behavioral variables (such as low, medium, and high performance of the behavior of concern). Regardless of the variables used to segment a larger market, the goal is to identify market segments, or subgroups, of people who share certain qualities such that they will relate to a given social marketing offer in a similar fashion (Maibach, Ladin, Maxfield, and Slater, 1996).

When social marketers identify reasonably homogeneous market segments with regard to the program's objectives, their ability to be consumer-oriented is improved in two important ways. First, social marketers can refine their use of audience and environmental research to generate critical insights about each market segment under consideration. Relevant benefits and barriers are far more easily, and more effectively, identified among properly defined market segments than among heterogeneous or poorly defined target markets. Second, this process can help to eliminate specific market segments from further consideration. For example, if a segment is too small, or if the resources available are not sufficient to develop an offer attractive to members of the segment, the marketing organization should focus its resources elsewhere.

Targeted Programs. By using segmentation, consumer research, and environmental assessment, social marketers are able to target marketing programs to the unique needs and circumstances of each segment. For example, to promote weight loss, the needs of one market segment might best be met through face-to-face counseling and group-based physical activity, another segment through self-help materials, and a third segment through the provision of prepackaged reduced-calorie foods. Rather than develop a "one size fits all" approach, social marketers create programs targeted to the specific needs of each market. If the resources available to the marketing organization are not sufficient to create a targeted program for each market under consideration, a decision must be made either to reduce the number of markets targeted or to make compromises in program design that leverage available resources across all markets.

Return on Investment as a Criterion for Decision Making

The dilemma posed in the preceding paragraph—focusing available resources on fewer people (or markets) versus making compromises in program design to accommodate more people—is one faced all too often in health promotion, because the resources available are rarely commensurate with the scope of the problem. Social marketers attempt to minimize this dilemma by making resource allocation decisions using return on investment (ROI) as the criterion for decision making. Because the bottom line for social marketing is behavioral influence, it provides a metric to measure the success of a programmatic investment, and thereby to determine ROI. Andreasen (1995) provides details for conducting these analyses.

Consider, as an example, a marketing program that seeks to promote physical activity among Medicare beneficiaries. After segments of the Medicare population have been identified, parameters can be estimated for each segment. These estimates might include size of the segment, current level of physical activity (and thus need for increased activity), cost of a tailored marketing program, and behavioral influence likely to result from the marketing program. Program managers can use the estimates to decide on which market segments to focus and how to allocate resources across those segments, based on maximizing ROI.

Maximizing ROI is not a static process based only on analyses during the planning phase of a program. Collecting feedback from target market members and program partners throughout all stages of program planning and implementation is an important attribute of social marketing. This allows marketing organizations to improve their performance on an ongoing basis, which further improves ROI (Maibach, 2000).

The Social Marketing Process as Informed by Behavioral Change Theory

As a discipline that approaches the management of voluntary behavior through the use of self-interested exchanges and positive reinforcement, the social marketing process draws heavily on behavioral change theory. Specifically, theories of human behavior and behavioral change play at least two important roles in social marketing. First, behavioral theory elucidates our understanding, at the conceptual level, of why people behave as they do. Thus, the insights from behavioral theory provide social marketers with a major asset in understanding the dynamics of current behavior in a target market and what it might take to change that behavior. For example, Social Cognitive Theory informs social marketers that self-efficacy and outcome expectancies are influential in how people regulate their behavior (Bandura, 1986). This book is replete with information on other behavioral theories of relevance to social marketers in understanding the dynamics of behavior.

Second, behavioral theories provide social marketers with guidance on how best to conduct consumer research and environmental assessments. Social marketers use well-established behavioral theories to focus their questions to consumers and to form their interpretation of consumer's answers (Nowak and Siska, 1995).

Cultural Competence

Social marketing programs tend to be culturally sensitive or culturally appropriate because social marketing is a consumer-oriented process. Social marketing program managers begin their process by identifying market segments and conducting research to understand the benefits sought by and the barriers of concern to members of these target markets. Social marketers proceed to the creation of programs or offers only after they thoroughly understand the relevant behavioral and cultural considerations associated with a given target market. Moreover, because social marketing places considerable emphasis on reducing or eliminating price barriers to behavioral change, it is sensitive to the fact that target markets with fewer resources face more profound barriers to behavioral change than do target markets with more resources.

The Creation of Change in Organizations and Public Policy

The strength of social marketing is its ability to influence individual behavior. This strength can also be applied to create change at the organizational level and at the societal level, because organizations and societies are collections of individuals. The behavior of social networks (that is, how people interact), the behavior of organizations (that is, the policies of private, nonprofit, and public-sector organizations that influence the health of employees, customers, and constituents), and the behavior of communities, states, and nations (that is, through laws and policies that influence the health of citizens and residents) are all amenable to change through a marketing approach.

The full potential of social marketing to influence behavior at each of these levels is just beginning to be explored. The Campaign for Tobacco-Free Kids is one exciting example. Two of the campaign's interlocking goals are to create a social, political, legal, media, economic, and ethical environment conducive to reducing tobacco use and exposure among kids, and to develop and achieve public and private policies that support elimination of tobacco use and exposure among children. Environmental change objectives include raising awareness and stimulating outrage among public and policymakers toward the tobacco industry's behavior, curbing the industry's undue influence on the political process at all levels, and isolating the tobacco industry by pressuring its allied and other industries (entertainment, advertising and media, retail, sponsorships). The policy change goal calls for supporting state and local legislative and program initiatives, building support for enactment of effective national tobacco-control legislation, supporting FDA oversight over tobacco, and encouraging and supporting litigation that furthers tobacco control.

The campaign recognizes that environmental change is influenced by changes in public and private policies and that, in turn, a positive environment and altered social norms have an impact on policymakers and their decisions. Both of these social changes influence individual behaviors among adult smokers and children who are smoking or beginning to experiment with the habit.

The Scalability of Social Marketing

Borrowing from the parlance of e-commerce, social marketing is a "scalable" process. By that we mean social market concepts and practices can be used to improve both local and national programs, and both low- and high-resource programs. At several points throughout this chapter, we have mentioned that social marketing involves making decisions about improving products (increasing benefits) and controlling pricing (removing barriers) within the constraints of resources available to the marketing organization. Organizations with more resources have the ability to make larger investments in program development and delivery, but the basic social marketing processes are designed to improve ROI regardless of size of the program or resources available. To illustrate this point, the following section presents two social marketing programs, one developed for a national program operating in a high-resource situation, and the other a local program in a low-resource situation.

Applications: Large- and Small-Scale Social Marketing Programs

Large-Scale Program: The National High Blood Pressure Education Program

This broad-scale, public- and private-sector program was begun in 1972, when large portions of the American public were unaware of the prevalence and the consequences of high blood pressure, and the program continues to this date (National Heart, Lung and Blood Institute, 1997). Detection and vigorous treatment efforts were lacking at that time. To address these problems, the National Heart, Lung, and Blood Institute brought together numerous federal agencies, state health departments, over 150 private-sector organizations, pharmaceutical and insurance companies, and others to work at the national, state, and local levels. The overall objective was to reduce the morbidity and mortality attributable to high blood pressure.

Research at that time showed that the public harbored misconceptions and lacked important information about high blood pressure. Most members of the public believed that symptoms of high blood pressure were readily evident; few knew that there usually are no symptoms and therefore no way to detect high blood pressure without the help of a health professional. The prevailing view was that high blood pressure was not a serious disorder; few knew that the actual consequences could include stroke, heart disease, and kidney failure. Moreover, the public didn't expect that their blood pressure should be regularly checked by a health professional. And many people with hypertension didn't understand how important it was to follow their treatment regimens every day, no matter how they felt.

Audience research conducted with health care professionals showed that most physicians and other health care professionals were not routinely screening for high blood pressure when they saw patients. Moreover, there were no commonly accepted standards for diagnosis or treatment. Developing standards for diagnosis and treatment of high blood pressure therefore became one critical focus of the project (Roccella and Ward, 1984).

National High Blood Pressure Education Program (NHBPEP) planners decided to implement a "push-pull" marketing strategy (Roccella, 2002). The program was designed to simultaneously encourage the public to demand—or "pull"—detection and treatment into the health care system and to encourage and enable professionals to provide—or "push"—standardized detection and treatment methods to their patients. The behavioral change objective established for the public target market was to have them request a blood pressure check routinely from their health care provider; the behavioral objective for people with high blood pressure was adherence to their treatment regimen. The behavioral change objective for health care professionals was to have them routinely check the blood pressure of all patients and treat (or refer) patients with high blood pressure, all based on standardized detection and treatment guidelines. These synergistic approaches, along with later efforts targeting family members and friends of people with hypertension (to reinforce the need for compliance with treatment regimens) set in motion a powerful behavioral change dynamic that rapidly began to improve blood pressure control.

Segmentation played an important role from the inception of the program. During the initial years of the NHBPEP, when the focus was largely on detection of high blood pressure, age and ethnicity were important segmentation factors because the prevalence of the disorder is higher among older adults and among African Americans. Later, as awareness and detection rates improved, program managers segmented the target market of people with hypertension into four submarkets: those not treating their blood pressure at all, those who were treating their condition inadequately and were thus not in control, those recently detected who were about to begin or had just begun treatment, and those who were properly treating their blood pressure and could benefit from positive reinforcement and continued support. Targeted programs were created to manage the behavior of people in each of these segments.

The products developed for the public target market by the NHBPEP included blood pressure screenings and other enhancements to detection, improved use of medication (and eventually, improved medications), and a variety of approaches to enable people with hypertension to better control their weight and become more physically active. Products developed for the health care professional target included treatment guidelines to standardize the methods used to detect and treat high blood pressure, various approaches to educating and reinforcing health professionals for making detection and treatment a routine part of their practice, and, later, methods for improving patient management.

The pricing strategy focused simply on making every step in the process from detection through treatment maintenance easier and less expensive. For the public target markets, this included making it easier and cheaper to have a regular blood pressure check. Free public screenings were widely implemented by NHBPEP partner organizations. For people with hypertension, educational materials were created and widely distributed to improve patients' ease in talking to their doctor—and in asking the right questions—about their conditions. Reducing stigma associated with the condition (stigma associated with admitting having an illness and stigma associated with taking medication for a lifetime) was another method whereby costs were reduced for people with hypertension. For health care professionals, making the recommended behaviors easier and less expensive included developing reminder systems, record-keeping systems, and inexpensive (or free) patient education materials.

Placement strategies were used to reinforce the pricing strategies. Blood pressure screenings were taken out of the doctor's office and moved into the community and the workplace (and eventually into many pharmacies and large grocery stores). High-quality "best practice" treatment was moved out of academic medical centers and into community health centers, work-site medical clinics, and local doctors' offices.

Mass media were used extensively as part of the NHBPEP promotional strategy. During an early phase of the program, "Jimmy the Greek" Snyder, a popular television personality and oddsmaker, was featured in television, radio, and print messages. He explained the high odds of having high blood pressure and encouraged the public to get blood pressure checks. Message strategies evolved as research findings showed changes in public understanding and behaviors. Lack of personal susceptibility remained a persistent problem; many people with hypertension came to understand the nature and consequences of the disease, and were aware of their condition, but did not appear to feel (or admit to be) personally vulnerable. To combat this, messages were created around the theme, "Do it (in other words, follow your therapy) for the loved ones in your life." Special campaigns were directed at African American men, a segment particularly resistant to therapy, and efforts to reach this target market through community-level programs were extensive (Roccella and Lenfant, 1995).

Lifelong therapy for a condition that has no symptoms remains a difficult sell, but overall, the NHBPEP has made considerable progress in raising awareness, increasing understanding, and improving rates of detection and treatment through its behavioral change objectives for the public and for health professionals. Since the inception of the program, there has been a substantial decline in mortality rate from stroke—nearly 60 percent—and a considerable portion of this is attributed to the National High Blood Pressure Education Program (National Heart, Lung and Blood Institute, 1997).

Small-Scale Program: University of Wisconsin Binge Drinking Prevention

The University of Wisconsin has for many years been one of the leading campuses in the United States in terms of percentage of students regularly engaging in binge drinking. As the secondary effects of sexual abuse, property damage, and fighting increased, the administration sought ways to influence students' behavior so as to reduce the problem. The university developed a social marketing intervention (Brower, Ceglarek, and Crowley, 2001) in association with a larger multiuniversity antibinge drinking project coordinated by the American Medical Association (AMA) and the Robert Wood Johnson Foundation (American Medical Association, 2001).

Project planning began with audience research and segmentation. Data sources included campus and city police data, dorm and dean-of-student records, and nationally representative survey data collected by the Harvard School of Public Health in 1993, 1997, and 1999 to learn about alcohol consumption habits of students in four-year colleges. These survey data included the number and type of drinks consumed, time period during which the drinks were consumed, frequency of drinking occasions, location of drinking, negative results of drinking, reasons for drinking or not drinking, and student views of campus policies regarding drinking.

Survey data showed that whereas 70 percent of the freshman class engaged in binge drinking, by the senior year only 53 percent did so; similarly, freshmen and sophomores caused most of the secondary effects of binge drinking. As a result, the student body was first segmented based on year in school (Wechsler, Kuo, Lee, and Dowdall, 2000).

Survey data also showed that the problem behavior began for some students before matriculation: 40 percent of the freshman class was binge drinking in high school. Of the 60 percent of the freshman class that did not binge drink in high school, about half (or 30 percent) began to binge as freshmen, and most early in the year.

As a result of these insights, the social marketing staff further segmented the target market based on the continuum of "prone to behave as desired" to "resistant to behave as desired." Students who had not been binge drinking in high school and were not doing so in college were felt to be "prone," and deemed amenable to messages reminding them to continue their non- or light-drinking behavior. Students who had been bingeing in high school and who continued to do so were felt to be "resistant" and likely to change their behavior only in response to the force of law. The primary target market for the program was defined as those students who did not binge in high school, but who began to do so as college freshmen.

By understanding the causes of bingeing behavior among members of the target market, staff aimed to develop a marketing program through which to prevent the behavior. Additional consumer research was conducted to better understand the behavior. This research showed that when the students arrived on campus, they felt a variety of strong needs. These needs included the desire to feel a sense of belonging in their new environment, to be comfortable in social settings, to take risks, to explore opportunities for personal growth and self-expression, to assert independence from their previous life at home with parents, to blow off steam at the end of the study week, and to get drunk. While alternative products can't compete in terms of meeting the need to get drunk, they can compete to meet these other needs.

Thus, from a marketing perspective, "binge drinking" was a brand that was regularly purchased by 70 percent of the freshman class to fulfill one or more of a variety of needs they experienced. The strategy developed for the social marketing program was to introduce new competing brands into the marketplace and to strengthen poorly performing current brands, to take market share away from the market leader.

The concepts of motivation, opportunity, and ability influenced strategy (Rothschild, 1999). Motivation arises from perceptions of self-interest and group norms. For example, students have a strong need to belong and to conform to campus norms. Opportunity considers whether the environment allows for the desired behavior. For example, students often say that they binge because there is nothing else to do. Ability considers whether the target has the skill set to behave appropriately. For example, when ten students ask another to go out drinking, it can be difficult to say, "no, I'd rather play basketball." Alternative brands were developed based on their potential to motivate, provide opportunity, and enhance ability. Delivering benefits through the distribution channel calls for having the brand available not just in the right place but also at the right time. To succeed in taking market share away from binge drinking, alternative products needed to compete directly with drinking-related activities in the time slots during which the drinking took place. As a result, several new brands were put in the market for late-night use on Thursday, Friday, and Saturday. These included alcohol-free dance clubs, movies, and recreational sports. In addition, student organizations were offered grants to move existing alcohol-free activities into the prime drinking time slots.

Database development was used to promote these and other alcohol-free products to the specific students who were most likely to be interested. During summer orientation, incoming freshmen completed a survey to determine the activities they enjoyed during their free time. At the beginning of the first semester, they then received a personalized list of activities on campus that corresponded to the activities they said they enjoyed and a list of names of everyone in their dorm who also enjoyed these activities. Master lists were provided to house fellows to assist them in planning alternative activities and were provided to campus organizations so that they might more effectively recruit new members. Thus, this list helped students identify positive ways of spending free time and people with whom to share the activities; the list helped self-interested student organizations become more effective at designing activities for which there was a demand and in recruiting new participants.

To further promote positive uses of spare time, a print ad campaign consisting of about thirty ads was developed for placement in the freshman dorms. Each ad featured a student organization and concluded by telling students to join one of the 645 student organizations that existed on campus. Each ad began with a pun to draw the student into the ad, continued by urging membership in something, and concluded with a call to action by telling the student how to learn more or how to join. Figure 19.2 shows two of these ads.

The ads do not preach abstention or moderation and do not even mention binge drinking. They recognize the needs of the students to belong, to socialize, to explore their own identities, and to take risks. Much like ads for commercial products, these ads extol the benefits of the brand being sponsored and implicitly show how members of the target market can meet their needs.

Through work with the student organizations, numerous partnerships were developed that served to benefit the program. These partners are the salesforce,

FIGURE 19.2. ADS FROM THE BINGE DRINKING PREVENTION PROGRAM.

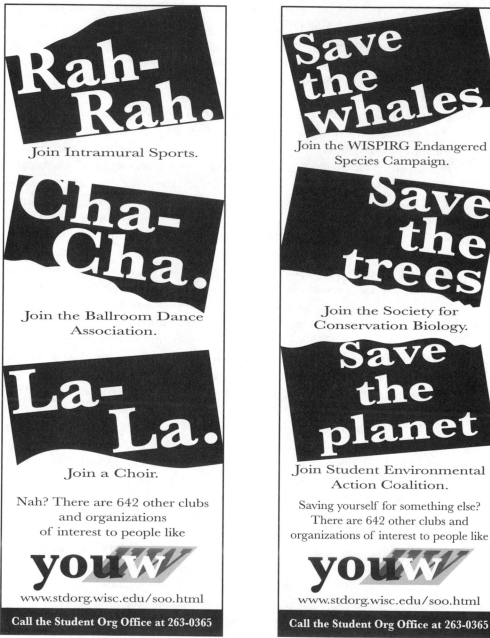

part of a system of retailers who provide the brand that is being marketed. In return, each organization receives a list of prospective members and many receive exposure through the ads.

In addition to the ad campaign, there is an e-mail campaign wherein each freshman receives a weekly e-mail with a listing of all nonalcoholic activities taking place on campus in the following week. There is no mention made of the lack of alcohol, but the listing shows numerous ways in which the student can explore his or her self-identity.

The project is still under way and the results are so far unknown. It is clear, though, that many of the new brands are thriving: hundreds of students attend each alcohol-free dance event and use the recreational sports facilities at times when the facilities had in the past been closed. Data regarding project outcomes will come from follow-up surveys that are being conducted as part of an independent evaluation of the larger AMA project. However, these data will not unequivocally answer questions of causality due to other events in the campus environment. These include changes in law enforcement (for example, underage consumption violations have gone up considerably), other educational programs, and general environmental changes in the perception of underage alcohol consumption.

Conclusion

This chapter has introduced the reader to a number of marketing concepts. In beginning to use marketing as a strategic framework, it is important to keep in mind target market members' perspectives about their own self-interests. To influence the behavior of target market members, social marketers must develop a timely exchange that heightens benefits and reduces barriers, and does so better than the currently available competitive choices. While the objective of social marketing is to change individual behavior, it can pursue this objective both directly and indirectly by changing the environment with respect to benefits and barriers and by changing the culture with respect to expectations and norms.

We hope this chapter has helped to enrich the reader's understanding of what social marketing is and isn't, and in the process reduced the potential for future misunderstandings about the concept. Many programs currently implemented under the banner of social marketing are not consistent with the approaches we have described; the reader should not confuse the name "social marketing" with its bona fide application. Conversely, programs conducted under other banners (for example, health communication, health education, health promotion) may well feature some of the marketing-based approaches we have described. We see this as normal and healthy for all disciplines involved; the most important innovations within a discipline often come from outside. While this may lead to confusion among some people as to the differences between disciplines, careful explications of each—as is clearly the objective of this book—can eliminate such confusion.

References

American Academy of Pediatrics AAP Task Force on Infant Positioning and SIDS. "Positioning and SIDS: Update, 1996–1997." May 10, 2001. Available at http://www.aap.org/new/sids/sids.htm.

American Medical Association. "A Matter of Degree: The National Effort to Reduce High-Risk Drinking Among College Students." September 7, 2001. Available at http://www.ama-assn.org/ama/pub/category/3558.html.

Andreasen, A. R. *Marketing Social Change: Changing Behavior to Promote Health, Social Development, and the Environment.* San Francisco: Jossey-Bass, 1995.

Bandura, A. *Social Foundations of Thought and Action: A Social Cognitive Theory.* Englewood Cliffs, N.J.: Prentice Hall, 1986.

Brower, A., Ceglarek, S., and Crowley, S. *A Matter of Degree: Quarterly Report to Robert Wood Johnson Foundation.* Madison, Wisc.: University of Wisconsin, January 2001.

Centers for Disease Control AIDS Community Demonstration Projects Research Group. "Community-Level HIV Intervention in Five Cities: Final Outcome Data from the CDC AIDS Community Demonstration Projects." *American Journal of Public Health,* 1999, *89,* 336–345.

Cohen D., and others. "Implementation of Condom Social Marketing in Louisiana, 1993 to 1996." *American Journal of Public Health,* 1999, *89,* 204–208.

French, S., and others. "Pricing and Promotion Effects on Low-Fat Vending Snack Purchases." *American Journal of Public Health,* 2001, *91,* 112–118.

Hornik, R. (ed.). *Public Health Communication: Evidence for Behavior Change.* Mahwah, N.J.: Erlbaum, forthcoming.

Kotler, P., and Andreasen, A. R. *Strategic Marketing for Nonprofit Organizations* (5th ed.). Englewood Cliffs, N.J.: Prentice Hall, 1996.

Kotler, P., and Armstrong, G. *Principles of Marketing.* (6th ed.) Englewood Cliffs, N.J.: Prentice Hall, 1994.

Kotler, P., and Roberto, E. L. *Social Marketing Strategies for Changing Public Behavior.* New York: Free Press, 1989.

Lefebvre, R. C., and Rochlin, L. "Social Marketing." In K. Glanz, F. M. Lewis, and B. K. Rimer (eds.), *Health Behavior and Health Education: Theory, Research, and Practice.* (2nd ed.) San Francisco: Jossey-Bass, 1996.

Lefebvre, R. C., and others. "Use of Database Marketing and Consumer-Based Health Communication in Message Design." In E. Maibach and R. Parrott (eds.), *Health Message Design.* Thousand Oaks, Calif.: Sage, 1995.

Maibach, E. "Five Strategies for Encouraging a Marketing Orientation in Social Change Organizations." *Social Marketing Quarterly,* 2000, *6,* 25–27.

Maibach, E. W., Ladin, K., Maxfield, A., and Slater, M. "Translating Health Psychology into Effective Health Communication: The American Healthstyles Audience Segmentation Project." *Journal of Health Psychology,* 1996, *3,* 261–278.

Marcus, A. C., and others. "Increasing Fruit and Vegetable Consumption Among Callers to the CIS: Results from a Randomized Trial." *Preventive Medicine,* 1998, *27,* S16–S28.

National Heart, Lung and Blood Institute. "The Sixth Report of the Joint National Committee on Prevention, Detection, Evaluation, and Treatment of High Blood Pressure." NIH Publication No. 98–4080. Washington, D.C.: November 1997.

Novelli, W. D. "Applying Social Marketing in Health Promotion and Disease Prevention." In K. Glanz, F. M. Lewis, and B. K. Rimer (eds.), *Health Behavior and Health Education: Theory, Research, and Practice.* San Francisco: Jossey-Bass, 1990.

Nowak, G., and Siska, M. "Using Research to Inform Campaign Development and Message Design. In E. Maibach and R. Parrott (eds.), *Designing Health Messages.* Thousand Oaks, Calif.: Sage, 1995.

Roccella, E. J. "The Contribution of Public Education Toward the Reduction of CVD Mortality: Experience from the National High Blood Pressure Education Program." In R. Hornik (ed.), *Public Health Communication: Evidence for Behavior Change.* Mahwah, N.J.: Erlbaum, 2002.

Roccella, E. J., and Lenfant, C. "Using Data to Focus Communication to Minority Populations." *Journal of Human Hypertension,* 1995, *9,* 53–57.

Roccella, E. J., and Ward, G. "The National High Blood Pressure Education Program: A Description of Its Utility as a Generic Program Model." *Health Education Quarterly,* 1984, *11,* 225–242.

Rothschild, M. L. "Carrots, Sticks, and Promises: A Conceptual Framework for the Management of Public Health and Social Issue Behaviors." *Journal of Marketing,* 1999, *63,* 24–37.

Slater, M. D. "Choosing Audience Segmentation Strategies and Methods for Health Communication." In E. Maibach and R. Parrott (eds.), *Designing Health Messages.* Thousand Oaks, Calif.: Sage, 1995.

Smith, W. A. "The Future of Social Marketing." Speech to the Marketing Conference on Creating Successful Partnerships, Carleton University, Ottawa, Canada, 1993.

Soumerai, S., Ross-Degnan, D., and Kahn, J. "Effects of Professional and Media Warnings About the Association Between Aspirin Use in Children and Reye's Syndrome." *The Millbank Quarterly,* 1992, *70,* 155–182.

Stables, G., and others. "Changes in Fruit and Vegetable Consumption and Awareness of U.S. Adults: Results of the 1991 and 1997 5 a Day for Better Health Program Surveys." *Journal of the American Dietetic Association* (under review).

Wechsler, H., Kuo, M., Lee, H., and Dowdall, G. "Underage College Drinkers Have Easy Access to Alcohol, Pay Less, and Consume More Per Occasion than Older Students." *Preventive Medicine,* 2000, *19*(1), 24–29.

Weinreich, N. K. *Hands-On Social Marketing.* Thousand Oaks, Calif.: Sage, 1999.

Wiebe, G. D. "Merchandising Commodities and Citizenship on Television." *Public Opinion Quarterly,* 1951–52, *15,* 679–691.

CHAPTER TWENTY

ECOLOGICAL MODELS OF HEALTH BEHAVIOR

James F. Sallis
Neville Owen

This chapter describes ecological models of health behavior and their conceptual antecedents. Because ecological models and their terminology may not be familiar to readers, we provide working definitions of key terms in Table 20.1. Also in this chapter, we propose principles that are derived from ecological models. These are intended to guide research efforts and to inform the systematic development and evaluation of more comprehensive health behavior change interventions. Finally, we present examples of applications of ecological models that are drawn from research on nutrition and physical activity.

What Are Ecological Models and Environmental Variables?

As described by Stokols (1992, 1996), the term *ecology* is derived from biological science and refers to the interrelations between organisms and their environments. The *ecological perspective,* as it has evolved in behavioral sciences and public health, focuses on the nature of people's transactions with their physical and sociocultural surroundings (Stokols, 1992, p. 7). Thus, *ecological* refers to models, frameworks, or perspectives, rather than to specific constructs or variables.

Because ecological models consider the connections between people and their environments, it is important to clarify the term *environment.* In ecological models of behavior, environment simply means the space outside of the person. Many models

TABLE 20.1. GLOSSARY OF TERMS.

Term	Definition
Behavior setting	Social and physical situations in which behaviors take place
Ecological models of health behavior	Models proposing that behaviors are influenced by intrapersonal, sociocultural, policy, and physical-environmental factors; these variables are likely to interact, and multiple levels of environmental variables are described that are relevant for understanding and changing health behaviors
Ecological perspective	Approaches to understanding health behavior by focusing on the nature of people's transactions with their physical and sociocultural surroundings
Ecological psychology	Study of the influence of the outside environment on the person
Environment	The space outside the person, contrasted with intrapersonal variables
Health promotive environment	Environmental factors that may facilitate or hinder health behavior changes
Policy	Legislative, regulatory, or policymaking actions that have the potential to affect health behaviors, sometimes unintentionally; policies are sociocultural influences that can alter physical environments
Social ecology	Study of the influence of the social context on behavior, including institutional and cultural variables

of behavior change acknowledge the importance of the internal and social environments, but fewer have specified explicitly the role of the physical environment.

Behavior setting is another term that we believe to be very helpful in understanding how environments influence behaviors. Behavior settings are those social and physical situations in which behaviors take place (Barker, 1968; Wicker, 1979).

We emphasize the environmental domain because its inclusion distinguishes ecological models from other models and theories, and because relatively little is known empirically about environmental correlates of, and influences on, health behaviors. "The purpose of an ecological model is to focus attention on the environmental causes of behavior and to identify environmental interventions" (McLeroy, Bibeau, Steckler, and Glanz, 1988, p. 366). However, ecological models are also distinguished by their multilevel nature. Because ecological models typically lack specificity at each level, other models can be integrated to enhance the specificity of treatment of intrapersonal, interpersonal, and community levels of influence, as well as influences in the environmental domain (Smedley and Syme, 2000).

Historical and Conceptual Background of Ecological Models

The current interest in ecological approaches to health behavior has developed out of several historical trends that have been reviewed previously (McLeroy, Bibeau, Steckler, and Glanz, 1988; Stokols, 1992, 1996). The most relevant conceptual traditions are drawn from public health and psychology. In the field of public health, environmental influences on disease have been recognized for centuries. The host-agent-environment model—clearly an ecological framework—is basic to public health analyses of infectious diseases. It can also be applied to understanding the roles of behavior in the causation and prevention of lifestyle-related chronic diseases (McLeroy, Bibeau, Steckler, and Glanz, 1988).

There are several traditions of ecological analysis of behavior within psychology. Skinner's (1953) position that antecedent and consequent events in the observable environment directly controlled behavior is an influential forerunner of current ecological models. Skinner's approach is in sharp contrast to theories asserting that causation of behavior arises primarily from perceptions and feelings within the individual.

Kurt Lewin (1936) coined the term *ecological psychology* to describe the study of the influence of the outside environment on the person. In Lewin's model, the role of the environment was limited in that only *perceptions* of the external environment were deemed to be important. Although the predominant contemporary explanations of behavior focus on cognitively mediated determinants, there is a strong stream of psychological theory and research documenting direct, automatic environmental control of behavior (Bargh and Chartrand, 1999).

Roger Barker (1968) conducted long-term observational studies of children in their everyday environments. From his studies, Barker came to believe that behaviors could be predicted more accurately from knowing the situations that people were in than from knowing about their individual characteristics (see Wicker, 1979, p. 6).

The work of Urie Bronfenbrenner (1979) focused on understanding the multiple levels of influence on behavior. Bronfenbrenner described three levels of environmental influences that interact with individual variables. The *microsystem* consists of interpersonal interactions in specific settings, such as with family members, social acquaintances, and work groups. The *mesosystem* refers to the interactions among the various settings, such as family, school, and work. The *exosystem* is the larger social system that can affect individuals and settings through economic forces, cultural beliefs and values, and political actions.

Albert Bandura's (1986) influential Social Cognitive Theory (see Chapter Eight) shares some features with ecological models. The structure of the theory specifies that behavior is influenced by personal and environmental factors. In the environmental realm, social aspects such as modeling have been most thoroughly studied. Although Bandura's writings rarely explicate the role of physical environments, models of health behaviors have been based on Social Cognitive Theory that posit multiple influences of the physical environment (Sallis and Hovell, 1990; Winett, King, and Altman, 1989).

Rudolph Moos (1980) developed a social ecological model of health-related behavior. Moos specified four categories of environmental factors that are relevant for health. The first is *physical settings*, which can include features of the natural environment, such as geography and weather, as well as features of the built environment, such as buildings and urban designs. The second is *organizational;* the size and function of organizations such as worksites, schools, and churches affect a wide range of behaviors. The third category is the *human aggregate*, which can be thought of as sociodemographic or sociocultural characteristics of the people inhabiting a given environment. The fourth category of environmental factors is *social climate*, the perceived aspects of the social environment that relate to such influences as the supportiveness of a social setting for particular behavioral choices or the clarity of expectations about what are appropriate or inappropriate behaviors.

Ecological Models of Health Behavior

McLeroy, Bibeau, Steckler, and Glanz (1988) proposed an ecological model of health behaviors that identified multiple levels of influence. The model was designed to guide researchers and practitioners to systematically assess and intervene on each of those levels of influence. The five levels of influence are *intrapersonal factors, interpersonal processes and primary groups, institutional factors, community factors,* and *public policy.* This model identifies specific levels of analysis that are most relevant for explaining and changing health behaviors.

Stokols (1992, 1996) provided a detailed exposition of the need for a social ecological approach to health behavior research and health promotion, and outlined four assumptions. The first is that health is influenced by multiple facets of physical and social environments. The role of personal attributes is also acknowledged. The second assumption is that environments themselves are multidimensional. Environments can be described as social or physical, actual or perceived; as discrete attributes (such as temperature or spatial arrangements); or as constructs (such as behavior setting or social climate). The third assumption recognizes that human-environment interactions can be described at varying levels of aggregation: individuals, families, work and cultural organizations, communities, or whole populations. Stokols' fourth assumption is that there is feedback across different levels of environments and aggregates of persons. Person-environment transactions occur in cycles in which people influence their settings, and these changed aspects of settings then act to influence health behaviors.

Stokols' *health-promotive environment* construct (1992, 1996) is an extension of some of the key concepts in the "Ottawa Charter for Health Promotion" (1986) and is consistent with the PRECEDE-PROCEED model of health promotion planning (Green, Richard, and Potvin, 1996; see Chapter Eighteen). Stokols argues that health promotion interventions should alter the environmental factors that facilitate or hinder positive health behaviors. In addition to indirect environmental effects on health through health behaviors, social and physical environments are thought to have *direct* effects on health through emotional well-being and social cohesion. For example, there appear to be salutary health effects of contact with the natural environment (Frumkin, 2001).

Theoretical and conceptual advancement is a critical step in the development of ecologically-based approaches to health behavior change. Before research can proceed, it is necessary to hypothesize the specific environmental variables that may influence behavior. Several theorists have provided valuable perspectives on how broad ecological models can be applied to more specific domains of health behavior research and interventions (Baranowski, 1989; Ewart, 1990; Green, Richard, and Potvin, 1996; Elder, Geller, Hovell, and Mayer, 1994; Winett, 1995).

A framework for integrating public health and psychological approaches to create more effective health behavior interventions was developed by Winett, King, and Altman (1989). The authors applied the model and provided a wealth of ideas on how to create more health-promoting environments and how to integrate environmental approaches with individual and small-group interventions to improve health behaviors.

Cohen, Scribner, and Farley (2000) proposed a structural model based on the proposition that health behaviors are influenced by the attributes of individuals and also by the conditions under which people live. The four categories of structural variables they proposed to guide intervention are (1) availability of protective or harmful consumer products, (2) physical structures (or physical characteristics of products), (3) social structures and policies, and (4) media and cultural messages. They also discuss the social distribution of environmental factors, risk behaviors, and adverse health outcomes, arguing, as do Lynch, Smith, Kaplan, and House

(2000), that socioeconomic disparities in health are largely attributable to differences in the material conditions of people's lives.

Multilevel Approaches

There is emerging evidence that the multilevel approaches derived from ecological models may be essential to bring about population improvements in health. A recent review identified key elements of successful social change efforts targeting tobacco, seatbelt and car seat use, recycling, and breastfeeding (Economos and others, 2001). Success elements included government involvement, mass communication, environmental and policy change, and direction by a coalition. This combination of elements is consistent with a multilevel approach of ecological models.

The most impressive application of multilevel intervention approaches is to tobacco control. Individual-level interventions have made limited contributions to the decline in smoking in industrialized nations. It is now believed that extensive multilevel interventions targeting individuals, social norms, policy and regulatory initiatives, and environmental change by reducing availability of cigarettes have led to long-term changes in smoking rates (Centers for Disease Control and Prevention, 1999; Warner, 2000). Other evidence of the importance of interventions at multiple levels can be found in the area of substance abuse among adolescents (Kumpfer and Turner, 1990) and adults (Goodman, Wandersman, Chinman, Imm, and Morrissey, 1996), as well as for cardiovascular diseases (Schmid, Pratt, and Howze, 1995).

A general acceptance of the need for multilevel interventions can now be seen in documents such as *Healthy People 2010* (U.S. Department of Health and Human Services, 2000) and the Institute of Medicine's recent report on promoting healthy behavior (Smedley and Syme, 2000). Despite the many calls for ecological approaches to intervention, reports of planned and formal implementation of ecologically informed multilevel approaches are rare. An assessment of funded health promotion programs in Canada showed that only 25 percent had clearly identified multilevel strategies (Richard, Potvin, Kishchuk, Prlic, and Green, 1996).

In summary, there is substantial interest among those in the health behavior and public health fields in the development of comprehensive multilevel interventions that are guided by ecological frameworks. There is also a general agreement that they are promising and necessary. The challenge now is to operationalize and apply ecological frameworks more specifically to health behavior change and to evaluate the effectiveness of multilevel interventions.

Principles of Ecological Approaches to Health Behavior Change

Using the ecological concepts and models from the preceding review, we developed a list of principles to guide ecological approaches to research and interventions. Some of the principles are common features of ecological models, and others reflect our focus on environmental influences and our belief that it will prove worthwhile to strengthen the specific application of ecological models to the design of interventions to influence particular health behaviors.

1. *Multiple levels of factors influence health behaviors.* Ecological models specify that intrapersonal factors, sociocultural factors, policies, and physical environments can influence health behaviors. Inclusion of all these types of influence distinguishes the potential contributions of ecological models from those of theories that primarily focus on intrapersonal and interpersonal influences. All levels of factors can influence behavior simultaneously, to varying degrees. Well-developed ecological models would specify not only that different types of variables interact but also *how* they interact.

2. *Multiple types of environmental influences affect health behavior.* Within the environmental category, ecological models specify multiple types of environmental influences. Ecological models posit that environmental factors influence behavior directly and also indirectly through individual perceptions. Characteristics of the natural environment, such as weather, climate, geography, and food production and distribution may affect behavior. Characteristics of built environments may also affect behavior. Examples include architectural features; community design and resources; commercial environments that affect access to foods, alcohol, and tobacco; information environments; entertainment environments; and technological environments.

3. *Behavior-specific ecological models can be useful.* Specific ecological models can guide research and interventions for different health behaviors. Environmental variables are often behavior specific. The availability of condoms in nightclubs has little relevance to dietary behaviors, and the presence of cycling trails in suburban neighborhoods is unlikely to affect alcohol intake. In other words, while broad constructs that operate across types of behaviors can be described, the specific variables must be more precisely articulated in applications of ecological models.

Early ecological models were general statements that multiple levels of variables influenced outcomes related to human health and welfare. Operationalizing the general principles of ecological models for specific behaviors is a challenging but essential step.

4. *Multilevel interventions may be most effective.* A critical assumption of ecological models is that single-level interventions are unlikely to have powerful or sustained effects. While the evidence in support of this contention is scarce, it is a testable proposition. Educational interventions designed to change beliefs and behavioral skills would be expected to work better when policies and environments support the targeted behavior changes. Similarly, environmental changes by themselves may be insufficient to change behavior. For example, building more sidewalks may not be adequate without programs to motivate people to use them. There is a growing recognition that combined individual, community, and environmental interventions are likely to be needed for effective behavior change, but the vast majority of interventions continue to target only the individual level.

The difficulty of implementing multilevel approaches should not be underestimated. An important barrier to multilevel interventions is that health professionals are usually familiar with individually focused programs but unfamiliar with strategies for policy and environmental change. The fact that it may take years to change policies and environments is a strong deterrent to program planners who are called on to achieve some impact in a short time or who work within a limited-funding time frame.

5. *Multilevel interventions are most easily implemented by multisectoral groups.* Due to the complexity of multilevel interventions, the involvement of multiple disciplines and sectors may be needed to plan, implement, and evaluate these programs. Participants from multiple sectors of society often must be engaged for long periods of time to implement the types of solutions suggested by ecological models. Implementation can be facilitated by engaging groups that control the policies and environments that are targeted for change. Within the academic sector, geographers may contribute methods of analyzing the physical environment, economists may provide data on the monetary costs and benefits of policy initiatives, and political scientists may advise on effective methods of creating political change. Early involvement of government agencies may be critical for successful implementation and funding of interventions. Representatives of the business sector can be recruited when proposed solutions will affect their interests.

Creating effective multisectoral collaborations requires large amounts of energy, creativity, and patience. However, they are likely to be worthwhile for successfully creating interventions (Bracht, 1999).

6. *To evaluate ecological interventions, monitor implementation and change in mediators at multiple levels.* Multilevel interventions are complex, and periodic feedback on the extent to which each intervention component is being implemented is useful. This is often referred to as assessing the process of implementing the intervention (McGraw and others, 2000). A particular challenge with this process is

the number of intervention components to be measured in multilevel interventions. A further complication is the lack of established measures for many environmental and policy variables, in contrast to the availability of a variety of measures for psychosocial variables.

Behavioral change interventions are effective when they change variables believed to control the behavior, or mediators. By definition, multilevel interventions attempt to change psychological, sociocultural, policy, and physical-environmental mediators. Determining whether the intervention changed the mediator can help explain why the intervention was a success or a failure and can guide improvements (Baranowski, Lin, Wetter, Resnicow, and Davis, 1997). A challenge in evaluating mediators is that environmental and policy variables can be conceptualized to have both direct effects that are not mediated *and* indirect effects that are mediated through individual perceptions.

7. *Political dynamics can limit ecological interventions.* Ultimately, health behaviors are affected by the political process. Unfavorable laws, inadequate enforcement of policies, negative corporate behaviors, lobbying by industry groups, and inability to put a given health behavior on the political agenda are important contributors to a wide variety of unhealthful behavioral patterns. Examples include poor enforcement of youth tobacco and alcohol access laws, subsidies for unhealthful food products, lack of funding for pedestrian facilities, and prohibition of needle exchange programs to prevent HIV. Political change is a necessary component for the success of many multilevel behavioral change interventions.

The climate for political change is dynamic. A change in government or organizational leadership may dramatically alter the priority placed on a given health behavior. Public opinion may shift due to publicity about new studies. Unexpected events, such as the tobacco settlement in the United States, may create opportunities for rapid political change. Political changes that are impossible at one time may become priorities, and health groups need to be ready to act when the time is right. Concerted and sustained effort by multisectoral groups can contribute to change in the political climate.

Applications of Ecological Models to Health Behavior

In the following sections, we describe examples of ecological models applied to eating and physical activity behaviors. These models help to explain the behaviors and to create effective interventions. Selected examples of empirical support for the principles outlined above are cited, but the review is not intended to be comprehensive.

Application to Obesity Prevention

There is increasing recognition that multilevel interventions are needed to solve some of the world's most pressing health problems (Smedley and Syme, 2000). This emerging consensus is exemplified by the various calls for a comprehensive response to the worldwide epidemic of obesity (World Health Organization, 1998).

Individually-based approaches to obesity prevention and treatment are widely viewed as ineffective by themselves, because they do nothing to alter the environmental factors believed to contribute to populationwide overeating and inadequate physical activity. Hill and Peters (1998) proposed numerous environmental factors that are contributing to the obesity epidemic, and Koplan and Dietz (1999) called for government policy changes to combat obesity. Nestle and Jacobson (2000) identified specific policy solutions, including taxes on food products with "empty" calories.

Egger and Swinburn (1997; Swinburn, Egger, and Raza, 1999) proposed an ecological model of obesity. For both eating and physical activity, they identified sociocultural factors and influences in the physical, economic, and political environments. The influences can be found in behavior settings, such as neighborhoods and schools, as well as in sectors of society including technology (labor-saving devices), the food industry, and transportation. The International Obesity Task Force (Kumanyika, Jeffery, Morabia, Ritenbaugh, and Antipatis, 2000) developed a comprehensive ecological model to guide worldwide efforts to prevent obesity. These models are an important step in developing multilevel approaches to the solution of the international health problem of obesity. It should be noted that these approaches have been outlined in some detail, but at present no data are available to demonstrate that the approaches are effective.

Another example of a behavior-specific and intervention-focused ecological model is the framework developed by Booth and others (2001) targeting physical activity and eating behavior. At the individual level, psychobiological, cultural, social, and environmental perception variables were specified in a hierarchical order. Health behavior represents the interaction of individuals and their environments, and three levels of environmental and policy variables were proposed. First, behavior settings were posited as having the most direct effects on behavior. Second, the behavior settings were viewed as being under the direct control of "microenvironmental" agents, who could also be considered leverage points for effecting change in that behavior setting. For example, restaurant offerings are controlled by owners, and school policies and practices are most directly controlled by school administrators. Third, the final layer of the model consists of "macroenvironmental" agents who exert indirect yet potentially powerful control over one or more behavior settings, typically through policies and regulations. Any given variable in a behavior setting likely has multiple indirect influences. For example, the availability of snack foods in the home is most directly influenced by family members, but it can be influenced indirectly by grocery stores, food manufacturers, advertising policies, health news, and policies affecting nutrition counseling in health care. The model assumes that various government agencies can be identified that directly or indirectly influence all behavior settings. This model can be used to identify the environmental characteristics, behavior settings, and influential agents that need to be targeted in intervention programs.

Application to Eating Behaviors

Unhealthful eating practices are linked to five of the top ten diseases in industrialized nations: heart disease, some cancers, stroke, diabetes, and atherosclerosis (U.S. Department of Health and Human Services, 1988). Changes in dietary habits of individuals of all ages have been recommended, but recent data indicate that dietary goals are not being met (U.S. Department of Health and Human Services, 2000). For simplicity, in this section we focus primarily on the target behavior of fat consumption, with additional examples related to fruit and vegetable intake. An expanded discussion of an ecological approach to nutrition and a literature review was published by Glanz and others (1995).

Multiple Types of Influence on Behaviors. There is evidence that each type of influence makes unique contributions to eating behavior (Capaldi, 1996). Intrapersonal correlates of intake, such as individual differences in taste preferences, health beliefs, mood, and perceived ability to change have been studied, as have social influences. At a higher level of social integration, culture is often expressed through food.

Multiple aspects of the physical environment can be influential. The effects of droughts and floods on availability of foods are clear, but inadequate distribution systems can also affect the availability of foods. An excellent study documented an association between availability of food products and their consumption (Cheadle and others, 1991). Percentages of shelf space devoted to low-fat dairy foods and red meat in grocery stores were strongly correlated with the frequency of consumption of these items by people living in the area. A similar study showed that availability of juice and vegetables in restaurants near the homes of African American boys was related to their consumption of those foods (Edmonds, Baranowski, Baranowski, Cullen, and Myres, 2001).

The interactions of influences across types of environmental and individual factors can be illustrated with a case example. We conducted a study of an intervention that was designed to teach behavioral change skills to low-income families so they could make dietary improvements. In general, middle-income European American families changed their diets, and low-income Mexican Americans made few changes (Nader and others, 1989). To help us understand this difference, we surveyed the availability of a long list of low-fat and low-sodium foods in areas where these families lived. The small corner stores in the neighborhoods where the Mexican American families lived simply did not have most of the items that we were promoting (Sallis, Nader, Rupp, Atkins, and Wilson, 1986). It appeared that families were more successful in making changes if healthful foods were conveniently available.

Multiple Types of Environmental Influences. French, Story, and Jeffery (2001) provided many examples of environmental correlates of eating. For example, a 147 percent increase in the number of fast-food restaurants between 1972 and 1995 mirrors a 200 percent increase in the proportion of all meals and snacks eaten at such restaurants. Portion sizes of packaged foods have increased over time. Twelve-ounce sodas were "king size" in the 1950s, but these are considered "child size" now. Food companies spent $11 billion in the United States in 1997 on mass media advertising, compared with the $1 million spent in 1999 by the National Cancer Institute to promote the 5 A Day for Better Health program (French and others, 2001). Student stores in middle schools stock mainly high-fat or high-sugar foods and no fresh fruits or vegetables (Wildey and others, 2000). Intervention studies show that price is a powerful environmental influence. Lowering prices of fruits and vegetables stimulated large increases in purchases in a high school cafeteria (French and others, 1997). Reducing the price of low-fat snacks in vending machines by 50 percent increased sales by 93 percent (French and others, 2001). Although few environmental and policy variables have been associated with eating behavior, many such variables have the potential to promote overconsumption.

Behavior-Specific Ecological Models. Significant progress in developing behavior-specific ecological models has occurred recently. The model described by Booth and others (2001) lists potential dietary influences in psychobiological, sociocultural, and environmental policy dimensions and has some similarities with the Egger and Swinburn model (Egger and Swinburn, 1997; Swinburn, Egger, and Raza, 1999). The model proposed by Booth and others (2001) identifies twelve behavior settings in which eating commonly occurs, ranging from home and work to automobiles and shopping malls. A multidisciplinary panel proposed sixty-three environmental influences in these behavior settings that could affect eating. The capacity of this model to assist researchers and practitioners to set priorities is enhanced by consensus ratings of the expected impact of each influence on behavior and the perceived difficulty of changing the influence in a healthful direction. Because of the large number of potential influences on eating behavior, models that help to set priorities for action and that can place a large array of diverse variables in a coherent framework are likely to be particularly helpful.

Multilevel Interventions. Although it was not possible to find examples of comprehensive ecologically-based nutrition interventions, several well-known multilevel nutrition interventions have been implemented. These include the California 5-a-Day for Better Health program (Foerster and others, 1995) and the National Cholesterol Education Program (Cleeman and Lenfant, 1998). Unfortunately, rigorous evaluations of the multiple levels of intervention of those large efforts are not available.

There are few examples of multilevel interventions that have been carefully evaluated in controlled studies, but two investigations illustrate the feasibility of implementing and evaluating multilevel nutrition interventions. The CATCH study randomized ninety-six primary schools to intervention or control conditions. The nutrition intervention included a classroom curriculum, a family component, and a cafeteria program to change the foods sold. This program that intervened at the individual, family, and school levels was effective in changing students' overall dietary intake (Luepker and others, 1996). The Australian National Workplace Health Project (Simpson and others, 2000) experimentally tested a multilevel model in a randomized trial targeting multiple behaviors including eating (see Chapter Fourteen). A 2×2 design was used to compare the separate and combined effects of sociobehavioral and environmental interventions, and the project planners hypothesized that the combined intervention would be most effective. This type of design is particularly needed to test hypotheses about the benefits of multilevel interventions.

Multilevel Interventions and Multisectoral Groups. The people and sectors that can be involved in collaborations to develop and implement nutrition interventions include dietitians, health scientists, social and behavioral scientists, economists, food industry representatives, advertising representatives, consumer advocates, and government representatives from health, agriculture, education, and legislative agencies. All may be needed to achieve the substantial and long-term changes in eating behavior needed to reduce the many serious nutrition-related diseases. The Partnership to Promote Healthy Eating and Active Living is an example of such a multisectoral collaboration (Booth and others, 2001).

Monitoring Implementation and Change at Multiple Levels. There are many existing instruments that assess potential nutrition-related mediators at the intrapersonal and interpersonal levels. There are few published measures of nutrition-related environmental variables that can be used to monitor implementation of environmental components of interventions. Cheadle, Wagner, Koepsell, Kristal, and Patrick (1992) described measures that could be used to evaluate environmental variables at worksites (recipe analysis), at grocery stores (percentage of shelf space for healthful foods), at restaurants (recipe analysis, number of fast food restaurants per capita), and at the policy level (food labeling regulations by state or country). Measures of the school's food environment were recently reviewed by Richter and others (2000). Because of the limited range of available measures, researchers are encouraged to develop indicators of the environmental and policy variables targeted in interventions.

Political Dynamics. Although the general public is very interested in nutrition, this interest has not translated into school meals that meet dietary guidelines, regulation of the nutritional content of fast food, reduction in portion sizes, restrictions on food advertising aimed at children, economic incentives to choose healthful foods at workplaces or restaurants, reimbursement for nutrition counseling in health care, or elimination of government subsidies for unhealthful foods. Health professionals and multisectoral groups can work to change political receptivity for nutrition change. Consumer advocacy groups, most notably the Center for Science in the Public Interest, have changed some practices in the U.S. food industry through media advocacy and have contributed to governmental policy changes through effective lobbying. Their work is a good model for creating political change (Nestle and Jacobson, 2000).

Application to Physical Activity

Physical inactivity significantly increases the risk of several chronic diseases (U.S. Department of Health and Human Services, 1996). Over half of the adult populations of industrialized nations are insufficiently active for health benefits (Owen and Bauman, 1992; U.S. Department of Health and Human Services, 1996). Despite extensive study, the full range of influences on physical activity is not well understood, and interventions have not produced impressive or long-term increases in physical activity (Sallis and Owen, 1999).

Multiple Types of Influence on Behaviors. Ecological models may be used to integrate the many known modifiable correlates of physical activity (Dzewaltowski,

1997). Findings from some three hundred studies of adults' physical activity showed that variables in all categories of correlates were consistently related to physical activity (Sallis and Owen, 1999, Chapter Seven). At the intrapersonal level, consistent associations with physical activity were found for biological factors; psychological, cognitive, and emotional factors; and several behavioral attributes and skills. At the level of social and cultural variables, three had consistent positive associations with physical activity: physician influence, social support from peers, and social support from one's spouse or family. At the physical-environmental level, climate and seasonal factors had a consistent association with physical activity. However, perceived access to physical activity facilities and cost of physical activity programs and home equipment had inconsistent associations.

Multiple Types of Environmental Influences. A wide range of environmental influences on physical activity have been proposed, and data are emerging to support many of them (Sallis and Owen, 1999; Sallis, Bauman, and Pratt, 1998). In the natural environment, season of the year was related to physical activity levels, and several studies showed that the best correlate of young children's physical activity was time spent outdoors. In an unanticipated finding, residing near the coast was associated with higher activity level, after controlling for socioeconomic status (Bauman, Smith, Stoker, Bellew, and Booth, 1999). Access to physical activity programs and facilities seems to be important for both young people (Sallis, Prochaska, and Taylor, 2000) and older adults (Booth, Owen, Bauman, Clavisi, and Leslie, 2000). There are mixed findings about whether living near exercise facilities enhances physical activity (Sallis, Bauman, and Pratt, 1998). The combination of physical and social environmental variables explained 40 to 60 percent of the variance in student physical activity at school (Sallis and others, 2001). A sizable literature in the transportation field shows that urban designs combining moderate density with mixed residential and commercial land use are consistently associated with more walking and cycling for transport (for example, Cervero and Gorham, 1995; Frank and Pivo, 1995).

Behavior-Specific Ecological Models. The need for specific ecological models for specific types of physical activity is particularly great because different physical activity behaviors are often performed in distinct settings (Owen, Leslie, Salmon, and Fotheringham, 2000). For example, vigorous fitness training is often done in health clubs, walking is most often done in one's neighborhood, and children are likely to play on park playgrounds. Each behavior setting has characteristics that appear to be relevant to specific types or purposes of physical activity. Owen, Leslie, Salmon, and Fotheringham (2000) proposed that specific models of the correlates of sedentary behavior are required, given that sedentary choices such as television viewing or computer and Internet use can compete with physical activity (Fotheringham, Wonnacott, and Owen, 2000).

Multilevel Interventions. The most powerful physical activity interventions are expected to provide communities, facilities, and programs that make activity convenient and to motivate people to use those resources. Several studies have evaluated multilevel interventions that combine educational, environmental, and policy change efforts. A good example is the effective program in rural Missouri that built walking trails and promoted their use through community coalitions and mass media (Brownson and others, 2000). In the school setting, both the CATCH (Luepker and others, 1996) and SPARK (Sallis and others, 1997) programs included a classroom behavioral change curriculum, family involvement, and policies to change physical education. Additional opportunities for school environment interventions have been identified (Wechsler, Devereaux, Davis, and Collins, 2000). An effective statewide intervention in Australia featured a mass media campaign plus a multilevel approach to change environments and policies (Bauman, Bellew, Owen, and Vita, 2001). Although studies to date show the promise of multilevel interventions, they do not unequivocally demonstrate that multilevel interventions are more effective than single-level approaches.

Multilevel Interventions and Multisectoral Groups. Sallis, Bauman, and Pratt (1998) proposed a model of ecological physical activity interventions that recommended the active involvement of many sectors of society, including public health, fitness industry, parks and recreation, criminal justice, transportation agencies, schools, employers, sports organizations, churches, urban planners, architects, mass media, and health insurance. The broad range of these relevant sectors suggests the extent to which physical activity influences are dispersed throughout society.

There are a few good examples of functioning multisectoral collaborations targeting physical activity change. The most well-developed is the New South Wales Physical Activity Task Force in Australia (described in Sallis, Bauman, and Pratt, 1998). The state premier (equivalent to the governor) instructed all government departments to participate in a long-term effort to develop, implement, and evaluate a statewide physical activity promotion initiative. In addition to the multiagency governmental leadership, health professionals, voluntary health agencies, and the fitness industry were involved. In the United States, the National Coalition for Promoting Physical Activity, the Partnership for a Walkable America (see Sallis, Bauman, and Pratt, 1998), and the Partnership to Promote Healthy Eating and Active Living (Booth and others, 2001) are multisectoral groups promoting environmental and policy change.

In specific settings, it is important to tailor the composition of the multi-sectoral groups to the situation. For worksite initiatives, the health insurance industry, unions, and company management control important resources and incentives that are essential for effective worksite physical activity programs (Veitch, Clavisi, and Owen, 1999).

Monitoring Implementation and Change at Multiple Levels. There are existing measures for many hypothesized mediators of physical activity in the psychological and social domains. Measures needed to monitor changes in activity-related environmental and policy variables are much less developed (Richter and others, 2000). Baker, Brennan, Brownson, and Houseman, (2000) proposed three types of measures that could be used to monitor intervention effects on community-level mediators. First, environmental enablers and barriers, such as perceived access to exercise facilities, can be collected from individuals and aggregated to the community level. The second type is objective, unobtrusive measures of environmental variables. Of particular relevance are Geographic Information Systems (GIS) (Korte, 1997) that can be used to obtain and manipulate objective measures of diverse environmental variables. GIS are commonly used in transportation and urban planning research (see for example, Frank and Pivo, 1995) but can be applied to study environmental correlates of health behaviors. A third type of assessment would define policies that could influence physical activity and evaluate people's perception of and support for those policies. Additional environmental variables may need to be assessed, such as amount of exposure to television (Salmon, Bauman, Crawford, Timperio, and Owen, 2000).

Political Dynamics. Many laws and policies may have indirect or unintended effects on physical activity. For example, budget cuts for parks and recreation departments may be rationalized on the basis of preserving health care for the poor, and cuts in school physical education may reflect a priority on strengthening core academic programs, without consideration of the effects on physical activity. Policies that provide massive funding for roads and highways but little for walking and bicycle trails may create barriers to physical activity.

Transportation funding in the United States is a good example of how political opportunities can change. There was a long tradition of spending virtually no federal transportation funds on walking and cycling facilities. Due to effective lobbying efforts, the 1991 Intermodal Surface Transportation Efficiency Act in the United States included substantial funding for walking and cycling projects that resulted in more than 3000 new cycling or pedestrian facilities over six years (Sallis, Bauman, and Pratt, 1998).

As research proceeds to document the effects of environmental characteristics, laws, and private sector policies on physical activity, the results may stimulate change in the political climate. Studies showing that older people are more active when their local communities have facilities and programs (MacDougall, Cooke, Owen, Willson, and Bauman, 1997) may contribute to political change. Policy change may be facilitated by evidence of public support for environmental interventions (Brownson and others, 1998).

Conclusion

Ecological models of behavior have been described for more than fifty years, but only recently have they begun to have a serious impact on health behavior research and health education practice. In the previous edition of this book, our chapter identified the need for more specific ecological models to identify variables that could guide research. Now in this third edition, we can report substantial progress in developing behavior-specific ecological models. A consensus seems to be emerging that multilevel interventions based on ecological models are promising approaches in health behavior research and for disease prevention and health promotion efforts (Smedley and Syme, 2000). There has been modest progress in demonstrating the utility of ecological models and the feasibility of conducting relevant studies. We believe the time is right for rapid progress in research to improve understanding of environmental and policy correlates of health behaviors. Multilevel interventions may be our best hope for reducing the toll of lifestyle-related diseases that continue to be epidemic in developed nations and that are rising in developing nations, but interventions should be based on research that identifies the critical intrapersonal, sociocultural, and environmental policy correlates of health behavior (Sallis, Owen, and Fotheringham, 2000). A high priority for research is to test the hypothesis that multilevel interventions are more effective than single-level approaches, and to determine under which conditions multilevel interventions are superior.

The evidence base on environmental and policy correlates of health behaviors will be incomplete in many areas for years to come. This raises the important question of whether health promotion practitioners should work to alter environmental variables and policies that behavior-specific ecological models suggest should influence health behaviors or wait for empirical documentation of the effects of a particular influence before acting. Although we advocate empirically-based health promotion practice, we think it would be shortsighted to discourage attempts to create more health-promotive environments just because no specific data exist on the relation between the environmental variable (or policy) and behavior. However, these attempts should be carefully monitored and evaluated as they unfold. Ongoing dialogue between researchers and practitioners on these issues is essential. We hope that improved ecological models will lead to a better understanding of the multiple levels of factors that influence health behaviors. This increased understanding should lead to more effective health behavior change efforts that have wide-reaching and long-lasting effects on public health.

References

Baker, E. A., Brennan, L. K., Brownson, R., and Houseman, R. A. "Measuring the Determinants of Physical Activity in the Community: Current and Future Directions." *Research Quarterly for Exercise and Sport*, 2000, *71*, 146–158.

Bandura, A. *Social Foundations of Thought and Action: A Social Cognitive Theory.* Englewood Cliffs, N.J.: Prentice Hall, 1986.

Baranowski, T. "Reciprocal Determinism at the Stages of Behavior Change: An Integration of Community, Personal, and Behavioral Perspectives." *International Quarterly of Community Health Education*, 1989, *10*, 297–327.

Baranowski, T., Lin, L. S., Wetter, D. W., Resnicow, K., and Davis, M. "Theory as Mediating Variables: Why Aren't Community Interventions Working as Desired?" *Annals of Epidemiology*, 1997, *7*, 589–595.

Bargh, J. A., and Chartrand, T. L. "The Unbearable Automaticity of Being." *American Psychologist*, 1999, *54*, 462–479.

Barker, R. G. *Ecological Psychology.* Stanford, Calif.: Stanford University Press, 1968.

Bauman, A., Bellew, B., Owen, N., and Vita, P. "Impact of an Australian Mass Media Campaign Targeting Physical Activity in 1998." *American Journal of Preventive Medicine*, 2001, *21*, 41–47.

Bauman, A., Smith, B., Stoker, L., Bellew, B., and Booth, M. "Geographical Influences Upon Physical Activity Participation: Evidence of a 'Coastal' Effect." *Australia and New Zealand Journal of Public Health*, 1999, *23*, 322–325.

Booth, M. L., Owen, N., Bauman, A., Clavisi, O., and Leslie, E. "Social-Cognitive and Perceived-Environment Influences Associated with Physical Activity in Older Australians." *Preventive Medicine*, 2000, *31*, 15–22.

Booth, S., and others. "Environmental and Societal Factors Affect Food Choice and Physical Activity: Rationale, Influences, and Leverage Points." *Nutrition Reviews*, 2001, *59*(3), 21–39.

Bracht, N. (ed.). *Health Promotion at the Community Level: New Advances.* (2nd ed.) Thousand Oaks, Calif.: Sage, 1999.

Bronfenbrenner, U. *The Ecology of Human Development.* Cambridge, Mass.: Harvard University Press, 1979.

Brownson, R., and others. "Promoting Physical Activity in Rural Communities: Walking Trail Access, Use and Effects." *American Journal of Preventive Medicine*, 2000, *18*, 235–241.

Brownson, R. C., and others. "Support for Policy Interventions to Increase Physical Activity in Rural Missouri." *American Journal of Health Promotion*, 1998, *12*, 263–266.

Capaldi, E. D. (ed.). *Why We Eat What We Eat: The Psychology of Eating.* Washington, D.C.: American Psychological Association, 1996.

Centers for Disease Control and Prevention. "Best Practices for Comprehensive Tobacco Control—August 1999." Atlanta: Office on Smoking and Health, 1999.

Cervero, R., and Gorham, R. "Commuting in Transit Versus Automobile Neighborhoods." *Journal of the American Planning Association,* 1995, *61,* 210–225.

Cheadle, A., Wagner, E., Koepsell, T., Kristal, A., and Patrick, D. "Environmental Indicators: A Tool for Evaluating Community-Based Health-Promotion Programs." *American Journal of Preventive Medicine,* 1992, *8,* 345–350.

Cheadle, A., and others. "Community-Level Comparisons Between the Grocery Store Environment and Individual Dietary Practices." *Preventive Medicine,* 1991, *20,* 250–261.

Cleeman, J. I., and Lenfant, C. "The National Cholesterol Education Program: Progress and Prospects." *Journal of the American Medical Association,* 1998, *280,* 2099–2104.

Cohen, D. A., Scribner, R. A., and Farley, T. A. "A Structural Model of Health Behavior: A Pragmatic Approach to Explain and Influence Health Behaviors at the Populations Level." *Preventive Medicine,* 2000, *30,* 146–154.

Dzewaltowski, D. "The Ecology of Physical Activity and Sport: Merging Science and Practice." *Journal of Applied Sport Psychology,* 1997, *9,* 254–276.

Economos, C. D., and others. "What Lessons Have Been Learned from Other Attempts to Guide Social Change?" *Nutrition Reviews,* 2001, *59*(3), 40–56.

Edmonds, J., Baranowski, T., Baranowski, J., Cullen, K. W., and Myres, D. "Ecological and Socioeconomic Correlates of Fruit, Juice, and Vegetable Consumption Among African-American Boys." *Preventive Medicine,* 2001, *32,* 476–481.

Egger, G., and Swinburn, B. "An 'Ecological' Approach to the Obesity Pandemic." *British Medical Journal,* 1997, *315,* 477–480.

Elder, J. P., Geller, E. S., Hovell, M. F., and Mayer, J. A. *Motivating Health Behavior.* Albany, N.Y.: Delmar, 1994.

Ewart, C. K. "Social Action Theory for a Public Health Psychology." *American Psychologist,* 1990, *46,* 931–946.

Foerster, S. B., and others. "California's '5 a Day—For Better Health!' Campaign: An Innovative Population-Based Effort to Effect Large-Scale Dietary Change." *American Journal of Preventive Medicine,* 1995, *11,* 124–131.

Fotheringham, M. J., Wonnacott, R. L., and Owen, N. "Computer Use and Physical Inactivity in Young Adults: Public Health Perils and Potentials of New Information Technologies." *Annals of Behavioral Medicine,* 2000, *22,* 269–275.

Frank, L. D., and Pivo, G. "Impacts of Mixed Use and Density on Utilization of Three Modes of Travel: Single-Occupant Vehicle, Transit, and Walking." *Transportation Research Record,* 1995, *1466,* 44–52.

French, S. A., Story, M., and Jeffery, R. W. "Environmental Influences on Eating and Physical Activity." *Annual Review of Public Health,* 2001, *22,* 309–325.

French, S. A., and others. "Pricing Strategy to Promote Fruit and Vegetable Purchase in High School Cafeterias." *Journal of the American Dietetic Association,* 1997, *97,* 1008–1010.

French, S. A., and others. "Pricing and Promotion Effects on Low-Fat Vending Snack Purchases: The CHIPS Study." *American Journal of Public Health,* 2001, *91,* 112–117.

Frumkin, H. "Beyond Toxicity: Human Health and the Natural Environment." *American Journal of Preventive Medicine,* 2001, *20,* 234–240.

Glanz, K., and others. "Environmental and Policy Approaches to Cardiovascular Disease Prevention Through Nutrition: Opportunities for State and Local Action." *Health Education Quarterly*, 1995, *22*, 512–528.

Goodman, R. M., Wandersman, A., Chinman, M., Imm, P., and Morrissey, E. "An Ecological Assessment of Community-Based Interventions for Prevention and Health Promotion: Approaches to Measuring Community Coalitions." *American Journal of Community Psychology*, 1996, *24*, 33–61.

Green, L. W., Richard, L., and Potvin, L. "Ecological Foundations of Health Promotion." *American Journal of Health Promotion*, 1996, *10*, 270–281.

Hill, J. O., and Peters, J. C. "Environmental Contributions to the Obesity Epidemic." *Science*, 1998, *280*, 1371–1374.

Koplan, J. P., and Dietz, W. H. "Caloric Imbalance and Public Health Policy." *Journal of the American Medical Association*, 1999, *282*, 1579–1581.

Korte, G. B. *The GIS Book: Understanding the Value and Implementation of Geographic Information Systems.* Sante Fe, N.M.: Onword Press, 1997.

Kumanyika, S. K., Jeffery, R. W., Morabia, A., Ritenbaugh, C., and Antipatis, V. J. "Obesity Prevention: The Case for Action. A Report of the Public Health Approaches to the Prevention of Obesity Working Group of the International Obesity Task Force." www.iotf.org (viewed November 2000)

Kumpfer, K. L., and Turner, C. W. "The Social Ecology Model of Adolescent Substance Abuse: Implications for Prevention." *The International Journal of the Addictions*, 1990, *25*, 435–463.

Lewin, K. *Principles of Topological Psychology.* (Trans. by F. Heider and G. Heider). New York: McGraw-Hill, 1936.

Luepker, R. V., and others. "Outcomes of a Field Trial to Improve Children's Dietary Patterns and Physical Activity: The Child and Adolescent Trial for Cardiovascular Health (CATCH)." *Journal of the American Medical Association*, 1996, *275*, 768–776.

Lynch, J. W., Smith, G. D., Kaplan, G., and House, J. S. "Income Inequality and Mortality: Importance to Health of Individual Income, Psychosocial Environment, or Material Conditions Interpretation." *British Medical Journal*, 2000, *320*, 1200–1204.

MacDougall, C., Cooke, R., Owen, N., Willson, K., and Bauman, A. "Relating Physical Activity to Health Status, Social Connections and Community Facilities." *Australia and New Zealand Journal of Public Health*, 1997, *21*, 631–637.

McGraw, S. A., and others. "Measuring Implementation of School Programs and Policies to Promote Healthy Eating and Physical Activity Among Youth." *Preventive Medicine*, 2000, *31*, S86–S97.

McLeroy, K. R., Bibeau, D., Steckler, A., and Glanz, K. "An Ecological Perspective on Health Promotion Programs." *Health Education Quarterly*, 1988, *15*, 351–377.

Moos, R. H. "Social-Ecological Perspectives on Health." In G. C. Stone, F. Cohen, and N. E. Adler (eds.), *Health Psychology: A Handbook.* San Francisco: Jossey-Bass, 1980.

Nader, P. R., and others. "A Family Approach to Cardiovascular Risk Reduction: Results from the San Diego Family Health Project." *Health Education Quarterly*, 1989, *16*, 229–244.

Nestle, M., and Jacobson, M. F. "Halting the Obesity Epidemic: A Public Health Policy Approach." *Public Health Reports*, 2000, *115*, 12–24.

"Ottawa Charter for Health Promotion." Ottawa: Canadian Public Health Association, 1986.

Owen, N., and Bauman, A. "The Descriptive Epidemiology of a Sedentary Lifestyle in Adult Australians." *International Journal of Epidemiology*, 1992, *21*, 305–310.

Owen, N., Leslie, E., Salmon, J., and Fotheringham, M. J. "Environmental Determinants of Physical Activity and Sedentary Behavior." *Exercise and Sport Sciences Reviews*, 2000, *28*, 153–158.

Richard, L., Potvin, L., Kishchuk, N., Prlic, H., and Green, L. W. "Assessment of the Integration of the Ecological Approach in Health Promotion Programs." *American Journal of Health Promotion*, 1996, *10*, 318–328.

Richter, K. P., and others. "Measuring the Health Environment for Physical Activity and Nutrition Among Youth: A Review of the Literature and Applications for Community Initiatives." *Preventive Medicine*, 2000, *31*, S98–S111.

Sallis, J. F., Bauman, A., and Pratt, M. "Environmental and Policy Interventions to Promote Physical Activity." *American Journal of Preventive Medicine*, 1998, *15*, 379–397.

Sallis, J. F., and Hovell, M. F. "Determinants of Exercise Behavior." *Exercise and Sports Sciences Reviews*, 1990, *18*, 307–330.

Sallis, J. F., Nader, P. R., Rupp, J. W., Atkins, C. J., and Wilson, W. C. "San Diego Surveyed for Heart-Healthy Foods and Exercise Facilities." *Public Health Reports*, 1986, *101*, 216–219.

Sallis, J. F., and Owen, N. *Physical Activity and Behavioral Medicine.* Thousand Oaks, Calif.: Sage, 1999.

Sallis, J. F., Owen, N., and Fotheringham, M. J. "Behavioral Epidemiology: A Systematic Framework to Classify Phases of Research on Health Promotion and Disease Prevention." *Annals of Behavioral Medicine*, 2000, *22*, 294–298.

Sallis, J. F., Prochaska, J. J., and Taylor, W. C. "A Review of Correlates of Physical Activity of Children and Adolescents." *Medicine and Science in Sports and Exercise*, 2000, *32*, 963–975.

Sallis, J. F., and others. "Effects of a Two-Year Health-Related Physical Education Program (SPARK) on Physical Activity and Fitness in Elementary School Students." *American Journal of Public Health*, 1997, *87*, 1328–1334.

Sallis, J. F., and others. "Environmental Characteristics Are Associated with Youth Physical Activity at School." *American Journal of Public Health*, 2001, *91*, 618–620.

Salmon, J., Bauman, A., Crawford, D., Timperio, A., and Owen, N. "The Association Between Television Viewing and Overweight Among Australian Adults Participating in Varying Levels of Leisure-Time Physical Activity." *International Journal of Obesity*, 2000, *24*, 600–606.

Schmid, T. L., Pratt, M., and Howze, E. "Policy as Intervention: Environmental and Policy Approaches to the Prevention of Cardiovascular Disease." *American Journal of Public Health*, 1995, *85*, 1207–1211.

Simpson, J. M., and others. "The Australian National Workplace Health Project: Design and Baseline Findings." *Preventive Medicine*, 2000, *31*, 249–260.

Skinner, B. F. *Science and Human Behavior.* New York: Macmillan, 1953.

Smedley, B. D., and Syme, S. L. (eds.). *Promoting Health: Intervention Strategies from Social and Behavioral Sciences.* Washington, D.C.: National Academy Press, 2000.

Stokols, D. "Establishing and Maintaining Healthy Environments: Toward a Social Ecology of Health Promotion." *American Psychologist*, 1992, *47*, 6–22.

Stokols, D. "Translating Social Ecological Theory into Guidelines for Health Promotion." *American Journal of Health Promotion*, 1996, *10*, 282–298.

Swinburn, B., Egger, G., and Raza, F. "Dissecting Obesogenic Environments: The Development and Application of a Framework for Identifying and Prioritizing Environmental Interventions for Obesity." *Preventive Medicine,* 1999, *29,* 563–570.

U.S. Department of Health and Human Services. "The Surgeon General's Report on Nutrition and Health." DHHS Publication No. PHS 91–50213. Washington, D.C.: U.S. Government Printing Office, 1988.

U.S. Department of Health and Human Services. "Physical Activity and Health: A Report of the Surgeon General." Atlanta: Centers for Disease Control, 1996.

U.S. Department of Health and Human Services. "Healthy People 2010." (Conference edition in two volumes). Washington, D.C.: Department of Health and Human Services, 2000.

Veitch, J., Clavisi, O., and Owen, N. "Physical Activity Initiatives for Male Factory Workers: Gatekeepers' Perceptions of Potential Motivators and Barriers." *Australia and New Zealand Journal of Public Health,* 1999, *23,* 505–510.

Warner, K. "The Need for, and Value of, a Multi-Level Approach to Disease Prevention: The Case of Tobacco Control." In B. D. Smedley and S. L. Syme (eds.), *Promoting Health: Intervention Strategies from Social and Behavioral Research.* Washington, D.C.: National Academy Press, 2000.

Wechsler, H., Devereaux, R. S., Davis, M., and Collins, J. "Using the School Environment to Promote Physical Activity and Healthy Eating." *Preventive Medicine,* 2000, *31,* S121–S137.

Wicker, A. *An Introduction to Ecological Psychology.* Monterey, Calif.: Brooks-Cole, 1979.

Wildey, M. B., and others. "Fat and Sugar Levels Are High in Snacks Purchased from Student Stores in Middle Schools." *Journal of the American Dietetics Association,* 2000, *100,* 319–322.

Winett, R. A. "A Framework for Health Promotion and Disease Prevention Programs." *American Psychologist,* 1995, *50,* 341–350.

Winett, R. A., King, A. C., and Altman, D. G. *Health Psychology and Public Health: An Integrative Approach.* New York: Pergamon, 1989.

World Health Organization. "Obesity: Preventing and Managing the Global Epidemic." Geneva: World Health Organization, 1998.

CHAPTER TWENTY-ONE

APPLYING THEORY TO CULTURALLY DIVERSE AND UNIQUE POPULATIONS

Ken Resnicow
Ronald L. Braithwaite
Colleen DiIorio
Karen Glanz

The notion of *generality,* or broad application, is basic to the definition of *theory.* Theories are by their nature *abstract* (Glanz and Rimer, 1995) and take on concrete meaning only when applied to specific situations, behaviors, or populations. Therefore, to apply theories of health-related behavior, one needs to operationalize—or clearly define—the key constructs so they can be measured and empirically tested.

In the process of operationalizing theoretical constructs, health professionals and health educators should develop an understanding of an individual or group's characteristics (ethnicity, socioeconomic status, gender, age, geographical location) and refine those constructs into *variables.* Thus, it is axiomatic that the application of theory to design health behavior change interventions requires an understanding of the intended audience and their problems, assets, perceptions, cultural milieu, and social environments (see Chapters One and Two; Green and Kreuter, 1999). Indeed, one of the most fundamental principles of the fields of contemporary health education and health promotion involves "starting where the people are." Because theories are abstract, they take on meaning when applied

Development of this manuscript was supported by National Cancer Institute grant # CA-69668, National Heart, Lung, Blood Institute grants # HL-64959 and # HL-62659, and funding from the U.S. Center for Substance Abuse Prevention grant # 8602, to the first author.

to a given content or topic area and when imbued with both dimensions of cultural sensitivity: *surface structure* and *deep structure.*

Attention to the unique characteristics of culturally and socioeconomically diverse populations has been revitalized in recent years, as health disparities persist despite advances in modern medicine (U.S. Department of Health and Human Services, 2000; House and Williams, 2000). Increasingly, diversity is a hallmark of American and international communities. More than ever before, we are aware of the many so-called "special populations" based on race or ethnicity, socioeconomic status, gender, sexual orientation, age, location, or language, to name but a few.

This chapter addresses the challenges of applying theories for understanding and influencing health behavior in culturally diverse and other sociodemographically unique populations. Much of the discussion centers around the notion of cultural sensitivity as it relates to developing health behavior change programs for racial and ethnic minority populations. The chapter begins with a rationale for targeted and tailored health behavior change programs and then presents key concepts to consider in developing culturally sensitive interventions. Finally, specific examples of how interventions can be tailored for racial and ethnic populations are provided, along with future research priorities.

Rationale for Understanding Unique Populations

There has been an assumption that programs must be adapted to fit the needs of minorities and other underserved populations. The rationale for targeted and culturally tailored health behavior change programs derives from four observations: (1) the growing ethnic and racial diversity in the U.S. population, (2) health disparities in diseases and mortality across racial and ethnic groups, (3) differences in the prevalence of behavioral risk factors across racial and ethnic groups, and (4) differences in the predictors of health behaviors across groups. Whereas the first three factors provide the rationale for *targeted* interventions (that is, delivery of programs to specific populations), it is the latter that provides the basis for *cultural tailoring* (Pasick, D'Onofrio, and Otero-Sabogal, 1996; Kreuter and Skinner, 2000).

Cultural differences described in this chapter are not meant to stereotype but are intended to illustrate, and should be seen as guideposts and possible opportunities for tailoring. Researchers and program planners should routinely conduct formative "diagnostic" research in their target population to determine the extent to which such differences (or others not noted here) may or may not apply to the group they will serve.

1. Ethnic and Racial Diversity

The United States is more racially diverse than ever before. Nonwhite residents constitute 30.9 percent of the total population, up from 24.4 percent in 1990 (U.S. Census Bureau, 2001). Minority racial and ethnic groups grew at a rate of 43.2 percent during the past decade, more than three times faster than the overall 13.1 percent rate of population growth and more than ten times faster than the 3.5 percent increase in whites (U.S. Census Bureau, 2001). The fastest rates of growth are among Hispanic and Asian groups. Those who report being multiracial are an emerging ethnic or racial group that numbered about 7 million people in the 2000 Census (U.S. Census Bureau, 2001). The proportion of whites in the United States is projected to continue decreasing, so that by the middle of the next century, there will be no single majority racial group in the country. Whereas this chapter focuses on the application of theory to various ethnic and other subgroups within the context of the U.S. demographics, many of the conceptual issues and research priorities discussed here are applicable to other societies around the world that have different ethnocultural and demographic compositions.

Socioeconomic Indicators and Racial or Ethnic Minority Status. Racial differences are often associated with differences in socioeconomic status between majority and minority groups. Minority groups tend to be less educated, more often living in poverty, and less likely to have adequate access to health care. The proportion of persons below the poverty level is higher for all minority races than for whites, and has been ever since these statistics were first tracked (National Center for Health Statistics, 2000). In 1998, 26 percent of blacks and 26 percent of persons of Hispanic origin were below poverty, compared to 11 percent of whites (National Center for Health Statistics, 2000). Levels of educational attainment are also lower: although the percentage of high school graduates among all U.S. groups increased from 77.6 percent to 84.1 percent between 1990 and 2000, nearly all minority groups (with the exception of Asian Americans) had significantly lower rates of high school graduation (U.S. Census Bureau, 2001).

Another social indicator of great importance to health status and health behavior is access to health care, which is usually measured by the availability of health insurance and a regular source of care. Although between 85 and 90 percent of Americans have a regular source of health care (National Center for Health Statistics, 2000), rates tend to be lower among racial minorities and in particular among immigrants. Other barriers to care, including language, long travel distances for rural residents, and the absence of culturally sensitive practitioners and programs, tend to disadvantage minorities, recent immigrants, and residents of rural areas. Many of the differences in health status and access to health care can be attributed to socioeconomic rather than racial, ethnic, or cultural factors. However, as the effects of culture, poverty, racial discrimination, and limited culturally appropriate health services are often interrelated in complex ways, it is difficult to disentangle the relative contribution of these factors on these observed differences.

Heterogeneity. Although discussions of cultural diversity usually emphasize differences between racial and ethnic groups, there is often as much heterogeneity *within* racial and ethnic groups. Failure to appreciate the heterogeneity *within* ethnic groups can lead to what has been called "ethnic glossing" (Trimble, 1990–1991) and ultimately to insensitive and ineffective interventions. This has significant implications for the development of culturally appropriate health behavior interventions. Differences in socioeconomic status, geography, and rural or urban residence are only a few of the factors that may lead to important intragroup differences.

American Indians are a case in point for within-group variation. The 2000 census indicates that there are 2.48 million self-identifying American Indians or Alaska Natives in the United States. An additional 1.6 million people reported Native American plus at least one other race (U.S. Census Bureau, 2001). There are 550 federally recognized American Indian tribes (Indian Health Service, 2001) as well as dozens of other tribes with just state-only recognition. The most populous tribes are Cherokee (369,000), Navajo (225,000), Sioux (107,000), and Chippewa (106,000) (U.S. Census Bureau, 1995). American Indians live on both rural reservations and in urban areas. Clearly, the identification of individuals or families as "American Indian" by itself fails to convey many important details about them. The same is true for Hispanic-Latino subgroups (such as Mexican American, Puerto Rican, Central American, and Cuban American), Asian Americans, who self-identify by one of the many Asian countries of origin, and even African Americans, who may have varied ethnic backgrounds (for example, Caribbean, North African, or East African).

2. Health Disparities: Mortality and Disease Rates

The recognition of differences in disease and mortality rates across ethnic and racial groups has led to increasing efforts to reduce or eliminate such health disparities (U.S. Department of Health and Human Services, 2000). It has long been known that African Americans die at earlier ages than do whites. As of 1998, life expectancy for African American males was 67.6 years compared with 74.5 years for white males. The difference is slightly less for African American women, 74.8

versus 80 for white women, but still alarmingly discrepant (National Center for Health Statistics, 2000). Infant mortality rates also reveal large disparities: infant mortality among whites was only 5.8, but it was 14.6 for blacks (Kochanek, Smith, and Anderson, 2001). African Americans have higher rates of heart disease, stroke, most cancers, pneumonia, influenza, chronic liver disease, diabetes, HIV, unintentional injuries, and homicide than do whites (Pamuk, Makuc, Heck, Reuben, and Lochner, 1998; Winkleby, Robinson, Sundquist, and Kraemer, 1999).

Many chronic diseases vary substantially across racial and ethnic groups in the United States, including heart disease, cancer, and diabetes. Most minority groups in the United States have higher rates of Type 2 (non-insulin-dependent) diabetes than do white persons: diabetes prevalence is 5.9 percent among adults in the United States as a whole, but is 10.8 percent in African Americans, 10.6 percent in Hispanics and Latinos, 12.2 percent in Native Americans, and 21.5 percent in Native Hawaiians (Carter, Pugh, and Monterrosa, 1996; Mau and others, 1997).

Similarly, the burden of cancer is not distributed equally in the United States. Many racial and ethnic minority groups suffer from higher incidence, higher mortality, and poorer survival rates than do white Americans (Miller and others, 1996; Glanz, Croyle, Chollette, and Pinn, forthcoming; seer.cancer.gov). While overall cancer incidence and mortality rates declined through the 1990s in both men and women, and in most minority populations, minority groups have still not gained equal ground (Howe and others, 2001; Haynes, Smedley, and Committee, 1999). For example, among women, white women have the highest overall cancer incidence rates across groups, but age-adjusted mortality rates for all cancers combined are much higher for African Americans than for white women. Also, African American, Mexican American, Native Hawaiian, and Alaska Native women have higher mortality rates for breast cancer, and African Americans, Native Hawaiians, and Alaska Native women had excessive lung cancer mortality (National Cancer Institute, 2000). While differences in mortality and survival are often attributed to cancers being diagnosed at a later stage, it is increasingly evident that late diagnosis and poor cancer outcomes are often due to poverty and inferior medical care (Lannin and others, 1999; Dignam and others, 1999; Hodgson, Fuchs, and Ayanian, 2001).

3. Behavioral Risk Factors

Where differences in well-known behavioral risk factors and in use of proven early detection strategies contribute to disparate disease and mortality rates, there is a clear need for interventions addressing those health-related behaviors. Tobacco use, certain dietary practices, obesity, and the use of early detection tests may explain some ethnic disparities in health problems. Cigarette smoking is a major cause of preventable disease and death in all ethnic groups, and men are more likely to smoke than women across all groups (U.S. Department of Health and Human Services, 1998). Among adults, American Indians, Alaska Natives, Native Hawaiians, and African American and Southeast Asian men have a high prevalence of smoking (U.S. Department of Health and Human Services, 1998; Kolonel and others, 2000). Asian American and Hispanic women have the lowest prevalence (U.S. Department of Health and Human Services, 1998).

Obesity is a risk factor for diabetes and cardiovascular disease and appears to play a role in cancer incidence and mortality for some cancer sites. Rates of obesity among women are higher for Hispanic, African American, Native Hawaiian, American Indian, and Alaska Native women than for whites. Among the largest minority groups, only Asian American women are less often overweight and obese than are white women (National Center for Health Statistics, 2000; Kolonel and others, 2000). Suboptimal dietary patterns and low rates of physical activity contribute to these rates of obesity. In fact, for many ethnic minorities, acculturation to an "American diet" means increasing their intake of animal fat and "junk foods," whereas traditional Asian, Hispanic, and Native Hawaiian dietary patterns are high in complex carbohydrates and relatively low in fat, and thus consistent with current dietary guidelines for good health.

The differences described here are but a few of the many differences in health-related behaviors that have been found among minority populations in the United States. While these examples address adults' behavioral risks, similar patterns have been noted among adolescents with regard to health risk behaviors (Healton and others, 2000). Even so, recent findings from one of the largest studies of adolescent health to date found that race, ethnicity, income, and family structure account for only a small percentage of the variance in adolescent risk behaviors including smoking, alcohol use, violence, and sexual activity (Blum and others, 2000).

4. Differences in Predictors of Health Behaviors Across Groups

Differences in mortality, disease, and risk factor prevalence provide the rationale for targeting interventions to certain racial and ethnic minority and other sociodemographic subgroups. However, these observations provide little guidance for cultural tailoring of promising interventions, or "how" to effect health-enhancing changes. This derives from understanding the correlates and predictors of health behaviors as they may differ across racial and ethnic populations—and from a close examination of how various theories can be applied to changing behavior across subpopulations.

The Theory of Planned Behavior suggests that a person's perceptions of whether important referent individuals approve or disapprove of performing a behavior, weighted by his or her motivation to meet the expectations of those referents, will contribute significantly to predicting his or her behavior (see Chapter Four). The theory does not, however, specify the relative importance of those influential persons, which may vary across age, gender, and ethnic groups. For example, there are ethnic differences in the relative effects of peers and parents on adolescents' substance-use behavior. Several studies have found that peers exert a stronger influence on cigarette and other drug use among whites and Hispanics than among African Americans (Gottfredson and Koper, 1996; Landrine, Richardson, Klonoff, and Flay, 1994). Conversely, parents appear to have a greater impact on the use of alcohol, tobacco, and other drugs among African Americans than among white youths (Clark, Scarisbrick-Hauser, Gautam, and Wirk, 1999; Robinson, Klesges, Zbikowski, and Glaser, 1997). Smoking among African American youths is inversely associated with parental disapproval, whereas no such association is evident in whites (Gritz and others, 1998). One explanation for the stronger impact of parental factors can be found in the work of Clark (Clark, Scarisbrick-Hauser, Gautam, and Wirk, 1999), who found that African American parents were far more likely than white parents to believe they could influence their children's smoking behavior and more likely to establish clear rules and expectations regarding smoking in the household. Thus, while the Theory of Planned Behavior might predict tobacco use among both African American and white youths, the relative contribution of key factors appears to differ between the groups.

In a different context, a survey of 756 parents with young children found that parents' sun-protection habits were the single most important predictor of children's sun-protection practices, across several ethnic groups (White, Asian American, Native Hawaiian, and mixed race) (Glanz, Lew, Song, and Cook, 1999). Given a different type of health behavior, a younger group of children, and families living in a highly multiethnic social environment (that is, Hawai'i), the intergroup differences in predictors of behavior are not so pronounced.

Theories of social support and social networks (see Chapter Nine) have often been examined in relation to women's health practices. A survey of more than two thousand Hispanic-origin women from eight U.S. regions examined the role of social networks and social integration in predicting whether women obtained mammography screening and Pap smears. The results showed that the effect of social integration on mammography was modest among Mexican, Cuban, and Central American women and that there was no effect among Puerto Rican women (Suarez and others, 2000). However, social integration had a strong effect on Pap smear screening for Mexican Americans, a modest effect among Central American women and Cuban women, and no effect for Puerto Rican women. These findings suggest the importance of recognizing different Hispanic subgroups, and also of understanding the group differences in social network characteristics and their potential to be useful in improving screening behavior (Suarez and others, 2000). Of equal importance, the findings of this particular study do not imply that such racial or ethnic subgroup differences occur across all relevant attitudes and psychosocial factors.

Appraisals of stressors and coping responses (see Chapter Ten) are often rooted in cultural experiences and may vary with minority and socioeconomic status. Racial or ethnic differences in the prevalence of socioeconomic and environmental risk factors associated with health behavior are also evident. For example, compared with whites, African Americans experience a greater number of negative stressful events, and they experience different types of stressors and employ different types of coping strategies in response to stress (Airhihenbuwa and Cole, 1988; Fitzpatrick and Boldizar, 1993). They also derive social support, a buffer against stress, from different sources (Thomas, Bethlehem, and Holmes, 1992). African American adolescents are more likely than their white counterparts to be victims of or witnesses to violence, to experience death of a parent or sibling, to be involved in the criminal justice system, and to have parents whose income has recently decreased (Fitzpatrick and Boldizar, 1993). Thus, they tend to rate the impact of stressful events differently than do white adolescents. Another important source of stress for African Americans and other minority racial groups is racism, which can increase feelings of anger, hostility, alienation, and helplessness, all of which have been associated with negative health outcomes (Barefoot, Dahlstrom, and Williams, 1983; Scherwitz and others, 1992). The higher levels of risk would appear inconsistent with the lower rates of tobacco use that have been found among African American youths (Healton and others, 2000). One explanation for this apparent paradox may be that the predictors of substance use, both risk and protective factors, in fact function differently across racial and ethnic subgroups.

Cultural Sensitivity: Definitions, Dimensions, and Application

Cultural sensitivity (CS) is one of the most widely accepted principles among health behavior researchers and practitioners. How to achieve it, however, and its impact on psychosocial and behavioral outcomes, have not been adequately described or empirically examined.

This section presents a conceptual framework for developing culturally sensitive interventions. It begins with some basic definitions, introduces the key dimensions of CS, and discusses the practical implications of applying CS to theories of health behavior and behavior change. Next, some strategies for developing culturally sensitive interventions are described.

What Is Cultural Sensitivity?

The term *cultural sensitivity* goes by many names, including cultural competence, culturally relevant, culturally appropriate, culturally consistent, multicultural, culturally legitimate, ethnically sensitive, cultural diversity, cultural pluralism, cultural tailoring, and cultural targeting (Marin and others, 1995). Although definitions and distinctions for these terms have been offered (Sue and Sue, 1999; Pasick, D'Onofrio, and Otero-Sabogal, 1996), the terminology has no accepted standards. In response to this need, the following definitions are proposed:

Cultural sensitivity: The extent to which ethnic or cultural characteristics, experiences, norms, values, behavior patterns, and beliefs of a target population, and relevant historical, environmental, and social forces are incorporated in the design, delivery, and evaluation of targeted health interventions, including behavioral change materials and programs.

Cultural competence: The capacity of individuals to exercise interpersonal cultural sensitivity (Marin and others, 1995). Culturally competent refers to practitioners, whereas culturally sensitive relates more to intervention programs, materials, and messages.

Multicultural: Incorporating and appreciating perspectives of multiple racial and ethnic groups without assumptions of superiority or inferiority. In this sense, culturally competent individuals and culturally sensitive interventions are implicitly multicultural. *Cultural pluralism* is a synonym.

Culturally-based: Programs and messages that use culture, ethnicity, history, and core values as a medium to engage participants and motivate behavior change.

Ethnic identity: The extent to which individuals identify with and gravitate toward their racial or ethnic group. Ethnic identity includes racial and ethnic pride, affinity for in-group culture (for example, food, media, and language), attitudes toward majority culture, involvement with group members, experience with and attitudes about racism, attitudes toward intermarriage, and the importance of preserving one's culture and aiding others of like background (Resnicow and Ross, 1997). For immigrant groups in particular, ethnic identity often includes acculturation, or adoption of values and practices of the host country (Sue and Sue, 1999).

Dimensions of Cultural Sensitivity

Cultural sensitivity can be conceptualized in terms of two primary dimensions: *surface structure* and *deep structure* (Resnicow, Braithwaite, Ahluwalia, and Baranowski, 1999). Surface structure involves matching intervention materials and messages to observable social and behavioral characteristics of a target population. For print and audiovisual materials, surface structure may involve using people, places, language, music, foods, brand names, locations, and clothing familiar to and preferred by the target audience. Surface structure includes identifying the channels (such as media outlets) and settings (such as churches or schools) that are most appropriate for delivery of messages and programs. It also entails understanding characteristics of the behavior in question, for example, the product brands that are used and the context in which the health behavior occurs. Surface structure refers to the extent to which interventions fit with the culture, experience, and behavioral patterns of the audience. In this sense, surface structure is analogous to face validity of psychological measures: a necessary but not sufficient prerequisite for construct validity. Like face validity, surface structure is generally achieved through expert and community review as well as the involvement of the target population in the intervention development process (Resnicow, Braithwaite, Ahluwalia, and Baranowski, 1999).

The second dimension of cultural sensitivity, *deep structure,* is less readily visible. Deep structure reflects how cultural, social, psychological, environmental, and historical factors influence health behaviors differently across racial and ethnic populations (Marin and others, 1995; Pasick, D'Onofrio, and Otero-Sabogal, 1996). This includes understanding how members of the target population perceive the cause, course, and treatment of illnesses as well as how they perceive the determinants of specific health behaviors, and involves appreciation for how religion, family, society, economics, and the government, both in perception and in fact, influence the target behavior. For example, many African Americans believe that the U.S. government may be covertly encouraging the spread of HIV/AIDS, guns, and drugs in their communities (Cochran and Mays, 1993). Including messages that incorporate, though not necessarily accept or refute these beliefs, may enhance program acceptance and effectiveness in communities in which such beliefs are prevalent.

Although many, if not all cultures share common values regarding issues such as the importance of family, there are cross-cultural differences in some core values that may influence how health behavior interventions are tailored for certain populations. For example, some cultures place greater importance on social harmony, interdependence (versus independence), religiosity, and a holistic view of health. Additionally, similar values may manifest uniquely across racial and ethnic groups based on their collective experience, communication style, and language.

Core cultural values for African Americans are often described as including communalism, religion or spiritualism, expressiveness, respect for verbal communication skills, connection to ancestors and history, commitment to family, and intuition and experience versus empiricism (Cochran and Mays, 1993). African

American culture is also characterized by a unique sense of time, rhythm, and communication style (Hecht, Collier, and Ribeau, 1993). The use of oral communication and stories, religious or spiritual themes, and historical references to convey messages should be considered when developing health behavior change programs for African Americans.

For Hispanics, core cultural values typically include respect for elders (*respeto*), fatalism, and the importance of positive social interactions (*simpatía*) (Sabogal, Otero-Sabogal, Pasick, Jenkins, and Perez-Stable, 1996). Native Hawaiian culture places strong emphasis on social harmony, well-ordered social relationships, and interdependence (Mokuau and Brown, 1994; McLaughlin and Braun, 1998). Affirmation of traditional values such as *'ohana* (family), *kokua* (cooperation), *mana* (oneness with all things), *lokahi* (harmony and unity), and *ho'oponopono* (group-based problem solving) is a central part of efforts to invoke inherent cultural resources to improve health and well-being in Native Hawaiian communities (McLaughlin and Braun, 1998).

The preceding examples of "core cultural values" are based on evidence from studies of persons in these ethnic and racial groups, but they are neither universal among all persons of these races nor exclusive to these groups. As mentioned earlier, there is no substitute for formative research for developing an understanding of the intended audience for a health communication or health promotion program.

Whereas surface structure generally increases the receptivity, comprehension, or acceptance of messages, deep structure conveys *salience*. Surface structure establishes the feasibility and acceptability of an intervention, whereas deep structure is believed to contribute to program impact.

Practice Implications of Cultural Sensitivity for Applying Theory

How does this model of cultural sensitivity affect our understanding and application of current theories of behavior change? The numerous epidemiological and psychosocial differences between ethnic or racial minorities and other unique populations—at both the surface and deep structure levels—raise a key question: Are existing models of health behavior change applicable to these audiences, or are new models and theories needed?

The answer is determined by philosophical and political orientation, not only empirical factors. If we reexamine the definition of "theory" and consider the examples discussed earlier in this chapter regarding predictors of health behaviors, it would appear that available models can indeed be adapted to racial or ethnic and other sociodemographic subpopulations. As described in Chapter Two and at the beginning of this chapter, a theory is a set of interrelated concepts, definitions, and propositions that present a *systematic* view of events or situations by specifying relations among variables, to *explain* and *predict* the events or situations; the notion of *generality,* or broad application, is important. Because theories are abstract, they take on meaning when applied to a given content or topic area and when imbued with both dimensions of cultural sensitivity: surface structure and deep structure.

Some models of health behavior are culturally sensitive, by their very nature and foundations. Community organization models emphasize community-driven actions (see Chapter Thirteen). One model of community organization that puts special emphasis on culturally relevant practice is the Community Organization and Development (COD) model for health promotion in communities of color (Braithwaite and others, 1989). This model involves a community-controlled coalition board undertaking its own community assessment and designing culturally relevant interventions through community problem solving (Braithwaite, Bianchi, and Taylor, 1994). The PRECEDE-PROCEED Planning Model also relies on the fundamental principle of participation of the audience in identifying problems and defining solutions and programs (Green and Kreuter, 1999; see Chapter Eighteen). With a strong emphasis on audience analysis, social marketing is another model that is inherently culturally sensitive (see Chapter Nineteen).

For some theories, the link between theory and culturally sensitive application is less obvious; indeed, the dilemma is more likely in the application than in the theory. In one clear example of applying mainstream theoretical models to culturally competent community interventions for adults with Type 2 diabetes, Gilliland and others (1998) describe how they translated constructs from Social Learning Theory into program methods and strategies for Native Americans and Native Hawaiians. Their programs, led by minority professionals, explicitly incorporate both surface structure components (such as familiar materials and settings) and deep structure elements (problem-solving approaches, family involvement) that fit the minority audiences' circumstances and values (Gilliland and others, 1998). Recently published results from one of these intervention studies showed that the new culturally-based intervention increased movement along stages of change for fat intake and physical activity (Mau and others, 2001).

In direct contrast to the approach of Gilliland and others, Oomen and others concluded that established health behavior models do not adequately address the unique needs of the older female Hispanic population, and that a new, culturally sensitive model must be used (Oomen, Owen, and Suggs, 1999). They contend that overemphasis on individual responsibility, failure to appreciate the role of socioeconomic deprivation, disregard for cultural aspects of dietary patterns, and lack of appreciation of the role of religion in Hispanics' perceptions of disease were all inadequately addressed by existing health behavior models. This raised concern about the lack of both surface *and* deep structure adaptations in available, empirically evaluated programs. This concern seems to reflect problems in application, not problems with the available models per se.

These two contrasting scenarios can be repeated with different racial and ethnic minorities. For example, some Afrocentric scholars contend that conceptual models developed from a Eurocentric perspective fail a priori to adequately incorporate the social, psychological, cultural, historical, and genetic characteristics of African Americans (Nobles, 1972). For example, Social Cognitive Theory (SCT) emphasizes individual-based determinants such as self-efficacy, personal goals, self-evaluative expectations, self-management, and assertiveness skills (Bandura, 1986; Bandura, 1997), which are rooted in what has been considered Eurocentric, predominantly male values of competitiveness, materialism, personal achievement, impulse control, and self-determinism (Nobles, 1972). Such individual-centered models, it has been argued, are too mechanistic and fail to adequately account for environmental determinants such as stress, racism, and poverty, and the high availability of guns and drugs and low availability of recreational, educational, and health facilities that for many African Americans may be more influential than individual motivation (Cochran and Mays, 1993).

The Afrocentric view asserts, to some degree, that individual and social learning principles may operate differently in African Americans, not only in degree but in kind. Proponents contend that a "one size fits all" application of SCT, even with culturally sensitive adaptation, may be less effective than developing a uniquely Afrocentric paradigm. However, the concept of collective efficacy can also be seen as a mode of human agency that is consistent with Social Cognitive Theory (Bandura, 2001), and this more inclusive reading of SCT is sometimes overlooked in Afrocentric writings. This is similar to the Hispanic viewpoint put forth by Oomen, Owen, and Suggs (1999), in the example of women with Type 2 diabetes.

In the contrasting approach, it is assumed that the fundamental determinants of behavior operate similarly in all populations, and that psychological and behavioral models, such as SCT, can be successfully adapted for a range of sociodemographic, racial, and ethnic populations (Bussey and Bandura, 1999; Bandura, 2001). It is this perspective that guides the remainder of this chapter. However, successful adaptation requires an integrative understanding of the unique personal and environmental characteristics of the target population, of the surface and deep structure determinants of behavior that can be translated into culturally sensitive messages and behavior change strategies.

The adaptation process requires practitioners and researchers to examine ethnocentric (or socioeconomically or professionally centered) assumptions inherent in their methods and to attempt to incorporate alternative conceptualizations of human experience. This mandates a worldview wherein researchers and program planners approach a community not from a deficit model, which assumes one-way assistance, but rather with the assumption that they too will learn and benefit from their experiences as much as the audience. It further means embracing the view that the community has resources, wisdom, solutions, and energy that can be mobilized to improve its health status.

Developing Culturally Sensitive Interventions

As we mentioned at the beginning of this chapter, it is not the theories but their application for developing interventions that requires careful adaptation to the audience with which one is working. As articulated in the PRECEDE-PROCEED Planning Model, the process of developing health behavior change programs that are culturally sensitive and appropriate for unique populations should begin with an analysis of the social environment, disease and behavioral risk factors, and the unique behavioral patterns and determinants in the target population (Green and Kreuter, 1999; see Chapter Eighteen). These data may come from the scientific literature, but information obtained directly from the community is also important. Direct information can be especially useful for elucidating predictors of behavior and can be obtained from both quantitative surveys and qualitative methods. Qualitative data collection can include exploratory focus groups, interviews with key informants, and pretesting results.

Focus groups are a potentially valuable means for developing culturally sensitive intervention messages. During the formative phase of intervention planning, members of the target audience are convened to explore thoughts, feelings, experiences, associations, language, assumptions, and environmental enabling and constraining factors in regard to the health behavior issues of interest and their context. Specific guidelines for conducting focus groups can be found elsewhere (Basch, 1988; Krueger, 1988).

Exploratory focus groups also provide an opportunity to examine the possible role of culturally-based messages. Although potentially costly, when developing interventions for minority groups, it can also be valuable to conduct a few groups with white audiences. Though some might view this as culturally *insensitive* (by establishing white values and practices as the norm) or simply a waste of resources, contrasting responses from racial and ethnic populations with those of the majority culture can help crystallize the extent of tailoring required. Such groups can also draw out the unique language used around a particular topic. For example, focus groups we conducted with African American smokers in Harlem revealed the term "loosies," which referred to single cigarettes purchased generally for twenty-five cents at newspaper stands. Focus groups with overweight African American teenage girls revealed terms such as "thick" and "nasty fat." Incorporating such terminology can increase the surface structure sensitivity of an intervention. It can also be useful to explore how the target population perceives that the prevalence, expression, and determinants of the target health behavior may differ in their community relative to whites or to the population as a whole.

When conducting exploratory focus groups, another strategy that can be used to delineate cultural differences is what we have called "ethnic mapping" (Resnicow, Braithwaite, Ahluwalia, and Baranowski, 1999). This entails having participants rate aspects of the target behavior along a visual continuum, ranging from "mostly a black (or Hispanic, and so on) thing" to "equally a black and white thing" to "mostly a white thing." This process begins by presenting several anchors for which responses have been generally consistent across the minority population. For example, rap music and Kwanzaa are rated "mostly black things," skiing and caviar are generally rated "mostly white things," and Christmas and television are generally rated "equally black and white things." Once participants become comfortable with the classification schema, elements of the target behavior can be classified using the same categories. In a recent series of four focus groups conducted to help develop an intervention to increase fruit and vegetable consumption among African American adults, participants were asked to rate 25 foods using this schema (Resnicow, Braithwaite, Ahluwalia, and Baranowski, 1999). If more than half the group rated an item in one of the three categories, it was considered a consensus. As shown in Table 21.1, results of the ethnic mapping exercise indicated that foods such as asparagus, tomato juice, pumpkin pie, and artichokes should probably not be emphasized in the proposed program. Or, if these foods are included, they should be introduced as foods that many participants may not have eaten or that are not usually consumed. Table 21.2 presents the results of ethnic mapping for various forms of physical activity from four focus groups conducted with adults from black churches in the Atlanta area. This process provided information that was not found in available quantitative data sources. The ethnic mapping technique may also be useful for examining other health behaviors such as smoking (for example, to determine brand preferences, quitting techniques, and perceptions about smokers), HIV/AIDS, cancer, and substance abuse.

Examples of Cultural Tailoring and Adaptation of Health Behavior Theory

In this section we present examples of the application of culturally sensitive approaches to developing theory-based health behavior intervention strategies. These examples highlight situations in which a culturally unique application of theory

TABLE 21.1. RESULTS OF ETHNIC MAPPING OF FRUIT AND VEGETABLE INTAKE FROM FOUR FOCUS GROUPS.

Mostly Black	Equally Black and White		Mostly White
Turnip greens	Apples	Pears	Artichoke
Collards	Bananas	Peaches	Asparagus
Sweet potato pie	Grapes	Pineapple	Beets
Watermelon	Oranges	Raisins	Bean salad
			Tomato juice
			Pumpkin pie
			Apricots

Note: N = 33.

TABLE 21.2. RESULTS OF ETHNIC MAPPING OF PHYSICAL ACTIVITY FROM FOUR FOCUS GROUPS.

Mostly Black	Equally Black and White		Mostly White
Basketball	Jogging	Aerobics at home	Aerobics at club
Housework for job	Jazz dancing	Walking	Square dancing
Jump rope or	Biking	Gardening	Hiking
Double Dutch	Bowling	Tennis	Squash
	YMCA	Swimming in pool	Swimming at beach
	Weights	Football	Ice skating

Note: N = 29.

is indicated. However, there are many examples of interventions, such as reminder systems for mammograms, that work equally well for minority and nonminority populations. These interventions may be boosted by access-enhancing strategies for low-income, ethnic minority populations (Legler and others, 2002).

The first two examples focus on issues that are often identified in relation to minority versus majority values: individualism versus communalism, and the role of religiosity. The third example concerns complementary approaches to reducing tobacco use among American Indians through implementation of smoking policies and smoking cessation programs.

Appealing to Attitudes Toward Individualism Versus Communalism

A Social Cognitive Theory framework would suggest that interventions could be tailored to account for communal motivation (Bandura, 2001). For example, when working with African Americans rather than focusing exclusively on individual efficacy, emphasis could be placed on social outcome expectations related to communal benefits, community versus individual efficacy, inter- rather than *intra*personal motivation, and collective rather than personal goals. Thus, appropriate messages for black adolescents developed from this perspective might include "Do it for yourself, your family, and your people;" "We need more healthy Brothers for the struggle;" and "Do it *with* a friend." In the context of SCT-based health behavior intervention strategies, these messages could be adapted to encourage various positive health behaviors related to substance use, exercise, diet, and sexual practices.

Hispanic culture has also been characterized as having a strong sense of collectivism (*colectivismo*), which includes high levels of personal interdependence, conformity, and sacrifice for the communal good (U.S. Department of Health and Human Services, 1990). Based on the observation that Hispanic youth appear less self-centered than other Americans, an emphasis on communal rather than self-centered motivation for healthful behavior may also be appropriate for this population.

Religiosity

Several studies of adults and adolescents have found higher levels of religiosity among blacks than whites (Levin, Taylor, and Chatters, 1994; Chatters, Levin and Ellison, 1998). Blacks are more likely to attend church, to place a higher value on religion, and to use religion as a coping strategy. The salience of religion in African American life is supported by the finding that religiosity is a stronger predictor of life-satisfaction for blacks than for whites, and that among black adolescents, religion appears more protective of substance abuse than among whites (Thomas, Bethlehem, and Holmes, 1992). Also, the church serves different functions in black and white communities. Beyond spiritual sustenance, black churches provide a forum for social discourse and political activism. Many black churches also provide social and medical services such as health screenings, voter registration campaigns, and feeding programs for the disadvantaged (Thomas, Bethlehem, and Holmes, 1992; Chatters, Levin, and Ellison, 1998).

Religiosity relates to the influence of social referents and thus may be viewed as analogous to constructs from the Theory of Planned Behavior (Ajzen, 1991; see Chapter Four). Linking health messages to religious or spiritual themes, or using religious leaders as messengers or influential referents, may be appropriate motivational strategies for African Americans. This can involve manipulation of social effects—for example, linking health behaviors to specific biblical commandments or using the norms of the faith community as a source of positive or negative sanctions. Also, invoking attitudes toward health practices—for example, emphasizing personal feelings of spiritual or religious pride or shame—can be used to encourage positive health behaviors or discourage health risk behaviors (Campbell and others, 1999).

Increased involvement in religion may also be associated with an increased responsiveness to fear-arousing messages among African Americans. Preaching in black religious institutions is often evangelical, replete with passionate messages of salvation versus damnation and virtue versus sin. As a result, African Americans may be more receptive to messages emphasizing their personal vulnerability to health problems, particularly when tied to religious themes. Such messages might be derived from the Precaution Adoption Process Model (Weinstein, 1988; see Chapter Six). Up to now, however, the question of whether the use of "fear" messages in the church reflects a motivational predisposition that may also operate outside of the context of faith-based institutions has not been empirically examined. Research is needed to determine the effectiveness of fear-arousing messages conveyed to African Americans and the degree to which responsiveness to such messages is related to religiosity.

Reducing Tobacco Use in American Indian Communities

Because tobacco use is unusually high among American Indian (AI) populations, and because American Indians' tobacco use may be tied to long-standing cultural traditions, efforts to improve health by reducing smoking are particularly challenging in AI communities. Over the past decade, two projects have taken different paths in attempting to reduce the deleterious health effects of tobacco among AIs (Hodge and Glover, 1999). Both interventions involve working with existing tribal and reservation structures, and include native staff or organizations (Hodge and Glover, 1999; LeMaster and Connell, 1994). Although the intervention strategies are derived from a number of different theoretical models, they consistently emphasize cultural relevance—for example, having tribal members as part of the research team and using familiar tribal icons in the message or design of education materials.

An intervention program working with the Northwest Indian Tribes was developed to enhance tobacco control policies. The program involved consultation interventions with Tribal representatives including a kickoff workshop, tobacco policy workbooks, follow-up visits, and telephone consultations (Lichtenstein and Lopez, 1999). The Indian Health Board was integral to the policy change approach, and it focused on and respected the political independence of the Tribes. As a result of this endeavor, several tribes developed smoke-free workplaces and curtailed the sale of cigarettes in their communities. Qualitative research findings showed that there were significant improvements in tobacco-use policies as a result of this project (Lichtenstein and Lopez, 1999).

A clinic-based intervention study was designed to help Indian adults in urban and rural communities in California to quit smoking. Using the physician "Quit for Life" smoking cessation model—which draws on Social Cognitive Theory— the team modified some aspects of the intervention so that it would be more culturally relevant for use in this Indian population. The model included an Indian culture–oriented teaching guide and a video in addition to follow-up and counseling by community health workers (trained paraprofessionals). It emphasized responsibility to family and tribe, and cultural respect for tobacco products. The evaluation showed that the cessation was more effective than a "standard care" control, and that it achieved an overall 6.8 percent quit rate, with a higher rate of 7.2 percent in those who were contemplating quitting before the cessation program was offered (Hodge and Casken, 1999).

Research Needs: Cultural Tailoring as an Application of Theory

Numerous empirical questions regarding the process and impact of cultural tailoring remain unanswered. With regard to surface structure, some assumptions are a priori valid. For example, it is largely self-evident that interventions should be written in the language of a population and at an appropriate reading level. However, other surface structure issues such as whether materials should portray role models exclusively from the target audience or from mixed racial and ethnic backgrounds, or if images should reflect the same socioeconomic background as the audience rather than a higher income bracket, require empirical examination. In some cases, racial and ethnic populations may prefer audiovisual materials that represent or are designed for multiple racial and ethnic or socioeconomic groups, instead of purely targeted materials. Indeed, many minority groups may perceive targeted interventions as singling out or casting an unfavorable light on their ethnic community. Similarly, it cannot always be assumed that racial and ethnic groups prefer, or are more responsive to, ingroup practitioners. And some bilingual populations may prefer interventions in English while others may prefer a mix of languages. Program developers may need to explore these issues each time they plan to introduce an intervention into a racial or ethnic subpopulation.

Little is known about how racial and ethnic groups may respond differentially to health behavior interventions or about how much tailoring is needed (Dent and others, 1996). Multicultural approaches have seldom been compared to strategies tailored specifically for one type of audience. More research is needed to examine this question.

Even less is known about the efficacy of deep structure messages. Controlled trials comparing the efficacy of culturally sensitive versus standard (non–culturally sensitive) materials are needed. In fact, it is largely unknown if culturally sensitive programs are truly more effective (Dent and others, 1996). To investigate the efficacy of culturally sensitive materials with a high degree of internal validity, it is important to use comparison materials that are similar in as many dimensions as possible to the culturally sensitive materials. For example, it may be possible to hold constant key scientific content and health education messages and the length of video or print interventions, and only vary the method of conveying content; that is, the tailored elements of the intervention.

Similarly, despite the inherent appeal of using culture to enhance self-esteem and motivate positive behavioral change, relatively little is known about the acceptance or efficacy of culture-based interventions. Many programs have incorporated culture-based themes, but they have rarely been isolated experimentally, so the unique impact of the culture-based components is not well understood. It should be noted that some might contend the need for controlled research to document the efficacy of such interventions is in fact an ethnocentric (and perhaps unnecessary) requirement to document what is intuitively known and inherently valuable. Others might argue that to withhold culturally sensitive interventions from one group for the purpose of an experimental research design would be unethical. Nonetheless, given the range of ethnic diversity among major minority racial and ethnic groups, it is possible that programs that use culture-based messages may be not only ineffective, but, somewhat paradoxically, even culturally insensitive for certain population subgroups.

Additional research issues include determining how surface and deep structure messages may function differently across racial, ethnic, and sociodemographic subgroups; which populations are more or less responsive to culturally-based messages; and which elements of ethnicity and culture are dependent and independent of socioeconomic factors. We hope that the rationale and framework for developing culturally sensitive interventions described in this chapter will assist program planners and researchers in their efforts to address these issues and to continue to improve the effectiveness of health behavior change interventions for diverse audiences.

Conclusion

There are clearly many unanswered research questions regarding the application of theory to culturally diverse and unique populations. However, the evidence suggests that the most debatable questions concern *application* and not the fundamental construction or utility of theories and models of health behavior. Measures of theoretical constructs often need to be different for unique racial and ethnic groups. The relationships uncovered in tests of theory to explain behavior may also vary between populations—not only culturally different populations, but audiences of different genders, ages, religions, and educational backgrounds.

In the end, it is the choice of promising theories, and the translation of theory into research and practice, that deserves the careful attention of researchers and program planners alike. Most professionals *do* pay attention to population differences but often at only a superficial level, and most of us can do so more carefully and thoroughly—making it possible to better grasp elements of deep structure in the communities with whom we work. Both researchers and practitioners should be encouraged, supported, and rewarded for developing substantive relationships with the populations they choose to study and serve. This, after all, will open the door to understanding how to measure, interpret, and apply theory more effectively.

References

Airhihenbuwa, C., and Cole, G. "Results of a Pilot Study of the Relationships of Psychosocial Measures Among Black Adolescent Students." *Western Journal of Black Studies*, 1988, *12*, 204–209.

Ajzen, I. "The Theory of Planned Behavior." *Organizational Behavior and Human Decision Processes*, 1991, 50, 179–211.

Bandura, A. *Social Foundations of Thought and Action. A Social Cognitive Theory.* Englewood Cliffs, N.J.: Prentice Hall, 1986.

Bandura, A. *Self-Efficacy: The Exercise of Control.* New York: Freeman, 1997.

Bandura, A. "Social Cognitive Theory: An Agentic Perspective." *Annual Review of Psychology*, 2001, *52*, 1–26.

Barefoot, J., Dahlstrom, W., and Williams, R. "Hostility, CHD Incidence, and Total Mortality: A 25-Year Follow-Up Study of 255 Physicians." *Psychosomatic Medicine*, 1983, *45*, 59–63.

Basch, C. "Focus Group Interview: An Underutilized Research Technique for Improving Theory and Practice in Health Education." *Health Education Quarterly*, 1988, *14*, 411–448.

Blum, R. W., and others. "The Effects of Race/Ethnicity, Income, and Family Structure on Adolescent Risk Behaviors." *American Journal of Public Health*, 2000, *90*, 1879–1884.

Braithwaite, R. L., Bianchi, C., and Taylor, S. E. "Ethnographic Approach to Community Organization and Health Empowerment." *Health Education Quarterly*, 1994, *21*, 407–419.

Braithwaite, R. L., and others. "Community Organization and Development for Health Promotion Within an Urban Black Community: A Conceptual Model." *Health Education*, 1989, *2*, 56–60.

Bussey, K., and Bandura, A. "Social Cognitive Theory of Gender Development and Differentiation." *Psychological Reviews*, 1999, *106*, 676–713.

Campbell, M. K., and others. "Fruit and Vegetable Consumption and Prevention of Cancer: The Black Churches United for Better Health Project." *American Journal of Public Health*, 1999, *89*, 1390–1396.

Carter, J. S., Pugh, J. A., and Monterrosa, A. "Non-Insulin-Dependent Diabetes Mellitus in Minorities in the United States." *Annals of Internal Medicine*, 1996, *125*, 221–232.

Chatters, L. M., Levin, J. S., and Ellison, C. G. "Public Health and Health Education in Faith Communities." *Health Education and Behavior*, 1998, *25*, 689–699.

Clark, P. I., Scarisbrick-Hauser, A., Gautam, S. P., and Wirk, S. J. "Anti-Tobacco Socialization in Homes of African-American and White Parents, and Smoking and Nonsmoking Parents." *Journal of Adolescent Health*, 1999, *24*, 329–339.

Cochran, S., and Mays, V. "Applying Social Psychological Models to Predicting HIV-Related Sexual Risk Behaviors Among African Americans." *Journal of Black Psychology*, 1993, *19*, 142–154.

Dent, C. W., and others. "Is Current Drug Abuse Prevention Programming Generalizable Across Ethnic Groups?" *American Behavioral Scientist*, 1996, *39*, 911–918.

Dignam, J., and others. Outcomes Among African-Americans and Caucasians in Colon Cancer Adjuvant Therapy Trials: Findings from the National Surgical Adjuvant Breast and Bowel Project. *Journal of the National Cancer Institute*, 1999, *91*, 1933–1940.

Fitzpatrick, K., and Boldizar, J. "The Prevalence and Consequences of Exposure to Violence Among African-American Youth." *Journal of the American Academy of Child & Adolescent Psychiatry*, 1993, *32*, 424–430.

Freeman, H. P. "The Meaning of Race in Science: Considerations for Cancer Research." *Cancer*, 1998, *82*, 219–225.

Gilliland, S. S., and others. "Recommendations for Development and Adaptation of Culturally Competent Community Health Interventions in Minority Populations with Type 2 Diabetes Mellitus." *Diabetes Spectrum*, 1998, *11*, 166–174.

Glanz, K., Croyle, R. T., Chollette, V. Y., and Pinn, V. W. "Cancer-Related Health Disparities Among Women." *American Journal of Public Health*, forthcoming.

Glanz, K., Lew, R. A., Song, V., and Cook, V. A. "Factors Associated with Skin Cancer Prevention Practices in a Multiethnic Population." *Health Education and Behavior*, 1999, *26*, 344–359.

Glanz, K., and Rimer, B. K. *Theory at a Glance: A Guide for Health Promotion Practice.* NIH Publication No. 95–3896. Bethesda, Md.: National Institutes of Health, National Cancer Institute, 1995.

Gottfredson, D. C., and Koper, C. S. "Race and Sex Differences in the Prediction of Drug Use." *Journal of Consulting & Clinical Psychology*, 1996, *64*, 305–313.

Green, L. W., and Kreuter, M. W. *Health Promotion Planning: An Educational and Ecological Approach.* (3rd ed.) Mountain View, Calif.: Mayfield, 1999.

Gritz, E. R., and others. "Cigarette Smoking in a Multiethnic Population of Youth: Methods and Baseline Findings." *Preventive Medicine*, 1998, *27*, 365–384.

Haynes, M. A., Smedley, B. D., and Committee on Cancer Research Among Minorities and the Medically Underserved, Institute of Medicine. (eds.). *The Unequal Burden of Cancer: An Assessment of NIH Research and Programs for Ethnic Minorities and the Medically Underserved.* Washington, D.C.: National Academy Press, 1999.

Healton, C., and others. "Tobacco Use Among Middle and High School Students: United States, 1999. *Morbidity and Mortality Weekly Report*, 2000. *49*, 49–53.

Hecht, L., Collier, M., and Ribeau, S. *African American Communication—Ethnic Identity and Cultural Interpretation.* (Vol. 2) Thousand Oaks, Calif.: Sage, 1993.

Hodge, F. S., and Casken, J. "Characteristics of American Indian Women Cigarette Smokers: Prevalence and Cessation Status." *Health Care for Women International*, 1999, *20*, 455–469.

Hodge, F. S., and Glover, C. S. "The National Cancer Institute's Research Efforts in Native American Communities: Approaches Used and Lessons Learned." In C. S. Glover and F. S. Hodge (eds.), *Native Outreach: A Report to the American Indian, Alaska Native, and Native Hawaiian Communities*. NIH Publication 98–4341. Bethesda, Md: National Cancer Institute, 1999.

Hodgson, D. C., Fuchs, C. S., and Ayanian, J. Z. "Impact of Patient and Provider Characteristics on the Treatment and Outcomes of Colorectal Cancer." *Journal of the National Cancer Institute*, 2001, *93*, 501–515.

House, J. S., and Williams, D. R. "Understanding and Reducing Socioeconomic and Racial/Ethnic Disparities in Health." In B. D. Smedley and S. L. Syme (eds.), *Promoting Health: Intervention Strategies from Social and Behavioral Research*. Washington, D.C.: National Academy Press, 2000.

Howe, H. L., and others. "Annual Report to the Nation on the Status of Cancer, 1973 Through 1998, Featuring Cancers with Recent Increasing Trends." *Journal of the National Cancer Institute*, 2001, *93*, 824–842.

Indian Health Service. *Indian Health Service Fact Sheet*. *www.ihs.gov*, 2001.

Kochanek, K. D., Smith, B. L., and Anderson, R. N. "Deaths: Preliminary Data for 1999." *National Vital Statistics Reports*, 2001, *49*(3), 1–48.

Kolonel, L. N., and others. "A Multiethnic Cohort in Hawai'i and Los Angeles: Baseline Characteristics." *American Journal of Epidemiology*, 2000, *151*, 346–357.

Kreuter, M. W., and Skinner, C. S. "Tailoring: What's in a Name?" *Health Education Research*, 2000, *15*, 1–4.

Krueger, R. A. *Focus Groups: A Practical Guide for Applied Research*. Thousand Oaks, Calif.: Sage, 1988.

Landrine, H., Richardson, J., Klonoff, E., and Flay, B. "Cultural Diversity in the Predictors of Adolescent Cigarette Smoking: The Relative Influence of Peers." *Journal of Behavioral Medicine*, 1994, *17*, 331–346.

Lannin, D. R., and others. "Influence of Socioeconomic and Cultural Factors on Racial Differences in Late-Stage Presentation of Breast Cancer." *Journal of the American Medical Association*, 1999, *279*, 1801–1807.

Lavery, L. A., and others. "Mortality Following Lower Extremity Amputation in Minorities with Diabetes Mellitus." *Diabetes Research and Clinical Practice*, 1997, *37*, 41–47.

Legler, J., and others. "The Effectiveness of Interventions to Promote Mammography Among Women with Historically Lower Rates of Screening." *Cancer, Epidemiology, Biomarkers, and Prevention*, 2002, *11*(1), 59–71.

LeMaster, P. L., and Connell, C. M. "Health Education Interventions Among Native Americans: A Review and Analysis." *Health Education Quarterly*, 1994, *21*, 521–538.

Levin, J. S., Taylor, R. S., and Chatters, L. M. "Race and Gender Differences in Religiosity Among Older Adults: Findings from Four National Surveys." *Journal of Gerontology*, 1994, *49*, S137–S145.

Lichtenstein, E., and Lopez, K. "Enhancing Tobacco Control Policies in Northwest Indian Tribes." In C. S. Glover and F. S. Hodge (eds.), *Native Outreach: A Report to the American Indian, Alaska Native, and Native Hawaiian Communities*. NIH Publication 98–4341. Bethesda, Md.: National Cancer Institute, 1999.

Marin, G., and others. "A Research Agenda for Health Education Among Underserved Populations." *Health Education Quarterly*, 1995, *22*, 346–363.

Mau, M. K., and others. "The Insulin Resistance Syndrome in Native Hawaiians. Native Hawaiian Health Research (NHHR) Project. *Diabetes Care*, 1997, *20*, 1376–1380.

Mau, M. K., and others. "Mediators of Lifestyle Behavior Change in Native Hawaiians: Initial Findings from the Native Hawaiian Diabetes Intervention Program." *Diabetes Care,* 2001, *24,* 1770–1775.

McLaughlin, L. A., and Braun, K. L. "Asian and Pacific Islander Cultural Values: Considerations for Health Care Decision Making." *Health and Social Work,* 1998, *23,* 116–126.

Mokuau, N., and Brown, C. "Life Themes of Native
ian Female Elders: Resources for Cultural Preservation." *Social Work,* 1994, *39,* 43–49.

Miller, B. A., and others. (eds.). *Racial/Ethnic Patterns of Cancer in the United States 1988–1992.* NIH Publication No. 96–4104. Bethesda, Md.: National Cancer Institute, 1996.

National Cancer Institute. *Surveillance, Epidemiology, and End Results Data.* SEER 3.0, Public Use CD-ROM, August 1999 submission; 2000.

National Center for Health Statistics. *Health, United States, 2000. With Adolescent Chartbook.* Hyattsville, Md.: 2000.

Nobles, W. "African Philosophy Foundations for Black Psychology." In R. Jones (ed.), *Black Psychology.* (2nd ed.) New York: HarperCollins, 1972.

Oomen, J. S., Owen, L. J., and Suggs, L. S. "Culture Counts: Why Current Treatment Models Fail Hispanic Women with Type 2 Diabetes." *The Diabetes Educator,* 1999, *25,* 220–225.

Pamuk, E., Makuc, D., Heck, K., Reuben, C., and Lochner, K. (1998). *Health, United States 1998: Socioeconomic Status and Health Chartbook.* DHHS no. 98–1232. Hyattsville, Md.: National Center for Health Statistics.

Pasick, R., D'Onofrio, C., and Otero-Sabogal, R. "Similarities and Differences Across Cultures: Questions to Inform a Third Generation for Health Promotion Research." *Health Education Quarterly,* 1996, *23*(Supplement), S142–S161.

Resnicow, K., Braithwaite, R., Ahluwalia, J., and Baranowski, T. "Cultural Sensitivity in Public Health: Defined and Demystified." *Ethnicity and Disease,* 1999, *9,* 10–21.

Resnicow, K., and Ross, D. "Development of a Racial Identity Questionnaire for African American Adults." *Journal of Black Studies,* 1997, *23,* 239–254.

Robinson, L. A., Klesges, R. C., Zbikowski, S. M., and Glaser, R. "Predictors of Risk for Different Stages of Adolescent Smoking in a Biracial Sample." *Journal of Consulting & Clinical Psychology,* 1997, *65,* 653–662.

Sabogal, F., Otero-Sabogal, R., Pasick, R., Jenkins, C., and Perez-Stable, E. "Printed Health Education Materials for Diverse Communities: Suggestions Learned from the Field." *Health Education Quarterly,* 1996, *23*(Supplement), S123–S141.

Scherwitz, L., and others. "Hostility and Health Behaviors in Young Adults: The Coronary Artery Risk Development in Young Adults (CARDIA) Study. *American Journal of Epidemiology,* 1992, *136,* 136–145.

Suarez, L., and others. "Social Networks and Cancer Screening in Four U.S. Hispanic Groups." *American Journal of Preventive Medicine,* 2000, *19,* 47–52.

Sue, D. W., & Sue, D. *Counseling the Culturally Different: Theory and Practice.* (3rd ed.) New York: Wiley, 1999.

Thomas, M., Bethlehem, L., and Holmes, B. "Determinants of Satisfaction for Blacks and Whites." *Sociological Quarterly,* 1992, *33,* 459–472.

Trimble, J. "Ethnic Specification, Validation Prospects, and the Future of Drug Use Research." *The International Journal of the Addictions,* 1990–1991, *25*(2A), 149–170.

U.S. Census Bureau. *Top 25 American Indian Tribes for the United States: 1990 and 1980.* Release date: August 1995.

U.S. Census Bureau. *U.S. Census 2000: Overview of Race and Hispanic Origin, Census Brief.* March 2001.

U.S. Department of Health and Human Services. *Alcohol and Other Drug Use Among Hispanic Youth.* DHHS no. 90–1726. Rockville, Md.: Office of Substance Abuse Prevention, 1990.

U.S. Department of Health and Human Services. *Tobacco Use Among U.S. Racial/Ethnic Minority Groups: A Report of the Surgeon General.* Atlanta: U.S. Department of Health and Human Services, Centers for Disease Control and Prevention, Office on Smoking and Health, 1998.

U.S. Department of Health and Human Services. *Healthy People 2010: Understanding and Improving Health.* Washington, D.C.: U.S. Government Printing Office, 2000.

Weinstein, N. D. "The Precaution Adoption Process." *Health Psychology,* 1988, *7,* 355–386.

Winkleby, M. A., Robinson, T. N., Sundquist, J., and Kraemer, H. C. "Ethnic Variation in Cardiovascular Disease Risk Factors Among Children and Young Adults: Findings from the Third National Health and Nutrition Examination Survey, 1988–1994." *Journal of the American Medical Association,* 1999, *281,* 1006–1013.

CHAPTER TWENTY-TWO

COMMUNICATION TECHNOLOGY AND HEALTH BEHAVIOR CHANGE

Neville Owen
Michael J. Fotheringham
Bess H. Marcus

The availability of new communication and information technology has opened up an unprecedented range of strategies for health behavior change programs and research. Advances in computer software have made the production of attractive printed materials widely accessible and have made it easier to produce tailored or personalized materials. The Internet, e-mail, mobile telephones, and handheld computers make it possible to reach audiences quickly and conveniently. Interactive communication via wireless systems and portable computers provides new opportunities to assess, guide, remind, and monitor health-related behavior.

Communication technology is also fertile ground for applying theories and models of health behavior to guide the development of educational and behavioral interventions. A number of interventions that apply Social Cognitive Theory (Chapter Eight) and The Transtheoretical Model (Chapter Five) have already been reported. Other theories and models at all levels can also be applied to communication technology. Online support groups may apply theories of social support and social networks, especially for people with diseases viewed as stigmatizing (for example, alcoholism, AIDS, breast cancer) (Davison, Pennebaker, and Dickerson, 2000; Reeves, 2000). Community organizing can occur via Internet-based civic journalism projects (Wallack, 2000). Message development for technological interventions may be informed by social marketing, consumer information processing, and Diffusion Theory.

This chapter describes some of the recent developments in and the attributes of communication technology that are most relevant to research and practice in health behavior change. A particular challenge is to use successfully with new media behavior change theories that have been developed primarily in the contexts of face-to-face, print, or broadcast media interventions. New communication technologies provide both opportunities and limitations. It is a priority to apply the most relevant theory and research methods in this new context, to build a sound base of evidence and conceptual guidelines to support the development and delivery of innovative and effective programs (Kreuter, Farrell, Olevitch, and Brennan, 2000).

Specifically, we consider new applications of communication technology for health-related behavior change, including tailored print, telephones, the Internet, and handheld computers. Our account of these innovations and some of their potential applications is counterbalanced by consideration of some of the barriers that can limit the use of these technologies, including cost, equity of access, security, and quality control.

Communication Technology Capacities for Health Behavior Change

In the recent past, strategies to promote health-related behavior change have most often used printed educational and behavioral-skills-based materials, telephone counseling, and campaigns using television and other print and broadcast media, in addition to in-person counseling and group education methods. Table 22.1 presents a broad timeline of the recent history of the uses of communication media in health behavior and health education. Programs that use new communication technology build on the earlier methods and can draw usefully from the theories and models on which they are based.

The face-to-face, conventional print, and broadcast media behavior change approaches listed in Table 22.1 remain valid and useful now, as in the past. New and emerging communication media are beginning to supplement, or in some cases replace, established uses of other media to deliver health education and health behavior change programs (see Rakowski, 1999). However, they will do so successfully and on a wide scale only if their efficacy and effectiveness can be established, and if they are both acceptable and accepted in practice. The theories and models that have been applied and the body of evidence on the efficacy and effectiveness of programs delivered using print and broadcast media can inform current and future uses of new communication media for health behavior change (Marcus, Owen, Forsyth, Cavill, and Fridinger, 1998).

TABLE 22.1. TIMELINE OF ESTABLISHED, NEWER, AND EMERGING COMMUNICATION MEDIA FOR HEALTH BEHAVIOR CHANGE PROGRAMS.

1970s	Individual and group behavioral counseling Self-help books and booklets Telephone counseling
1980s	Mass media (particularly television and radio) broadcast programs Computer-supported mailouts and linked telephone counseling Videotaped health behavior counseling Telephone counseling Targeted print communications
1990s	Multimedia CD-ROM programs Web site delivery of behavioral content Interactive e-mail advice Automated telephone counseling Tailored print communications
2000s	Interactive Web sites Mobile telephones with enhanced capacities Personal digital assistant (PDA) delivery of programs Device portability via wireless application protocols Integrated, secure database linkages Web television, with tailoring to consumer preferences

There has been recent and rapid growth in the use of communication technology. For example, in March 2001, some 170 million adults in the United States were estimated to be active users of the Internet (CyberAtlas, 2001a). It has been estimated that each month more than half of the Internet users in the United States access health-related information on the Internet (Fox and Rainie, 2000). These developments make it possible for mass-reach information and advice programs to be targeted more precisely to the needs and interests of particular consumer groups and at-risk populations (Noell and Glasgow, 1999). In settings in which established patterns of communication technology use exist, programs can be personally tailored and efficiently delivered to members of a variety of different social groups (Fotheringham and Owen, 2000). For example, relevant settings include communities, workplaces, and primary health care settings. In addition, new technologies can be used to extend both the reach and depth of mass media (Barbara K. Rimer, personal communication, 2001).

The vision for the future of information technology innovation in health behavior and health education is exciting. However, the realization of what is possible within that vision presents considerable challenges (Patrick, 2000). There are significant obstacles to the use of new communication technologies to enhance health that will need to be overcome. Although the "digital divide" between those who have and those who do not have access to information technology is believed to be narrowing, access continues to be a major barrier for disadvantaged social groups (U.S. Department of Commerce, 2000). The costs of developing, disseminating, and accessing health-related applications are prohibitive for many groups. Culturally appropriate content still lags behind need (Children's Partnership, 2000). There is also the problem of "information overload" (Rudd and Glanz, 1990)—new communication media, particularly the Internet, provide ready access to unprecedented volumes of information, but the formidable quantity and variable quality of such information can themselves be barriers.

Relevant Attributes of New Communication Technologies

Some characteristics of new communication technologies that can provide potential advantages over other media are outlined in Table 22.2, along with examples of theories and models that may be relevant to understanding and making use of these attributes. Economies of scale, dissemination of expert knowledge, and independence from time and space restrictions can be strengths of conventional mass media. Newer communication media add capacities for tailoring information to the needs and interests of particular groups or individuals. For example, it is possible to provide program participants with appropriate information at a time of their convenience rather than being restricted to mass delivery of a uniform message at one time, as with television or radio (Anderson, Bikson, Law, and Mitchell, 1995). Programs may be more attractive due to their novelty. Dynamic graphics and sound in these new multimedia technologies may further enhance their appeal.

A fundamental distinction to be kept in mind is the difference between media-based programs that are "there for the taking" versus those that are delivered as planned interventions, intended to be tested in controlled studies or to be used in controlled settings in a systematic fashion. This distinction can be illustrated by comparing, for example, Web sites that are publicly available on the Internet with Web sites that are available only to registered participants or on a workplace or health care intranet system. The studies to be described in the following sections fall mainly into this latter category.

Health behavior interventions using new media potentially can assist users to tailor program content to better suit their own needs. In highly interactive applications, users can access the information or program as often as they wish, making their particular version of a program more or less intensive. This can be of

TABLE 22.2. CAPACITIES, ADVANTAGES, AND THEORETICAL FOUNDATIONS OF NEW COMMUNICATION TECHNOLOGIES FOR HEALTH BEHAVIOR CHANGE.

New Capacities	Advantages	Theoretical Foundations
Interactivity		
Tailoring	Individualized and tailored program delivery, according to responses of the person accessing the program	Social Cognitive Theory The Transtheoretical Model Precaution Adoption Process Model Health Belief Model
Instantaneous feedback	Immediate feedback provided through Web sites; presented material dictated by participant responses	Social Cognitive Theory Theory of Reasoned Action and Theory of Planned Behavior Diffusion Theory
Appeal		
Convenience	Eliminates time restrictions on access to material	Consumer Information Processing
Channel preference	Some target groups may prefer computer-delivered information	Communication Theory
Flexibility	Recipients choose what material they receive, when, and how often	Social Marketing
Engagement		
Credible simulations	Participants role-play and explore "virtual" environments without risks inherent in actual activities	Social Cognitive Theory Communication Theory
Openness of communication	More open responses to sensitive questions, more willingness to explore sensitive issues	Diffusion Theory Interdependence Theory
Multimedia interfaces	Still and video graphics and recorded sound files reduce literacy requirements for material	Social Marketing

Note: Theories listed are examples only. Both the capacities and advantages may be articulated as applications of a variety of theories. For example, "tailoring" is a method that can be an application of any theory or of no theory at all.

benefit, for example, to those with busy schedules who cannot commit to regular engagements (Schneider, Schwartz, and Fast, 1995). The use of graphical and audio interfaces can allow users with limited reading skills or visual limitations to receive material that may have been inaccessible through conventional print media (Robinson, Patrick, Eng, and Gustafson, 1998).

A further advantage of these new technologies is interactivity—the capacity both to gather data from users and provide personalized feedback (Dirkin, 1994). Program participants can be asked to respond to online or telephone questions, and the data can be used to generate personally relevant advice. Data can be recorded to document how interventions are accessed and used. Computer-mediated communication allows "virtual"' environments and social situations to be portrayed and explored by users. The use of online role plays can avoid some of the inhibitions or risks that may be inherent in taking part in the activities themselves. In these contexts, the social modeling, shaping, and reinforcement constructs from operant learning models and Social Cognitive Theory (Chapter Eight) may be operationalized in ways that tend to be less feasible using more traditional communication and behavioral change media. There are several other domains in which more formal linkages can be developed between the capacities described in Table 22.2 and the theories that can guide their use.

Applications of Communication Technology in Health Behavior Change

For health behavior change programs, new communication technologies have the potential to support important innovations in program delivery, particularly in providing feedback to participants. The major types of feedback that can be provided are *personal feedback*, *normative feedback* and *ipsative feedback*. These types of feedback are not unique to programs delivered using information technology, nor are they mutually exclusive. They can be delivered in face-to-face settings and via more traditional media. However, as examples in the following sections show, feedback can be more efficient, rapid, and complex through the use of new communication technology.

Personal feedback refers to the information that respondents obtain about the answers that they have provided. This type of feedback can provide information, for example, on respondents' current behavioral status, motivational levels, or beliefs and attitudes.

Normative feedback refers to the information respondents obtain when comparing their responses with the responses of another group, for instance a group of comparable age or comparable in motivational level. Giving people feedback about their personal fat-intake level, as compared with their peer group's average intake, is an example of normative feedback (Brug, Glanz, van Assema, Kok, and van Breukelen, 1998; Brug and others, 1999). This type of feedback relates to social comparison theory, and also draws on a key construct in the Theory of Reasoned Action (see Chapter Four).

Ipsative feedback (sometimes called *iterative feedback*) refers to a comparison between a person's most recent status and that found at previous assessments (Brug, Glanz, van Assema, Kok, and van Breukelen, 1998). This type of feedback thus allows respondents to review their progress, lack of progress, or even relapse regarding, for example, level of risk behavior, motivational level, or changes in relevant cognitions. It may be especially well-suited to the process of incremental goal setting as a way to improve self-efficacy, based on Social Cognitive Theory (see Chapter Eight).

Computer Tailoring of Print Media Interventions

Potential recipients of health behavior change programs have a wide range of personal attributes, interests, and circumstances. Including all possibly relevant information and advice options in a conventional printed format (a brochure or a booklet, for example) would result in long and involved messages that include inappropriate material (Kreuter, Farrell, Olevitch, and Brennan, 2000). Computer tailoring of print-based interventions makes it feasible to design and implement multiple, individually relevant versions of printed materials, in contrast to delivering a single standardized generic version for all recipients (De Vries and Brug, 1999). One of the advantages of individually tailoring print communications is that it may increase the probability of the material being read, retained, and considered (Brinberg and Axelson, 1990; Brug, Steenhuis, van Assema, and De Vries, 1996; Rimer, 2000; Skinner, Strecher, and Hospers, 1994; Skinner and others, 1999).

Tailoring can be based on age, sex, educational attainment, and other sociodemographic attributes. This is a strategy that may not implicate any health behavior theory, *or* it may be closely reflective of an established theory or theories. Published studies of computer tailoring have used constructs from Social Cognitive Theory (see Chapter Eight) and The Transtheoretical Model (see Chapter Five) to shape the structure and the content of interventions. Other theoretical models have also been used, including the Precaution Adoption Process Model, the Theory of Planned Behavior, the Health Belief Model, and Protection Motivation Theory (see Rakowski, 1999).

Brug, Steenhuis, van Assema, and De Vries (1996) examined the effectiveness of computer-tailored nutrition education to reduce fat intake and increase fruit and vegetable consumption. The tailoring process was implemented using three interrelated computerized elements: (1) an assessment instrument to assess dietary intake and factors associated with behavior change, (2) a source file containing all of the message segments to be combined into tailored messages—including segments appropriate for all possible screening responses, and (3) a program that selects relevant message segments based on the assessment results. This third element is sometimes referred to as an *expert system*, as it takes the role of a quasi-"expert," making preprogrammed decisions about which message segments to include in the tailored message.

Data from the initial assessment instrument are used to create and store a profile of each participant. This is then used as the basis for decisions about which message segments are most appropriate for a particular individual. A 121-item self-administered questionnaire assessed fat, fruit, and vegetable consumption, as well as likely psychosocial correlates of dietary intake, based on the Theory of Planned Behavior (see Chapter Four). Using these data, participants were classified in terms of their dietary behaviors, awareness levels, and attitudes. Message segments, focused on reduced fat intake and increased fruit and vegetable consumption, were tailored according to intake levels and to related attitude and awareness factors. For example, different message segments about fat consumption were composed for application to three categories of participant: those consuming appropriate amounts of fat, those consuming greater than recommended amounts of fat, and those eating amounts of fat that were greater than recommendations and also greater than the average person of their gender. The tailoring algorithm—the element of the program that applies theory-based decisions about which assessment instrument responses should elicit which specific message segments—was a series of "if"-"then" logic statements controlling the selection of message segments. The assessment results were read into a computer, and appropriate message segments were selected from the message file and placed in a logical order in a personalized, individually addressed letter.

Brug, Steenhuis, van Assema, and De Vries (1996) evaluated this program in a study with employees at a large worksite. Two weeks after completing the screening instrument, half of the participants received tailored feedback, while the other half received general nutritional information, formatted in the same manner as the tailored letters. The tailored letters were between four and nine pages in length; the generic letters were five pages long. Three weeks after receiving the letters, participants were mailed a second screening questionnaire. Compared with those receiving the generic material, participants who received tailored letters had significantly more positive attitudes toward dietary changes, were significantly more likely to subsequently report intentions to change their dietary intake, and had significantly lower fat-consumption levels. Taken at face value, this finding would seem to support the utility of providing tailored feedback shaped by health-behavior theory. However, a later study by Brug and others (1999) compared the effects of feedback on participants' diets, with and without feedback based on theoretically derived variables. They found that it was no more effective to include feedback based on psychosocial factors that, theoretically, should be related to behavioral change.

Studies addressing other behaviors such as physical activity (Marcus and others, 1998; Pinto and others, 2000), nutrition (Brug, Campbell, and van Assema, 1999; Campbell and others, 1999), smoking cessation (Dijkstra, De Vries, and Roijackers, 1998; Strecher and others, 1994), and attendance at mammography screenings (Rakowski and others, 1997) have included, to varying degrees, feedback based on theoretically derived variables. But most of the study designs used have not allowed explicit comparisons of theoretically versus nontheoretically derived programs to be made. Given the findings of Brug and others (1999), it will be important for future studies to include such comparisons. While the tailoring of message content may increase the likelihood that the print materials will be attended to, it is not yet certain that theoretically derived message content will be a more effective guide to behavior change than are more basic forms of tailoring generic print materials.

Broader challenges in developing tailored print interventions include identifying the relevant domains to assess and the types of messages that will most effectively address those domains. It is assumed that using constructs from behavior change theories to guide tailored health behavior communications will enhance the efficacy of interventions (Kreuter, Farrell, Olevitch, and Brennan, 2000; Kreuter and Strecher, 1996; Marcus and others, 1998; Rimer and Glassman, 1999; Velicer and Prochaska, 1999). While it seems plausible that this will be the case, further evidence from carefully designed studies with relevant control groups is needed before more definite conclusions can be drawn about the efficacy of theoretically derived tailoring strategies.

Computer-Assisted Interventions via Telephone

Use of the telephone to deliver advice and support has been found to promote behavior change (McBride and Rimer, 1999; Soet and Basch, 1997). Telephone contact, in particular, can be effective for promoting the adoption and maintenance of physical activity in healthy and clinical populations (see, for example, King and others, 1995). Telephone-based programs may be particularly relevant for working adults who may find it more difficult to attend face-to-face programs on a regular basis.

Real-time data collection and feedback can be provided via telephone using computer-controlled speech generation. Users communicate either by using a

Touch-Tone telephone keypad or voice recognition. These systems can interact with each individual at close intervals and may be more likely to provide a contact when the participant is at an opportune time in the behavioral change process. It is likely that some people may be more responsive to spoken material, either due to literacy level or to personal preference. A further advantage of computer-delivered telephone technology is that participants can initiate interactions with the telephone system whenever they experience a need for assistance, rather than waiting for a counselor to call them.

Researchers are examining whether telephone-based interventions are more effective than tailored print-based interventions. In one study, print alone was found to be more effective (Lipkus, Lyna, and Rimer, 1999). Other studies have examined the effectiveness of telephone-based interventions delivered by a computer-generated voice (Ramelson, Friedman, and Ockene, 1999). In addition, there are studies examining whether, for some complex topics such as decision making about mammography, combinations of tailored print and tailored telephone may be more effective than delivery by either medium alone (McBride and Rimer, 1999).

Lipkus, Rimer, Halabi, and Strigo (2000) examined tailored interventions to increase mammography use among women members of a health maintenance organization. Women aged fifty and older were randomized to usual care, to tailored print communications, or to tailored telephone counseling. After one year, a significantly higher proportion of the women who received telephone counseling had mammograms on schedule, compared with those who received tailored print or usual care but only after the first year of intervention. For women off-schedule for their mammograms, telephone counseling rather than tailored print might be the preferred first-line intervention.

In a recently completed clinical trial (Delichatsios and others, 2001), members of a large managed care organization were randomized to receive either physical activity counseling or dietary counseling, during weekly calls made into an interactive telecommunication system. Participants receiving physical activity counseling were significantly more likely to meet physical activity criteria at three months than were those in the comparison group receiving dietary counseling. However, group differences were no longer significant at six months.

Internet Delivery of Health Behavior Change Programs

The computer-generated personalized print interventions described above are innovative communication technology applications that will be subject to further development. Brug and others (1999) have described this development in terms of the *First Generation* of computer-tailored health advice delivery (via print) and the emerging *Second Generation* (interactive applications with immediate feedback, using screen-based delivery, particular via the Internet). As Table 22.1 suggests, print-based delivery can be augmented by the new and emerging capacities of interactive communication technologies summarized in Table 22.2.

Internet technologies allow direct delivery of tailored health behavior communications without the use of print on paper as the medium with which participants interact (as has been the case for the programs described in the preceding section on print-media interventions). However, it should be recognized that reliance solely on electronic transmission of information, with no capacity for printed copy to be retained, could act to limit the impact of a program. Provision of an option to generate "printer-friendly" versions of the tailored information may facilitate retention.

The more immediate and live aspects of Web site delivery can support innovative strategies based on constructs from relevant theory. Social Cognitive Theory (see Chapter Eight), while emphasizing behavioral performance and direct reinforcement as the major pathways to change, identifies a significant role for social modeling—vicarious learning by observing the behaviors of others. Program participants might, for example, access visual or audiovisual presentations of particular and specifically relevant "models" of their own age and gender performing new behaviors. Multiple options for each personalized intervention component can be stored and presented as appropriate. These are accessed according to a relevant tailoring algorithm, cued by participant responses or by requests.

Lieberman (1997) has considered how Web-deliverable interactive multimedia instructional methods can be used in health promotion interventions targeted to children and adolescents. Lieberman argues that such methods can enhance attention to and active processing of health promotion messages, motivation to learn about health, knowledge about prevention and self-management, perceived self-efficacy for healthy behaviors, and communication about health with others who can provide social support.

The mechanics of Web sites and Web site programming can be advantageous for integrating data collection, self-monitoring, and interventions. The costs of data collection and analysis can be reduced by the use of Web-based surveys (Sheehan and Hoy, 1999). Outside of high startup costs for equipment and Web page design, the actual implementation of a survey can be significantly reduced, with no costs for paper or postage. Direct transfer from forms to the analysis software can simplify data management and only limited data cleaning would be necessary (Fotheringham, Owies, Leslie, and Owen, 2000).

Social support (elements of which include informational support, emotional support, and instrumental support) is an important element of health behavior change programs (see Chapter Nine). Internet-based programs that focus on social support may be of particular relevance to assisting those with chronic health conditions such as diabetes (Gustafson and others, 1999) or for assisting with weight loss (Tate, Wing, and Winett, 2001).

Palmtop Computers and Personal Digital Assistants

A recent development in information and communication technologies is the rapid diffusion of palmtop computers. The more sophisticated versions of such tools are referred to as personal digital assistants (PDAs)—lightweight, pocket-sized devices often including software through which information can be synchronized with desktop computers or network mainframes. Some PDAs are provided with wireless capabilities to remotely connect to desktop computer systems or are connectable in conjunction with telephone (including mobile telephone) networks. In effect, this is the convergence of palmtop computer and mobile-telephone technologies.

To date, the use of palmtop computers and PDAs in health behavior and health education programs has been limited. One study reported the use of palmtop computers for cognitive-behavioral treatment of panic disorders (Newman, Kenardy, Herman, and Taylor, 1997). It was found that the integrated use of palmtop computers for self-monitoring and cognitive-behavioral therapy was acceptable to users, and that users were highly adherent to self-monitoring recommendations. Similar findings were reported in an early study investigating the use of palmtop computers in the treatment of obesity (Agras and others, 1990).

Whalen, Jamner, Henker, and Delfino (2001) used PDAs (as "electronic diaries") to examine smoking and mood in adolescents. Risk of smoking, urges to smoke, and alcohol intake were found to be elevated in those identifying frequent negative moods. Whalen and associates argue that the electronic diary methods that were tested hold promise for the development of targeted preventive interventions such as affect-regulation training.

There is a range of studies now under way examining the use of PDAs in health education and health behavior change. For example, the National Institutes of Health established the Women's Health Initiative in 1991 to examine the risk factors for death, disability, and impaired quality of life in postmenopausal women. Approximately 160,000 women of different racial and ethnic backgrounds from communities across the United States are participating. Various substudies are being conducted, including a study to evaluate the use of computerized dietary assessment and tailored feedback using PDA technology for real-time dietary monitoring and assessment. The PDA system is linked to a feedback program via the Internet or a modem. Data received are analyzed based on dietary goals for fat grams, fruit and vegetables, and grain servings. Online feedback provides motivational messages and assists participants in reaching their daily dietary goals (Karen Glanz, personal communication, 2002).

PDA applications may be relatively expensive if the handheld devices are provided to people. They may also be hard for elderly participants to use (Wright and others, 2000). The ongoing refinement of these devices is likely to see their increased use for the delivery of health behavior change programs. A broad range of potential applications appears to be feasible. The potential capacities for PDAs to support real-time data collection and to provide immediate feedback and guidance to program participants remain to be developed and tested.

Limitations of New Communication Technology

Costs of Developing and Delivering Internet-Based Applications

Screen-based programs delivered to large audiences have different cost structures from those that apply to print-based approaches. Although economies of scale operate such that the *per unit* cost of print materials decreases as the scale of production increases, the total cost of print-based interventions nevertheless increases per unit reached. In contrast, the cost of Internet-based interventions, after development, is held constant. In effect, the more people a print-based intervention reaches, the more it costs to deliver (acknowledging that economies of scale do operate). The cost of an Internet-based intervention does not increase with increased reach in the same manner. Most of the cost of implementation of the software for Internet-based applications is incurred in starting up, and there are costs associated with ongoing system maintenance. However, in the longer term, automated communication systems may be less expensive than retraining or hiring new staff (Paperny, 1997). Minimal professional time is required for any interaction, due to the efficiency of these systems, even when the number of participants is very large (Schneider, Schwartz, and Fast, 1995).

The cost structures for implementing programs are certainly changed by the use of new technologies. The costs of development and installation are high. For example, the volume of content that is necessary to be created for use in tailored interventions is considerably greater than that required for generic print materials. An additional consideration is the development and testing of tailoring algorithms. However, the incremental unit costs of delivery are ultimately reduced, so large numbers of participants can access a program or service without increasing the costs of delivery. The initially higher costs of hardware and software purchase and programming should be weighed against the ongoing cost of health professionals' consultation time or ongoing program delivery through face-to-face, print, or telephone media.

Although there are increasing opportunities for free Internet access through libraries and kiosks, lack of Internet access remains a barrier for many people. However, recent surveys indicate that the profile of Internet users may be becoming more representative of the general population (Pew Research Center for the People and the Press, 1999). Nevertheless, the socially disadvantaged or those who lack health insurance coverage may be less likely to have access to such technologies (Eng and others, 1998; Science Panel on Interactive Communication and Health, 1999). Residents of rural areas, inner cities, and lower socioeconomic status neighborhoods tend to have less access to computer and communications infrastructure than do persons in other areas (U.S. Department of Commerce, 1995).

Applications based on providing palmtop computers to individuals do have unit costs associated with delivery. However, as these devices become more ubiquitous and the technology merges with that of mobile telephones, it may be reasonably anticipated that this cost will decrease. Similarly, while some research has suggested that palmtop devices may be difficult to use for some elderly users (Wright and others, 2000), the ongoing refinement of these devices is likely to see their increased use in health behavior change programs. The rapid diffusion of both palmtop computers and mobile telephone technologies is likely to continue and will create opportunities for health behavior change initiatives.

Access to Internet-Based Programs—The "Digital Divide"

Widespread adoption of Internet-based services will be impeded as long as a substantial proportion of the population (including low-income, rural, and inner-city families, certain racial or ethnic groups, disabled persons, and the elderly) lack access to the relevant technology infrastructure (see Chapter Sixteen). Such people may also lack the ability to use applications because of lower literacy levels, language barriers, or other factors (Eng and others, 1998). However, an increasing proportion of the populations of industrialized countries has Internet access. Differences in access rates according to gender, ethnicity, educational attainment, and income in the United States appear to be shrinking. In 2000, the U.S. Department of Commerce published the fourth report in its "Falling Through the Net" series, which indicated that 51 percent of the U.S. population had home computers, and 41.5 percent had Internet access from their homes. These figures represent an increase from 42.1 percent and 26.2 percent, respectively, in 1998—home Internet access nearly doubling in two years (U.S. Department of Commerce, 2000). Further, the Pew Internet Project reported that by December 2000, 56 percent of adults in the United States had home Internet access (Rainie and others, 2001). It has been argued that, if this pattern continues, home Internet access may reach saturation more rapidly than has any preceding technology (U.S. Department of Commerce, 2000). In the near future, it should become clear whether access to these new communication technologies is becoming more socially equitable.

Information Excess and Information Quality

Information is critical to health-related decisions. Consumers actively seek information about health-related products, services, and therapeutic regimens (Rudd and Glanz, 1990). Access to relevant and accurate knowledge is a necessary but not sufficient basis for health behavior change. The rapid growth and development of information technologies is changing the ways in which consumers acquire this type of information.

From the perspective of Consumer Information Processing Theory, the most important characteristics of the consumer choice environment are the quantity and quality of information available (Rudd and Glanz, 1990). The quantity of information available through new media technologies, particularly the Internet, is seemingly boundless (Shenk, 1998; Johnson, 1997). Increasingly, information-processing and selection strategies are playing pivotal roles in the decision making of individuals (Castells, 1993). The overabundance of information and uncertainty of the quality of information available through the Internet have led to initiatives such as the (unsuccessful) lobbying for "health" domain names with World Health Organization–certified quality health content (Illman, 2000).

There is no editorial control of information on the Internet. Literally anyone with control of a Web site can claim to be a health expert (Sonnenberg, 1997). This means that the quality of sites cannot be guaranteed, and for many consumers, it may be difficult or impossible to determine whether a site is of good quality. A recent study (CyberAtlas, 2001b) indicated that among those who used the Internet to seek health information, 65 percent did so using general search engines such as Yahoo! or Google, whereas only 24 percent used health portals such as WebMD or DrKoop. Further, 11 percent used sites that were built to provide information about specific health topics, such as Oncology.com. This finding suggests that consumers of Internet health resources may not be using information-seeking strategies that are likely to optimize the quality of the information and advice that they receive.

The Internet is a crowded and cluttered medium. Drawing people's attention to good quality health information is a major challenge. A further, and significant, challenge for health behavior change programs is how to get people to pay attention to what program providers want to help them to do. It seems likely that Internet delivery of health behavior change programs will require a range of supplementary strategies, if the attention of more than just a few people is to be drawn to such programs and if those drawn are to be induced to make use of them. For example, it is likely that more traditional broadcast and print media or telephone recruitment strategies may be required to attract people's attention. In workplaces, the use of intranet systems and communication channels such as staff newsletters or targeted e-mails may be required.

Conclusion

The uses of new communication technology capacities in health behavior interventions are in early stages of development. The broader acceptability and effectiveness of programs delivered using this technology have yet to be demonstrated. While some interventions using new communication technologies have been shown to be effective, much more research evidence on outcomes is needed. Nevertheless, it seems highly likely that the use of new information technologies will soon enable a significantly larger proportion of the population to use effective behavioral programs for health promotion and disease prevention. Such programs have the potential to result in a substantial public health impact (Ramelson, Friedman, and Ockene, 1999).

The theories and models of health behavior described in other chapters will be central to the creative and disciplined development of innovative programs using new communication technology. There is the potential for the capacities described in Table 22.2 to significantly enhance how behavioral change programs are developed and delivered. Health behavior theories provide the tools by which this potential may be conceptualized and analyzed more formally. Controlled studies comparing theoretically derived elements of programs to standard elements will be particularly informative.

Communication technologies undoubtedly show great promise in providing new ways to develop and deliver health behavior change initiatives. The central challenges are to be attentive to access and equity issues, to critically apply relevant health behavior theories and models, and to evaluate carefully the outcomes of innovative strategies and programs.

References

Agras, W. S., and others. "Developing Computer-Assisted Therapy for the Treatment of Obesity." *Behavior Therapy*, 1990, *21*, 99–109.

Anderson, R., Bikson, T., Law, S., and Mitchell, B. *Universal Access to E-mail: Feasibility and Societal Implications.* Santa Monica, Calif.: RAND, 1995.

Brinberg, D., and Axelson, M. L. "Increasing the Consumption of Dietary Fiber." *Health Education Research*, 1990, *5*, 409–420.

Brug, J., Campbell, M., and van Assema, P. "The Application and Impact of Computer-Generated Personalized Nutrition Education." *Patient Education and Counseling,* 1999, *36,* 145–156.

Brug, J., Glanz, K., van Assema, P., Kok, G., and van Breukelen, G. "The Impact of Computer-Tailored Feedback and Iterative Feedback on Fat, Fruit and Vegetable Intake." *Health Education and Behavior,* 1998, *25,* 517–531.

Brug, J., Steenhuis, I., van Assema, P., and De Vries, H. "The Impact of a Computer-Tailored Nutrition Intervention." *Preventive Medicine,* 1996, *25,* 236–242.

Brug, J., and others. "Computer-Tailored Nutrition Education: Differences Between Two Interventions." *Health Education Research,* 1999, *14,* 249–256.

Campbell, M. K., and others. "Varying the Message Source in Computer-Tailored Nutrition Education." *Patient Education & Counseling,* 1999, *36,* 157–169.

Castells, M. "The Informational Economy and the New International Division of Labor." In M. Carnoy, M. Castells, S. S. Cohen, and F. H. Cardoso (eds.), *The New Global Economy in the Information Age: Reflections on Our Changing World.* University Park, Pa.: Pennsylvania State University Press, 1993.

Children's Partnership. *Online Content for Low-Income and Underserved Americans.* Santa Monica, Calif.: The Children's Partnership, 2000. Available at *http://www.childrenspartnership.org/pub/low_income/.* Viewed September 1, 2001.

CyberAtlas. *March 2001 Internet Usage Statistics.* CyberAtlas, 2001a. Available at *http://cyberatlas.internet.com/big_picture/traffic_patterns/print/0,,5931_747041,00.html.* Viewed May 1, 2001.

CyberAtlas. *Online Health Consumers More Proactive About Healthcare.* CyberAtlas, 2001b. Available at *http://cyberatlas.internet.com/markets/healthcare/article/ 0,,10101_755471,00.html.* Viewed May 1, 2001.

Davison, K. P., Pennebaker, J. W., and Dickerson, S. S. "Who Talks? The Social Psychology of Illness Support Groups." *American Psychologist,* 2000, *55,* 205–217.

Delichatsios, H. K., and others. "Randomized Trial of a 'Talking Computer' to Improve Adults' Eating Habits." *American Journal of Health Promotion,* 2001, *15,* 215–224.

De Vries, H., and Brug, J. "Computer-Tailored Interventions Motivating People to Adopt Health-Promoting Behaviors." *Patient Education and Counseling,* 1999, *36,* 99–105.

Dijkstra, A., De Vries, H., and Roijackers, J. "Computerized Tailored Feedback to Change Cognitive Determinants of Smoking: A Dutch Field Experiment." *Health Education Research,* 1998, *13,* 197–206.

Dirkin, G. "Technological Supports for Sustaining Exercise." In R. Dishman (ed.), *Advances in Exercise Adherence.* Champaign, Ill.: Human Kinetics, 1994.

Eng, T. R., and others. "Access to Health Information and Support: A Public Highway or a Private Road?" *Journal of the American Medical Association,* 1998, *280*(15), 1371–1375.

Fotheringham, M. J. and Owen, N. "Section Editors' Introduction: Interactive Health Communication in Preventive Medicine." *American Journal of Preventive Medicine,* 2000, *19,* 111–112.

Fotheringham, M. J., Owies, D., Leslie, E., and Owen, N. "Interactive Health Communication in Preventive Medicine: Internet-Based Strategies in Teaching and Research." *American Journal of Preventive Medicine,* 2000, *19,* 113–120.

Fox, S., and Rainie, L. *The Online Healthcare Revolution.* Washington, D.C.: Pew Internet and American Life Project, 2000. Available at *http://www.pewinternet.org.* Viewed April 18, 2001.

Gustafson, D. H., and others. "Impact of a Patient-Centered, Computer-Based Health Information/Support System." *American Journal of Preventive Medicine*, 1999, *16*, 1–9.

Illman, J. "WHO's Plan to Police Health Websites Rejected." *British Medical Journal*, 2000, *321*, 1308.

Johnson, S. *Interface Culture: The Way We Create and Communicate.* New York: Basic Books, 1997.

King, A. C., and others. "Long-Term Effects of Varying Intensities and Formats of Physical Activity on Participation Rates, Fitness, and Lipoproteins in Men and Women Aged 50 to 65 Years." *Circulation*, 1995, *9*, 2596–2604.

Kreuter, M. W., Farrell, D., Olevitch, L., and Brennan, L. *Tailoring Health Messages.* Mahwah, N.J.: Erlbaum, 2000.

Kreuter, M. W., and Strecher, V. J. "Do Tailored Behavior Change Messages Enhance the Effectiveness of Health Risk Appraisal? Results from a Randomized Trial." *Health Promotion Research*, 1996, *11*(1), 97–105.

Lieberman, D. A. "Interactive Video Games for Health Promotion: Effects on Knowledge, Self-Efficacy, Social Support, and Health." In R. L. Street, W. R. Gold, and J. Manning (eds.), *Health Promotion and Interactive Technology: Theoretical Applications and Future Directions.* Mahwah, N.J.: Erlbaum, 1997.

Lipkus, I. M., Lyna, P. R., and Rimer, B. K. "Using Tailored Interventions to Enhance Smoking Cessation Among African-Americans at a Community Health Center." *Nicotine & Tobacco Research*, 1999, *1*, 77–85.

Lipkus, I. M., Rimer, B. K., Halabi, S., and Strigo, T. S. "Can Tailored Interventions Increase Mammography Use Among HMO Women?" *American Journal of Preventive Medicine*, 2000, *18*, 1–10.

Marcus, B. H., Owen, N., Forsyth, L. H., Cavill, N. A., and Fridinger, F. "Interventions to Promote Physical Activity Using Mass Media, Print Media and Information Technology." *American Journal of Preventive Medicine*, 1998, *15*, 362–378.

Marcus, B. H., and others. "Efficacy of an Individualized, Motivationally-Tailored Physical Activity Intervention." *Annals of Behavioral Medicine*, 1998, *20*, 174–180.

McBride, C. M., and Rimer, B. K. "Using the Telephone to Improve Health Behavior and Health Service Delivery." *Patient Education and Counseling*, 1999, *37*, 3–18.

Newman, M. G., Kenardy, J., Herman, S., and Taylor, C. B. "Comparison of Palmtop-Computer-Assisted Brief Cognitive-Behavioral Treatment to Cognitive-Behavioral Treatment for Panic Disorder." *Journal of Consulting and Clinical Psychology*, 1997, *65*, 178–183.

Noell, J., and Glasgow, R. E. "Interactive Technology Applications for Behavioral Counseling." *American Journal of Preventive Medicine*, 1999, *17*, 269–274.

Paperny, D.M.N. "Computerized Health Assessment and Education for Adolescent HIV and STD Prevention in Health Care Settings and Schools." *Health Education and Behavior*, 1997, *24*, 54–70.

Patrick, K. "Information Technology and the Future of Preventive Medicine: Potentials, Pitfalls and Policy." *American Journal of Preventive Medicine*, 2000, *19*, 132–135.

Pinto, B., and others. "Physical Activity Promotion Using a Computer-Based Telephone Counseling System." *Annals of Behavioral Medicine*, 2000, *22*, S212.

Pew Research Center for the People and the Press. *Online Newcomers More Middle-Brow, Less Work-Oriented: The Internet News Audience Goes Ordinary.* Washington, D.C.: The Pew Research Center for the People and the Press, 1999. Available at: http://www.people-press.org/tech98sum.htm. Viewed May 1, 2001.

Rainie, L., and others. *More Online, Doing More.* Pew Internet and American Life Project, 2001. Available at http://www.digitaldividenetwork.org. Viewed March 30, 2001.

Rakowski, W. "The Potential Variances of Tailoring in Health Behavior Interventions." *Annals of Behavioral Medicine,* 1999, *21,* 284–289.

Rakowski, W., and others. "A Stage-Matched Intervention for Screening Mammography." *Annals of Behavioral Medicine,* 1997, *19,* S63.

Ramelson, H. Z., Friedman, R. H., and Ockene, J. K. "An Automated Telephone-Based Smoking Cessation Education and Counseling System." *Patient Education and Counseling,* 1999, *36,* 131–144.

Reeves, P. M. "Coping in Cyberspace: The Impact of Internet Use on the Ability of HIV-Positive Individuals to Deal With Their Illness." *Journal of Health Communication,* 2000, *5*(Supplement), 47–59.

Rimer, B. K. "Foreword." In M. Kreuter, D. Farrell, L. Olevitch, and L. Brennan (eds.), *Tailoring Health Messages.* Mahwah, N.J.: Erlbaum, 2000.

Rimer, B. K., and Glassman, B. "Is There a Use for Tailored Print Communications in Cancer Risk Communication?" *Journal of the National Cancer Institute. Monographs,* 1999, *25,* 140–148.

Robinson, T. N., Patrick, K., Eng, T. R., and Gustafson, D. "An Evidence-Based Approach to Interactive Health Communication." *Journal of the American Medical Association,* 1998, *280,* 1264–1269.

Rudd, J., and Glanz, K. "How Individuals Use Information for Health Action: Consumer Information Processing." In K. Glanz, F. M. Lewis, and B. K. Rimer (eds.), *Health Behavior and Health Education: Theory, Research, and Practice.* San Francisco: Jossey-Bass, 1990.

Schneider, S. J., Schwartz, M. D., and Fast, J. "Computerized, Telephone-Based Health Promotion." *Computers in Human Behavior,* 1995, *11,* 135–148.

Science Panel on Interactive Communication and Health (SPICH). *Wired for Health and Well-Being: The Emergence of Interactive Health Communication.* Washington, D.C.: Office of Disease Prevention and Health Promotion, U.S. Department of Health and Human Services, 1999.

Sheehan, K. B., and Hoy, M. G. "Using E-Mail to Survey Internet Users in the United States." *Journal of Computer-Mediated Communication,* 1999, *4.* Available at http://www.ascusc.org/jcmc/vol4/issue3/sheehan.html. Viewed July 20, 1999.

Shenk, D. *Data Smog: Surviving the Information Glut.* San Francisco: HarperCollins, 1998.

Skinner, C. S., Strecher, V. J., and Hospers, H. "Physician's Recommendations for Mammography: Do Tailored Messages Make a Difference?" *American Journal of Public Health,* 1994, *84,* 43–49.

Skinner, C. S., and others. "How Effective Is Tailored Print Communication?" *Annals of Behavioral Medicine,* 1999, *21,* 290–298.

Soet, J. E., and Basch, C. E. "The Telephone as a Communication Medium for Health Education." *Health Education and Behavior,* 1997, *24,* 759–772.

Sonnenberg, F. A. "Health Information on the Internet." *Archives of Internal Medicine,* 1997, *157,* 151–152.

Strecher, V. J., and others. "The Effects of Computer-Tailored Smoking Cessation Messages in Family Practice Settings." *Journal of Family Practice,* 1994, *39,* 262–270.

Tate, D. F., Wing, R. R., and Winett, R. A. "Using Internet Technology to Deliver a Behavioral Weight Loss Program." *Journal of the American Medical Association,* 2001, *285,* 1172–1177.

U.S. Department of Commerce. *Falling Through the Net: A Survey of the "Have Nots" in Rural and Urban America*. Washington, D.C.: National Telecommunications and Information Administration, 1995.

U.S. Department of Commerce. *Falling Through the Net: Toward Digital Inclusion*. Washington, D.C.: National Telecommunications and Information Administration, 2000.

Velicer, W. F., and Prochaska, J. O. "An Expert System Intervention for Smoking Cessation." *Patient Education and Counseling*, 1999, *36*, 119–129.

Wallack, L. "The Role of Mass Media in Creating Social Capital: A New Direction for Public Health." In B. D. Smedley and S. L. Syme (eds.), *Promoting Health: Intervention Strategies from Social and Behavioral Research*. Washington, D.C.: National Academy Press, 2000.

Whalen, C. K., Jamner, L. D., Henker, B., and Delfino, R. J. "Smoking and Moods in Adolescents with Depressive and Aggressive Dispositions: Evidence from Surveys and Electronic Diaries." *Health Psychology*, 2001, *20*, 99–111.

Wright, P., and others. "Text Entry on Handheld Computers by Older Persons." *Ergonomics*, 2000, *43*, 702–716.

CHAPTER TWENTY-THREE

EVALUATION OF THEORY-BASED INTERVENTIONS

The RE-AIM Model

Russell E. Glasgow

This chapter focuses on issues in and approaches to the evaluation of theory-based health education and health behavior interventions. Given the breadth of this general topic, this chapter will be restricted to what has been termed *impact* or *outcome* evaluation. Readers may refer to separate and important literatures on *process* and *formative* evaluation, which are beyond the scope of this chapter but are important to coordinate with outcome evaluation. In addition, entire texts are available on issues of clinical trial design and statistical analyses that also are beyond the scope of this chapter. This chapter, after discussing general issues in evaluating health promotion and health education interventions, will focus specifically on evaluation questions that are especially important for informing the translation of research results into practice.

Key Evaluation Issues

Internal and Construct Validity

Internal validity refers to the extent to which outcomes of a study can be attributed to an experimental factor (for example, an intervention) rather than to extraneous or confounding factors. *Construct validity* in evaluation refers to the ability to attribute differences between conditions (usually an intervention versus a control or comparison condition) to the "active ingredient" or factor theoretically of most interest. (This is not the same as *construct validity of a measure.*) Many of these issues involve research design and methodological procedures to ensure that the differences between conditions are restricted only to those about which one wants to make interpretive statements and to collection of appropriate process measures of the hypothesized mediating mechanisms of therapeutic change. A subset of process measures that is directly relevant to this chapter is the consistent measurement of intervention delivery, or implementation. Such measures assess the extent to which the intervention(s) are actually delivered as intended. This is important for avoiding the commission of "type III errors," or concluding that an intervention is ineffective when in fact it was not delivered or implemented as intended (Basch, Sliepcevich, and Gold, 1985). As discussed in the section on efficacy and effectiveness, it is also important to assess possible negative or iatrogenic effects of interventions as well as positive consequences.

External Validity

External validity refers to the extent to which we can generalize or apply the results of a study to other contexts, settings, and situations outside of the specific situations studied in a given investigation. External validity also concerns the representativeness of the intervention settings, intervention agents, and participants in a study.

Balancing Internal and External Validity

A key issue is the balance between internal and external validity characteristics of a study. Designs that produce higher internal validity may lead to lower levels of external validity. This is because enhanced internal validity is usually accomplished by simplifying and restricting the conditions studied, and such activity by definition makes the study results less broadly applicable. To assess an intervention's efficacy, internal validity should be maximized. But to ensure relevance and disseminability, external validity is critical. The tension between internal and external validity issues is discussed in more detail under the section on stages of intervention research. Fortunately, there are strategies that can be used to enhance external validity without sacrificing internal validity, and that is the focus of much of this chapter.

The ultimate goal of research is to gain sufficient knowledge about an intervention to answer the key question phrased so well over thirty years ago by Gordon Paul—"What treatment, for what population, delivered by whom, under what conditions, for what outcome, is most effective, and how did it come about?" (Paul, 1969).

Intervention Contexts and Intermediate Outcomes

To assess the impact of an intervention, we must understand the conditions under which it works and for whom, and both the immediate and longer-term effects it produces. For most health behavior and education studies, and especially those delivered within or by a setting or mediating agent such as a worksite, school, medical clinic, or community organization, it is also important to understand effects at both the setting and the individual levels. To facilitate understanding and to place the results of a study in appropriate context, it is often helpful to create a study schematic that outlines visually what happened to potential settings and individuals who could participate in the program. This often includes specification of recruitment inclusion or exclusion issues, intervention setting(s), participation rates and reasons for declining participation, intervention implementation issues, process or mediating mechanisms, and participant retention results. Figure 23.1 presents an example of such an intervention study schematic. Such schematics are now standard requirements for many journals.

When evaluating theory-based interventions, it is also particularly important to identify and measure mediating variables and to conduct analyses to assess the effects of mediating variables. Mediating variables represent hypothesized pathways or processes through which an intervention is expected to achieve its effects. For example, a program to reduce illicit substance use might be found to achieve reductions in frequency of use via increasing self-efficacy to resist peer pressure. In-depth discussions of analytic procedures to evaluate mediating variables can be found elsewhere (Baron and Kenny, 1986; MacKinnon and Dwyer, 1993). The point, however, is that it is critically important to identify how health behavior interventions work, both to increase our understanding of theoretical mechanisms and to create more efficient and effective interventions.

Phases of Research

Several research groups have proposed a series of "phases of research" that should guide the development of health behavior interventions and evaluations. Some of these, especially those of Greenwald and Cullen (1985) and Flay (1986) have been widely adopted and have been used by the National Cancer Institute, the National Heart, Lung, and Blood Institute, and many other agencies and organizations concerned with advancing the science of health promotion. The Greenwald and

FIGURE 23.1. HYPOTHETICAL WORKSITE INTERVENTIONS PARTICIPATION FLOW DIAGRAM.

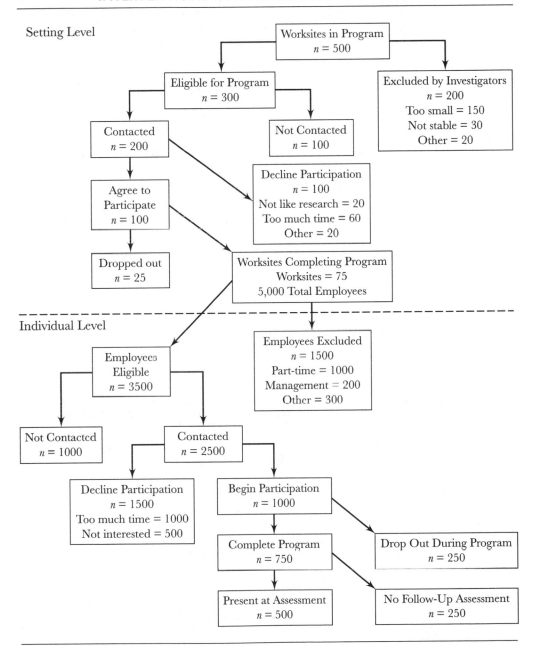

Cullen model of five phases of research is summarized in Table 23.1, with a health education example for each phase. The basic point shared by these conceptualizations is that there is a preferred sequence in which research should evolve, beginning with basic laboratory research and literature reviews to explore initial hypotheses, followed by "efficacy" studies designed to assess interventions under ideal or optimal conditions. These efficacy studies maximize internal validity to firmly establish the scientific basis of interventions, before proceeding to later "effectiveness" studies. Effectiveness studies then determine the impact of the intervention when conducted under more representative or applied field conditions and when applied to more representative or "defined populations" rather than highly screened and motivated, self-selected volunteers who are studied in efficacy research.

A final phase, but one which has received much less attention from both funding agencies and researchers, is that of demonstration or dissemination research. Such research investigates ways to enhance and factors that influence the widespread adoption of interventions proven to be efficacious and effective in previous stages of research. Several authors have contrasted the different goals, assumptions, and issues studied in efficacy research, which is concerned primar-

TABLE 23.1. GREENWALD AND CULLEN (1985) MODEL OF PHASES OF RESEARCH.

	Phase	Health Behavior Example
Phase 1	Hypothesis development	Identification of link in existing literature between sedentary behavior and obesity among adolescents
Phase 2	Methods development	Pilot testing of intervention to increase adolescent physical activity and validation of measures
Phase 3	Controlled intervention trials (Efficacy studies)	Small-scale randomized trial of physical activity intervention for adolescents
Phase 4	Defined population studies (Effectiveness)	Larger-scale trial of physical activity intervention when applied to all adolescents in participating middle schools
Phase 5	Demonstration (Dissemination)	Evaluation of results when physical activity program is provided to all middle schools in a given state

Source: Greenwald and Cullen, 1985.

ily with internal validity, with those of effectiveness and dissemination research, which are more concerned with external validity and public health impact issues (Lichtenstein and Glasgow, 1992; Flay, 1986; McKinlay, 1996).

Evaluation Models

Several separate but related models and frameworks have been proposed to help guide health promotion evaluations. Some of these are designed both to help develop and to evaluate interventions (Green and Kreuter, 1999; Biglan, Ary, and Wagenaar, 2000), and others are intended to help frame evaluation issues only (Lomas, 1997). Evaluation models help to focus attention on important issues and are useful to both researchers and practitioners. For practitioners, evaluation models identify key factors to consider when developing or selecting health behavior programs and when reading the research literature. For researchers, evaluation models identify important dimensions to be included in program evaluations. Two of the more comprehensive models that have heavily influenced the development of the RE-AIM framework discussed in this chapter are the PRECEDE-PROCEED model (Green and Kreuter, 1999; see also Chapter Eighteen) and Diffusion Theory (Rogers, 1995; Nutbeam, 1996; see Chapter Fourteen).

Other lines of research have stressed the importance of considering factors that will determine the "real world" impact of research and applicability in applied settings. These studies include research by Oldenburg and colleagues (Oldenburg, Sallis, French, and Owen, 1999; Oldenburg, French, and Sallis, 2000) on diffusion, dissemination, and institutionalization. Their work has documented the large gap between research and adoption (or use in applied, nonresearch settings) and the almost exclusive preoccupation of health promotion research with efficacy studies that emphasize internal validity. Important work by Goodman Steckler and colleagues has identified and measured factors related to the extent to which interventions are disseminated or become "institutionalized." A third line of research that has helped focus development of practical and feasible interventions has been that of Abrams and others (1996), who have proposed that we should evaluate the impact of interventions not solely by their efficacy (effects and magnitude of change related to internal validity) but also by their reach or the percentage of potentially eligible persons who have access to and participate in an intervention. Their proposal that the impact of an intervention was a multiplicative function of its reach times efficacy (Abrams and others, 1996) led most directly to the development of the RE-AIM evaluation framework used in this chapter.

The RE-AIM Evaluation Framework

RE-AIM is an acronym for Reach, Efficacy or Effectiveness (depending on the phase of research), Adoption, Implementation, and Maintenance (Glasgow, Vogt, and Boles, 1999; Glasgow, McKay, Piette, and Reynolds, 2001). *Reach* refers to the percentage of potential participants who are exposed to an intervention and how representative they are. Reach, Efficacy, and Effectiveness (see Table 23.2) are most often thought of as relating to individuals or groups (as in an experimental study in which subjects are assigned to groups). *Efficacy* and *Effectiveness* concern both the intended or positive impacts of an intervention and the possible negative or unintended consequences of the intervention on quality of life and related factors.

In the context of the RE-AIM evaluation framework, *Adoption* and *Implementation* operate mainly at the setting or contextual level. Adoption refers to the participation rate and representativeness of both the settings (such as worksites, medical offices, schools, communities) in which an intervention is conducted and the intervention agents (for example, teachers, physicians, health educators) who deliver the intervention. Although Adoption is as important as Reach (at the in-

TABLE 23.2. RE-AIM DIMENSIONS AND QUESTIONS IN EVALUATING HEALTH EDUCATION AND HEALTH BEHAVIOR PROGRAMS.

RE-AIM Dimension	Questions
Reach (Individual level)	What percentage of potentially eligible participants will take part and how representative are they?
Efficacy or Effectiveness (Individual level)	What impact did the intervention have on all participants who began the program, on process intermediate and primary outcomes, and on both positive and negative (unintended) outcomes including quality of life?
Adoption (Setting level)	What percentage of settings and intervention agents (such as worksites, schools or educators, medical offices or physicians) will participate and how representative are they?
Implementation (Setting or agent level)	To what extent are the various intervention components delivered as intended (in the protocol), especially when conducted by regular (nonresearch) staff in applied settings?
Maintenance (Both individual and setting level)	1. Individual level: What are the long-term effects (minimum in six to twelve months following intervention)? 2. Setting level: To what extent are different intervention components continued or institutionalized?

dividual level), far less attention has been devoted to it. Implementation refers to the extent to which various components of an intervention are delivered as intended in real-world evaluations. Implementation is often problematic, especially when conducted in applied settings by regular staff who have numerous other responsibilities beyond implementation of the research protocol.

Maintenance, the final dimension of the RE-AIM model, has indices at both the individual and setting levels. At the individual level, it refers to the long-term results of an intervention (defined as a minimum of six months following the last intervention contact). For most behaviors, long-term maintenance has proven challenging, and the factors that influence maintenance may be different than those that influence initial behavior change (Marlatt and Gordon, 1985; Orleans, 2000). An important practice when evaluating maintenance is to follow and characterize results for all participants who begin a program and not just for those who are present for follow-up. Attrition is often substantial or differential across conditions or participant subgroups.

At the setting level, Maintenance refers to the institutionalization of a program (Goodman and Steckler, 1987). This is the extent to which intervention settings continue a program (and which components of the intervention are used) once the formal research project and supports are withdrawn. Maintenance at the setting level is particularly important. As Patterson, Kristal, Biener, and others (Patterson and others, 1998) recently have demonstrated in their follow-up study of a worksite nutrition intervention, even well-designed and effective interventions are unlikely to be institutionalized if resources are not allocated for this purpose.

The relationships among various RE-AIM dimensions are as important as the results on any given dimension. Expanding upon the work of Abrams and colleagues (Abrams, Emmons, and Linnan, 1996; Abrams and others, 1996), who proposed that Impact = Reach × Efficacy, RE-AIM hypothesizes that the overall public health impact of an intervention is a function of all five RE-AIM dimensions. Thus, all five RE-AIM dimensions are equally important and equally in need of research attention. The implication is that to have a broad and major impact at the population level, an intervention must do reasonably well on all or most RE-AIM dimensions. It is not enough to have a highly efficacious intervention if that intervention has poor reach, is not likely to be adopted by many settings, and can only be implemented by a handful of highly trained specialists. While few health behavior programs to date have been shown to produce sustained behavioral change, the optimal intervention would also achieve successful Maintenance, or long-term behavioral change outcomes.

From a practical perspective, few current health behavior programs are strong on all five RE-AIM dimensions. The framework can also be helpful to decision makers in clarifying outcomes that are most important to them and in considering the pros and cons of different choices. For example, one may need to choose between a program with high efficacy but that is unlikely to be adopted by many practitioners and one that has demonstrated high Reach, but appears to have very low Efficacy.

Applications of RE-AIM to Health Education and Promotion

The two applications in this section illustrate the application of the RE-AIM framework to evaluation of two different health behavior change programs. For each program, the effects on Reach, Effectiveness, Adoption, Implementation, and Maintenance are addressed, followed by a summary discussion of the overall public health impact of the program, considering the pattern of results across the five RE-AIM dimensions. The first example comes from the health care setting and is a recent randomized trial of touchscreen computer-assisted diabetes self-management education (Glasgow and Toobert, 2000; Glasgow, Toobert, Hampson, and Strycker, forthcoming).

The Choosing Well Diabetes Self-Management Program

The purpose of this project was to evaluate the effectiveness of several different components and supplements to a basic touchscreen computer-assisted dietary goal setting and follow-up intervention that had been found efficacious in a previous randomized trial (Glasgow and others, 1997). The previous study had been conducted in the offices of two internists. The program produced encouraging results on both outcomes and cost effectiveness at both short-term (three-month) and longer-term (twelve-month) assessments relative to a computer-assessment-only condition. While these results were encouraging, we recognized that relatively few practices would have the resources to dedicate office staff to address dietary change issues during routine medical contacts. For this reason, and to study the adoption and generalization of intervention effects, we revised the program to be offered as a centralized resource for a hospital network provider system. Patients were contacted through their primary care providers, but services were provided at a central location, the Center for Healthy Living.

We secured the participation of all fourteen medical offices and forty of forty-two primary care providers approached (Adoption). The physicians sent out letters to all adult type 2 diabetes patients under their care to describe the program and invite participation. Research staff then followed up the letter with phone calls to answer questions and screen patients for eligibility and interest. Recruitment and participation are described in detail in Glasgow and Toobert (2000).

Seventy-six percent of eligible patients who were offered participation began the program (Reach). There were no differences between participants and decliners on any of a series of demographic or medical history variables. Participants were randomized to one of four conditions using a 2×2 factorial design, with the factors being (1) presence or absence of telephone follow-up support and (2) presence or absence of a community-resource-use enhancement condition. Patients in all conditions received a basic computer-assisted assessment, feedback, and dietary goal-setting intervention based on the successful 1997 study.

To study implementation and generalization factors, four different intervention staff delivered the various treatments and were assigned to see approximately equal numbers of participants in all conditions. These intervention staff were all familiar with diabetes but had vastly different types of training, expertise, and experience: one was a nurse and certified diabetes educator, one was a doctoral-level behavioral psychologist, one was a registered dietician, and one was a bachelors-level educator. Two came from research backgrounds, and the other two had not previously participated in formal research studies. All four interventionists consistently implemented all components of the various interventions, with no differences among intervention staff on either implementation or outcomes.

There was significant improvement overall on almost all measures. These included assessments of dietary behavior change, biological indices, and quality-of-life and process measures at the three-month follow-up (Efficacy or Effectiveness). There were few differences between conditions in level of improvements. There was generally good Maintenance at the twelve-month follow-up assessment. All conditions continued to show significant improvement from baseline on all measures. The telephone follow-up component enhanced long-term results on some measures, but there were few differences between conditions on most outcomes (Glasgow, Toobert, Hampson, and Strycker, forthcoming). We concluded that the overall public health impact of the basic intervention was fairly high, because all conditions produced good results on most of the five RE-AIM dimensions. However, the incremental effects of adding other components to the basic intervention were small and generally nonsignificant.

Planned Parenthood Smoking Cessation Study

The second illustration of the use of the RE-AIM evaluation framework comes from an effectiveness study of a brief smoking cessation intervention conducted by regular office staff during routine visits by patients to Planned Parenthood offices (usually for contraceptive, primary care, or family planning purposes) reported by Glasgow, Whitlock, Eakin, and Lichtenstein (2000).

This study was conducted in the offices of four Planned Parenthood offices in a large metropolitan area. All offices that were approached subsequently agreed to participate in the study (Adoption). This randomized trial evaluated the brief intervention, conducted by regular staff from the various clinics following training, compared with generic self-help control condition and an advice-to-quit pamphlet. The intervention was designed to take only one to two minutes of the clinician's time and approximately twelve to fifteen minutes of a staff assistant's time for follow-up counseling. It began with a nine-minute video developed specifically for young, low-income female smokers, followed by clinician advice to quit (this component was identical for both conditions), motivational interviewing-based staff assistance in developing a specific quit plan (Rollnick, Mason, and Butler, 1999), self-help materials, and attempts to make two follow-up telephone calls to review progress.

The Planned Parenthood system had an excellent process for assessing the smoking status of clients, and over 99 percent of clients had their smoking status identified. Of the smokers invited to participate in the study, 76 percent agreed. There were no differences on demographic or smoking history variables between participants and nonparticipants (Reach). At six-week assessment, the intervention produced significantly higher cessation rates (10 percent versus 7 percent, $p < .05$). At the six-month follow-up, although both self-reported quit rates (18 percent versus 15 percent) and biochemically validated results (6.4 percent versus 3.8 percent) favored the intervention condition, the differences did not reach significance (Effectiveness at six weeks and individual Maintenance at six months).

The Implementation results revealed possible reasons for the short-term success and ambiguous longer-term results. The clinicians and staff delivered almost all of the in-session treatment components consistently, given that this was a real-world effectiveness study (the video, advice to quit, and staff counseling and provision of self-help materials were each implemented between 85 and 96 percent of the time). However, it proved difficult to reach these low-income clients for follow-up phone calls: 42 percent received one call and only 10 percent received both follow-up phone calls. The extent to which the participating clinics continued the program after the study was completed (setting level Maintenance) is not known. Considering results across the RE-AIM dimensions, we concluded that the program had moderate public health benefits: it was strong on Reach and Adoption, moderate on Effectiveness, mixed on Implementation, and relatively weak on individual-level Maintenance.

A Caveat

Both of the described examples used the RE-AIM framework to evaluate Phase 3 or Phase 4 research trials. The RE-AIM measures collected therefore reflect this research context, and in some cases are proxies for what we ultimately would like to assess. For example, the measure of Reach involved willingness to participate in randomized research trials and assessment procedures. What we would really like to assess is willingness to participate in the intervention independent of the research requirements. Similarly, Adoption indices reported in these studies required organizations to participate in research as well as to deliver the interventions. The ultimate goal is to assess RE-AIM dimensions independent of participation in research.

Challenges to Conducting Theory-Based Health Behavior Research in Applied Settings

Table 23.3 summarizes several key challenges faced when delivering or evaluating health behavior interventions in applied settings. It uses the RE-AIM model to consider both common challenges and possible solutions. The chief challenge to Reach is that because of logistical and methodological difficulties, too often evaluations include only participants who are easy to reach and track. Another danger is of casting too narrow a net in evaluating results, focusing only on narrow outcomes and omitting measures of potential mediating variables and other process measures that can help us understand how intervention effects (or lack of effects) occur. Table 23.3 presents a list of ways to broaden this perspective.

With respect to adoption, too few health behavior research projects have been conducted in representative or challenged real-world settings. Researchers should pay equal attention to the recruitment and representativeness of settings as we do to the representativeness of individual participants. Another frequent problem is that of type III error (Basch, Sliepcevich, and Gold, 1995), inappropriately concluding that an intervention is not effective when in fact the program was not delivered or implemented as intended. Collection of implementation measures can greatly help to avoid this type of inferential error. Most challenging of all may be the almost universal lack of information on maintenance of health behavior programs at the setting level. We need much greater understanding of the extent to which settings continue or modify an intervention once the initial program or research is completed.

As illustrated in Table 23.3, many of these challenges can be anticipated and addressed by using the RE-AIM framework. The key to successfully overcoming the challenges in Table 23.3 is to develop and evaluate programs with the end goal of translation to practice (or policy) in mind. These issues can and should be addressed, using RE-AIM or other frameworks, regardless of the phase of a particular research study. From the outset of intervention design and development, it is important to consider the implications for, and whenever possible, to obtain measures of Reach, Effectiveness, Adoption, Implementation, and Maintenance.

TABLE 23.3. COMMON CHALLENGES ENCOUNTERED IN EVALUATING HEALTH BEHAVIOR INTERVENTIONS.

Challenge	Remedy
R: Not including a relevant, high risk, or representative sample	Use population-based recruitment or over-recruit high-risk subgroups Do not include too many exclusion criteria

E: Not thoroughly understanding outcomes or how they came about:
    No knowledge of mediators
    Conflicting or ambiguous results
    Inadequate control conditions to rule out alternative hypotheses
	Assess broad set of outcomes including possible negative ones
	Include measures of hypothesized mediators
	Conduct subgroup analyses or include different assessment points
	Select stringency of control condition to fit your question

A: Program not ever adopted or endorsed—only used in academic settings	Involve potential adoptees beginning with initial design phase Approach a representative or broad group of settings early on when revision is still possible
I: Protocols not delivered as intended (type III error)	Assess if treatment is too complicated, too intensive, or not compatible with other duties Involve potential (nonresearch) intervention agents in program design
M: Program or effects not maintained over time	Include maintenance phase both in protocol and in evaluation plan Leave treatment behind after study and plan for institutionalization

For many health behavior projects, the end goal is to produce practical programs that can be applied consistently in real-world settings in a way that makes a difference in the health behavior, health, and quality of life of participants. It is equally important to know how many persons are reached, including especially those who may be most at risk or segments of the population that bear disproportionate disease burdens. Although it may not be until Phase 5 research that one can definitely answer these important questions, these issues can and should be considered throughout the various phases of research. By using RE-AIM or similar evaluation frameworks to focus attention on these issues at *each* stage of research, we should be able to increase the chances that the programs we develop can be translated to and successfully implemented in applied settings.

References

Abrams, D. B., Emmons, K. M., and Linnan, L. A. "Health Behavior and Health Education: The Past, Present, and Future." In K. Glanz, F. M. Lewis, and B. K. Rimer (eds.), *Health Behavior and Health Education: Theory, Research, and Practice.* (2nd ed.) San Francisco: Jossey-Bass, 1996.

Abrams, D. B., and others. "Integrating Individual and Public Health Perspectives for Treatment of Tobacco Dependence Under Managed Health Care: A Combined Stepped Care and Matching Model." *Annals of Internal Medicine,* 1996, *18,* 290–304.

Baron, R., and Kenny, D. "The Moderator-Mediator Variable Distinction in Social Psychological Research: Conceptual, Strategic, and Statistical Considerations." *Journal of Personality and Social Psychology,* 1986, *51,* 1173–1182.

Basch, C. E., Sliepcevich, E. M., and Gold, R. S. "Avoiding Type III Errors in Health Education Program Evaluations." *Health Education Quarterly,* 1985, *12,* 315–331.

Biglan, A., Ary, D., and Wagenaar, A. C. "The Value of Interrupted Time-Series Experiments for Community Intervention Research." *Prevention Science,* 2000, *1,* 31–49.

Flay, B. R. "Efficacy and Effectiveness Trials (and Other Phases of Research) in the Development of Health Promotion Programs." *Preventive Medicine,* 1986, *15,* 451–474.

Glasgow, R. E., McKay, H. G., Piette, J. D., and Reynolds, K. D. "The RE-AIM Framework for Evaluating Interventions: What Can It Tell Us About Approaches to Chronic Illness Management?" *Patient Education and Counseling,* 2001, *44,* 119–127.

Glasgow, R. E., and Toobert, D. J. "Brief, Computer-Assisted Diabetes Dietary Self-Management Counseling: Effects on Behavior, Physiologic Outcomes, and Quality of Life." *Medical Care,* 2000, *38,* 1062–1073.

Glasgow, R. E., Toobert, D. J., Hampson, S. E., and Strycker, L. A. "Implementation, Generalization, and Long-Term Results of the "Choosing Well" Diabetes Self-Management Intervention." Forthcoming.

Glasgow, R. E., Vogt, T. M., and Boles, S. M. "Evaluating the Public Health Impact of Health Promotion Interventions: The RE-AIM Framework." *American Journal of Public Health,* 1999, *89,* 1322–1327.

Glasgow, R. E., Whitlock, E. P., Eakin, E. G., and Lichtenstein, E. "A Brief Smoking Cessation Intervention for Women in Low-Income Planned Parenthood Clinics. *American Journal of Public Health,* 2000, *90,* 786–789.

Glasgow, R. E., and others. "Long-Term Effects and Costs of Brief Behavioral Dietary Intervention for Patients with Diabetes Delivered from the Medical Office." *Patient Education and Counseling,* 1997, *32,* 175–184.

Goodman, R. M., and Steckler, A. "A Model for the Institutionalization of Health Promotion Programs." *Family and Community Health,* 1987, *11,* 63–78.

Green, L. M., and Kreuter, M. W. *Health Promotion Planning: An Educational and Ecological Approach.* (3rd ed.) Mountain View, Calif.: Mayfield, 1999.

Greenwald, P., and Cullen, J. W. "The New Emphasis in Cancer Control." *Journal of the National Cancer Institute,* 1985, *74,* 543–551.

Lichtenstein, E., and Glasgow, R. E. "Smoking Cessation: What Have We Learned Over the Past Decade?" *Journal of Consulting and Clinical Psychology,* 1992, *60,* 518–527.

Lomas, J. *Improving Research Dissemination and Uptake in the Health Sector: Beyond the Sound of One Hand Clapping.* (Rep. No. C97-1) Montreal: McMaster University Centre for Health Economics and Policy Analysis/Policy Commentary, November 1997.

MacKinnon, D., and Dwyer, J. "Estimating Mediated Effects in Prevention Studies." *Evaluation Review,* 1993, *17,* 144–158.

Marlatt, G. A., and Gordon, J. R. *Relapse Prevention: Maintenance Strategies in the Treatment of Addictive Behaviors.* New York: Guilford Press, 1985.

McKinlay, J. B. "More Appropriate Evaluation Methods for Community-Level Health Interventions." *Evaluation Review,* 1996, *20,* 237–243.

Nutbeam, D. "Achieving 'Best Practice' in Health Promotion: Improving the Fit Between Research and Practice." *Health Education Research,* 1996, *11,* 317–326.

Oldenburg, B., French, B. F., and Sallis, J. F. "Health Behavior Research: The Quality of the Evidence Base." *American Journal of Health Promotion,* 2000, *14,* 253–257.

Oldenburg, B. F., Sallis, J. F., French, M. L., and Owen, N. "Health Promotion Research and the Diffusion and Institutionalization of Interventions." *Health Education Research,* 1999, *14,* 121–130.

Orleans, C. T. "Promoting the Maintenance of Health Behavior Change: Recommendations for the Next Generation of Research and Practice." *Health Psychology,* 2000, *19,* 76–83.

Patterson, R. E., and others. "Durability and Diffusion of the Nutrition Intervention in the Working Well Trial." *Preventive Medicine,* 1998, *27,* 668–673.

Paul, G. L. "Behavior Modification Research: Design and Tactics." In C. M. Franks (ed.), *Behavior Therapy: Appraisal and Status.* New York: McGraw-Hill, 1969.

Rogers, E. M. *Diffusion of Innovations.* (4th ed.) New York: Free Press, 1995.

Rollnick, S., Mason, P., and Butler, C. *Health Behavior Change: A Guide for Clinicians.* New York: Churchill Livingstone, 1999.

CHAPTER TWENTY-FOUR

PERSPECTIVES ON USING THEORY

Past, Present, and Future

Karen Glanz

A recent television special featured an emotional meeting between a mother whose son died suddenly in an accident and four people who had been given a new chance at life by donation of her son's heart, kidneys, and lungs. One day earlier this month, my short drive to the office was slowed by the sound of sirens followed by a fire truck and a Hazmat crew, who had been called to check suspicious mail for the presence of anthrax (a false alarm). Last month, two sisters who visited a genetic counselor to receive results of genetic testing faced the news that one has a 90 percent chance of developing breast cancer in her lifetime, while the other has only the same risk as the general population (one in eight). Both the mutation-positive sister and the heart transplant recipient can now go online from their homes and join a support group with other people in their circumstances. The mutation-negative sister can choose from one of several interactive Web-based risk assessment tools.

As Rosenstock said in the first edition of *Health Behavior and Health Education*, "It would be the height of folly to predict the future needs of health education [and health behavior] research and practice, at least without the assistance of an outstanding California astrologer or the Great Kreskin" (Rosenstock, 1990, p. 405).

The author wishes to acknowledge Barbara K. Rimer for her significant contributions to this chapter.

545

What is certain is that times have changed and that scientific advances and new technology have dramatically altered our lives. They have changed the health risks we confront, the information we can obtain, our day-to-day priorities and worries, our relationships, and the ways we communicate.

The modern field of health behavior and health education dates back only about eighty years, and progress has accelerated most rapidly in the past thirty years. As the chapters in this book have shown, many of the early ideas of social and behavioral theorists remain as solid foundations for our work today. A review of the closing chapters in the first two editions of this book reveals gradual shifts in emphasis, as well as striking similarities in some persistent and important challenges (Rosenstock, 1990; Glanz, Lewis, and Rimer, 1990; Abrams, Emmons, and Linnan, 1996). To make progress, we need to stand on the shoulders of the pioneers in the field, equip ourselves to be explorers, address today's problems with new tools, and anticipate the challenges of the future.

Crosscutting Propositions About Using Theory

To begin, we offer some key crosscutting propositions to readers to put the use of health behavior theory in perspective. These ideas are germane to the review and discussion of each of the chapters in this section.

1. It is important not to confuse *using* or *applying* theory with testing theory or developing theory.
2. Testing the efficacy or effectiveness of theory-based interventions does not constitute testing a theory or theories per se.
3. When combining theories, systematic approaches should be used and the principle of parsimony, or selective inclusion of constructs, should be followed.
4. Rigorous tests of theory-based interventions, including measurement and analyses of mediator and moderators, are the building blocks of the evidence base in health education and health behavior (HEHB).
5. Theory, research, and practice are part of a continuum from understanding the determinants of behavior, through testing strategies for change, to disseminating successful interventions (Rimer, Glanz, and Rasband, 2001; Hiatt and Rimer, 1999; Sallis, Owen, and Fotheringham, 2000; National Center for Chronic Disease Prevention and Health Promotion, 2000; Flay, 1986).
6. There is as much to learn from failure as there is to learn from success.
7. There is no substitute for knowing the audience.

The authors of the six chapters in Part Five describe tools, strategies, models, and issues for applying theory in HEHB. This section of *Health Behavior and Health Education* tackles the complexity of health behavior and health promotion at its multiple levels. A basic theme is that if intervention strategies are based on a carefully researched understanding of the determinants of behavior and environments, and if systematic approaches to tailoring, targeting, implementation, and evaluation are used, the chances are good that programs will be effective. Two chapters, on the PRECEDE-PROCEED Planning Model (Chapter Eighteen) and on ecological models (Chapter Twenty), are updated versions of chapters from the preceding edition, written by the same authors. Two other chapters, "Social Marketing" (Chapter Nineteen) and "Applying Theory to Culturally Diverse and Unique Populations" (Chapter Twenty-One), are substantial revisions of chapters in the second edition, written by new authors. Finally, two completely new chapters are included: one on communication technology and health behavior change (Chapter Twenty-Two) and the other on the RE-AIM Model as a framework for evaluating theory-based interventions (Chapter Twenty-Three).

This chapter reviews highlights from each of the six chapters in this section, discusses emerging developments and challenges, and comments on the state of the art in the use of theory in HEHB theory, research, and practice. The discussion aims to provoke thought and debate and to stimulate further reading, rather than to provide definitive answers or prescriptions for the field.

The PRECEDE-PROCEED Planning Model

In Chapter Eighteen, Andrea Gielen and Eileen McDonald present an overview of PRECEDE-PROCEED, describe each of its phases, and apply the model in a case study of child injury prevention. They explicitly illustrate the ways that behavior change theories can be applied and incorporated into a systematic planning process. They further note the challenges of using PRECEDE-PROCEED, which, when fully applied, can be a demanding and laborious process for practitioners and community groups. But when mastered, it can lead to the development of effective, appropriate health education programs.

Although health behavior theories are critical tools, the health educator cannot substitute theory for planning or research. However, theories help us interpret problem situations and plan feasible and promising interventions. Theory also plays an important role in program evaluation. Because it identifies the assumptions behind intervention strategies, theory helps to pinpoint intermediate steps that should be assessed in evaluation. These "mediating factors" help to clarify

the reasons why programs achieve or fail to achieve our goals for success in changing behaviors or environments. The PRECEDE-PROCEED model has as its
raison d'etre the systematic application of theory and previous research to the assessment of local needs, priorities, circumstances, and resources (Green and others, 1994). It owes its robustness in part to the fact that it is intuitively appealing
and logical.

Theory is most likely to be informative during Step 4 of the planning process
suggested by PRECEDE-PROCEED, educational and organizational diagnosis.
This phase focuses on examining factors that shape behavioral actions and environmental factors. Theories help guide the examination of predisposing, enabling,
and reinforcing factors. For example, the constructs of the Health Belief Model
might help us understand why some women do not get mammograms (see Chapter Three). PRECEDE-PROCEED can also be used in conjunction with The
Transtheoretical Model to design stage-appropriate health education messages
(see Chapter Five and Chapter Twenty-Two). This type of analysis is used to focus
on specific leverage points that might best influence desired behaviors. Throughout the analysis, both literature reviews and information collected directly from a
community or program audience are important (Alciati and Glanz, 1996). Levers
are sought among predisposing factors such as motives, reinforcing factors such
as rewards, and enabling factors or barriers such as insurance or access to care.
The concepts of priority, changeability, and community preferences should be
considered along with analytical and empirical findings about health behavior determinants. These ideas are also consistent with concepts espoused in earlier chapters on community organization, diffusion of innovations, and organizational
change.

Recently, Bartholomew, Parcel, Kok, and Gottlieb (2001) have described Intervention Mapping as a framework for developing theory- and evidence-based
health education programs. Intervention Mapping is composed of five steps that
can be considered complementary to the planning phases of the PRECEDE-
PROCEED Model. Readers may find Intervention Mapping helpful in guiding
them toward explicit specification of how to use both theory and empirical findings to develop effective health education interventions.

Social Marketing

Social marketing is a process that promotes desired voluntary behaviors among
members of a target market, by offering attractive benefits and reducing barriers
associated with healthful choices. It involves the adaptation of commercial marketing technologies to promote socially desirable goals. Thus, the main beneficia-

ries of social marketing programs are the recipients (target market) or society at large, rather than the person or group who initiates the marketing program. In Chapter Nineteen, Maibach, Rothschild, and Novelli take a fresh look at social marketing. They place social marketing along a continuum of approaches to influence behavior—with education and law at two extremes and marketing in the middle. With social marketing, success is most likely when the marketers accurately determine the perceptions, needs, and wants of target markets and satisfy them through the design, communication, pricing, and delivery of appropriate, competitive, and visible offerings. The process is consumer-driven, not expert-driven. This orientation is consistent with principles of community organization, and its product development approach parallels the innovation development process of Diffusion Theory. At the same time, it shares an economic perspective with "behavioral economics," a field of inquiry that relates individual behaviors to economic variables (Bickel and Vuchinich, 2000). Concepts from behavioral economics, including the notion of tradeoffs considered when making decisions, deserve further attention along with social marketing and other theories of health behavior.

As with the PRECEDE-PROCEED model, social marketing provides a framework for identifying what drives and maintains behavior, and what factors might drive and maintain behavioral change. It also requires identification of potential intermediaries, channels of distribution and communication, and actual and potential competitors. As the authors indicate, theories of health behavior can help guide the analytical process in social marketing and aid in the formulation of intervention strategies and materials. Because of the focus on understanding consumers (or target audiences) from their own point of view, social marketing models are robust for use in diverse and unique populations, including disadvantaged groups and ethnic minorities. In fact, Maibach and his coauthors stress that social marketing programs tend to be inherently culturally sensitive because they follow a consumer-oriented process.

A new idea that the authors introduce to Chapter Nineteen is that social marketing is a "scalable" process and can be used in both low- and high-resource programs. They illustrate this by providing case examples of both a large-scale social marketing program—the National High Blood Pressure Education Program—and a small-scale university program for binge drinking prevention. The combination of motivation, opportunity, and ability was harnessed in designing the binge drinking prevention program. This combination, which includes providing social activities that are alternatives to binge drinking, is especially important in efforts to reduce a risky behavior that may be perceived as enjoyable by the audience. Process evaluation suggests that the program is being well received, but data are not yet available to determine whether the main aim is achieved (the reduction of binge drinking). Such evaluations should be included on health education's research agenda for the future, especially for small-scale programs that might be easily replicated.

Ecological Models

In Chapter Twenty, Sallis and Owen update their 1996 chapter and describe the aims and core concepts of ecological models for health education and health behavior change. As shown in Chapter One and emphasized in recent authoritative publications (Smedley and Syme, 2000), the basic tenets of ecological perspectives— of multilevel determinants of behavior and environments, and of transactions between individuals and their environments—are widely recognized as useful and appropriate orientations for contemporary health promotion. Although there is a shift toward lower-cost, broad-reach programs and away from intensive and costly face-to-face interventions for reducing risky health behaviors, much more work remains to be done (Orleans, Gruman, Ulmer, Emont, and Hollendonner, 1999).

Sallis and Owen outline the historical foundations of ecological models of human behavior. Ecological models also have a long tradition, and a controversial place, in the science of epidemiology, in which critiques of the "ecological fallacy" demonstrate the often-found lack of correspondence between individual-level and group-level associations of the same or similar variables. MacIntyre and Ellaway (2000) provide a thoughtful articulation that argues for the revitalization of an ecological perspective with links to epidemiology, medical geography, and sociology. New methods of statistical analysis, including multilevel modeling, make it possible to better understand people's relationships to their surroundings and to identify leverage points to improve population health (MacIntyre and Ellaway, 2000).

Further discussions of the issues discussed in Sallis and Owen's applications of ecological models to nutrition and physical activity may interest readers, especially those who seek an international perspective. McCarthy (1999) discusses the shift in thinking about transport and health, from an emphasis on safety to the opportunity for health benefits, and describes various categories of intervention that may reduce both chronic disease risk factors and unintentional injuries. Robertson, Brunner, and Sheiham (1999) analyze food as a political issue, arguing that reductions in diet-related diseases require international, national, community, and individual action.

An important point that deserves attention is that, despite many calls for multilevel interventions, proposed interventions are often based solely on data regarding cross-sectional associations between environmental factors and behaviors. We need to understand the *causes* of health behavior problems before we can design successful interventions. For example, childhood obesity has been linked to more hours of television viewing (Gortmaker and others, 1996). One reason this seemed to be true is that television watching might reduce levels of physical activity. Two randomized trials tested the effects of school-based interventions to prevent obesity through reduced television viewing. Each study found a lower prevalence of obesity among experimental subjects, though among only girls in one study (Gortmaker and others, 1999). Both studies found somewhat improved dietary behaviors (Robinson, 1999; Gortmaker and others, 1999). However, the Task Force on Community Preventive Services found insufficient evidence to recommend these programs for promotion of *physical activity,* because of their inability to demonstrate a link between less time watching television and increased physical activity (Centers for Disease Control and Prevention, 2001). It may be that the link between television viewing and physical activity needs to be more tightly controlled, as in the pilot study of contingent television viewing recently reported by Faith and others (2001). Paradoxically, then, such interventions would be more individually than environmentally focused.

The challenge to conduct better research on ecological interventions remains an important one for health education and health behavior. These studies are expensive and demanding and therefore require substantial collaboration across areas of expertise. Most likely, a combination of inductive and deductive approaches, using both qualitative and quantitative techniques, will reveal the rich texture of an ecological perspective while allowing assessment of their impact on valued outcomes.

Applying Theory to Culturally Diverse and Unique Populations

Chapter Twenty-One, by Resnicow, Braithwaite, DiIorio, and Glanz, addresses the challenges of applying theories of health behavior for understanding and influencing health behavior in culturally diverse and sociodemographically unique populations. The chapter, revised and written by new authors specifically for this edition, briefly addresses the rationale for targeted and tailored behavioral change programs and presents key concepts to consider in developing culturally sensitive interventions. The authors tread cautiously as they provide examples of culturally unique groups while trying to avoid stereotyping.

Relationships between socioeconomic status (SES) and racial or ethnic minority status receive special attention in this chapter. The graded association of SES with many health behaviors, conditions, and diseases is well-known. However, recent data suggest that reducing the prevalence of health risk behaviors (smoking, alcohol consumption, sedentary lifestyle, obesity) in low-income populations will reduce only a modest proportion of their excess mortality (Lantz and others, 1998). There are as well important interactions between intrapersonal factors and inequities in access to health care (Mustard and Frohlich, 1995), and impoverished social environments most likely also play a role (Adler and others, 1994; Emmons, 2000). In addition, there is still a large component of unexplained variance.

The study of culture, health, and illness is a fascinating branch of cultural anthropology that has much to offer to professionals in health education and health behavior (Helman, 2000). People usually acquire ideas about their bodies as part of growing up in a particular culture or society, and these concepts of body image, body functioning, illness, self-care, disability, and stigma affect their receptivity to health education messages. Social phenomena, such as family structure, gender roles, housing arrangements, and sanitation, also vary across cultural groups and have powerful impacts on many health-related behaviors (Helman, 2000). Readers who are unfamiliar with the literature on culture, health, and illness will find that basic texts such as Helman's provide a worthwhile orientation to these issues.

Chapter Twenty-One raises a critical question: Is it possible to use, or apply, general theories that involve the same constructs and relationships regardless of a person's ethnic background, economic status, or developmental stage? To answer this question, it is important to return to the definition of "theory" and to recall the distinction between using theory and developing or testing theories. Theories are by nature abstract and take on concrete meaning only when applied to specific situations, behaviors, or populations. Thus, to apply a theory—whether to describe or explain a situation, or to develop an intervention to address an identified problem—one needs to operationalize the key constructs so they can be measured and empirically tested. It is in the process of operationalizing theoretical constructs that one must develop an understanding of the person or group's characteristics (ethnicity, SES, gender, age, and so on) and refine constructs into variables. Indeed, the relationships uncovered may vary between groups—in fact, they probably will. This does not mean, however, that existing theories are not applicable or not useful. Few, if any, of the major theories of health behavior being used today are so highly specified and quantified that they precisely predict the relationships among constructs and hence variables. Also, we know of no data that show the mainstream theories included in this book to be less effective with minority groups than with majority racial and ethnic populations. Generally, it is in the application process that care must be taken to specify the theory's constructs for a particular group.

The authors of Chapter Twenty-One urge practitioners and researchers to go beneath the surface when working with culturally unique or other diverse populations. Their advice is sound and deserves to be heeded. Health education and health behavior experts need to learn *and adhere to* the basic principles of developing good health education programs—starting where the people are, stepwise design of interventions, pretesting, pilot testing, and adapting programs to fit their contexts. One size does not fit all.

Tailoring and Targeting in Health Behavior Change

Both Chapter Twenty-One, on culturally diverse and unique populations, and Chapter Twenty-Two, on communication technology, emphasize the importance and promise of targeted and tailored health education interventions. There has been some controversy and debate about the definitions of tailoring and targeting (Kreuter and Skinner, 2000; Rimer, 2000), and it is useful to distinguish between these strategies. On one hand, *targeting* involves identifying a specific population, such as a group with a high rate of a given illness, and designing a program or intervention that includes specific messages or materials intended for that group (Kreuter, Farrell, Olevitch, and Brennan, 2000). For example, if epidemiology suggests a high rate of stomach cancer among Japanese immigrants living in rural areas, a program that is targeted to that group might use rural organizations, Japanese language translations, and familiar faces on printed materials. This definition of targeting is consistent with Resnicow's description and involves a "surface structure" approach to cultural sensitivity (see Chapter Twenty-One). Targeted approaches have been used for a long time in HEHB.

Tailoring, on the other hand, usually refers to interventions created specifically for individuals, based on characteristics unique to them and usually based on data collected from them (Kreuter, Farrell, Olevitch, and Brennan, 2000). However, some authors have also used "tailoring" to describe adaptations of materials and interventions "that best fit the relevant needs and characteristics of a specific target population" (Pasick, 1996, p. 431). Resnicow and colleagues also discuss "cultural tailoring" as the development of programs that address differences in the determinants of health behaviors across unique groups, or programs incorporating a "deep structure" understanding of racial and ethnic minorities (see Chapter Twenty-One). While it is unlikely that a consensus can be reached about the meaning and implications of this terminology, readers may find it helpful to think of "targeted" interventions as strategies based on group-level variables and "tailored" interventions as strategies and messages that are customized based on individual-level variables (Kreuter and Skinner, 2000; Kreuter, Farrell, Olevitch, and Brennan, 2000; Rimer, 2000).

In Chapter Twenty-Two, Owen, Fotheringham, and Marcus focus attention on program strategies that are characterized by the provision of feedback. This is a common feature of tailored messages and interventions. These programs are sometimes referred to as "interactive," although the recipient may or may not experience them as truly interactive. For example, a letter received in the mail, even if it contains personal information based on a questionnaire completed by the recipient, is no more "interactive" than is a generic letter or brochure. The recipient may not even know who handled the assessment or produced the letter. Thus, it is important to recognize that interactivity may be transparent to the target audience, and that this feature depends more on the medium (mail, telephone, interactive Web site) than on the content or technology behind the message.

Tailored print communication has been subjected to sufficient empirical testing to conclude that it has great promise as an intervention modality (Skinner, Campbell, Rimer, Curry, and Prochaska, 1999). Tailored strategies can provide customized messages and reduce provider burden at the same time, by automating the processing of large amounts of information about individuals. But more study is needed. Tailored communications are not theory-specific, and different theories are best used as a basis for tailoring in relation to different behaviors and audiences. The quality, appearance, literacy level, and packaging of tailored communications can vary widely. Even Kreuter and Skinner's (2000) contention that "by tailoring materials, superfluous information is eliminated" is not necessarily a given. Few (if any) health behaviors have been the subject of enough rigorous theory-based research that we truly know what is superfluous and what messages comprise the "active ingredients." Moreover, tailored materials can be designed well or poorly. Tailoring holds great promise and great challenges as well.

Communication Technology and Health Behavior Change

The new chapter by Owen, Fotheringham, and Marcus, "Communication Technology and Health Behavior Change," describes the extraordinary opportunities and the substantial limitations of communication technology applications to HEHB. This chapter describes some recent studies of tailored health communications (see also the previous section), as well as telephone, Internet, and palmtop computer strategies for health behavior change. The opportunities are many and varied, and growing as new technologies become available.

The rapid evolution of interactive health communication was the focus of an important report recently released by the Department of Health and Human Services (Science Panel on Interactive Communication and Health, 1999). This report generated excitement, but it also raised concerns. These new media can be new forms of mass media, there for the taking, or they can be part of a planned and consciously delivered intervention strategy. In either form, they can be beneficial or harmful in their effects on self-care, formal health care, and time and money.

Readers are reminded to carefully consider the advantages, costs, and limitations of new communication technologies and to match the intervention to the problem and audience. A marriage of technology and applied theory has great potential to benefit public health and deserves further development.

The RE-AIM Model for Evaluating Theory-Based Health Behavior Interventions

In Chapter Twenty-Three, Glasgow describes the RE-AIM Model as a guide for impact or outcome evaluation of theory-based health behavior interventions. The acronym RE-AIM stands for Reach, Efficacy or Effectiveness, Adoption, Implementation, and Maintenance (Glasgow, Vogt, and Boles, 1999). A key idea behind the RE-AIM Model, and the message of its first two components (the "RE"), is that the public health impact of interventions is a function of both their efficacy and reach. This idea was also articulated by Abrams, Emmons, and Linnan (1996) in the previous edition of this book. Simply put, more intensive and individualized interventions may be more efficacious than are low-intensity approaches, but they cost more and usually reach a much smaller proportion of the population. Glasgow reminds us not only to consider this equation but to also take a traditional public health perspective that considers possible negative or unintended consequences on quality of life.

The second half of the RE-AIM Model emphasizes Adoption, Implementation, and Maintenance. These concepts invoke other theories such as diffusion of innovations and organizational change at the organizational level, as well as The Transtheoretical Model at the intrapersonal level. The RE-AIM Model as a whole also aligns well with various models of the phases of research (National Center for Chronic Disease Prevention and Health Promotion, 2000; Hiatt and Rimer, 1999; Flay, 1986; Sallis, Owen, and Fotheringham, 2000).

Glasgow provides two applications of the RE-AIM Model, one from a diabetes self-management program and the other from a Planned Parenthood smoking cessation study. These examples come from large and well-funded applied research programs, but readers who are working in the field of practice or in smaller programs should not dismiss them or the model. Rather, RE-AIM provides useful guideposts and reminders about how to maximize the potential success and eventual impact of HEHB change programs.

Chapter Twenty-Three does not attempt to provide a text on research design, measurement, or statistical analysis. Rather, it raises important issues for HEHB researchers and practitioners to incorporate into the "big picture" of their efforts to improve the health of specific risk groups and large populations.

Moving Forward

After becoming familiar with some contemporary theories of health behavior, the challenge is to use them within a comprehensive planning process. Planning systems such as PRECEDE-PROCEED and processes such as social marketing increase the odds of success by examining health and behavior at multiple levels. At a simplistic level, an ecological perspective emphasizes two main options: change people and change the environment. The most powerful approaches will use both of these options together (Smedley and Syme, 2000). The activities most directly tied to changing *people* are derived from individual-level theories such as the Health Belief Model, The Transtheoretical Model, and The Transactional Model of Stress and Coping. In contrast, activities aimed at changing the *environment* draw on community-level theories. In between are Social Cognitive Theory, social support and social networks, and interpersonal communication models. Each of these focuses on reciprocal relations among persons or between individuals and their environments.

Theoretical frameworks are guides in the pursuit of successful efforts, maximizing flexibility and helping to apply the abstract concepts of theory in ways that are most useful in diverse work settings and situations. A knowledge of theory and comprehensive planning systems offers a great deal. Other key elements of effective programs are a good program-to-audience match; accessible and practical information; active learning and involvement; and skill building, practice, and reinforcement. Theory helps you ask the right questions, and effective planning enables you to zero in on these elements in relation to a specific problem. Effective use of theory for practice and research requires practice, but can yield important dividends in efforts to enhance the health of individuals and populations.

References

Abrams, D. B., Emmons, K. M., and Linnan, L. A. "Health Behavior and Health Education: The Past, Present, and Future." In K. Glanz, F. M. Lewis, and B. K. Rimer (eds.), *Health Behavior and Health Education: Theory, Research, and Practice.* (2nd ed.) San Francisco: Jossey-Bass, 1996.

Adler, N., and others. "Socioeconomic Status and Health: The Challenge of the Gradient." *American Psychologist*, 1994, *49*(1), 15–24.

Alciati, M. H., and Glanz, K. "Using Data to Plan Public Health Programs: Experience from State Cancer Prevention and Control Programs." *Public Health Reports,* 1996, *111,* 165–172.

Bartholomew, L. K., Parcel, G. S., Kok, G., and Gottlieb, N. H. *Intervention Mapping: Designing Theory and Evidence Based Health Promotion Programs.* Mountain View, Calif.: Mayfield, 2001.

Bickel, W. K., and Vuchinich, R. E. (eds.). *Reframing Health Behavior Change with Behavioral Economics.* Mahwah, N.J.: Erlbaum, 2000.

Centers for Disease Control and Prevention. "Increasing Physical Activity: A Report on Recommendations of the Task Force on Community Preventive Services." *Morbidity and Mortality Weekly Report,* 2001, *50*(RR-18), 1–14.

Emmons, K. "Health Behaviors in Social Context." In L. F. Berkman and I. Kawachi (eds.), *Social Epidemiology.* New York: Oxford University Press, 2000.

Faith, M. S., and others. "Effects of Contingent Television on Physical Activity and Television Viewing in Obese Children." *Pediatrics,* 2001, *107,* 1043–1048.

Fishbein, M. "The Role of Theory in HIV Prevention." *AIDS Care,* 2000, *12,* 273–278.

Flay, B. "Efficacy and Effectiveness Trials (and Other Phases of Research) in the Development of Health Promotion Programs." *Preventive Medicine,* 1986, *15,* 451–474.

Glanz, K., Lewis, F. M., and Rimer, B. K. "Moving Forward: Research and Evaluation Methods for Health Behavior and Health Education." In K. Glanz, F. M. Lewis, and B. K. Rimer (eds.), *Health Behavior and Health Education: Theory, Research, and Practice.* San Francisco: Jossey-Bass, 1990.

Glasgow, R. E., Vogt, T. M., and Boles, S. M. "Evaluating the Public Health Impact of Health Promotion Interventions: The RE-AIM Framework." *American Journal of Public Health,* 1999, *89,* 1322–1327.

Gortmaker, S. L., and others. "Television Viewing as a Cause of Increasing Obesity Among Children in the United States." *Archives of Pediatric and Adolescent Medicine,* 1996, *150,* 356–362.

Gortmaker, S. L., and others. "Reducing Obesity Via a School-Based Interdisciplinary Intervention Among Youth: Planet Health." *Archives of Pediatric and Adolescent Medicine,* 1999, *153,* 409–418.

Green, L., Richard, L., and Potvin, L. "Ecological Foundations of Health Promotion." *American Journal of Health Promotion,* 1996, *10*(4), 270–281.

Green, L., and others. "Can We Build On, or Must We Replace, the Theories and Models in Health Education?" *Health Education Research,* 1994, *9,* 397–404.

Helman, C. G. *Culture, Health, and Illness.* (4th ed.) Oxford, U.K.: Butterworth-Heinemann, 2000.

Hiatt, R. A., and Rimer, B. K. "A New Strategy for Cancer Control Research." *Cancer, Epidemiology, Biomarkers and Prevention,* 1999, *8,* 957–964.

Kreuter, M., Farrell, D., Olevitch, L., and Brennan, L. *Tailoring Health Messages: Customizing Communication With Computer Technology.* Mahwah, N.J.: Erlbaum, 2000.

Kreuter, M., and Skinner, C. S. "Tailoring: What's in a Name?" *Health Education Research,* 2000, *15,* 1–4.

Lantz, P. M., and others. "Socioeconomic Factors, Health Behaviors, and Mortality: Results from a Nationally Representative Prospective Study of U.S. Adults." *Journal of the American Medical Association,* 1998, *279,* 1703–1708.

MacIntyre, S., and Ellaway, A. "Ecological Approaches: Rediscovering the Role of the Physical and Social Environment." In L. F. Berkman and I. Kawachi (eds.), *Social Epidemiology.* New York: Oxford University Press, 2000.

Marmot, M. "Multilevel Approaches to Understanding Social Determinants." In L. F. Berkman and I. Kawachi (eds.), *Social Epidemiology.* New York: Oxford University Press, 2000.

McCarthy, M. "Transport and Health." In M. Marmot and R. G. Wilkinson (eds.), *Social Determinants of Health.* New York: Oxford University Press, 1999.

Mustard, C., and Frohlich, N. "Socioeconomic Status and the Health of the Population." *Medical Care,* 1995, *33*(12), DS43-DS54.

National Center for Chronic Disease Prevention and Health Promotion. "Setting the Agenda, CDC Research in Chronic Disease Prevention and Health Promotion." Atlanta: Centers for Disease Control and Prevention, September 2000.

Orleans, C. T., Gruman, J., Ulmer, C., Emont, S. L., and Hollendonner, J. K. "Rating Our Progress in Population Health Promotion: Report Card on Six Behaviors." *American Journal of Health Promotion,* 1999, *14,* 75–82.

Pasick, R. J. "Socioeconomic and Cultural Factors in the Development and Use of Theory." In K. Glanz, F. M. Lewis, and B. K. Rimer (eds.), *Health Behavior and Health Education: Theory, Research, and Practice.* (2nd ed.) San Francisco: Jossey-Bass, 1996.

Rimer, B. K. "Response to Kreuter and Skinner." *Health Education Research,* 2000, *15,* 503.

Rimer, B. K., Glanz, K., and Rasband, G. "Searching for Evidence About Health Education and Health Behavior Interventions." *Health Education and Behavior,* 2001, *28,* 231–248.

Robertson, A., Brunner, B., and Sheiham, A. "Food as a Political Issue." In M. Marmot and R. G. Wilkinson (eds.), *Social Determinants of Health.* New York: Oxford University Press, 1999.

Robinson, T. N. "Reducing Children's Television Viewing to Prevent Obesity: A Randomized Controlled Trial." *Journal of the American Medical Association,* 1999, *282,* 1561–1567.

Rosenstock, I. M. "The Past, Present, and Future of Health Education." In K. Glanz, F. M. Lewis, and B. K. Rimer (eds.), *Health Behavior and Health Education: Theory, Research, and Practice.* San Francisco: Jossey-Bass, 1990.

Sallis, J. F., Owen, N., and Fotheringham, M. J. "Behavioral Epidemiology: A Systematic Framework to Classify Phases of Research on Health Promotion and Disease Prevention." *Annals of Behavioral Medicine,* 2000, *22,* 294–298.

Science Panel on Interactive Communication and Health. *Wired for Health and Well-Being: The Emergence of Interactive Health Communication.* Washington, D.C.: U.S. Department of Health and Human Services, U.S. Government Printing Office, April 1999.

Skinner, C. S., Campbell, M. K., Rimer, B. K., Curry, S., and Prochaska, J. O. "How Effective Is Tailored Print Communication?" *Annals of Behavioral Medicine,* 1999, *21,* 290–298.

Smedley, B. D., and Syme, S. L. (eds.). *Promoting Health: Intervention Strategies from Social and Behavioral Research.* Washington, D.C.: National Academy Press, 2000.

NAME INDEX

A

Abelson, R. P., 67
Abrams, A. B., 170
Abrams, D. B., 107, 108, 148, 166, 167, 535, 537, 546, 555
Adams, J., 339
Adams, R. J., 249
Adhikari, G., 285
Adler, N., 14, 552
Affleck, G., 216
Ahluwalia, J., 493, 494, 499
Aida, Y., 255
Airhihenbuwa, C., 492
Ajzen, I., 27, 42, 68, 72, 74, 75, 76, 128, 145, 147, 425, 501
Akiyama, H., 188
Albarracin, D., 74, 76
Alciati, M. H., 353, 354, 355, 394
Alinsky, S. D., 281, 283, 286, 287, 299
Allen, A. J., 336
Alter, C., 344, 345, 346
Altman, D. G., 465, 466
Ammerman, A., 31
Ammerman, R. T., 379
Andersen, B. L., 228

Andersen, R. E., 266
Anderson, C., 152, 346
Anderson, C. A., 127
Anderson, D. M., 112
Anderson, D. R., 108
Anderson, R., 513
Anderson, R. E., 266
Anderson, R. N., 489
Andreasen, A. R., 438, 439, 449, 450
Antipatis, V. J., 471
Antoni, M. H., 56, 226
Antonovsky, A., 211, 212, 221
Antonucci, T. C., 188, 195
Apanovitch, A. M., 154
Appleyard, J., 72, 93
Arean, P., 298
Argyris, C., 340, 342
Aristotle, 22
Armistead, L. P., 56, 58
Armsden, G., 14
Arnold, R., 290, 294
Aron, A., 243
Aron, E. N., 243
Artz, L. M., 166, 167
Ary, D., 253, 535
Ashforth, S. J., 341
Aspinwall, L. G., 187, 217

Atkins, C. J., 473
Audrain, J., 228
Avery, B., 282
Aveyard, P., 108, 109
Axelson, M. L., 516
Ayanian, J. Z., 489

B

Babbie, E., 28
Bachman, J., 348
Backus, C. A., 58
Baider, L., 219
Baker, E. A., 478
Baker, S. P., 423, 424
Bakker, A. B., 255
Balshem, A., 223
Bandawe, C. R., 74
Bandura, A., 26, 30, 31, 47, 50, 51, 76, 103, 123, 151, 156, 165, 166, 167, 168, 170, 172, 173, 174, 187, 217, 266, 296, 382, 397, 416, 450, 465, 497
Baranowski, J., 472
Baranowski, T., 152, 165, 166, 167, 168, 170, 177, 179, 180, 466, 469, 472, 493, 494, 499

SUBJECT INDEX

A

Action: cues to, in Health Belief Model (HBM), 49, 50, 55, 58, 61, 145; defined, 101, 102; delayed action effect, 111–112; in Precaution Adoption Process Model (PAPM), 125, 128–129; in Transtheoretical Model (TTM), 101, 102, 105, 113

Action planning, defined, 342–343

Action research, defined, 342–343, 347

Administrative assessment, in planning model, 414, 419–420, 428–430

Adolescent Social Action Program (ASAP), 301–304, 305, 391

Adoption: defined, 315; in diffusion of innovation, 317, 319, 321–322, 326; of organizational change, 347, 349–350, 351, 352; in RE-AIM evaluation framework, 536–537, 538, 540, 541

Advisers: in social relationship interventions, 198. *See also* Lay health advisers (LHAs)

African Americans: breast cancer prevention for, 55–56, 202–204; communities of, 283; heterogeneity among, 488; life expectancy for, 14, 488–489; Motivational Interviewing to change eating behaviors of, 255–257; religiosity among, 501–502

Agenda setting, media studies on, 368, 372–374

AIDS/HIV prevention: and diffusion of innovations, 313; Health Belief Model (HBM) applied to, 56–58; and Precaution Adoption Process Model (PAPM), 121–122; theories underlying school curricula for, 12

Alcohol use/abuse prevention: binge drinking prevention program for, 455–459; influence and communication for, 257–259; social cognition for, 176–177. *See also* Substance use/abuse prevention

Alternative medicine, and patient-provider communication, 250

American Academy of Pediatrics, 424; AAP Task Force on Infant Positioning and SIDS, 441; Committee on Public Education, 378

American Indians: heterogeneity of tribes of, 488; tobacco-use reduction program for, 502–503

American Medical Association, 455

American Social Health Associate Panel, 77

Appraisal bias, in coping with stress, 213, 215–216

Appraisal support, defined, 186, 187

Asian Americans, heterogeneity among, 488

The Aspen Institute, 297

Assessment: in planning model, 411, 412–419, 423–430; of stages in Precaution Adoption Process Model (PAPM), 138–139. *See also* Evaluation; Measurement

Attitude: defined, 68; and planned behavior, 85–86, 87, 88, 89; and reasoned action, 70, 72

Attribution Theory, 35